AF332983

Pharmacological Basis of
Large Animal Medicine

DEDICATION

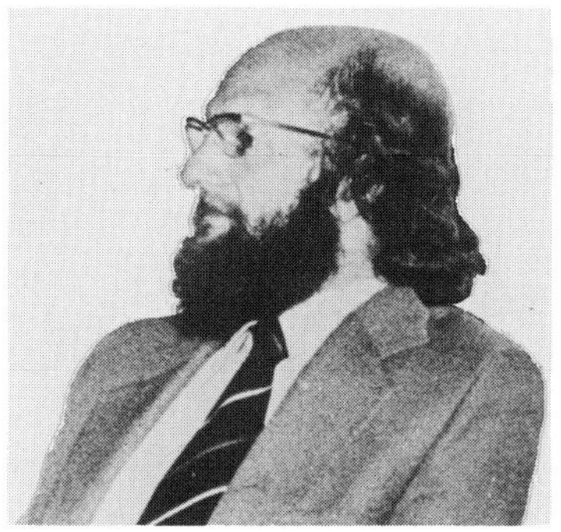

This book is dedicated to the memory of one of the
co-editors, Andrew T. Yoxall, who died during
preparation of the text. A graduate of the Cambridge
Veterinary School, Andrew's infectious enthusiasm and
skills as author, editor and innovator have done much to
advance Veterinary Pharmacology in Europe. He was
founder member and first Secretary of the British
Association for Veterinary Clinical Pharmacology and
Therapeutics. He was also the first President of the
European Association for Veterinary Pharmacology
and Toxicology. With Alan Teale, he organised the 1978
refresher course on which this book is based. His vision
led to the introduction of the *Journal of Veterinary
Pharmacology and Therapeutics* which, with Charles
Short, he edited for a number of years. As an enthusiast
and as a friend he will be sadly missed by his co-editors.

Pharmacological Basis of Large Animal Medicine

EDITED BY

J. A. BOGAN
BSc MSc PhD
Department of Veterinary
Pharmacology
University of Glasgow

P. LEES
BPharm PhD
Department of Physiology
Royal Veterinary College
Field Station, Hatfield

AND

A. T. YOXALL
MA VetMB MRCVS DVA

Blackwell Scientific Publications

OXFORD LONDON EDINBURGH
BOSTON MELBOURNE

©1983 by
Blackwell Scientific Publications
Editorial offices:
Osney Mead, Oxford OX2 0EL
8 John Street, London WC1N 2ES
9 Forrest Road, Edinburgh EH1 2QH
52 Beacon Street, Boston, Massachusetts
  02108, USA
99 Barry Street, Carlton, Victoria 3053,
  Australia

All rights reserved. No part of this
publication may be reproduced, stored in a
retrieval system, or transmitted, in any form
or by any means, electronic, mechanical,
photocopying, recording or otherwise
without the prior permission of the
copyright owner

First published 1983

Set by Southline Press Ltd., Ferring, West
Sussex.
Printed in Great Britain by Henry Ling Ltd.,
Dorchester

DISTRIBUTORS

USA
  Blackwell Mosby Book Distributors
  11830 Westline Industrial Drive
  St. Louis, Missouri 63141

Canada
  Blackwell Mosby Book Distributors
  120 Melford Drive, Scarborough
  Ontario M1B 2X4

Australia
  Blackwell Scientific Book Distributors
  214 Berkeley Street, Carlton
  Victoria 3053

British Library
Cataloguing in Publication Data

Pharmacological basis of large animal
medicine
  1. Veterinary Pharmacology
  I. Bogan, J. A.   II. Lees, P.
  III. Yoxall, A. T.
  636. 089′5′1   SF915

ISBN 0–632–01055–X

Contents

PART 3   IMMUNOLOGY AND PARASITOLOGY

PART 4   REPRODUCTION

PART 5   NUTRITION, METABOLISM AND FLUID BALANCE

PART 6   OTHER PHARMACOLOGICAL AGENTS

Contributors

W. EDWARD ALLEN MVB PhD MRCVS
Department of Surgery & Obstetrics, The Royal Veterinary College,
Hawkshead Lane, Hatfield

J. ARMOUR PhD MRCVS
Department of Veterinary Parasitology, University of Glasgow

J. D. BAGGOT MVM PhD DSc MRCVS MACVSc
School of Veterinary Medicine, University of California, Davis

J. A. BOGAN BSc MSc PhD
Department of Veterinary Pharmacology, University of Glasgow

R. BOMFORD
Department of Experimental Immunobiology, Wellcome Research
Laboratories, Beckenham, Kent

R. J. BYWATER MSc PhD BVMS MRCVS
Beecham Pharmaceuticals Research Division, Animal Health Research
Centre, Tadworth, Surrey

P. M. DIXON MVB PhD MRCVS
Veterinary Field Station, University of Edinburgh

J. L. DUNCAN BVMS PhD MRCVS
Department of Veterinary Parasitology, University of Glasgow

D. L. FRAPE BSc PhD Dip Agric MIBiol
Dalgety-Spillers Nutritional Research Centre, Kennet, Newmarket

E. L. GERRING BVetMed PhD MRCVS
Department of Surgery and Obstetrics, Royal Veterinary College,
Hawkshead Lane, Hatfield

R. J. HEITZMAN
Institute for Research on Animal Diseases, Compton, Berkshire

J. R. HOLMES MVSc PhD MRCVS
Department of Veterinary Medicine, University of Bristol

R. HOPES BVMS MRCVS
Beaufort Cottage Stables, Newmarket, Cambridge

D. L. HUDD BVetMed MRCVS
Lilly Research Centre, Windlesham, Surrey

M. J. MEREDITH BSc BVetMed PhD MRCVS
Department of Animal Husbandry, Royal Veterinary College, Boltons Park Farm, Hatfield

P. LEES BPharm PhD
Department of Physiology, Royal Veterinary College, Hawkshead Lane, Hatfield

A. H. LINTON PhD DSc FRCPath
Department of Microbiology, University of Bristol

SUSAN E. MARRINER BVMS MRCVS
Department of Veterinary Pharmacology, University of Glasgow

P. A. MULLEN MRCVS PhD BSc
Union International Co., West Smithfield, London

C. D. MUNRO BVM&S PhD MRCVS
Department of Veterinary Surgery, Royal (Dick) School of Veterinary Studies, Edinburgh

S. W. RICKETTS BSc BVSc FRCVS
Beaufort Cottage Stables, Newmarket, Cambridge

J. SANFORD BVSc PhD MRCVS
Wyeth Laboratories, Maidenhead, Berkshire

J. SCARNELL BVSc MRCVS
Veterinary Biologicals Service Department, The Wellcome Foundation, Beckenham

D. H. SNOW BVSc(Syd) BSc(Syd) PhD
Department of Veterinary Pharmacology, University of Glasgow
Veterinary School

A. J. TEALE MA VetMB MSc MRCVS
Veterinary Research Department, Kenya Agricultural Research Institute,
Kikuyu, Kenya

JILL R. THOMSON BVSc(Pret)
Veterinary Investigation Centre, East of Scotland College of Agriculture

W. M. VANDAELE Dr VetMed Lic Zoot
Director of Technical Development, Smith Kline Animal Health
Laboratories, Brussels

C. L. WRIGHT MSc BVSc MRCVS DTVM
Veterinary Investigation Centre, Auchincruive, Ayr

Preface

This volume, a companion to *Pharmacological Basis of Small Animal Medicine*, provides a guide to the scientific principles underlying the rational use of drugs as therapeutic and managemental agents in large animal medicine.

Twenty years ago the idea of such a book would have been unlikely; the paucity of knowledge of even the mode of action of most drugs and their fate in the body, the often empirical way in which they were used, and the poor efficacy of many drugs available at that time made any study of their proper use impossible. During the last 20 years, however, the pharmaceutical industry has provided the clinician with a valuable array of potent and effective agents, and it is now essential that veterinarians should have some knowledge of their properties if these agents are to be used safely and effectively. It should no longer be acceptable for a practitioner merely to read the data sheet provided with a product or to use the drug without further thought for any of the indications mentioned therein, relying only on the notoriously fickle 'clinical judgement' for assessment of efficacy. There are now sufficient published data describing the basic and clinical pharmacology and therapeutic efficacy in most areas of veterinary therapy on which to base a reasoned approach concerning the drug of first choice for most disease conditions.

The book should be of value to practitioners, to students in their preclinical years who wish to understand the relevance of much of the background pharmacology they are asked to learn, and especially to students in their clinical years. Because of the history of the courses in the veterinary schools, it has been difficult to introduce therapeutics to students in their later years. While diagnostic medicine must remain of paramount importance for students, it must be recognised that many of the control measures for diseases and animal management increasingly involve the use of drugs and vaccines.

This book was conceived following a refresher course on Large Animal Therapeutics held at Guildford in 1978 and it has therefore had a long gestation period. One of the editors (A.T.Y.) was ill for a considerable period and has subsequently died. Because of this and also as a result of further administrative problems, the book has taken longer to publish than any of us envisaged. We are extremely grateful to the authors of the chapters for their forbearance first in writing and then updating their chapters on two occasions. However, we believe that this updating exercise has had some considerable benefit in providing a more polished final version.

Inevitably in a book such as this, which is essentially a new venture, there are few gaps in coverage but we feel that most of the major topics of modern large animal therapy are covered. We are grateful to Jony Russell and his colleagues at Blackwell Scientific Publications for their continued support of the book and for their help and encouragement.

PART 1
PHARMACOKINETICS

1

Absorption and distribution

J.A. BOGAN

Pharmacokinetics is an important area in the understanding of the action of drugs in animals. However, it is only in the last decade that sufficient pharmacokinetic studies have been made in large animals to make us realise that many of the therapeutic failures in large animals and many of the variations in effect between species are due more to different pharmacokinetics of the drug than to lack of intrinsic activity.

The aim of drug therapy is to provide a sufficient concentration of a drug at the site of action and to maintain this concentration for a certain period of time. The subject of pharmacokinetics defines all the different processes involved in maintaining these concentrations which are represented diagramatically in Fig. 1.1.

Passage of drugs through biological membranes

Drugs are transported within the animal's body dissolved in the aqueous phase of blood plasma. The ability of drugs to be absorbed into plasma or to

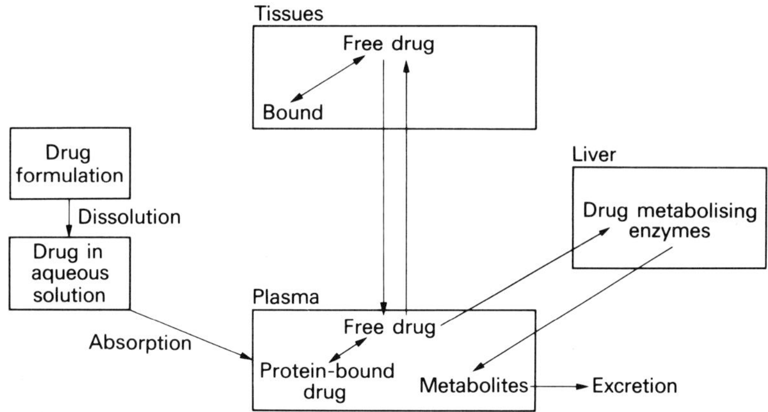

Fig. 1.1 Scientific representation of the processes involved in the absorption, distribution, and excretion of a drug in the body.

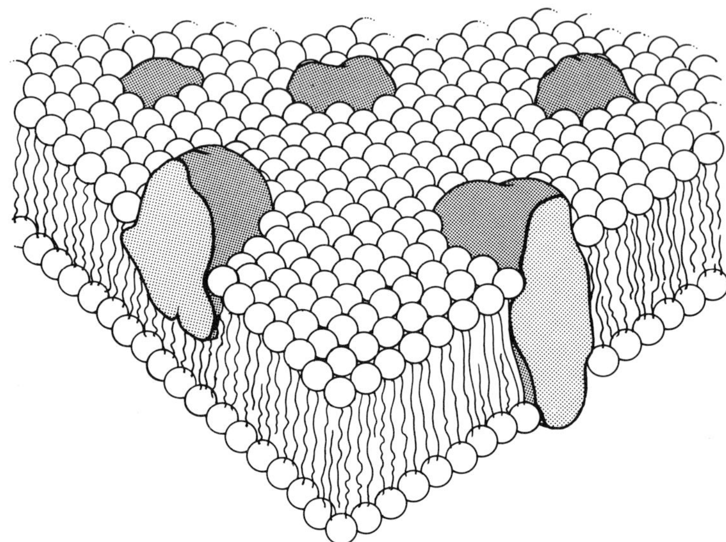

Fig. 1.2   The lipid-globular protein mosaic of the cell membrane. The phospholipids form a bilayer with their ionic, polar groups (represented by circles) in contact with water and their fatty acid chains (represented by wavy lines) within the bilayer. The solid bodies represent globular proteins embedded in the bilayer. (After Singer S. J. & Nicholson G. L. (1972) *Science* **175**, 720–31.)

distribute out of plasma to their site of action and to other tissues is dependent on their ability to cross biological membranes.

Cell membranes can be considered as simple bimolecular layers of phospholipid (Fig. 1.2) and, although they greatly vary in complexity (e.g. gastrointestinal epithelium, capillary walls, etc.), nevertheless, from a pharmacokinetic standpoint, they function as bimolecular layers of phospholipid of differing thickness. Since these membranes are essentially lipid, the *rate* at which drug molecules cross this barrier by passive diffusion is dictated by their lipid solubility — more lipid-soluble molecules crossing the barrier more rapidly. For example, the rate of onset of anaesthesia after rapid intravenous administration of a barbiturate is dictated by the rate of drug transfer across the blood–brain barrier and this rate is proportional to its lipid solubility (Table 1.1).

The other important factor which determines the ability of a drug to cross membrane barriers is the degree of its ionisation. Most drugs are weak acids or weak bases and exist in body fluids partly in an ionised and partly in an un-ionised state. Only un-ionised molecules can pass readily through cellular membranes and the passage of a drug will continue until equilibrium is achieved between the amounts of un-ionised drug on either side of the membrane. However, the *total* amount of drug on either side of the

Table 1.1 Onset of anaesthesia after i.v. administration of barbiturates.

Barbiturate	$\dfrac{\text{Lipid (arachis oil)}}{\text{water}}$ solubility	Approximate time to onset of anaesthesia after i.v. injection (min.)
Thiopentone	580	0.2
Pentobarbitone	39	0.8
Phenobarbitone	3	12.0

membrane may be vastly different since the ratio of un-ionised to ionised drug varies markedly with pH according to the Henderson–Hasselbalch equation:

$$\text{for an acid}\qquad \log\left(\frac{\text{un-ionised}}{\text{ionised}}\right)= \text{pKa}-\text{pH}$$

$$\text{for a base}\qquad \log\left(\frac{\text{ionised}}{\text{un-ionised}}\right)= \text{pKa}-\text{pH}$$

In these equations the pKa or acidic dissociation constant value for the drug is a known constant. For example, Fig. 1.3 demonstrates the distribution of meclofenamic acid between gastric juice and plasma in the horse. At equilibrium, for every 100 un-ionised molecules of meclofenamic acid in the gastric juice, there will be 100 un-ionised molecules in plasma; however, *in total* there will be 100 000 molecules in plasma for every 101 in the stomach. Equilibrium, therefore, is very much in favour of absorption out of the stomach.

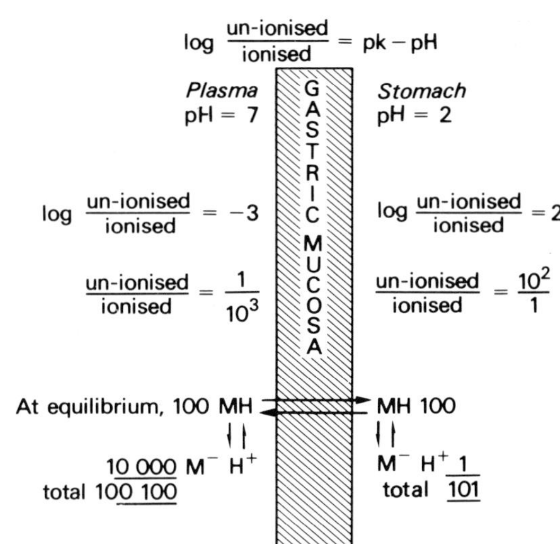

Fig. 1.3 Distribution of meclofenamic acid (pKa=4) between gastric juice and plasma, in the horse.

In general, acidic drugs are well absorbed from acidic environments such as the stomach and upper small intestine and accumulate in alkaline environments, while basic drugs are well absorbed from alkaline environments such as the lower small intestine and accumulate in acid environments. Thus in the horse acids such as meclofenamic acid and phenylbutazone are well and rapidly absorbed from the acid stomach and upper small intestine while basic drugs such as morphine, tetracyclines, and all the common anthelmintics are not absorbed until they reach the more alkaline environment of more distal regions of the small intestine. It should be realised that this process of *passive diffusion*, in which only lipid-soluble, non-ionised drugs pass through membranes, is not uni-directional and that drugs administered to the systemic compartment readily achieve significant concentrations in the gastro-intestinal tract. For example, levamisole is as effective against gastro-intestinal nematodes when given subcutaneously as when given orally. Being a weak base, the concentrations achieved in the relatively acidic horse stomach or ruminant abomasum are higher than those in plasma (Bogan *et al* 1981).

Distribution of drugs in the systemic compartment

Tissues and fluids in the systemic compartment are normally about pH 7·4 and it might be expected that drugs would be distributed equally throughout the tissues. However, in plasma many drugs are bound to plasma proteins, mainly albumin, and in many tissues drugs may be bound to proteins and other tissue constituents such that an unequal distribution often prevails. Protein- and tissue-bound drug is unavailable for further distribution to the liver for metabolism or to the glomerular filtrate for excretion and, generally the bound component serves as a reservoir for drug. The extent of binding varies from none to very high for different drugs but usually is of the same order in different species (Table 1.2). Individual or species differences in drug activity are rarely a result of binding differences.

The process of passive diffusion is the method by which the great majority of drugs distribute in the animal's body. There are a few exceptions where drugs are transported against a concentration gradient by active transport mechanisms. Active transport of drug molecules requires energy and is mediated by carrier substances which complex with the drug and transport it through the membrane. The two sites where active transport mechanisms are of most importance are in the renal tubular epithelium and in the choroid plexus. There are many active transport mechanisms known for endogenous compounds and it is probable that drugs which are actively

Table 1.2 Extent of binding of drugs to plasma protein in different species.

	Horse	Cow	Dog	Human
Benzylpenicillin	54[a]	49[b]	–	65[c]
Oxytetracycline	50[d]	50[d]	–	24–64[e]
Chloramphenicol	45–50[e]	45–50[e]	39[f]	25[e]
Ampicillin	8[a]	–	–	18[g]
Phenylbutazone	98	–	97[h]	98[h]
Digitoxin	–	87[i]	89[i]	92[i]

References. a Durr (1976); b Keen (1965); c. Kunin (1967a); d Pilloud (1973a); e Kunin (1967b); f Baggot (1966); g Howell *et al* (1972); h Perel *et al* (1964); i Baggot & Davis (1973).

transported bear a structural similarity to a natural substrate. Active transport mechanisms are important for the penicillins and account both for their low concentrations in the CNS and their rapid renal excretion. Other drugs for which active transport mechanisms have been demonstrated are some sulphonamides and phenylbutazone.

Routes of administration

Oral administration

Before a drug is available for absorption from the gastrointestinal tract and other sites, it must first dissolve. Although many drugs, such as albendazole, are said to be insoluble they must dissolve to some extent to have an action.

Particle size affects the rate of drug uptake: the smaller the particle size, the greater the surface area and thus the more rapidly the drug is dissolved. Particle size has been shown to markedly affect the activity and toxicity of the anthelmintic phenothiazine and various proprietary brands of digoxin have caused problems in digitalisation because of considerable differences in their rates of dissolution. Drugs inactivated to a large extent in the gut, such as benzylpenicillin and insulin, are not administered by the oral route.

Drugs which are mainly ionised at gut pH (e.g. tubocurarine and the trypanocidal 'dye-type' drugs homidium and isometamidium) are not absorbed and must be given by the parenteral route.

Ruminant animals

Ruminant animals are characterised by the presence of a large fermenting

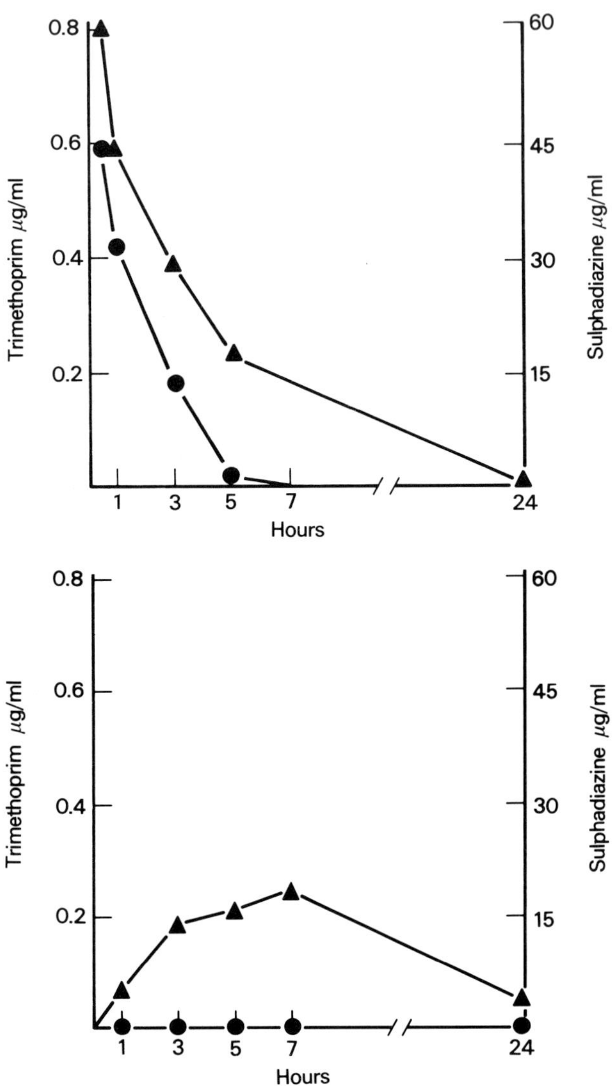

Figs. 1.4 & 1.5 The concentration of sulphadiazine and trimethoprim in the plasma of sheep after administration of 25 and 5 mg/kg, respectively, by the intravenous (upper) and oral (lower) routes. (From Piercy 1978.) ▲ = sulphadiazine. ● = trimethoprim.

bulk in the ruminoreticulum which occupies about 20% of the body mass (Warner & Flatt 1955) and forms the anterior portion of the alimentary canal. Posterior to the ruminoreticulum the abomasum (pH 1–3) and small and large intestines appear to function similarly to the stomach and intestine of simple-stomached animals with respect to drugs, i.e. drugs are absorbed by passive diffusion, only lipid-soluble, un-ionised drugs being well absorbed. However the characteristics of drug passage across the highly specialised ruminal epithelium are still not well established. Drugs given orally are initially markedly diluted by the contents of the fore-stomachs. Drugs are known to be absorbed by the passive diffusion of un-ionised, lipid-soluble molecules through the ruminal epithelium and the process is pH dependent. This has been demonstrated for thiabendazole (McManus *et al* 1966), sulphonamides (Austin 1967), amphetamine (Baggot *et al* 1973), and pentobarbitone, salicylate, antipyrine and quinine (Jenkins *et al* 1975). It does appear, however, that the rate of transfer is slow compared with other portions of the gut with the result that, for many drugs, only a small amount will be absorbed before the contents have been passed on into the abomasum and small intestine. Thus for many drugs, oral administration to ruminants is impractical. If the rate of systemic metabolism and/or excretion is rapid, then the drug may not achieve useful systemic concentrations. For example, Piercy (1978) has shown that trimethoprim does not achieve measurable plasma levels after oral administration to sheep while sulphadiazine (the other component of some potentiated sulphonamide preparations and which has a slower metabolism and/or excretion) does achieve measurable concentrations (Figs. 1.4 and 1.5). Thomson & Black (1978) have also shown with ampicillin that administration to the rumen by stomach tube in calves does not result in measurable plasma levels.

On the other hand, this property of the rumen acting to slow the absorption of drugs may be used to advantage. The benzimidazole anthelmintics, mebendazole and flubendazole (and it would seem reasonable to suggest that all benzimidazole anthelmintics act similarly (Coles 1977)) have been shown to exert their effects by preventing glucose uptake by helminths (Van den Bossche 1972). They do this by initially causing the disappearance of microtubular structures in the intestinal cells of the nematodes (or tegumental cells of tapeworms), followed by accumulation of secretory granules and autolysis (Borgers & de Nollin 1975, Borgers *et al* 1975a, Borgers *et al* 1975b) (Fig. 1.6). Because glycogen depletion is slow (Van den Bossche 1976), the challenge to the parasites must be maintained for a long period. The current hypothesis (Coles 1977) is that the benzimidazoles act in the same way but that differences in their activities are due to differing pharmacokinetics. Thus the more active compounds, such as fenbendazole, mebendezole, oxfendazole and albendazole, are more water-insoluble than the less active thiabendazole and cambendazole (Fig. 1.7). This low water solubility combined with the effect of the rumen slowing their absorption serves to maintain concentrations of the more active compounds in plasma (and presumably in the gastrointestinal tract) for long periods (Marriner & Bogan 1980). This mode of action also explains why mono-gastric

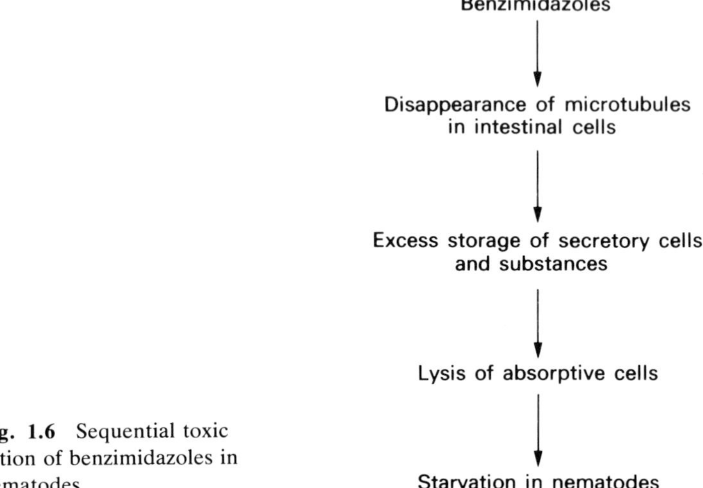

Fig. 1.6 Sequential toxic action of benzimidazoles in nematodes.

	Position 2	Position 5	UK trade names	Decreasing water solubility	Dose (mg/kg) for >95% control of sheep/cattle gut parasites
Thiabendazole	(S, N ring)	H–	Thibenzole Equizole Thiprazole		50–100
Cambendazole	''	$(CH_3)_2CHCO_2NH-$	Bovicam		25
Parbendazole	$CH_3\overset{O}{\overset{\|}{C}}-O-NH-$	$CH_3CH_2CH_2CH_2-$	Brentic Helmatac		20–30
Oxibendazole	''	$CH_3CH_2CH_2O-$	Rycovet Widespec		10–20
Mebendazole	''	(phenyl)$-\overset{O}{\overset{\|}{C}}-$	Telmin		15
Fenbendazole	''	(phenyl)$-S-$	Panacur		5
Oxfendazole	''	(phenyl)$-\overset{O}{\overset{\|}{S}}-$	Systamex Synanthic		5
Albendazole	''	$CH_3CH_2CH_2S-$	Valbazen		5

Fig. 1.7 Structure of the benzimidazoles marketed as anthelmintics in the UK. Decreasing water solubility down the series is probably the cause of increased spectrum of activity and increased potency.

animals such as the dog require daily dosing for five days with mebendazole while a single dose is active in ruminants. Even in ruminants, however, divided doses would appear to be more effective than single doses.

It may be that little improvement in potency or spectrum of activity of the benzimidazoles is possible, since with increasing insolubility, the concentrations of dissolved drug achieved in the gut may be insufficient for activity and the majority of the drug will be excreted in the faeces undissolved.

An additional feature unique to ruminant animals is that some orally administered liquids and suspensions may be delivered directly to the abomasum by closure of a specialised structure, the reticular (often called oesophageal) groove. This mechanism, greatest in young animals, decreases with age but adult animals often retain some activity. We have found that, in adult sheep, this reflex occurs consistently to a similar extent in individual animals but varies markedly between animals (Marriner 1980). McEwan & Oakley (1978) have also shown that the commonly used anthelmintic drenches, fenbendazole, thiabendazole, and levamisole, may all be delivered directly to some extent to the abomasum with little differences between the different anthelmintics. Closure of the oesophageal groove is probably behavioural and much of the early work implicating salt solutions (Wester 1930) as a stimulus for closure of the groove is probably incorrect (Ørskov 1972).

Fig. 1.8 shows the concentration of meclofenamate in plasma after administration of meclofenamic acid as a slurry orally and intraruminally to

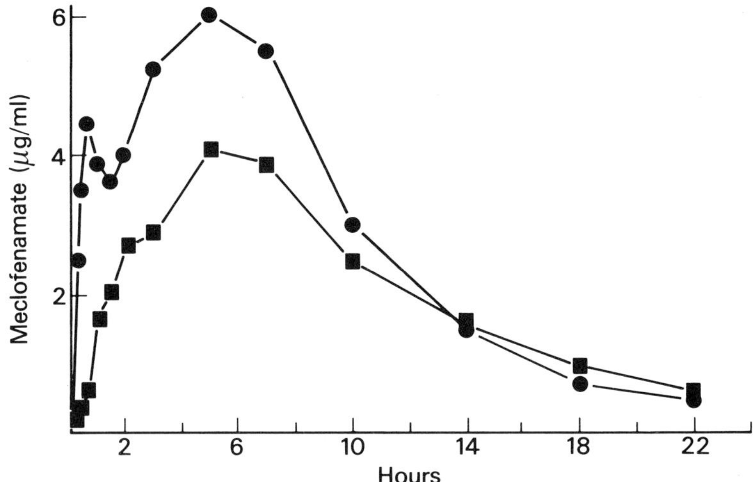

Fig. 1.8 Mean concentrations of meclofenamate in plasma after administration of meclofenamic acid orally and via a ruminal fistula in the same three sheep (Marriner & Bogan 1979). ● = oral, ■ = intraruminal.

sheep. Meclofenamic acid has a pKa of 4 and is not absorbed to any great extent from the rumen. The initial peak at 30 minutes is due to the proportion of drug delivered directly to the abomasum by closure of the oesophageal groove.

Passive diffusion involves transfer into as well as absorption from the gastrointestinal tract, and drugs such as levamisole are as effective against gastrointestinal parasites when given subcutaneously as by the oral route. Indeed, with the anthelmintics levamisole, pyrantel and piperazine, unlike the benzimidazoles, it is the peak concentration in the gastrointestinal tract which is important since they exert their effects at ganglia and neuromuscular junctions in the helminths (Van den Bossche 1976).

Horse

In the horse, the pharmacokinetic role of the enlarged caecum, which functions as a fermentation vat similar to the reticulorumen, and that of the modified large intestine are unknown. To some extent the gastrointestinal tract of the horse appears to function similarly to that in simple-stomached animals. Acidic drugs such as meclofenamic acid and phenylbutazone are well and rapidly absorbed from the horse stomach (pH 1.1–6.8 (Schwarz *et al* 1926)) and weakly basic drugs are absorbed from the small intestine. Nevertheless, the caecum may play a role in slowing the kinetics of insoluble drugs since in the horse, like the ruminant and unlike other simple-stomached animals, benzimidazole anthelmintics are effective in single oral doses.

The presence of food in the gastrointestinal tract may affect the absorption of drugs. It may do this by slowing gastric emptying time and/or by adsorption of the drug to food particles. It is well recognised in man that with many drugs, such as ampicillin, food will delay the time it takes to reach peak concentrations and that the bioavailability (area under the plasma concentration/time curve) of the drug may be reduced. Surprisingly, in large animal species, little consideration has been given to this aspect. Sullivan & Snow (Pers. Commun.) have shown that, in ponies, the absorption of phenylbutazone is markedly impaired by food. The peak plasma concentration and the bioavailability were both reduced by more than 50% when the ponies were fed prior to oral administration as compared with overnight fasting. Gerring *et al* (1981) have also observed marked differences in absorption of phenylbutazone in the horse, presumably due to feed intake. The potential for impaired absorption would seem to be greater in the herbivorous animal, the surface area of the food and the adsorptive capacity of cellulose fragments being considerably greater than in carnivorous animals.

Intravenous administration

The administration of drugs directly into the bloodstream usually provides a more rapid pharmacological effect in the systemic compartment, since the drug does not have to be absorbed. In veterinary medicine, this route is often used unnecessarily when it confers little therapeutic advantage and runs the risk of an adverse reaction since these are much more common when drugs are given by this route. In the horse, for example, we have frequently seen hyperexcitability, hypertension, and tachycardia when the narcotic analgesics morphine and pethidine or the tranquillisers azaperone and acepromazine have been given intravenously but rarely when administration was intramuscular. Hypersensitivity reactions, such as those seen infrequently with penicillin and more commonly with tetracyclines, tend to be more severe after intravenous administration. (It should be noted that when formulations are designed for intramuscular and subcutaneous routes, the kinetics may be adversely affected by using the intravenous route.) For the injectable anaesthetics, this route does provide a method for giving an appropriate dose to effect, since equilibration between plasma and brain tissue occurs rapidly.

Intramuscular and subcutaneous administration

Intramuscular and subcutaneous sites provide drug to the bloodstream more slowly and maintain concentrations for longer than intravenous administration. They have the added advantages of being more convenient and less hazardous than intravenous administration.

Absorption from subcutaneous or intramuscular sites can be slowed by the use of relatively insoluble salts or the use of formulations in water-immiscible, oily vehicles. Salts such as procaine or benzathine penicillin result in slower absorption of the penicillin moiety (Fig. 1.9): on solution, the acid and base radicals of the salt function as if they had been injected separately, i.e. benzylpenicillin in sodium, procaine and benzathine penicillin functions in *exactly* the same way, while the procaine radical may exert a local analgesic action. (Procaine from procaine penicillin may be detected as a prohibited substance in the urine of racing animals.)

The rate of uptake of drug from intramuscular or subcutaneous sites is proportional to the blood flow at the site. In general, absorption from subcutaneous sites is said to be less rapid than the more highly perfused muscle sites. Some recent work (Palmer 1978) using ampicillin and amoxycillin administered subcutaneously and intramuscularly to calves showed only small differences in the rate of absorption between the routes, and intramuscular administration in the neck region resulted in faster absorption

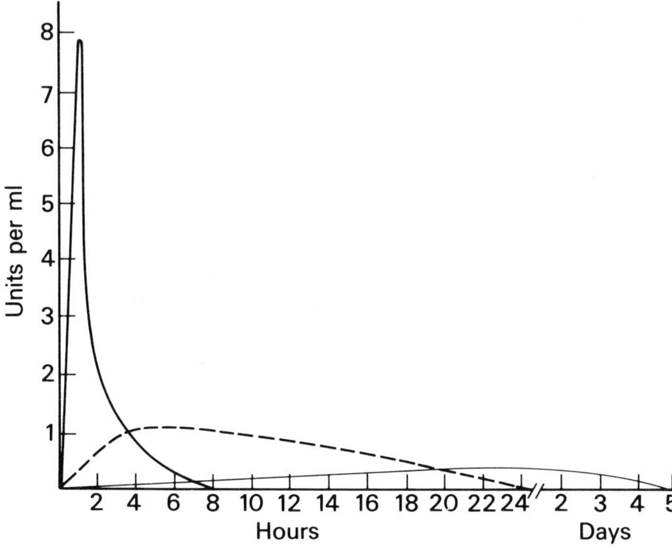

Fig. 1.9 Concentration of penicillin in blood after administration of equivalent doses of sodium, procaine, and benethamine or benzathine penicillins (Glaxo Veterinary Research Newsletter 1975). — = sodium penicillin, ---- = procaine penicillin, — = benzathine or benethamine penicillin.

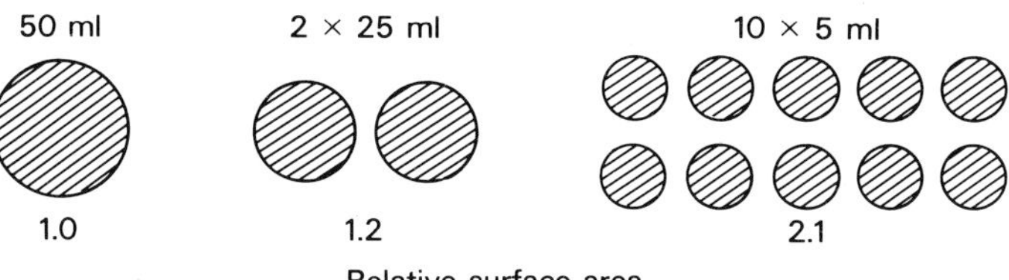

Fig. 1.10 Relation of bolus size to surface area.

than in the rump region. Bogan *et al* (1981) have shown no difference in absorption of levamisole from subcutaneous sites in the neck, gluteal, and thoracic regions of sheep. Groothuis *et al* (1978) have also shown that a febrile response induced by *E. coli* endotoxin resulted in reduced absorption after oral and intramuscular administration of amoxycillin and ampicillin.

The size of the injection bolus may be important in large animal therapeutics. It is surprising that, even in experiments measuring drup uptake from intramuscular or subcutaneous sites, no mention is usually made of the size of the injection and the number of sites used. For insoluble oily boluses, drug uptake is proportional to the surface area of the bolus and dividing the dose into aliquots may increase drug uptake markedly (Fig. 1.10). However, even with water-miscible injection boluses such as procaine penicillin, it is probable that more intimate contact between the salt crystals and blood or interstitial fluid will occur with small injection size. Bogan *et al* (1981) have shown that dividing the dose of levamisole between five subcutaneous sites in the thoracic region of sheep resulted in higher peak plasma concentrations at one hour than when the same dose was given at a single thoracic site. Therefore, it one wants the same response to occur to a drug in, say, a 50 kg calf and a 500 kg cow, then the injection volume should be kept constant. This factor may explain why normally recommended dosages of some antibiotics (in particular oxytetracycline (Pilloud 1973a) and chloramphenicol (Pilloud 1973b, Sisodia *et al* 1973)) do not provide adequate therapeutic concentrations in the plasma of cattle and horses when given intramuscularly.

Intramammary administration (see also Chapter 5)

Intramammary infusion is commonly used in cattle — approximately 10–15 million antibiotic intramammary tubes are used annually in the UK. The milk:plasma tissue barrier functions like other cellular barriers, drugs being transferred by passive diffusion. Drugs may pass into the milk following systemic administration and into the circulation following intramammary infusion, passage in both directions depending on the drug's lipid-solubility and acid-base properties. Milk is slightly more acidic (pH 6.5–6.9, mastitic milk pH 6.9–7.2) than blood plasma and the theoretical ratio for milk: plasma concentrations at equilibrium will thus be greater than one for the basic antibiotics (all the major groups with the exception of penicillins and cephalosporins) and less than one for acids such as penicillins and cephalosporins. For a number of reasons, including tissue binding, the observed milk:plasma ratios vary slightly from those predicted theoretically but in general most of the commonly used antibiotics achieve reasonable duration of minimum inhibitory concentrations (MICs) for sensitive organisms in milk after intramuscular administration (Table 1.3). Systemic chloram-

Table 1.3 Duration of minimal inhibitory concentrations (MIC) of antibiotics in milk after a single intramuscular injection. (Abstracted from Ziv 1975.)

	Observed milk plasma ratio	MIC in milk (μg/ml)	Dose rate (mg/kg)	Duration of MIC in milk (hours)
Benzylpenicillin sodium	0.12–0.20	0.05	11	6.0
Benzylpenicillin procaine	0.12–0.20	0.05	10	24.0
Ampicillin	0.22–0.30	0.05	10	6.0
Cloxacillin	0.20–0.24	0.05	25	12.0
Dihydrostreptomycin	0.20–0.80	0.10	40	12.0
Oxytetracycline	0.75–0.95	0.50	11	12.0

phenicol provides adequate mammary concentrations only when given as the succinate salt (Ziv 1980). The low penetration of dihydrostreptomycin and other aminoglycosides into milk is related to their low lipid/water partition coefficients and slow passage through tissue barriers. In this field, the excellent work of Rasmussen (1966) and Ziv (1975) is recommended. From a therapeutic point of view, in acute mastitis, systemic treatment provides more reliable concentrations throughout the udder than intra-mammary infusion, especially when the udder is inflamed and/or fibrosed (Fünke 1975).

The intramammary treatment of cows with antibiotics at the beginning of the dry period requires the use of very long-acting formulations. These formulations utilise both methods of producing long-acting preparations, i.e. the use of insoluble salts and of water-immiscible (usually oily) bases. The effect of combining these two approaches is demonstrated in Fig. 1.11.

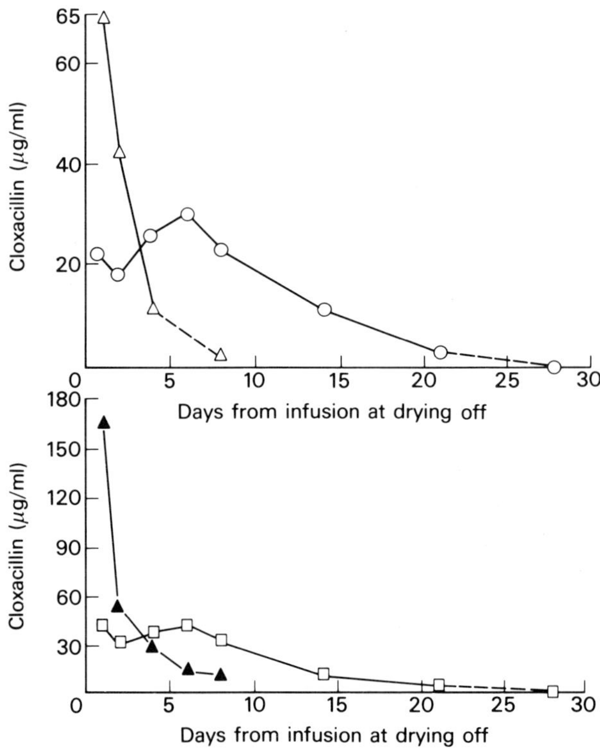

Fig. 1.11 Concentration of cloxacillin in the udder secretions of dry cows obtained using different formulation bases (*top*) and different cloxacillin salts (*below*). (From Smith *et al* 1967.) ○ = 0.5 g benzathine cloxacillin in 3% aluminium monostearate base (SR), Δ = 0.5 g benzathine cloxacillin in quick release paraffin base (QR), ▲ = 1.0 g sodium cloxacillin in 3% aluminium monostearate base (SR), □ = 1.0 g benzathine cloxacillin in 3% aluminium monostearate base (SR).

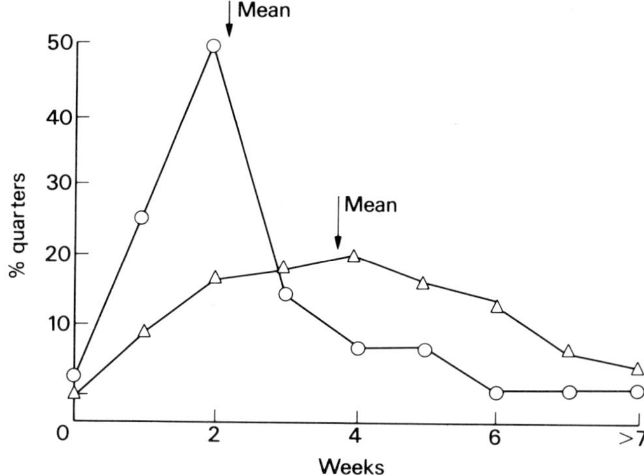

Fig. 1.12 Persistence of cloxacillin in the secretions of 29 infected and 55 uninfected quarters of 21 cows treated with 0.5 g benzathine cloxacillin in 3% aluminium stearate mineral oil base after the final milking of lactation. The distributions are of the number of weeks before the concentration fell below 0.5 μg/ml of secretion. (From Smith *et al* 1968.) ○ = infected, Δ = uninfected.

It should be noted, however, that these preparations maintain MICs in udder *secretions* for a very long period but it is unlikely, indeed impossible, that they maintain MICs throughout the udder since free drug will diffuse to the systemic circulation. However, maintenance of the MICs may not be necessary since the initial high concentrations throughout the udder will remove existing infections and, subsequent to this, any new infections which enter via the teat canal will be eliminated where sufficient concentration will be maintained by the injection bolus. There is probably an optimum period of 3–4 weeks to the length of action required of an intramammary preparation for the dry cow period, since over 97% of all new infections occur in the first 21 days after drying off (Dodd & Griffin 1975). This compromise is required to keep the size and cost of the injection bolus reasonable. The presence of infection can also affect the elimination of the antibiotic from the quarter, infection usually resulting in faster elimination (Smith *et al* 1968) (Fig. 1.12).

Topical treatment

Many drugs penetrate intact skin surprisingly rapidly. The absorption rate may be increased by incorporating the drug in certain formulations, especially with the solvent dimethylsulphoxide. This route is convenient for the treatment of large animals, especially cattle, and it is to be expected that an

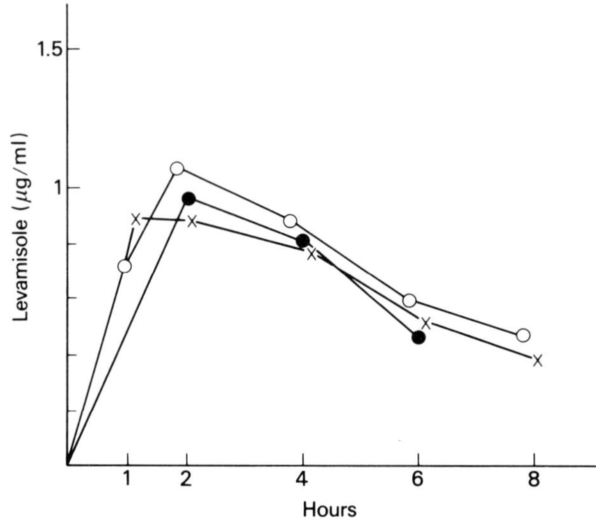

Fig. 1.13 Blood concentrations of levamisole after administration by the topical ('spot-on')
route at the dose rate of 10 mg/kg compared with 10 mg/kg orally and 8 mg/kg subcutaneously.
(From Dorn & Federmann 1976.) ○ = spot-on, ● = orally, × = subcutaneously.

increasing number of veterinary drugs will be applied in this way. Fig. 1.13
shows the concentrations of levamisole in blood after topical ('spot-on')
application of a commercial preparation compared with subcutaneous and
oral administration.

The application of organophosphorus preparations for systemic warble-
cide activity is now most conveniently done by 'pour-on' techniques using
small volumes.

Percutaneous absorption may pose dangers to the user, especially with
highly potent compounds such as etorphine — the narcotic analgesic component of Immobilon — and prostaglandin preparations in females of child-
bearing age.

Principles of drug dosage

The concentrations of a drug in plasma after intravenous injection usually
follow a biphasic pattern (Fig. 1.14), the initial rapid fall, or α phase, being
due to distribution and the slower, or β phase, being due to elimination. In
the β phase, blood levels fall exponentially and the time taken for the
concentration to fall by 50% is called the half-life. When the half-life of a
drug is quoted without further clarification, it usually refers to that in plasma
in the β phase. A knowledge of the half-life of the drug is essential to

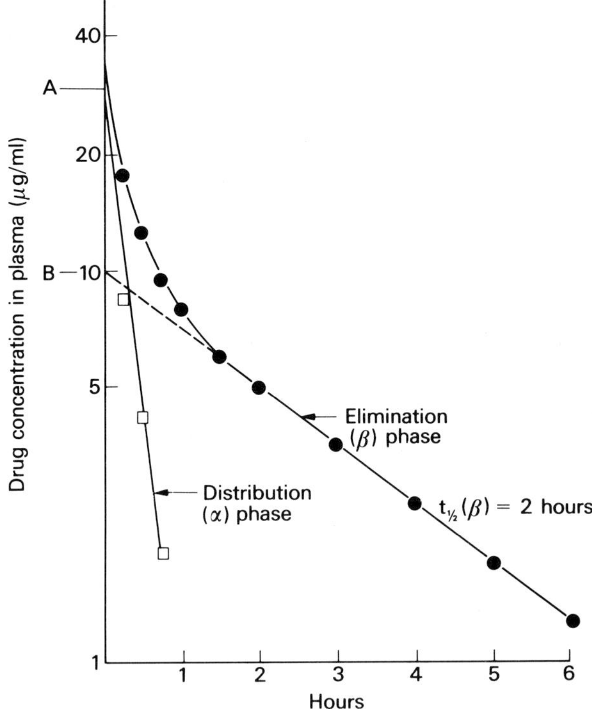

Fig. 1.14 Typical time course of the concentration of a drug in plasma after intravenous administration of a single dose. The half-life of the elimination (or β) phase is two hours. (From Baggot 1977.)

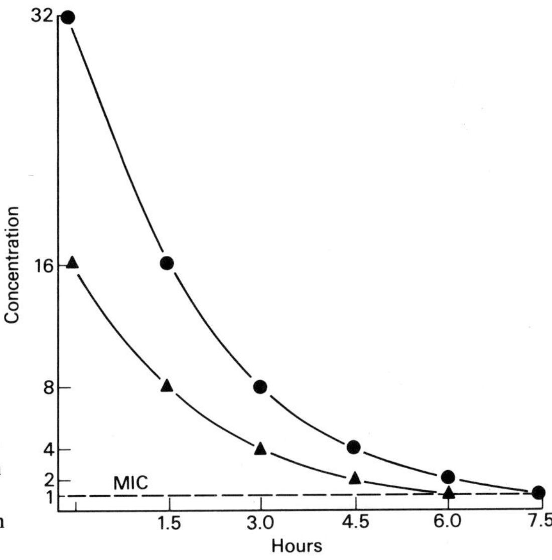

Fig. 1.15 Plasma concentrations of ampicillin (half-life 1.5 hours) in the horse required to maintain a minimum inhibitory concentration at dosage intervals of six hours.

calculate dosage regimens. For example, with ampicillin which, in the horse, has a half-life of 1.5 hours (Dürr 1976), an intravenous dose is required which will provide a plasma concentration 16 times the therapeutic concentration (MIC) to provide therapeutic concentrations for six hours. Dosing intervals can be increased by increasing the dose level but doubling the dose only increases the dosage interval by 1.5 hours (Fig. 1.15). In this case, an initial high ('loading') dose would be of little value, whereas for drugs with longer half-lives such as oxytetracycline (β phase half-life in cattle 9.1 hours) there is value in using an increased loading dose in short interval regimens. In cattle, an initial loading dose of oxytetracycline of 3.5 mg/kg followed by 2.1 mg/kg twelve hourly will maintain plasma concentrations of > 0.13 μg/ml — the MIC for organisms considered highly susceptible to oxytetracycline (Pilloud 1973a).

The limiting factors to increasing the dose to extend dosage intervals are that initially high concentrations may cause toxicity and that the cost of treatment becomes prohibitive. If dosing intervals are extended by forming slow-release formulations, it is important to realise that long-acting preparations do not provide adequate concentrations readily (see Fig. 1.9) and that there are advantages in combining a quick- and slow-release preparation, such as sodium and procaine penicillin.

References

Austin F. H. (1967) Absorption, distribution and excretion of sulphonamides in ruminants. *Fed. Proc.* **26,** 1001–1005.

Baggot J. D. (1966) In *Principles of Drug Disposition in Domestic Animals,* W. B. Saunders, Philadelphia.

Baggot J. D. & Davis L. E. (1973) Plasma protein binding of digitoxin and digoxin in several mammalian species. *Res. Vet. Sci.* **15,** 81–7.

Baggot J. D., Davies L. E. & Reuning R. H. (1973) The disposition kinetics of amphetamine in the ruminant animal. *Arch. Int. Pharmocodyn. Ther.* **202,** 17–27.

Bogan J. A., Marriner S. E. & Galbraith E. A. (1981) Pharmacokinetics of levamisole in sheep. *Res. Vet. Sci.* **32,** 124–6.

Borgers M. & De Nollin S. (1975) Ultrastructural changes in Ascaris suum intestine after mebendazole treatment in vivo. *J. Parasit.* **61,** 110–122.

Borgers M., De Nollin S., De Brabander M. & Thienpont D. (1975a) Influence of the anthelmintic mebendazole on microtubules and intracellular organelle movement in nematode intestinal cells. *Am. J. Vet. Res.* **36,** 1153–1166.

Borgers M., De Nollin S., Verheyen A. *et al* (1975b) Effects of new anthelmintics on the microtubular system of parasites. In *Microtubules and Microtubule Inhibitors* Borgers M. & De Brabander M. (eds) pp. 497–508. North Holland, Amsterdam.

Coles G. C. (1977) The mechanism of action of some veterinary anthelmintics In *Perspectives in the control of parasite disease in animals in Europe* Jolly D. W. & Somerville J. M. (eds) pp. 53–63. Royal College of Veterinary Surgeons, London.

Dodd F. H. & Griffin T. K. (1975) The role of antibiotics treatment at drying-off in the control of mastitis. In *Proc. of Seminar on Mastitis Control* Dodd F. H. *et al* (ed) pp. 282–302. International Dairy Federation, Brussels.

Dürr A. (1976) Comparison of the pharmacokinetics of penicillin G and ampicillin in the horse. *Res. Vet. Sci.* **20**, 24–29.

Fünke (1975) In *Proc. of seminar on mastitis control* Dodd F. H. *et al* (ed) pp. 311–312. International Dairy Federation, Brussels.

Gerring E. L., Lees P. & Taylor J. B. (1981) Pharmacokinetics of phenylbutazone and its metabolite in the horse. *Equine Vet. J.* **13**, 152–157.

Groothuis D. G., Van Miert A.S.P.A.M., Ziv G. *et al* (1978) Effect of experimental *Eschericia coli* endotoxaemia on ampicillin: amoxycillin blood levels after oral and parenteral administration in calves. *J. Vet. Pharm.* **1**, 81–84.

Howell A. *et al* (1972) Effect of protein-binding on levels of ampicillin and cloxacillin in synovial fluid. *Clin. Pharm. Ther.* **13**, 152–7.

Jenkins W. L., Davis L. E. & Boulos B. M. (1975) Transfer of drugs across the ruminal wall in goats. *Am. J. Vet. Res.* **36**, 1771–1776.

Keen P. M. (1965) The binding of three penicillins to plasma protein of several mammalian species as studied by ultrafiltration at body temperature. *Br. J. Pharmacol.* **25**, 507–14.

Kunin C. M. (1976a) Clinical significance of protein-binding of penicillins. *Ann. N.Y. Acad. Sci.* **145**, 282–90.

Kunin C. M. (1976b) A guide to use of antibiotics in patients with renal disease. *Ann. Intern. Med.* **67**, 151–8.

Marriner S. E. & Bogan J. A. (1979) The influence of the rumen on the absorption of drugs: studies using meclofenamic acid administered by various routes to sheep and cattle. *J. Vet. Pharmacol. Therap.* **2**, 109–115.

Marriner S. E. & Bogan J. A. (1980) Pharmacokinetics of albendazole in sheep. *Am. J. Vet. Res.* **41**, 1126–1129.

Marriner S. E. (1980) The Pharmacokinetics of Drugs in the Ruminant Animal. PhD thesis, University of Glasgow.

McEwan A. D. & Oakley G. A. (1978) Anthelmintics and closure of the oesophageal groove in cattle. *Vet. Rec.* **102**, 314.

McManus E. C., Washko F. V. & Tocco D. J. (1966) Gastrointestinal absorption and secretion of thiabendazole in ruminants. *Am. J. Vet. Res.* **27**, 849–855.

Ørskov E. R. (1972) Technology of feeding so that the rumen is by-passed following artificial rearing. In *Proc. World Congress on Animal Feeding*, pp. 627–640. Madrid.

Perel J. M. *et al* (1964) A study of structure–activity relationships in regard to species difference in the phenylbutazone series. *Biochem. Pharmacol.* **13**, 1304–17.

Piercy D. W. T. (1978) Distribution of trimethoprim/sulfadiazine in plasma, tissue and synovial fluids. *Vet. Rec.* **102**, 523.

Pilloud M. (1973a) Pharmacokinetics, plasma protein binding and dosage of oxytetracycline in cattle and horses. *Res. Vet. Sci.* **15**, 224–230.

Pilloud M. (1973b) Pharmacokinetics, plasma protein binding and dosage of chloramphenicol in cattle and horses. *Res. Vet. Sci.* **15**, 231–238.

Rasmussen F. (1966) *Studies on the mammary excretion and absorption of drugs.* Carl Fr. Mortensen, Copenhagen.

Sisodia C. S. *et al* (1973) A pharmacological study of chloramphenicol in cattle. *Am. J. Vet. Res.* **34**, 1147–1151.

Schwarz C. *et al* (1926) Die H-Ionenkonzentration im Mageninhalt des Pferdes. *Arch. Ges. Physiol.* **213**, 595–601.

Smith A. *et al* (1967) The persistence of cloxacillin in the mammary gland when infused immediately after the last milking of lactation. *J. Dairy Res.* **34**, 47.

Smith A. *et al* (1968) Report, National Institute for Research in Dairying, Reading, UK p. 63.

Thompson S. M. R. & Black W. D. (1978) A study of the influence of the method of oral administration of ampicillin upon plasma drug levels in calves. *Can. J. Comp. Med.* **42**, 255–259.

Van den Bossche H. (1972) Biochemical effects of the anthelmintic drug mebendazole. In *Comparative Biochemistry of Parasites* Van den Bossche H. (ed) pp. 139–157. Academic Press, New York.

Van den Bossche H. (1976) The molecular basis of anthelmintic action. In *Biochemistry of parasites and host-parasite relationships* Van den Bossche H. (ed) p. 564. Elsevier, Amsterdam.

Warner R. G. & Flatt W. P. (1965) Anatomical development of the ruminant stomach. In *Physiology of Digestion in the Ruminant,* Dougherty R. W. (ed) p. 24. Butterworths, London

Wester I. (1930) *Berl. Tierarztl. Wschr.* **46**, 1.

Ziv G. (1975) Pharmacokinetic concepts for systemic and intramammary antibiotic treatment in lactating and dry cows. In *Proc. of seminar on mastitis control* Dodd F. H. pp. 314–240. International Dairy Federation, Brussels.

Ziv G. (1980) *Proc. Inter. Meet. Vet. Pharm.* Cambridge, England

2

Drug elimination

D.H. SNOW

Species differences

As there are marked species differences in both the dose rate and frequency of drug administration required to obtain a particular response, it is usually not possible to extrapolate data from one species to another. These species differences can arise for a number of reasons: for example, the dose of xylazine required in horses is ten times greater than in cattle for a similar effect; this is probably due to it having different inherent potencies in the two species. In the majority of cases, however, differing dose rates and frequency of administration are related to differing rates of elimination. For example, phenylbutazone must be administered more frequently in the horse than in man because of markedly different elimination rates. It is therefore the purpose of this chapter to discuss those factors that determine the rate of drug elimination.

Drug half-life

The elimination of an active drug from the body is dependent on the processes of metabolism (also referred to as biotransformation), and excretion. It is the rate at which one or both of the mechanisms operate for a specific drug, together with the apparent volume of distribution and protein binding of a drug, that largely determines the duration of activity of that compound. Once a steady state of distribution has been attained following drug administration, it is the processes of elimination which determine the rate of decrease of circulating plasma levels of the drug. This rate is used to obtain the plasma half-life ($t_{\frac{1}{2}}$ of a drug, which is the time taken for the plasma (or serum) concentration of the drug to decline by 50%. Information on the half-life of a drug in a particular species is very important in determining a rational dosage regimen as it is generally assumed that the duration of pharmacological activity of a drug in the tissues is related to its plasma concentration. There are a few notable exceptions to this rule, corticosteroids for example.

Research studies

Although a great deal is known about the metabolic fate of drugs in man and various laboratory animals, studies in the larger domestic species have been rather limited until recently. However, during the last decade or so increased research on the pharmacodynamics and metabolism of drugs in these species has taken place. Such investigations have been instituted for a number of reasons. The finding by Pilloud (1973a, 1973b) that the recommended dosage schedules for a number of antibiotics were insufficient to attain adequate blood concentrations has led to a more detailed examination of the dose rates required. Stricter legislation both in EEC countries and the USA on the requirements for information about the level of residues of drugs and metabolites in tissues of feed animals has also meant that more detailed research on the fate of drugs is needed. In the horse the main impetus for this research has arisen from the need to detect drugs (or their metabolites) which could be used for illegal purposes in racing and performance events. Many of the studies carried out in the horse have been reviewed by Moss (1976).

It is not intended in this chapter to deal with the complex models and mathematical considerations involved in the studies of pharmacokinetics, details of which can be obtained from the texts by Notari (1975) and van Rossum (1977). Baggot (1977) considers both of the above aspects with special reference to domestic animals, while La Du *et al* (1971) disuss factors influencing drug disposition and biotransformation.

Drug biotransformation (metabolism)

For the majority of compounds administered therapeutically, the most important route of elimination is by metabolism in the body, but within and between individuals the extent of metabolism varies widely, even for drugs which are closely related structurally. In general the purpose of biotransformation is to make a compound more readily excreted. If this process did not occur, drugs could persist and exert their activity for a long time. The metabolites arising from biotransformation are therefore always more polar and less lipid-soluble than the parent drug; they normally are inactive or have reduced activity. However, metabolism may also produce an active compound from an inactive or less active one and in this case the administered drug is referred to as a pro-drug.

The majority of biotransformation reactions occur within the parenchymal cells of the liver. In addition, varying degrees of metabolism can occur within other tissues of the body, such as kidney, lung, intestine, and plasma. Metabolism of compounds in organs other than the liver appears to depend upon whether the drug is similar to endogenous compounds which undergo metabolism in the relevant organ.

Within the hepatic cell, biotransformation can proceed in the soluble, the mitochondrial, or the microsomal fractions, although the last is by far the most important location. A group of fairly non-specific enzymes which are referred to as the drug-metabolising enzymes (DMES) and whose activity can be altered by a number of factors are found in association with the microsomal or smooth endoplasmic fraction of the cell. This enzyme system, as well as having the capacity to metabolise exogenous compounds, also contributes to the metabolism of certain endogenous compounds such as the sex steroids. However, there are other more specific steroid hydroxylases in the hepatic cell which are considered to play a much more important role in the inactivation of these steroids. The role of DMES in drug metabolism and factors influencing this system are discussed by Remmer (1970).

Compounds can undergo a large number of reactions to convert them from a lipid-soluble form to less lipid-soluble metabolites. For convenience the metabolism of compounds can be divided into two phases:

Phase I reactions — metabolic transformations, resulting from oxidation, reduction, etc.

Phase II reactions — synthetic reactions resulting in the addition of a conjugate to a drug or metabolite which has a suitable chemical group attached.

Phase I and II reactions can occur separately or sequentially, and a drug may undergo metabolism by a variety of routes, resulting in the formation of a large number of metabolites. Thus, in the case of the phenothiazine tranquilisers, numerous metabolites have been identified, and in the horse the types of phenothiazine metabolites excreted are influenced by the structure of the drug, the route of administration and, to a lesser extent, the individual animal (Weir & Sanford 1972). Large variations in the metabolism of the same compound can also occur between species as a result of both qualitative and quantitative differences in metabolic pathways. This is well illustrated in the case of amphetamine, which has been shown (Baggot & Davis 1973) to give rise to different metabolites in different species.

Phase I reactions

Oxidation

By far the most frequent metabolic pathway is oxidation which takes place in the hepatic microsomes and is brought about by the mixed function oxidases of the DMES. The system requires the presence of NADPH (reduced nicotinamide adenine dinucleotide phosphate) and a cytochrome, P-450, which reacts with molecular oxygen. Increased activity of this pathway is

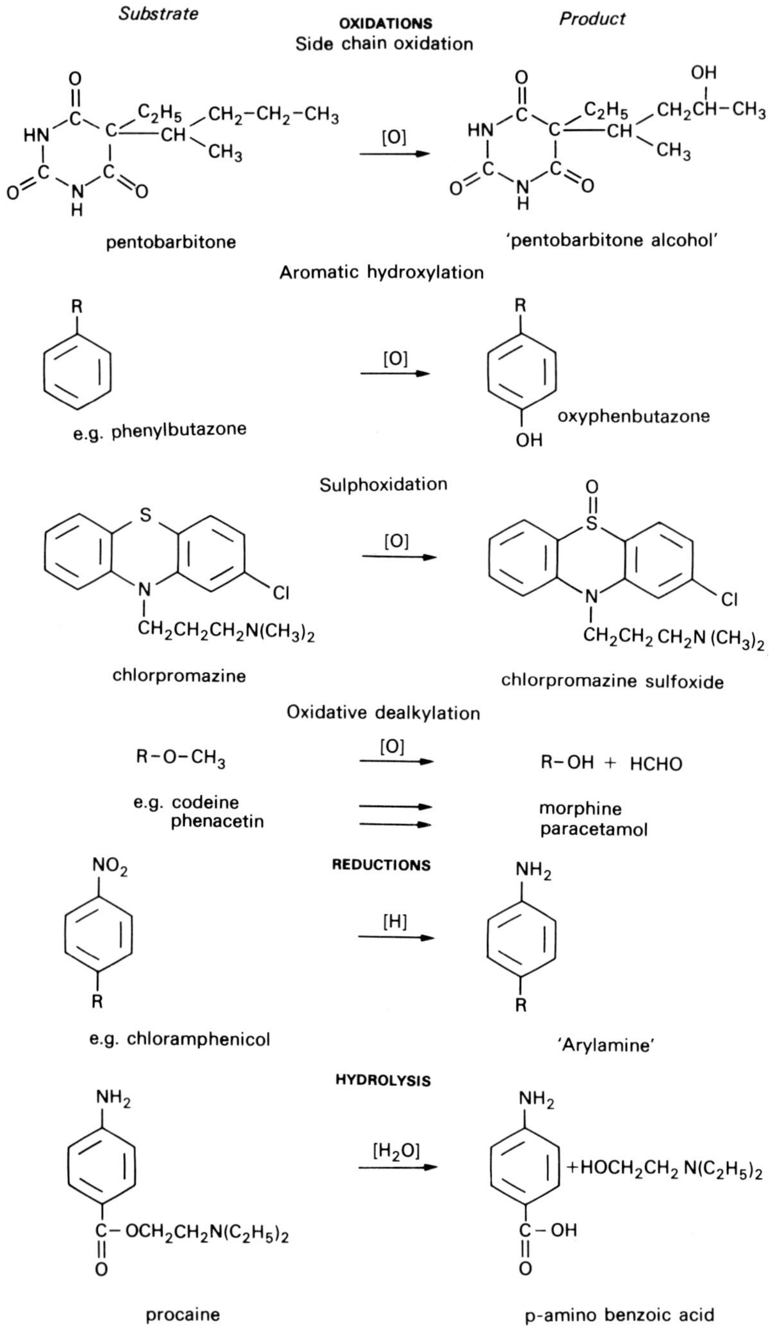

Fig. 2.1 Examples of phase I reactions.

associated with an increase in the amount of cytochrome P-450. Some of the more important types of oxidation reactions are shown in Fig. 2.1. In addition, but to a considerably lesser degree, non-microsomal oxidation can also occur, e.g. oxidation of alcohols by alcohol dehydrogenase, and deamination of catecholamine-related compounds by monoamine oxidase.

Reduction

Within the microsomes, reduction of nitro- and azo-compounds to amines can occur, e.g. chloramphenicol is converted to an amine (Fig. 2.1).

Hydrolysis

This is an important metabolic process for inactivating a large number of compounds which possess either an ester (i.e $-\overset{\text{O}}{\underset{}{\text{C}}}-\text{O}-$) or an amide (i.e. $-\overset{\text{O}}{\underset{}{\text{C}}}-\text{NH}-$) linkage. Esterases, a large group of enzymes of varying specificity, are found not only in association with the liver drug metabolising enzyme system but also in a number of other tissues including the plasma. One of the esterases found in plasma is pseudocholinesterase (butyrylcholinesterase) which is responsible for the metabolism of a number of therapeutic agents, including the local anaesthetic procaine and the muscle relaxant succinylcholine. Blood-borne esterases are also important in activating those compounds which have been esterified to prolong their rate of absorption from intramuscular sites, e.g. corticosteroid and anabolic steroid preparations. Amides (e.g. the local anaesthetic lignocaine) are hydrolysed by amidases which are found mainly in the soluble fraction of the liver.

Activation

In addition to inactivating drugs, phase I reactions are also responsible for the conversion of inactive pro-drugs to active compounds. Some of the more important therapeutic agents that are used and are dependent on conversion to an active compound are shown in Table 2.1. The conversion of an inactive to an active compound can sometimes be used to advantage in therapeutics. Thus, the semi-synthetic penicillin, hetacillin, being a pro-drug, does not adversely affect the ruminal flora when administered orally to ruminants, but once absorbed through the hepatic vein it enters the liver and is converted to the active drug, ampicillin. The fasciolicide, diamphenethide, which is effective against immature flukes, depends for its activity on being deacetylated in hepatic cells to a compound which is active against the fluke and attains high concentrations in the hepatocyte (Harfenist 1973). On the other hand, diamphenethide is probably less efficacious against mature

Table 2.1 Examples of transformation of inactive pro-drugs into active metabolites.

Pro-drug	Metabolite
Chloral hydrate	Trichloroethanol
Parathion	Paraoxon
Malathion	Malaoxon
Carbon tetrachloride	Active radical
Hetacillin	Ampicillin
Diamphenethide	De-acetylated derivative

forms which feed off blood, as much lower concentrations of the active form are found in the blood (Harfenist 1973).

Sometimes drugs which require liver activation can become toxic. This may arise when enzyme induction has occurred, leading to more rapid formation of the active compound. Carbon tetrachloride hepatoxicity has been attributed to excessively rapid formation of the active free radical which leads to parenchymal damage, starting in the endoplasmic reticulum (Remmer 1970). Seawright *et al* (1972) have shown that pretreatment of sheep with DDT or phenobarbitone caused an increase in liver microsomal enzyme activity and this was associated with marked increase in susceptibility, while the reverse occurred on a protein-deficient diet (Hunt 1971). Although the effect of a high protein diet is also thought to be due to induction of the drug metabolising enzymes, Seawright *et al* (1972) were unable to demonstrate an increase in microsomal enzyme activity as indicated by aminopyrine N-demethylase. High-fat diets also increase carbon tetrachloride toxicity because they increase its rate of absorption from the gastrointestinal tract.

In the case of the phosphorothionates (e.g. parathion and malathion), enzyme induction may either increase or decrease the toxicity of these organophosphorus insecticides depending on the structure of the compound and the possibilities offered for competing activation and inactivation reactions (Menzer & Best 1968).

Table 2.2 Major conjugations in animals.

Main source of conjugating agent	Conjugate	Major target groups
Carbohydrate	Glucuronic acid	$-OH$, $-COOH$, $-NH_2$ $>NH$, $-SH$
Amino acids	Glycine	aromatic$-COOH$, aromatic alkyl$-COOH$
Miscellaneous	Sulphate	aromatic$-OH$, aromatic$-NH_2$
	Acetylation	

Phase II (synthetic or conjugation) reactions

These reactions occur when the drug or phase I metabolite contains a group — usually OH, COOH, NH_2 or SH — which is suitable for combining with an endogenous compound to form readily excreted, water-soluble, polar metabolites (Williams 1971). The conjugated forms are invariably pharmacologically inactive. The important conjugating agents and their sources are shown in Table 2.2. These agents do not combine directly with the drug or metabolite but require the presence of a nucleotide and a transferring enzyme, as shown below for glucuronic acid, one of the commonest conjugating agents.

1 Activation of glucuronic acid to uridine diphosphate glucuronic acid (UDPGA):

$$\text{Glucose-1-phosphate} + \text{UTP} \xrightarrow{\text{pyrophosphorylase}} \text{UDR glucose} + \text{pyrophosphate}$$

$$\text{UDR glucose} + 2NAD^+ + H_2O \xrightarrow[\text{dehydrogenase}]{\text{UDPG}} \text{UDP-glucuronic acid} + 2NADH + ZH^+.$$

2 Transfer of conjugating agent from nucleotide UDPGA to drugs:

$$\text{UDP-glucuronic acid} + \text{RZH} \xrightarrow[\text{transferase}]{\text{glucuronyl}} \text{RZ-glucuronic acid} + \text{UDP}$$

where Z = O, COO, NH, or S.

There are some species variations in the conjugation reactions that can take place. For example, in the cat, glucuronic acid conjugation and, in the pig, sulphate conjugation, are absent. This absence can arise from a defect in the occurrence of the conjugating agent, in the ability to form the necessary nucleotide, or in the amount of the transferring enzyme present.

Factors affecting the rate of biotransformation

A large number of factors have been shown to influence the rate of drug metabolism (Table 2.3). Of those listed some are of much greater impor-

Table 2.3 Factors that can influence drug metabolism.

Species	Diet
Strain/Breed	Stress
Age	Temperature
Sex	Time of day
Chronic administration	Route of excretion
Presence of other foreign compounds	Gut flora
Route of administration	Season
Size of dose	Altitude
Disease	

tance than others. Most of the information on the influence of these factors has been derived from investigations in laboratory animals, especially the rat. Because of the lack of investigations in large animals, the relevance of some of these factors has not yet been ascertained.

Species

Although the general pattern of drug metabolism is common to all species and follows the processes outlined previously, variation in the plasma half-life of a drug in different species and the metabolites formed indicate that both quantitative and qualitative species differences occur. Usually no generalisation about relative rates of degradation for a certain drug between species can be applied, although it appears, from the drugs so far studied, that ruminants have a very efficient metabolising system. A knowledge of the rate of metabolism in a particular species is important for instituting correct therapy, especially when a repeated dosage regimen is to be used.

Important differences between species in the plasma half-life of drugs occur with a large number of antibacterial agents such as trimethoprim (Table 2.4), an antimetabolite used synergistically with a sulphonamide. These differences are important when considering the dosage frequency required to maintain adequate blood levels. Also of importance is the fact that, as this drug is given together with sulphonamides in a ratio of 1:5, a sulphonamide should be selected which has a similar half-life to trimethoprim in the species concerned, in order to maintain this ratio in the animal. However, Piercy (1978) has indicated that trimethoprim exists in a reservoir in tissue fluids and therefore the period of its bioavailability extends for a longer time than is indicated by its plasma half-life. The same consideration applies also for other drug combinations and is one of the main reasons why commercial fixed-dose preparations of multiple drugs should be considered undesirable.

Table 2.4 Plasma half-life values (hours) for some drugs in different species.

Drug	Horse/ Pony	Cow	Goat	Pig	Dog	Man
Trimethoprim	3.0–6.0[a]	1.0[b]	0.5[c]	2.0[d]	3.0[a]	9.0–12.0[e]
Chloramphenicol	0.9[f]	3.5[g]	2.0[f]	1.3[f]	4.2[f]	1.5–3.5[h]
Oxytetracycline	10.5[i]	9.1[i]	–	–	6.0[j]	9.6[h]
Quinidine	4.4[k]	–	0.85[k]	5.4[k]	5.6[k]	–

a Alexander & Collett 1975; b Davitiyananda & Rasmussen 1974; c Nielsen & Rasmussen 1972; d Nielsen & Rasmussen 1975; e Kaplan *et al* 1970; f Davis *et al* 1972; g Pilloud 1973b; h Kunin 1967; i Pilloud 1973a; j Baggot *et al* 1978; k Neff *et al* 1972.

Important species differences in half-life for some other commonly used drugs are also indicated in Table 2.4. Most of these differences result from variations within the hepatic drug metabolising enzyme systems. However, another important cause of species variation is seen in drugs that rely on plasma butyrylcholinesterase for their metabolism. Ruminants have negligible amounts of this enzyme in their plasma, whereas in the horse, pig, and dog much larger quantities are found (Voss 1974). These differences are generally considered to account for the differing dose requirements for succinylcholine in different species.

Intraspecies variation (breed or strain)

In rats it has been well established that differences occur in the rate of metabolism between different strains (Quinn *et al* 1958). In the rabbit, Siegart *et al* (1964) and Cram *et al* (1965) also found differences between strains, especially in their response to hepatic enzyme inducing agents (see below). Siegart *et al* (1964) also suggested that individual variations in oxidation of drugs by dogs in their experiments were due to breed differences. Unfortunately the effects of any breed differences have not been studied to a great extent in domestic animals. From studies carried out in various ruminant species, rates of drug metabolism have generally been found to be similar, indicating that if there is little between species variation there is unlikely to be a significant intraspecies variation. In the horse, no detailed comparative studies have been carried out; however there are indications that breed differences may exist. In the pony, the half-life for antipyrine was found to be 118 minutes (Argenizio & Hintz 1970) whilst, in the thoroughbred, it was 70 minutes (Powis & Snow 1978). As these studies were carried out in different laboratories and locations, other factors may also have contributed to these differences. However, if breed differences do exist, they are of potential importance, especially in reference to 'dope testing', as many of the studies have been carried out in ponies and may therefore be inapplicable to the racing animal.

Sex

The influence of sex on drug metabolism has been well established in the rat (Quinn *et al* 1958) although less indication of this is found in other species. However, Davis & Wolff (1970) reported a significant sex difference in the plasma half-life of the central muscle relaxant glyceryl guaicolate in the horse — the half-lives in males and females being 84.4 and 59.6 minutes respectively.

Table 2.5   Effect of age on plasma half-life of trimethoprim in the goat. (Data from Nielsen & Rasmussen 1976.)

Age	$T_\frac{1}{2}$(min)
2 days	182
3 weeks	115 ± 12
6 weeks	48 ± 3
16 weeks	33 ± 3
Adults	40 ± 5

Age

In both the very young (neonate) and the very old, decreases in the rate of drug elimination are found. In the neonate, this is due mainly to a decreased rate of biotransformation; however, a reduction in renal excretion, especially by active processes, may also occur. As indicated in Table 2.5, in the neonatal goat it takes approximately 30 days for microsomal drug metabolising enzymes to develop progressively to levels found in the adult. Similar findings have been made in the pig (Short & Davis 1970). Therefore, in the neonate, to prevent drug accumulation and possible toxicity, the interval between successive doses has to be extended. In old animals, decreased elimination may occur as a result of pathological changes in tissues involved in metabolism or excretion. Although this latter point is unlikely to be a problem in most farm animals, it may be important in the horse which has attained an advanced age.

Induction and inhibition of drug metabolism

Induction

Prior exposure of an animal to various compounds in the environment or treatment with certain drugs can bring about an increase in activity of the hepatic drug metabolising enzymes (Conney 1967). This increased activity is due to an increase in the concentration of drug metabolising enzymes which is reflected as an increase in the smooth endoplasmic reticulum of hepatocytes and often an increase in liver weight as well. Compounds which bring about these changes are referred to as inducers. These inducers therefore can cause both auto-induction and also an increased rate of metabolism of other compounds both of exogenous and endogenous origin which may not be related pharmacologically or chemically to the inducer. Inducers can be either broad spectrum (e.g. phenobarbitone), stimulating increased biotransformation of a large number of substrates which undergo metabolic oxidation, reduction or glucuronide conjugation, or they can be narrow spectrum (e.g. carcinogenic polycyclic hydrocarbons), stimulating only a few metabolic pathways. The magnitude of induction caused by a compound is dependent on a number of factors. In neonates, much lower doses of phenobarbitone are required to produce induction than in adults. Inducing action is dose-dependent, many inducers only being effective at near toxic doses. The duration of exposure to the inducer is also important, a period of at least several days being required.

In the various species studied, mainly laboratory animals and man, several hundred compounds belonging to many chemical classes have been shown to be capable of stimulating the DMES. Fortunately in man it has been found that, of the therapeutic agents used, only a small number act as inducers, including barbiturates, phenylbutazone, phenytoin, and griseofulvin (Sher 1971, Conney & Burns 1972). Few investigations have been carried out on compounds which may act as inducing agents in farm animals. Cook & Wilson (1970) found that phenobarbitone treatment stimulates hepatic drug metabolising enzymes in the cow, sheep, goat, and pig. Phenylbutazone has been shown to cause enzyme induction in a number of species (Chen *et al* 1962, Welch *et al* 1967), leading to more rapid metabolism of a number of other drugs. In contrast, in the horse Piperno *et al* (1968) found that, following repeated administration of phenylbutazone, an increased half-life occurs and this effect has been attributed to the metabolite oxyphenbutazone inhibiting metabolism of phenylbutazone (Tobin *et al* 1977). This finding contrasts with that of a recent study in which administration of phenylbutazone to horses at a dose rate of 8.2 mg/kg/day for two weeks caused no alteration in the rate of metabolism of phenylbutazone or antipyrine (Snow *et al* 1981).

Organochlorine pesticides are well known inducing agents (Conney 1967) and they have been shown to exert this action in sheep and pigs (Street *et al* 1966). The possible significance of this effect is no longer as important as previously because the use and environmental concentrations of this class of compound have markedly declined due to legislation.

Diet has also been shown to affect the concentration of drug metabolising enzymes (Campbell & Hayes 1974). The dietary constituent most extensively studied is protein and, generally, it has been demonstrated that a reduction in either quantity or quality of protein leads to a depression of this system, while protein-rich diets can lead to increased activity.

Inhibition

Inhibition of metabolising enzymes can lead to delayed elimination of a drug and possible cumulative effects following repeated dosage or unexpected duration of pharmacological activity following single administration. Inhibition can occur in a number of ways.

Inhibition of DMES. Some compounds, although probably far fewer in number than inducing agents, cause inhibition of the drug metabolising enzymes. Examples include the experimental compound SKF 525A, chloramphenicol, piperonyl butoxide, and some organophosphates. The effect of chloramphenicol is of some importance because, in a number of species, prior administration has been shown to result in a prolongation of barbiturate anaesthesia (Adams & Dixit 1970, Adams 1970). Interestingly, in the horse, Tobin *et al* (1977) reported that chloramphenicol did not increase the half-life of phenylbutazone. Piperonyl butoxide is used in fly-sprays to delay the metabolism of toxic pyrethrins by insects. In sheep, diphenylhydantoin and chlorcyclizine have been shown to decrease the rate of metabolism of pentobarbitone (Cooper & Hawk 1978).

Inhibition of non-microsomal enzymes. This can occur in the liver and other tissues. Of importance therapeutically is the effect seen with organophosphorus compounds which can form irreversible complexes with both butyryl and acetylcholinesterase in blood and tissues. Inhibition of the former enzyme decreases the ability of the animal to eliminate other drugs metabolised by this enzyme, and therefore leads to a prolonged effect. Fatalities following normal doses of succinylcholine can occur if the animal has had recent or concurrent exposure to an organophosphorus compound such as certain anthelmintic preparations. The return to normal rates of metabolism will depend on the de-novo synthesis of enzyme. Fig. 2.2 shows

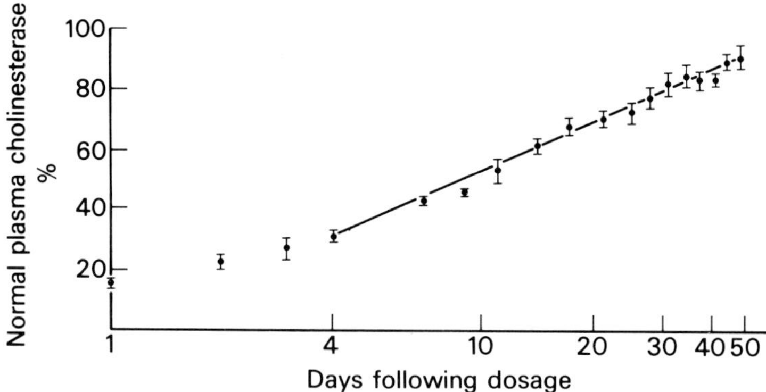

Fig. 2.2 Effect of the administration of the organophosphorous anthelmintic dichlorvos on plasma cholinesterase in the horse (Snow 1974).

the effects of the organophosphorus anthelmintic dichlorvos on equine plasma butyrylcholinesterase. As illustrated, even following a therapeutic dose a prolonged period of time is required for the enzyme to return to normal levels. In man a number of monoamine oxidase (MAO) inhibitors are used therapeutically and, since this enzyme is responsible for normal metabolism of catecholamines and other endogenous and exogenous amines, high dietary intake of certain amines in cheeses and meat extracts with an MAO inhibitor can lead to toxic manifestations.

Competitive inhibition. This may occur when two or more drugs, which depend upon the same metabolic pathway, are administered concurrently. However, this is considered to be of little therapeutic importance unless saturation of the metabolic pathway has occurred.

Pathological changes

Liver disease is the condition most likely to lead to decreases in rate of drug metabolism. Such alteration can be brought about in a number of ways; by altered hepatic blood flow, by decreased extraction of compounds from the blood by the parenchymal cells or, most commonly, by a decreased activity of the microsomal enzymes and other metabolic pathways. However, the presence of liver disease does not necessarily imply an altered rate of drug metabolism, and in man it was concluded that the effects of hepatic disease on metabolism varied with the nature and severity of the condition (Cookesley & Powell 1971). Generally, acute conditions will alter metabolism whilst chronic conditions have been shown to have little effect.

Metabolism in the gastrointestinal tract

The effect of gastrointestinal micro-organisms on drugs that are either orally administered or that penetrate into the tract following passive diffusion is an area that is receiving increasing attention (Scheline 1973). It has been shown that the metabolic capacity of these micro-organisms for foreign compounds can be very large, with many of the transformations that occur in the rest of the body also taking place in these micro-organisms. Because of the differences in digestive systems of the different domestic species, the possible importance of this type of metabolism can vary. In ruminants, chloramphenicol is rapidly metabolised by the ruminal flora (Baggot 1977) and therefore cannot be given orally, in addition to the obvious problems of the compound's effects on the ruminal flora.

Excretion of drugs and drug metabolites

The primary route of excretion for the majority of drugs and their metabolites is via the kidney. In addition, there are a number of other routes by which varying amounts of drugs and metabolites can be excreted, e.g. in bile, sweat, saliva and milk. The lungs are an important route of elimination for volatile anaesthetics. The degree of lipid solubility and the extent of ionisation in plasma are the main factors that determine the proportion of a drug eliminated by excretion.

Renal

Most drug metabolites as well as a number of polar drugs are excreted in the urine. Drugs that are eliminated mainly unchanged in the urine include many antibiotics. The renal clearance of a drug, which is defined as the volume (ml) of plasma water cleared of a substance per minute by both kidneys, is determined by 1 glomerular filtration, 2 active tubular secretion (carrier-mediated) in the proximal convuluted tubule, and 3 passive tubular re-absorption in the proximal and distal portion of the nephron.

Glomerular filtration is a non-selective process, the only limiting factor being the size and shape of the molecule; very high molecular weight compounds such as proteins are unable to pass through the pores in the glomerulus. Therefore most therapeutic agents pass readily into the filtrate, their rate of passage being dependent on the glomerular filtration rate (GFR) and the extent to which the drug is bound to plasma protein. Once the drug has entered the filtrate, the extent to which it is eliminated in the urine depends on the degree of tubular re-absorption.

Active secretion. This term implies the movement of molecules against an electrochemical gradient in or out of cells. It is an active process since it requires the expenditure of energy: either at the cell membrane or within the cell, the drug to be transferred is combined with a carrier that moves across the cell and then releases the drug into the lumen of the tubule. The most important features of this mechanism are a high velocity of passage, the ability to be inhibited by certain compounds and a maximal capacity. Binding of a drug to plasma protein does not prevent its excretion by this mechanism. Generally active secretion occurs in the proximal tubule. Some of the more important therapeutic agents that are excreted by the active process are penicillin, frusemide, salicylate, and trimethoprim. In addition, a number of conjugates are excreted in this manner. The carrier-mediated system can be inhibited by various compounds and the plasma half-life of a drug may be prolonged by this means. In the early days of penicillin G therapy, before longer-acting compounds were available, the agent probenicid, by competing for the transport mechanism responsible for penicillin excretion, was administered concurrently with this antibiotic to prolong its half-life. In a similar manner phenylbutazone will also prolong the rate of elimination of penicillin (Kampmann *et al* 1972).

Tubular re-absorption. Most molecules are able to move freely across the tubular cells but, because of the concentration gradient developed along the nephron as a result of the re-absorption of water, the general movement of solutes is from the lumen of the tubule to the blood rather than vice versa. Since this process occurs by simple diffusion, egress of highly lipid-soluble drugs from the tubular fluid is favoured. As lipid-soluble drugs have to be in the un-ionised state for re-absorption, the degree of ionisation also affects the extent of re-absorption. As in other tissues, the degree of ionisation is determined by the pKa of the compound and the pH of the environment. Therefore compounds which have low lipid solubility or which are highly ionised at tubular fluid pH will be excreted largely in the urine.

Since the pH of urine varies widely between different species, the degree of re-absorption of certain drugs will vary accordingly. This effect will only be of importance in prolonging the duration of activity of the compound if renal excretion is the major route of elimination of the drug. In carnivores urine pH is acidic, generally varying between 5.5 and 7.0, whilst in herbivores urine has an alkaline pH (7.0–8.5). However, urine pH in any species is also dependent on diet — a high protein content resulting in an acidic pH. Interestingly it has been found that the majority of horses in training for racing have an acidic urine (Moss 1976), although the exact reasons for this difference are unknown. For drugs that are weak acids and have a pKa between 3 and 7, raising the pH will increase the degree of ionisation and decrease the re-absorption. On the other hand, for basic compounds with pKa values between 7 and 11, an increase in urine acidity will increase excretion.

Effects of renal disease

Pathological conditions affecting the kidney can affect the elimination of drugs in a number of ways. In diseases which result in uraemia, the binding of drugs to albumin can be markedly altered, leading to an increased distribution of the drug and possibly a greater pharmacological response which may also lead to toxic manifestations. The effects of uraemia on drug disposition are discussed extensively by Baggot (1977). Not only may uraemia alter the expected response to a therapeutic agent, but a decreased excretory capacity of the kidney will also cause adverse effects. Reduced elimination of active compounds by the kidney can lead to a prolonged duration of action of the compound, and repeated dosage will lead to cumulation and possible toxic effects, e.g. with streptomycin. Impaired renal excretion will result in slower excretion of drugs in the urine, which makes the treatment of urinary tract infections more difficult.

Biliary excretion

A large number of drugs are excreted in small amounts via the bile following passive diffusion from the liver parenchyma into the bile canaliculi. For these compounds this route of elimination is of little significance. However, there are some compounds and conjugates, especially glucuronides, which can be excreted in higher concentrations in the bile, and it is thought that such excretion occurs by an active process. In general, factors that appear to facilitate biliary excretion are a molecular weight above 300 and the possession of polar groups (Plaa 1971). The species of animal also influences the extent to which a drug undergoes biliary excretion (Abou-el-Makarem *et al* 1967), especially of compounds with a molecular weight between 300 and 500. Williams (1971) has divided species into good, moderate, and poor biliary excretors. Of the larger domestic animals, only the sheep has been studied and it was classed as a moderate excretor. As stated by Williams (1971), there is a tendency for newer drugs to be of higher molecular weight than in the past, and therefore the extent of biliary excretion becomes more important. This suggests that studies should be carried out in the larger domestic animals to ascertain to which category of biliary excretion they belong.

Once a drug has been excreted in the bile into the small intestine it can undergo a number of fates. If it is excreted in a polar form it is generally excreted in the faeces. However, if a conjugated drug or its metabolite is excreted, it may be hydrolysed by the gut flora to yield the lipid-soluble parent compound or metabolite. This latter compound may then be excreted in the faeces, further degraded and excreted or, depending on conditions, be re-absorbed through the intestinal wall by passive diffusion. If this occurs an enterohepatic circulation of the drug is established as shown in Fig. 2.3. This recirculation is only of importance if large concentrations of the compound are excreted via the bile when it will contribute significantly to the overall elimination of the drug.

Saliva and sweat

Drugs are excreted in both of these secretions, although this amount is only a

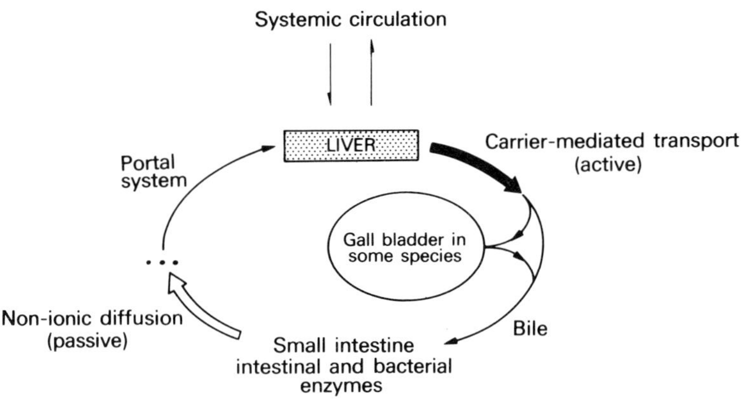

Fig. 2.3 Enterohepatic circulation of a lipid-soluble foreign or endogenous compound. (From Baggot 1977.) ● = Drug metabolising enzymes.

small fraction of the overall elimination of a drug. Drugs enter these secretions by passive diffusion. Those excreted in the saliva may be re-absorbed through the intestinal wall, thus establishing a similar cycle to that for biliary excretion. Because of the excretion of drugs in the saliva, it has been used as an alternative fluid to urine for the detection of illegal drug use in horses.

Milk

Drugs can also be excreted in varying but significant amounts via the mammary gland in lactating animals. A knowledge of the extent of such excretion is extremely important in considering appropriate mastitis therapy, and also in considering which drugs used for systemic treatment are likely to cause significant contamination of milk and render it unfit for human consumption. Factors affecting excretion of compounds, especially antibiotics into milk, are considered in Chapters 1, 3 and 5.

References

Abou-El-Makarem M. M., Milburn P., Smith R. L. *et al* (1967) Biliary excretion of foreign compounds. *Biochem. J.* **105,** 1289–93.

Adams H. R. (1970) Prolongation of barbiturate anaesthesia by chloramphenicol in laboratory animals. *J. Am. Vet. Med. Assoc.* **157,** 1908–1913.

Adams H. R. & Dixit B. N. (1970) Prolongation of pentobarbital anaesthesia by chloramphenicol in dogs and cats. *J. Am. Vet. Med. Assoc.* **156,** 902–905.

Alexander F. & Collett R. A. (1975) Trimethoprim in the horse. *Eq. Vet. J.* **7,** 203–206.

Argenzio R. A. & Hintz H. F. (1970) Glucose tolerance and effect of volatile fatty acid on plasma glucose concentration in ponies. *J. Anim. Sci.* **30,** 514–8.

Baggot J. D. & Davis L. (1973) A comparative study of the pharmacokinetics of amphetamine. *Res. Vet. Sci.* **14**, 207–215.

Baggot J. D. (1977) *Principles of Drug Disposition in Domestic Animals.* W. B. Saunders, Philadelphia.

Baggot J. D., Powers T. E., Powers J. D., Kowalski J. J. & Kerr K. M. (1978) Pharmacokinetics and dosage of oxytetracycline in dogs. *Res. Vet. Sci.* **24**, 77–81.

Campbell T. C. & Hayes J. R. (1974) Role of nutrition in the drug metabolising enzyme system. *Pharmac. Rev.* **26**, 171–197.

Chen W. Vrendten P. A., Dayton P. G. & Burns J. J. (1962) Accelerated aminopyrine metabolism in human subjects pretreated with phenylbutazone. *Life Science* **2**, 35–42.

Conney A. H. (1967) Pharmacological implications of microsomal enzyme induction. *Pharmac. Rev.* **19**, 317–366.

Conney A. H. & Burns J. J. (1972) Metabolic interactions among environmental chemicals and drugs. *Science* **178**, 576–586.

Cook R. M. & Wilson K. A. (1970) Metabolism of xenobiotics in ruminants. Phenobarbital induction of liver microsomal nitrogen demethylase. *J. Agr. Fd. Chem.* **18**, 441–442.

Cookesley W. G. E. & Powell L. W. (1971) Drug metabolism and interaction with particular reference to the liver. *Drugs* **2**, 177–189.

Cooper B. S. & Hawk H. W. (1978) Effect of liver microsomal enzyme-inducing drugs on blood serum pentobarbital clearance and sleeptime in sheep and rabbits. *Am. J. Vet. Res.* **39**, 649–651.

Cram R. L., Juchau M. R. & Fouts J. R. (1965) Differences in hepatic drug metabolism in various rabbit strains before and after pre-treatment with phenobarbital. *Proc. Soc. Exp. Biol. Med.* **118**, 872–75.

Davis L. E. & Wolff W. A. (1970) Pharmacokinetics and metabolism of glyceryl guaiacolate in ponies. *Am. J. Vet. Res.* **31**, 469–473.

Davis L. E., Neff C. A., Baggot J. D. & Powers T. E. (1972) Pharmacokinetics of chloramphenicol in domesticated animals. *Am. J. Vet. Res.* **33**, 2259–2266.

Davitiyananda D. & Rasmussen F. (1974) Half-lives of sulphadoxine and timethoprim after a single intravenous infusion in cows. *Arch. Vet. Scand.* **15**, 356–365.

Harfenist M. (1973) Diamphenithide — A new fasciolicide active against immature parasites. *Pestic. Sci.* **4**, 871–882.

Hunt E. R. (1971) Hepatotoxicity of carbon tetrachloride in sheep. 1. The influence of diet. *Aust. Vet. J.* **47**, 272–274.

Kampmann J., Molholm Hansen J., Siersboek-Nielsen K. T. *et al* (1972) Effect of some drugs on penicillin half-life in blood. *Clin. Pharmac. Ther.* **13**, 516–9.

Kaplan S. A., Weinfeld R. E., Cotlet S. *et al* (1970) Pharmacokinetics profile of trimethoprim in dog and man. *J. Pharm. Sci.* **59**, 358–363.

Kunin C. M. (1967) A guide to use of antibiotics in patients with renal disease. *Ann. Intern. Med.* **67**, 151–158.

La Du B. N., Mandel H. G. & Way E. L. (1977) *Fundamentals of Drug Metabolism and Drug Disposition.* Williams & Wilkins, Baltimore.

Menzer R. E. & Best N. H. (1968) Effect of phenobarbital on the toxicity of several organophosphorus insecticides. *Toxic Appl. Pharm.* **13**, 37–42.

Moss M. S. (1976) The metabolism of urinary and salivary excretion of drugs in the horse and their relevance to detection of dope. pp 263–280. In *Drug Metabolism from Microbe to Man,* Parke D. V. and Smith R. L. (eds.) Taylor & Francis, London.

Neff C. A., Davis L. E. & Baggot J. D. (1972) A comparative study of the pharmacokinetics of Quinidine. *Am. J. Vet. Res.* **33**, 1521–1525.

Nielsen P. & Rasmussen F. (1972) Elimination of trimethoprim in pigs and goats. *Acta Pharmac. Toxic.* (Suppl. 1) **31**, 94.

Nielsen P. & Rasmussen F. (1975) Half-life and renal excretion of trimethoprim in swine. *Acta Pharm. Toxic.* **36**, 123–131.

Nielsen P. & Rasmussen F. (1976) Influence of age on half-life of trimethoprim and sulphadoxine in goats. *Acta Pharm. Toxic.* **38,** 113–119.

Notari R. E. (1975) *Biopharmaecutics and pharmacokinetics. An introduction.* Marcel Dekker, New York.

Piercy D. W. T. (1978) Distribution of trimethoprim sulphadiazine in plasma, tissue and synovial fluids. *Vet. Rec.* **102,** 523–4.

Pilloud M. (1973a) Pharmacokinetics, plasma protein binding and dosage of oxytetracycline in cattle and horses. *Res. Vet. Sci.* **15,** 224–230.

Pilloud M. (1973b) Pharmacokinetics, plasma protein binding and dosage of chloramphenicol in cattle and horses. *Res. Vet. Sci.* **15,** 231–238.

Piperno E., Ellis D. J., Getty S. M. *et al* (1968) Plasma and urine levels of phenylbutazone in the horse. *J. Am. Vet. Med. Assoc.* **153,** 195–198.

Plaa G. L. (1971) Biliary and other routes of excretion of drugs. In *Fundamentals of Drug Metabolism and Drug Disposition.* La Du B. N. Mandel H. G. and Way E. L. (eds.) Williams & Wilkins, Baltimore.

Powis G. & Snow D. H. (1978) The effects of exercise and adrenaline infusion upon the blood levels of propranolol and antipyrine in the horse. *J. Pharmac. Exp. Ther.* **205,** 725–731.

Quinn G. P., Axelrod J. & Brodie B. B. (1958) Species strain and sex difference in metabolism of hexobarbitone, amidopyrine, antipyrine and aniline. *Biochem. Pharmac.* **1,** 152–159.

Remmer H. (1970) The role of the liver in drug metabolism. *Am. J. Med.* **49,** 617–629.

Scheline R. R. (1973) Metabolism of foreign compounds by gastrointestinal microorganisms. *Pharmac. Rev.* **25,** 451–523.

Seawright A. A., Skele D. P., Mudie A. W. *et al* (1972) The effect of diet and drugs on hepatic microsomal aminopyrine N-demethylase activity *in vitro* and susceptibility to carbon tetrachloride in sheep. *Res. Vet. Sci.* **13,** 245–250.

Sher S. P. (1971) Drug enzyme induction and drug interactions: literature tabulation. *Toxic. Appl. Pharmac.* **18,** 780–834.

Short C. R. & Davis L. E. (1970) Post-natal development of drug metabolizing activity in swine. *J. Pharmac. Exp. Ther.* **174,** 185–196.

Siegert M., Alaleben B., Liebenschutz W. *et al* (1964) Underschiede in der mikrosomalen oxydation und acetylierung von arzneimitteln bei vershciedenen arten and raasen. *Arch. Exp. Path. Pharmak.* **247,** 509–521.

Snow D. H. (1974) Studies on the action of an anthelmintic prepation of dichlorvos in horses. *Vet. Rec.* **95,** 231–233.

Snow D. H., Douglas T. A., Thompson H. *et al* (1981) Phenylbutazone toxicosis in equidae: a biochemical and pathophysiologic study. *Am. J. Vet. Res.* **42,** 1754–9.

Street J. C., Chadwick R. N., Wang M. *et al* (1966) Insecticide interactions affecting residue storage in animal tissues. *J. Agr. Fd. Chem.* **14,** 545–49.

Tobin T., Blake J. W. & Valentine R. (1977) Drug interactions in the horse; effects of chloramphenicol, quinidine, and oxyphenbutazone on phenylbutazone metabolism. *Am. J. Vet. Res.* **38,** 123–127.

Van Rossum J. M. (1977) *Kinetics of Drug Action.* Springer Verlag, Berlin.

Voss G. (1974) A contribution to the comparative biochemistry of vertebrate serum cholinesterases. *Arch. Toxic.* **32,** 181–7.

Weir J. J. R. & Sanford J. (1972) Urinary excretion of phenothiazine tranquillisers by the horse. *Equine. Vet. J.* **4,** 88.

Welch R. M., Harrison Y. E. & Burns J. J. (1967) Implications of enzyme induction in drug toxicity studies. *Toxic. Appl. Pharmac.* **10,** 340–351.

Williams R. T. (1971) Species Variations in Drug Biotransformations. In *Fundamentals of Drug Metabolism and Drug Disposition.* La Du B. N., Mandel H. G. and Way E. L. (eds.) p. 187. William & Wilkins, Baltimore.

PART 2
ANTIBACTERIAL DRUGS

3

Systemic antimicrobial therapy in large animals

J.D. BAGGOT

Pharmacokinetics

General Considerations

The absorption, distribution, and fate of antimicrobial agents in the body are largely determined by certain physicochemical properties of the drugs. The degree of lipid solubility and extent of ionisation in various body fluids are most important in this regard. Stability towards chemical and metabolic inactivation within the stomach and small intestine of mono-gastric animals or the reticulorumen and abomasum of ruminant species determines the amount of an oral dose which is potentially available for absorption. Dissolution often controls the rate of absorption of a drug substance from solid dosage forms. This applies to sustained-release preparations injected intramuscularly as well as to tablets and capsules which are given orally. Both absorption and distribution take place by passive diffusion, a process which is characterised by the movement of drug molecules down a concentration gradient without the expenditure of energy (see Chapter 1). Only lipid-soluble molecules can diffuse through the gastrointestinal mucosa, penetrate cell membranes, and enter transcellular fluids (such as cerebrospinal, synovial, and ocular fluid). Extensive binding (i.e. greater than 80%) to plasma albumin restricts the distribution of a drug, giving higher total concentrations in the plasma than are available for activity. Protein binding is reversible, so that it provides a reservoir of potentially active drug within the circulating blood. Binding also has the effect of delaying excretion by glomerular filtration. The fate of a drug can determine its potential value in treatment of a particular condition and must be taken into account when considering the influence of disease states (such as uraemia) on dosage. The term 'fate' comprises the distribution pattern as well as the biotransformation pathways and excretion mechanisms.

In antimicrobial therapy, it is essential that an effective level of drug be achieved and maintained for an adequate period of time at the site of infection. This depends on the plasma (or serum) concentration and the ability of the drug to diffuse into the infection site. Therapeutic plasma concentrations of antimicrobial agents must always be related to the sensitivity (or susceptibility) of the infecting micro-organisms.

Application of principles to antimicrobial agents

The majority of antimicrobial agents are organic bases, which include the aminoglycosides (streptomycin, neomycin, kanamycin, and gentamicin), the macrolide group (erythromycin, spiramycin and tylosin), lincomycin, clindamycin and spectinomycin. Chloramphenicol is a relatively simple molecule that diffuses freely across biological membranes. The polymyxins, which are cationic detergents, are basic peptides with molecular weights of about 1000. They readily form water-soluble salts with mineral acids.

The macrolide antibiotics, lincomycin and clindamycin, are lipid-soluble, whereas the aminoglycosides and spectinomycin (an aminocyclitol) are polar molecules. The low solubility of aminoglycosides and spectinomycin in a lipid medium severely limits their absorption from the gastrointestinal tract and decreases the extent of their distribution, which includes restricting their passage into the milk of lactating cows. Under steady state conditions, the milk ultrafiltrate:plasma ultrafiltrate concentration ratio for aminoglycoside antibiotics is approximately 0.6:1 (Ziv & Sulman 1973a, 1974a). They are, however, rapidly absorbed from intramuscular injection sites. The aminoglycosides and spectinomycin are bound to plasma proteins only to a negligible extent and are removed from the body by renal excretion (glomerular filtration). The macrolides, lincomycin and clindamycin, distribute widely throughout the body, enter cells, and attain high concentrations in the milk. The antibiotic concentrations in milk may be 3.5–7 times higher than those present in the serum (Ziv & Sulman 1973a, 1973b). Both lincomycin and clindamycin also penetrate well into bone. Erythromycin and lincomycin are excreted in active form in the bile and probably undergo enterohepatic circulation, which would decrease the rate of their elimination. Biotransformation is the principal process of elimination for clindamycin, the inactive metabolites being excreted in the urine and bile. In human beings, only about 10% of administered clindamycin is excreted unchanged in the urine and small quantities are found in the faeces.

Chloramphenicol is well absorbed from appropriate formulations given intramuscularly or orally, with the exception of oral administration in ruminant animals. It is widely distributed in body fluids, crosses the placental barrier, and reaches therapeutic concentrations in transcellular fluids. The extent of binding to plasma proteins is within the range 30–46% and is independent of drug concentration (Davis *et al* 1972). The drug is eliminated mainly by hepatic metabolism (glucuronide formation), with a small fraction of the dose being excreted unchanged in the urine of herbivorous species. Although the inactive metabolites are rapidly removed by the kidneys, a portion enters the bile and is conveyed into the small intestine. Hydrolysis of the glucuronide conjugate restores activity to the drug and increases lipid solubility. The latter property enables the drug to be re-absorbed, thereby establishing an enterohepatic cycle. Neonatal animals of all species are deficient in drug-metabolising enzymes and in these, as in mature animals with extensive liver damage, repeated dosing may lead to toxic levels of the drug by accumulation. Chloramphenicol is known to inhibit microsomal enzyme activity.

Absorption of polymyxins is slow from the gastrointestinal tract but takes place readily from subcutaneous and intramuscular sites. They are nephrotoxic and their parenteral administration is indicated only in severe urinary tract or systemic infections due to coliform bacteria or *Pseudomonas aeruginosa*. The polypeptide antibiotics are moderately bound to plasma proteins, diffuse poorly through biological membranes attaining low concentrations in transcellular fluids. Polymyxin B and colistimethate are excreted mainly by glomerular filtration.

The tetracyclines are amphoteric compounds, forming salts with acids or bases. They are incompletely absorbed from the gastrointestinal tract of omnivorous species. Tetracyclines form stable chelate complexes with metallic ions (calcium, magnesium) which decreases their absorption. Since they interfere with bacterial flora in the rumen, they should not be given orally to ruminant animals. The tetracyclines, being lipophilic compounds, can diffuse readily through cell membranes. Variation in the extent of distribution among tetracycline analogues is attributable to differences in the degree of lipid solubility. They are bound to plasma proteins in varying degree, the more lipophilic compounds (methacycline, doxycycline, and minocycline) being extensively bound. They are found in highest concentrations in highly perfused organs, penetrate the placental barrier, and attain relatively high concentrations in the milk. The milk:serum concentration ratio at equilibrium was 0.75:1 for oxytetracycline and 1.53:1 for doxycycline (Ziv & Sulman 1974b). Oxytetracycline undergoes enterohepatic circulation and is slowly eliminated by glomerular filtration. A small fraction of the dose, whether given orally or parenterally, is excreted in the faeces.

Antimicrobial agents, which are organic acids, include the penicillins, cephalosporins and sulphonamides. Penicillin G (benzylpenicillin), penicillin V (phenoxymethyl penicillin) and the semi-synthetic penicillins (cloxacillin, ampicillin, and amoxycillin) are predominantly ionised (99%) in the plasma. Binding of the penicillins to plasma albumin ranges from 16–22% for ampicillin to over 80% for cloxacillin. Penicillin G is 50–65% bound to plasma albumin in domestic animals. The systemic availability of amoxycillin following oral dosage clearly exceeds that of ampicillin. Penicillin V partially overcomes the instability of penicillin G in acid gastric contents and, when given on an equivalent oral dose basis, yields higher serum levels. Its antibacterial spectrum is identical to that of penicillin G. The penicillins distribute widely throughout the body, but they do not attain high concentrations within cells or in transcellular fluids. Because of the high susceptibility of many Gram-positive bacteria to penicillin, the level of antibiotic reached may be therapeutically effective. Fever increases the distribution of penicillin. This is manifested by an increase in the apparent volume of distribution, which reflects extent of distribution, and the higher concentration attained in cerebrospinal fluid. Ampicillin and, presumably, amoxycillin penetrate membranes (physiological barriers) more easily than penicillin G. These semi-synthetic penicillins are less ionised in the blood plasma and more lipid-soluble. The penicillins are eliminated almost entirely by the kidneys. The renal mechanisms involve both glomerular filtration and proximal tubular secretion. Only the unbound penicillin molecules in the plasma are available for filtration. However, protein binding does not interfere with tubular secretion, which is an active carrier-mediated process. Enterohepatic circulation may account for the slow elimination of ampicillin compared with penicillin G.

The sulphonamides are organic acids which are well absorbed from the gastrointestinal tract, except the enteric compounds. They are widely distributed throughout the body and penetrate cell membranes in accordance with their degree of ionisation and lipid solubility. Sulphamethazine (pKa 7.4), which is 50% non-ionised in the blood plasma, attains an equilibrium milk:plasma concentration ratio of 0.59:1 (Rasmussen 1958). The half-life, apparent volume of distribution, and extent of plasma protein (albumin) binding of various sulphonamides in cows are shown in Table 3.1. The percentage bound to plasma proteins decreases with increasing concentration of the sulphonamide (25–250 μg/ml) in the plasma. They are eliminated by a combination of renal excretion and biotransformation processes. The fate of sulphonamides in the kidneys involves glomerular filtration of the unbound molecules in the plasma, active carrier-mediated excretion (proximal tubule) of the ionised moiety, and re-absorption, by passive diffusion, of the lipid-soluble non-ionised fraction. The extent of re-absorption is determined by the pKa and lipid solubility of the sulphonamide and the pH of the tubular fluid. Urinary alkalinisation decreases re-absorption by promoting ionisation within tubular fluid, and increases the solubility of sulphonamides and their acetyl derivatives in the urine. The normal urinary reaction of herbivorous species is alkaline. The pathways of biotransformation include acetylation of the aromatic amino group, which takes place in reticuloendothelial cells of the liver and other tissues, and hydroxy-

Table 3.1 pKa, half-life, apparent volume of distribution and binding to plasma proteins of various sulphonamides in cows. (Data from Nielsen & Rasmussen 1977 and Boxenbaum *et al* 1977).

Compound	pKa	Half-life (min.)	Apparent volume of distribution (litre/kg)	Protein binding *in vivo* (%)
Sulphanilamide	10.4	370	1.08	<20
Sulphamethazine	7.4	680	0.44	70
Sulphadiazine	6.4	150	0.75	14
Sulphadoxine	6.1	650	0.37	48–66
Sulphamethoxazole	6.0	140	0.30	62
Sulphadimethoxine	6.0	750	0.31	80–85
Sulphachlorpyridazine	5.9	70	0.24	80–85
Sulphamethylphenazole	5.7	1010	0.60	85

Table 3.2 Relative concentrations of sulphonamides and their metabolites in urine of goats. (Data from Nielsen 1973 and Atef & Nielsen 1975.)

Sulphonamide	Plasma conc. (µg/ml)	Relative urine concentrations (%)		
		Unchanged drug	N⁴-acetyl-drug	Conjugated metabolites
Sulphanilamide	27–243	52	38	7
Sulphamethazine	31–180	33	4	30
Sulphadiazine	78	73	7	4
Sulphamethoxazole	30–171	82	13	5
Sulphadoxine	46–86	42	27	31

lation of the aromatic ring which may, in turn, be conjugated with glucuronic acid. Both oxidation and glycuronide formation are catalysed by hepatic microsomal enzymes. The unchanged drug and inactive metabollic products are excreted in the urine (Table 3.2).

Comparative aspects of absorption and distribution

When considering dosage levels of antimicrobial agents for large animals, one has to compare absorption and distribution of the drugs in the species concerned. The rate of elimination determines the interval between successive doses. Following oral dosage, the systemic availability, which depends on diffusion through the gastrointestinal or reticuloruminal mucosa and passage through the liver, can vary among large animal species. Chloramphenicol, given orally to ruminant animals, is inactivated by reduction of the nitro group within the ruminal environment (Theodorides *et al* 1968), consequently, it is not available for absorption (Davis *et al* 1972). Repeated oral dosage with antibiotics or sulphonamides may upset the normal bacterial flora in the rumen from where absorption of drugs does take place, though often at a slow rate.

In horses, both the extent and the rate of drug absorption from the gastrointestinal tract are unpredictable. Much of the variation in absorption can undoubtedly be attributed to binding of drug molecules to particulate matter in the stomach and to the rate of gastric emptying. Medication of the feed or drinking water is a common method of administering antimicrobial agents to pigs. In this species, absorption from the gastrointestinal tract, which takes place mainly in the small intestine, may be rapid and complete.

Non-physiological factors which influence absorption in all species are the release of drug from solid dosage forms and certain physicochemical properties (in particular lipid solubility) of the drug substance. Stability of the drug in a strongly acidic environment must also be considered: penicillin G, for example, is hydrolysed by gastric acid; penicillin V, oxacillin, nafcillin and cloxacillin are more acid-stable and are well absorbed from the small intestine. The systemic availability of orally administered ampicillin is low (20–40%), while amoxycillin, given as the trihydrate, is well absorbed (55–70% of the dose) from the gastrointestinal tract. The clinical efficacy of amoxycillin in the treatment of enteric conditions in calves was considered to be very satisfactory (Palmer *et al* 1977). Treatment consisted of 400 mg amoxycillin (trihydrate) dispersible powder which was given twice daly in milk or milk replacer and continued for 4–5 days. In almost half the calves treated, the initial dose was given by intramuscular injection of amoxycillin aqueous suspension (7 mg/kg). The high polarity of the aminoglycoside antibiotics and spectinomycin limits their absorption. Tylosin is not stable in solutions of pH less than 4; the drug is converted to an active product — desmycosin (Huber 1977).

Parenteral administration implies that the gastrointestinal tract is bypassed, the drug being given by injection. When the intravenous route of administration is used, absorption of the drug substance is instantaneous and complete systemic availability is assured. When other routes of injection are employed, the rate of absorption, though usually rapid, may vary among preparations of the same drug and absorption may not always be complete. Parenteral formulations which contain the bases of erythromycin, tylosin, and chloramphenicol solubilised in organic solvents produce much lower peak concentrations in the serum and lower milk levels than the respective water-soluble preparations. The concentrations of chloramphenicol in serum and milk of cows given a single intramuscular injection (50 mg/kg) of either chloramphenicol base solubilised in an organic solvent or an aqueous solution of chloramphenicol soldium succinate (Fig. 3.1) exemplify the difference in availability of chloramphenicol.

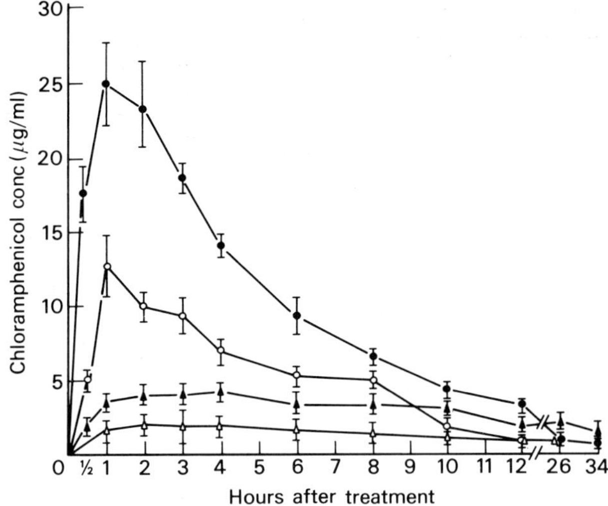

Fig. 3.1 Chloramphenicol levels (mean ± s.e.) in serum and milk, determined by the microbological assay method, after a single intramuscular injection (50 mg/kg) of chloramphenicol or cloramphenicol sodium succinate give to each of four cows with normal udders, at a three-week interval. (From Ziv *et al* 1973.) ● = Serum (after chloramphenicol sodium succinate), ○ = milk (after chloramphenicol sodium succinate), ▲ = serum (after cloramphenicol), Δ = milk (after chloramphenicol).

In any species of animal, it is conceivable that greater differences in drug absorption may occur between various muscle locations than between intramuscular and subcutaneous sites. Delayed absorption from certain parenteral formulations may be attributable to the effect of the vehicle on dissolution of the drug substance. The aim of sustained-release dosage forms, such as procaine penicillin G, is to maintain therapeutic levels of the drug for an extended period of time. Even though the half-life of penicillin G is 0.7 hour in the cow (Ziv *et al* 1973b), a single dose (30 000 units/kg) of procaine penicillin G in aqueous suspension given by intramuscular injection was shown to maintain the serum penicillin concentration above 0.05 unit/ml for 24 hours (Schipper *et al* 1971). An injectable formulation of oxetetracycline base (200 mg/ml) in 2-pyrrolidone represents an advance on previously developed sustained-release preparations of this antibiotic. A single dose (20 mg/kg) given by deep intramuscular injection to cattle maintained therapeutic (bacteriostatic) blood levels (i.e., > 1.0 μg/ml) for 48 hours (Hooke 1978). The recommended pre-slaughter withdrawal time (withholding period) for this drug preparation is 28 days as compared with 21 days for oxytetracycline hydrochloride. The convenience, in terms of frequency of dosage, offered by sustained-release dosage forms has to be balanced against the loss of flexibility in dosage. The rate of absorption from

Table 3.3 Passage of chemotherapeutic agents from the systemic circulation into milk.

Drug	pKa	Milk pH	Concentration ratio (milk ultr : plasma ultr) theoretical	Concentration ratio (milk ultr : plasma ultr) experimental	Reference
Organic acids					
Benzyl penicillin	2.7	6.8	0.20	0.13–0.26	a
Cloxacillin	2.7	6.8	0.20	0.25–0.30	a
Ampicillin	2.7, 7.2	6.8	0.26	0.24–0.30	a
Amoxycillin	2.7, 7.2	6.8	0.26		
Cephaloridine	3.4	6.8	0.25	0.24–0.28	a
Sulphadimethoxine	6.0	6.6	0.19	0.23	b
Sulphamethazine	7.4	6.6	0.55	0.59	c
Organic bases					
Erythromycin	8.8	6.8	6.1	8.7	d
Tylosin	7.1	6.8	3.0	3.5	e
Lincomycin	7.6	6.5–6.8	2.8	2.30–5.60	f
Trimethoprim	7.6	6.5–6.8	2.8–5.3	2.90–4.90	g
Aminoglycosides	(7.8)	6.5–6.9		0.20–0.80	h
Spectinomycin	8.8	6.8	7.5	0.4	e
Polymyxin B	10.0	6.8	8.0	0.3	i
Neutral and amphoteric compounds					
Chloramphenicol	–	6.5–7.1	(1.0)	1.1	k
Oxytetracycline	–	6.5–6.8		0.75	l
Doxycycline	–	6.5–6.8		1.53	l

Note. The individual references should be consulted for the design of each experiment. It is important to know the mode of drug administration as an equilibrium state will not be established by a single intravenous injection.

References. a Ziv *et al* 1973b; b Stowe & Sisodia 1963; c Rasmussen 1958; d Rasmussen 1959; e Ziv & Sulman 1973a; f Rasmussen 1966b; g Rasmussen 1970; h Ziv & Sulman 1974a; i Ziv & Sulman 1973c; k Ziv *et al* 1973a; l Ziv & Sulman 1974b.

intramuscular preparations must be adequate so as to allow therapeutic levels of antibiotic to be established at the site of the infection. In addition to formulation of the drug product, the properties of the drug substance which govern distribution — i.e. lipid solubility, degree of ionisation and protein binding — are important in this regard.

Although the intramuscular injection of erythromycin (12.5 mg/kg given at 24-hour intervals) yielded subtherapeutic levels in the serum for the majority of potentially susceptible Gram-positive bacteria, therapeutically effective levels (>1.0 μg/ml) were maintained in the milk (Baggot 1977). Studies on the penetration of antimicrobial agents from the systemic circulation into milk indicate that the mammary gland epithelium behaves as a lipoidal membrane which separates blood of pH 7.4 from milk, which has a somewhat lower pH value (normal pH range is 6.5–6.8). It has been shown that only the lipid-soluble, non-ionised moiety of an organic electrolyte in the water phase of blood plasma diffuses into milk (Rasmussen 1966a). In normal lactating cows, weak acids give milk ultrafiltrate:plasma ultrafiltrate concentration ratios less than or equal to unity; organic bases, excluding aminoglycosides and spectinomycin which are strong bases, attain concentration ratios greater than one (Table 3.3). This suggests that lipophilic weak bases have a certain advantage in parenteral antibiotic treatment when distribution into milk is desired. In animals with mastitis, the milk pH reaction is usually increased (up to 0.7 of a pH unit). Consequently, the concentration ratios of the lipid-soluble organic bases will be lower in mastitis as compared with normal cows (Table 3.4). The choice of chemotherapeutic agent for systemic therapy of mastitis should be based upon the susceptibility of the infecting micro-organism to the drug and upon the drug concentration in milk which can be attained with usual dosage.

The formulation of sustained-release parenteral preparations must be such that their intramuscular injection will cause neither tissue damage nor residual levels persisting at the site of administration. When injections of

Table 3.4 Influence of milk pH on the accumulation of organic bases in the milk.

Drug	pKa	Milk pH	Concentration ratio (milk ultr : plasma ultr)		Reference
			theoretical	experimental	
Tylosin	7.1	6.5	4.98	5.2	e
		6.8	3.00	3.5	
		7.1	1.00	1.0	
Lincomycin	7.6	6.5	5.42	5.5	m
		6.8	2.83	3.05	
		7.1	1.16	2.65	
Chloramphenicol		6.5–6.8		1.1	k
		7.1		1.1	
Spectinomycin*	8.75	6.5	7.66	0.5	e
		6.8	4.24	0.6	
		7.1	2.00	0.7	

* Passage of spectinomycin into milk is limited by its high degree of ionization in serum (95.8 per cent) and its low lipid solubility.
References. As Table 3.3 except: m Ziv & Sulman 1973b.

sulphonamide and/or trimethoprim preparations were given to pigs, macro- and microscopic lesions were produced, appearing mainly as areas of necrotic muscle tissue six days after the injection and as scar tissue at 30 days. The intramuscular injection of preparations containing tetracyclines, erythromycin, tylosin, and of the vehicles glycerol formal and propylene glycol caused similar tissue damage (Rasmussen & Hogh 1971, Rasmussen *et al* 1973, Rasmussen & Svendsen 1976). The addition of 22% polyvinyl pyrrolidone to sulphamethazine injection (20%), which is alkaline in reaction, did not diminish the tissue-damaging effect of the intramuscular injection (Rasmussen & Ladefoged 1974). Moreover sulphonamide residues were detected at injection sites 30 days after the administration of certain preparations (Rasmussen & Svendsen 1976). The amount of sulphonamide in the tissue constitutes a negligible residue when it is within the range of tolerance level — which, for sulphamethazine, is 0.1 parts/10^6 in the uncooked edible tissues of cattle and pigs (Booth 1977). The FDA recommendations on withdrawal times and tolerance levels of injectable antibiotics commonly used in pigs are shown in Table 3.5.

The unbound portion of an antimicrobial agent in the bloodstream is available for distribution, which includes passive diffusion into gastrointestinal fluids. This aspect of drug distribution can have considerable significance in ruminant animals and in the horse. The transfer process is similar to absorption, although it operates in the reverse direction. Physicochemical properties of organic electrolytes which influence passive diffusion are the degree of lipid solubility and the extent of ionisation of the drug in plasma (pH 7.4). Upon entering the reticuloruminal fluid (pH 5.5–6.5), organic bases (such as the macrolide antibiotics and lincomycin) and the tetracyclines can become 'trapped' by ionisation. This process has two

Table 3.5 Drug withdrawal times and tolerance levels of injectable drugs commonly used in swine. (Data from *Veterinary Pharmacology and Therapeutics* (1977) Courtesy of the Editors and Iowa State University Press.)

Drug	Pre-slaughter withdrawal time (days)	Tolerance level (parts/10^6)
Dihydrostreptomycin sulphate (DHS)	30	Zero
Erythromycin	7	0.1
Lincomycin hydrochloride monohydrate	2	0.1
Oxytetracycline	18	0.1
Procaine penicillin G	5	Zero
Procaine penicillin G and dihydro-streptomycin sulphate	30	Pen., zero; DHS, unpublished
Tylosin	4	0.2

important consequences. First, a significant fraction of the dose is contained in this location and, secondly, the antibiotic may interfere with activity of the normal bacterial flora. A similar process can be applied to the large intestine (colon) of horses. Disturbances of fermentation could result in the equine digestive system.

Comparative elimination mechanisms

Elimination includes both biotransformation and excretion. In all species of animals, the majority of antibiotics are eliminated mainly by renal excretion. The penicillins, cephalosporins, aminoglycosides, spectinomycin, oxytetracycline, tylosin, polymyxin B and colistin are excreted unchanged in the urine. Glomerular filtration is the principal mechanism of excretion but some antibiotics, notably the penicillins, are actively transported into urine by a carrier-mediated process in the proximal renal tubule. Ampicillin and amoxycillin undergo an enterohepatic circulation which extends their indications to treatment of intestinal infections and delays somewhat their rate of elimination. Oxytetracycline also undergoes a considerable degree of enterohepatic cycling and is slowly eliminated by glomerular filtration. Tylosin is probably excreted in both urine and bile. When the glomerular filtration rate is reduced, the rate of elimination of those antibiotics is decreased so that the usual interval between successive doses should be lengthened. This is particularly important in the case of aminoglycosides, which have a relatively narrow margin of safety, and for polymyxin B and colistin which are nephrotoxic. Due to high affinity binding of dihydrostreptomycin to kidney tissue, parenteral preparations containing this antibiotic have a pre-slaughter withdrawal time of 30 days and a zero tolerance level in food-producing animals.

The liver is the principal organ of elimination for erythromycin, lincomycin, clindamycin, minocycline, and chloramphenicol. Erythromycin and lincomycin undergo enterohepatic circulation and are slowly excreted unchanged in the bile. Clindamycin, minocycline, and chloramphenicol are inactivated by metabolism, the metabolites being excreted in urine and bile. In human beings, deoxycycline was shown to enter the small intestine by passive diffusion and, to a much lesser extent, by excretion in the bile (Whelton *et al* 1974). Chelation of the antibiotic by luminal contents renders it inactive, so that it is unlikely to interfere with the intestinal microflora.

Trimethoprim (a base (pKa 7.6)) and sulphadoxine (an acid (pKa 6.1)) are often combined for therapeutic use in farm animals. It is interesting to compare the rate and mechanisms of elimination of these two drugs. In cows and goats, the half-life of trimethoprim is 0.6–1.0 hour and the drug is eliminated mainly by hepatic metabolism (oxidative processes followed by glucuronide conjugation). The half-life of sulphadoxine is 11–12 hours in the ruminant animals and renal excretion (glomerular filtration, carrier-mediated tubular secretion, and passive back-diffusion) is the principal process of elimination (Davitiyananda & Rasmussen 1974, Nielsen & Rasmussen 1976a, 1976b). In swine, the half-life of trimethoprim is two hours and, while hepatic metabolism is the predominant metabolic pathway, renal excretion is relatively more important in this species than in ruminant animals. The half-life of sulphadoxine in swine is eight hours and, in contrast to ruminant animals, metabolism (N^4–acetylation which takes place in the lung, liver and kidney tissue) is the most prominent elimination process (Nielsen & Rasmussen 1975). The apparent volumes of distribution (l/kg) of trimethoprim and sulphadoxine are 1.3 and 0.3, respectively, in the different species. The values of the kinetic parameters ($t_\frac{1}{2}$ and V^1_d) remained the same whether the two drugs were given alone or in combinination. The fate of trimethoprim and sulphadoxine thus includes both biotransformation and renal excretion, the two drugs being metabolised by different pathways but having similar mechanisms of renal excretion. There is no competition between the drugs for carrier-mediated secretion in the proximal tubule as trimethoprim is an organic base and sulphadoxine is a weak acid. Urinary pH influences tubular re-absorption (passive diffusion) of the drugs in opposite ways. Under alkaline conditions, trimethoprim re-absorption is enhanced while sulphadoxine is more highly ionised and re-absorption is decreased.

Antimicrobial actions and therapy

Spectrum of antimicrobial activity

Antimicrobial agents can be classified according to their spectrum of activity. Antibiotics with a narrow range of activity can be divided into two groups. Those of the first group are active against Gram-positive bacteria and include penicillin G, penicillin V, methicillin and cloxacillin (which are penicillinase-resistant), erythromycin, tylosin, lincomycin and clindamycin. Bacitracin, a polypeptide antibiotic which inhibits bacterial cell wall synthesis, is active against a variety of Gram-positive cocci and bacilli.

The activity of antibiotics in the second group is mainly against, or in some cases restricted to, Gram-negative bacteria. This group includes streptomycin, dihydrostreptomycin, spectinomycin (which is not an aminoglycoside), polymyxin B and colistin. The aminoglycoside antibiotics may be considered to have a broad range of antibacterial activity but their use should, perhaps, be limited to therapy of infections due to susceptible Gram-negative micro-organisms. It is important to realise that there is often wide variation in sensitivity of susceptible micro-organisms or bacterial strains to an antibiotic. Consequently, a quantitative assessment of sensitivity narrows the choice of potentially suitable antibiotics for treatment of bacterial infections. Experience has often led to a certain antibiotic being considered the drug of choice for treatment of a particular condition. This knowledge takes into account not only the in-vitro sensitivity, but also the accessibility of the drug to the site of the infection.

Antimicrobial agents that are effective against both Gram-positive and Gram-negative bacteria are considered to have a broad spectrum of activity. They include ampicillin, amoxycillin, carbenicillin, cephalothin, cephalexin (acid-stable), kanamycin, neomycin, gentamicin, the tetracyclines, sulphonamides and chloramphenicol. The tetracyclines and chloramphenicol are highly effective against some micro-organisms that are innately insensitive to many antimicrobial agents, such as those of the rickettsiae and the psittacosis-lymphogranuloma group.

Type of antibacterial action

At therapeutic concentrations, the action of some antimicrobial agents is bactericidal while that of others is bacteriostatic (Table 3.6). Bactericidal antibiotics kill bacteria, while bacteriostatic agents suppress bacterial growth and depend upon the defence mechanisms of the host animal to overcome the infection. In view of the need for active humoral and cellular defence mechanisms, the simultaneous administration of corticosteroids and bacteriostatic antimicrobial agents appear to be irrational. Some antibiotics (such as erythromycin, chloramphenicol, and the tetracyclines) are primarily bacteriostatic, but may be bactericidal to certain strains under some conditions.

The dosage rates of antimicrobial agents selected for clinical use are related to antibacterial action but they are also influenced by the margin of safety and the probability of inducing resistant strains. It is desirable, at least with bacteriostatic agents, to maintain serum concentrations within the

Table 3.6 Antimicrobial agents grouped according to antibacterial action.

Bactericidal	Bacteriostatic
Penicillins	Tetracyclines
Cephalosporins	Chloramphenicol
Aminoglycosides	Macrolides
Bacitracin	Lincomycin
Polymyxin B	Spectinomycin
Trimethoprim/sulphonamide	Sulphonamides

therapeutic range throughout the course of therapy. For antibiotics with bactericidal activity, it is not clear whether the area under the serum concentration-time curve or the peak serum concentration is the more important. It seems likely that the maximimal serum concentration attained, which determines the level reached at infection sites, may be of greater chemotherapeutic significance.

Therapy with combined antimicrobial agents

Anitmicrobial drug interactions may be additive, synergistic, or antagonistic. In addition, the spectrum of activity may be increased.

Addition

The antibacterial action resulting from the simultaneous use of two antimicrobial agents frequently is additive. For example, when a sulphonamide is combined with other bacteriostatic agents, such as tetracyclines, it is likely that an additive effect will result. The antibacterial activity of a combined sulphonamide preparation is the sum of the activities of the component sulphonamides. An advantage associated with use of combined preparations is that each sulphonamide exhibits its own solubility in water, thus giving greater total sulphonamide solubility with reduced risk of causing crystalluria. Bacitracin and polymyxin B or neomycin (or both) are incorporated into a number of topical preparations. The purpose of combinations of this kind is to broaden the spectrum of antibacterial activity, as bacitracin affects only Gram-positive organisms and polymyxin activity is restricted to Gram-negative bacteria. The actions of bacitracin and polymyxin B are compatible in that bacitracin inhibits bacterial cell wall synthesis and polymyxin B is a surface-active agent which induces permeability changes in the bacterial cell membrane.

Synergism

Under some circumstances, certain antimicrobial drug combinations exert a so-called 'synergistic' effect. Synergism is said to be present when the combined effect of two or more drugs exceeds the algebraic sum of the effects produced by the drugs acting separately. The simultaneous administration of a sulphonamide and trimethoprim leads to a synergistic antimicrobial action. Sulphonamides inhibit bacterial growth by preventing para-aminobenzoic acid from being incorporated into the pteroylglutamic acid (folic acid) molecule. Trimethoprim is a powerful and selective inhibitor of microbial dihydrofolate reductase, the enzyme that reduces dihydrofolate to tetrahydrofolate. Consequently, the use of a sulphonamide with trimethoprim introduces sequential blocks in the pathway by which micro-organisms synthesise tetrahydrofolate from precursor molecules (Angehrn & Then 1973). In proprietary preparations, the drugs are combined in fixed proportions, which are based on optimum activity determined *in vitro,* and presumably take into account the extent of distribution and duration of action of the sulphonamide and trimethoprim. In human beings, a trimethoprim–sulphamethoxazole (1:5) combination is used clinically. The choice of sulphamethoxazole for the combined product is logical since both drugs have approximately the same half-life, so that any appropriate dosage interval will be similar for both drugs. Trimethoprim has a short half-life in domestic species of animal compared with that in the human, and a considerably small fraction of the dose is excreted unchanged in the urine (Table 3.6). Even though it is unlikely that a fixed combination of trimethoprim with any sulphonamide would maintain optimal concentrations of both drugs in domestic animals, the clinical effectiveness of the combined preparation (trimethoprim–sulphadiazine; trimethoprim–sulphadoxine) have proved their value.

The simultaneous presence at the site of infection of an aminoglycoside (streptomycin, kanamycin, or gentamicin) and penicillin results in a synergistic action against Enterococci. This action is manifested by a large increase in the rate of bactericidal action of the penicillin (Miles *et al* 1951). Moreover, ampicillin or penicillin G used simultaneously with streptomycin exerts a synergistic action against *Listeria monocytogenes* and carbenicillin can be synergistic with gentamicin for some strains of Pseudomonas (Sonne & Jawetz 1969, Smith *et al* 1969). Except for cases of severe bacterial infections in which the aetiology cannot be delineated and in which delay in treatment may be dangerous, the simultaneous administration (but not in the form of 'fixed-dose' mixtures) of two or more antibacterial drugs should

Table 3.7 Elimination of trimethoprim. (Data from Alexander & Collett 1974 and Kaplan *et al* 1970).

Species	Half-life (hours)	Percentage of dose excreted unchanged in 24-hour urine
Man	10.6	47
Pony	3.8	10
Dog	3.0	20
Pig	2–2.5	16
Cow	1.0	3
Goat	0.65	2

be restricted to diseases in which their superiority over single drugs has been proved clinically. When multiple drug therapy is employed, each agent must be administered in the same dose as that given when used alone (Weinstein 1975).

Antagonism

Antagonism may be defined as the circumstance in which the total effect of a combination of drugs is less than the algebraic sum of the effects of the individual drugs in the combination. The basis of antagonism can be related only in general terms to the mechanism of antibacterial action. The tetracyclines, chloramphenicol, and the macrolides act by inhibiting protein synthesis in bacteria. These antibiotics, which are all bacteriostatic in action, can antagonise penicillins (inhibition of cell wall synthesis) and aminoglycosides (inhibition of ribosomal protein biosynthesis). The treatment of brucellosis and glanders, which is caused by *Pseudomonas (Actinobacillus) mallei,* constitute exceptions in that the use of streptomycin together with a tetracycline leads to better results. The sulphonamides, which have a bacteriostatic action can also antagonise penicillins (Gunnison *et al* 1951). The penicillins exert their bactericidal action only against micro-organisms that are multiplying.

Factors influencing antibacterial activity

The activity of antimicrobial agents can be altered by pH of their environment, by the presence of tissue constituents, blood, and pus; while chemical inactivation (incompatibility) inevitably reduces activity. The influence of pH on antibacterial activity is of clinical significance in treating urinary tract infections and suppurative processes. The activity of aminoglycosides is much higher in an alkaline medium. There is a 20- to 80-fold increase in potency of streptomycin at pH 8.0 as compared to pH 5.8. Increase in local acidity secondary to tissue damage may be responsible for failure of the drug to eradicate sensitive micro-organisms at sites of injury or abscess formation. While the predominant action of macrolides and lincomycins is bacteriostatic, in an alkaline environment they can exert a bactericidal effect. Urinary alkalinisation increases the solubility of sulphonamides and their acetyl derivatives (major metabolite), and causes a greater fraction of the dose to be excreted unchanged in the urine. The antibacterial activity of nitrofurantoin is greater, while methenamine (hexamine) is effective only in acid urine. The antiseptic property of methenamine is due to its decomposition to formaldehyde in an acidic environment. It is to be noted that low pH alone is bacteriostatic.

Principles of dosage

Having decided that an antimicrobial agent is indicated, the choice of drug should be made only after certain features of the patient, apart from the site and nature of the infection, have been considered. It is necessary to take into account the species of animal, the functional state of the kidneys, the residue potential of drug in food-producing animals, and, because of passage of antimicrobial agents into milk, special consideration must be given to systemic therapy in dairy cows. The site of the infection or disease condition (e.g., mastitis, pneumonia, cystitis) may reduce, for therpeutic application, the number of antimicrobial agents to which the micro-organisms were found to be susceptible *in vitro*. In veterinary medicine, the dosage forms that are available and the cost of the course of therapy will also influence selection of the drug. Whichever drug product is selected, it must be given by the appropriate route and it is essential that dosage be adequate. A higher dosage level (mg/kg body weight) may be required for an oral as compared with a parenteral preparation of a drug.

The proper selection and effective dosage of antimicrobial agents can be based on a critical evaluation of the clinical response. This approach can only be gained by experience and, though valuable, it is empirical. The remission of an infectious disease during the course of antimicrobial therapy is, of course, reassuring and could be taken as suggesting that the dosage regimen and the drug preparation administered were highly satisfactory; however this evidence is inconclusive because the animal might have recovered without any treatment. The pharmacokinetic approach, which is based on well designed drug disposition studies, defines dosage more precisely and allows, at the very least, the plasma (or serum) levels to be predicted. One would anticipate optimum effectiveness with antimicrobial therapy when the dosage regimens based on clinical experience and those developed mathematically from disposition studies are in agreement.

The factors which determine dosage of an antimicrobial agent include the extent of distribution and rate of elimination of the drug, the range of therapeutic (i.e. effective and non-toxic) plasma concentrations, accessibility of the agent to the site of infection, and whether the action is bacteriostatic or bactericidal at therapeutic levels. The binding of antimicrobial agents to plasma proteins *in vivo* assumes clinical significance only when the levels of free drug are reduced to values below the minimum inhibitory concentrations for susceptible micro-organisms. When the route of administration is other than intravenous, the rate of absorption and the extent of systemic availability of the drug substance from the dosage form administered are complicating factors that must be taken into account.

A dosage regimen entails two variables: the size of each dose and the frequency with which it is repeated, usually expressed as a dosage interval. In treating bacterial diseases, it is always desirable to establish a therapeutic amount of drug in the body quickly and to maintain an effective level throughout the course of therapy. This objective is best accomplished by initiating therapy with a priming dose, usually given intravenously, and administering a series of maintenance doses at appropriate intervals. The margin of safety and the rate of elimination (expressed as half-life) of a drug are the factors which limit the size of each dose and the duration of effective plasma levels, respectively. For antimicrobial agents, with the notable exception of penicillins, increasing the size of the intravenous dose above that which will give an effective plasma concentration for a period exceeding twice the half-life of the agent is neither a safe nor an economical method for lengthening the interval between successive doses. Since the overall elimination of antimicrobial drugs follows first-order (i.e. exponential) kinetics, geometric increases in dose produce only linear increases in the duration of therapeutic levels. First-order elimination implies that 50% of the drug in the body is eliminated each half-life. Since the half-life value is based on intravenous dosage, drug administration in appropriate formulations by other parenteral routes or *per orum* can be an effective means for lengthening the dosage interval. Sustained-release preparations (such as procaine penicillin G) are particularly useful in this regard. When drug uptake (dissolution and absorption) is slower than elimination, the rate of uptake will determine the duration of action as long as sufficient is absorbed to maintain an effective level.

Applied aspects of dosage

The dosage regimens presented in Tables 3.8 to 3.11 inclusive are guidelines, based mainly on pharmacokinetic data derived from experiments performed in normal animals, for horses, cattle, calves, and pigs. The dosage level for each drug product represents the dose that should be effective in treatment of the majority of conditions for which the drug is indicated; bacterial diseases caused by highly and moderately susceptible micro-organisms would be expected to respond favourably. The dosage interval recommended is that which would be appropriate to use should a series of doses be given. For drugs that are eliminated mainly by renal excretion, in particular aminoglycoside antibiotics, the interval between successive doses should be lengthened in patients with reduced renal function. The route of administration takes into account the formulation of the preparation and the species of animal for which the drug is recommended. For various reasons certain preparations may not be available in some countries. Since chloramphenicol should not be used in food-producing animals, dosage regimens for this antibiotic are not given for cattle and pigs.

Table 3.8 Tentative dosage regimens for antimicrobial agents in horses.

Drug preparation	Route of administration	Dosage regimen Dose (mg/kg)	Interval (h)
Sodium penicillin G	i.v., i.m., s.c.	15–25 000 units/kg	6–8
Procaine penicillin G in buffered aqueous suspension	i.m.	20 000 units/kg	24
Ampicillin sodium	i.v., i.m., s.c.	10–20	8–12
Amoxycillin trihydrate aqueous solution	i.m., s.c.	6–8	12
Streptomycin sulphate	i.m.	8–12	8
Kanamycin sulphate	i.m.	4–6	8
Gentamicin sulphate	i.m.	2–4	8
Trimethoprim/sulphadoxine	i.v., i.m.	4–20	12

Drug preparation	Route of administration	*Priming*	*Maintenance*	Interval (h)
Oxytetracycline hydrochloride	i.v. (slowly)	5	3	12
Chloramphenicol sodium succinate	i.m.	50	25	8
Sulphadimethoxine sodium	i.v.	55	27.5	12
Sulphamethazine sodium	i.v.	110	55	12–24
Sulphamethazine	p.o.	150	75	24

Horses

Tentative dosage regimens for antimicrobial agents in horses are given in Table 3.8. The penicillins are considered to be the antimicrobial agents of choice for chemotherapy in the horse. It is desirable to administer certain injectable preparations (e.g. sulphonamides, tetracyclines) by the intravenous route to avoid irritation and tissue damage at the injection site. Intravenous injections should always be given slowly. Procaine penicillin G should never be injected intravenously, because this drug is formulated as an aqueous suspension, designed to provide slow uptake of penicillin G from the intramuscular site. The adverse pharmacological effects which procaine might induce (mainly interference with the cardiac conduction mechanism) constitute another important contraindication to intravenous administration of this preparation.

The aminoglycoside antibiotics are rapidly and completely absorbed from intramuscular injection sites. The short half-life of chloramphenicol in the horse, which is one hour (Davis *et al* 1972, Pilloud 1973), and unpredictable absorption from the gastrointestinal tract make intramuscular injection the only feasible route of administration for maintaining therapeutic levels of this drug. A sustained-release parenteral dosage form which would provide therapeutic levels of chloramphenicol (i.e. >5 μg/ml) in the plasma for 24 hours might be considered worth future development. Oral dosage, biliary excretion, and, possibly most important, passive diffusion from the systemic circulation represent ways in which antimicrobial agents might interfere with essential bacterial flora in the colon of the horse.

Adult cattle

In Table 3.9 recommendations for dosage rates of antimicrobial preparations in cattle are given. The same preparations and dosage regimens may be used in sheep and goats. Although one is reluctant to extrapolate pharmacokinetic data from one species of animal to another, there is no conclusive evidence to show that drug uptake from parenteral sites of administration, extent of distribution, or rate of elimination differ significantly between these three species of domestic ruminants. The total dosage given to a goat differs substantially from that given to a cow, this difference relating to the weight of the animals. Increasing the dose of sustained-release preparations (such as procaine or benzathine penicillin) above a certain level may prolong but will not elevate the serum concentrations of the drug. To avoid the persistence of residual levels at the intramuscular site of injection, the subcutaneous route may be used for some preparations. Oral dosage with antimicrobial agents is undesirable in adult ruminants because of the likelihood of interfering with the ruminal flora. Prolonged parenteral therapy with the weak bases erythromycin, lincomycin, and oxytetracycline (and even more so with doxycycline) could also affect the ruminal flora. The long pre-slaughter withdrawal times associated with the parenteral use of oxytetracycline preparations and streptomycin are worthy of note. Other aminoglycoside antibiotics (gentamicin, kanamycin, and neomycin), should they be used parenterally, would have a 30 day withdrawal time as well. Probably the most common way that milk becomes contaminated with penicillin is through intramammary infusion of the drug in the treatment of bovine mastitis (Eberhart *et al* 1963). In dairy cows, the time required for 'milk-out' varies with the formulation of the antibiotic preparations.

Calves

Dosage regimens of antimicrobial agents suitable for use in calves are presented in Table 3.10. Unlike the young of other mammalian species, calves apparently have an efficient renal function (Dalton 1968). This implies that the usual adult dosage intervals for those antimicrobial agents which are eliminated mainly by renal excretion can be utilised in the chemotherapy of calf diseases. Oral dosages with amoxycillin, given as the trihydrate in lactose, was found to be highly effective in the treatment of diarrhoea which was considered to be of complex aetiology (Palmer *et al* 1977). Chloramphenicol sodium succinate, given by intramuscular injection, was useful for the treatment of certain salmonella and fusiformis infections in calves. To maintain therapeutic plasma levels of the drug, a dosage regimen consisting of a priming dose (50 mg/kg) followed by a series of maintenance

Table 3.9 Tentative dosage regimens for antimicrobial agents in cattle.

Drug preparation	Route of administration	Dosage regimen			Pre-slaughter withdrawal time
		Dose (mg/kg)		Interval (h)	(days)
Sodium penicillin G	i.v., i.m., s.c.	10 000 units/kg		8	5
Procaine penicillin G in buffered aqueous suspension	i.m.	15 000 units/kg		24	5
Procaine penicillin G in oil with aluminum monostearate	i.m.	15 000 units/kg		48	*
Benzathine penicillin G	i.m.	20 000 units/kg		96	30
Ampicillin sodium	i.v., i.m., s.c.	6		8	5
Ampicillin trihydrate in aqueous suspension	i.m., s.c.	10		12	6
Dihydrostreptomycin sulphate	i.m.	10		8–(12)	30
Oxytetracycline base in 2-pyrrolidone	i.m.	20		48	28
		Priming	*Maintenance*		
Oxytetracycline hydrochloride in propylene glycol and water	i.m.	10	7.5	24	21
Lincomycin hydrochloride	i.v., i.m.	10	6	12	*
{ Erythromycin lactobionate	i.v.	10			
{ Erythromycin base (20%) in organic solvent	i.m.	10	6	12	14
{ Tylosin tartrate buffered	i.v., i.m.	10			
{ Tylosin base (20%) in 50% propylene glycol	i.m.	10	6	8	8
Sulphamethazine sodium	i.v.	110	55	24	10
Sulphadimethoxine sodium	i.v.	55	27.5	24	10

*Not approved for use.

Table 3.10 Tentative dosage regimens for antimicrobial agents in calves.

Drug preparation	Route of administration	Dosage regimen Dose (mg/kg)		Interval (h)
Sodium penicillin G	i.v., i.m., s.c.	15 000 units/kg		6–8
Procaine penicillin G in buffered aqueous suspension	i.m.	15 000 units/kg		24
Ampicillin sodium	i.v., i.m., s.c.	6–10		8–12
Amoxycillin aqueous suspension	i.m.	7		8–12
Amoxycillin trihydrate	p.o.	7		8–12
Streptomycin sulphate	i.m.	8		8–12
Kanamycin sulphate	i.m.	6		8–12
Trimethoprim/sulphadoxine	i.v., i.m.	8/40		24
Trimethoprim/sulphadiazine	i.v., i.m.	8/40		24
		Priming	*Maintenance*	
Chloramphenicol sodium succinate	i.m.	50	25	12
Sulphamethazine sodium	i.v.	110	55	24
Tylosin base (20%) in 50% propylene glycol	i.m.	10	6	8–12

Table 3.11 Parenteral dosage regimens for antimicrobial agents in pigs.

Drug preparation	Route of administration	Dosage regimen Dose (mg/kg)		Interval (h)
Sodium penicillin G	s.c., i.m.	20 000 units/kg		8
Procaine penicillin G in buffered aqueous suspension	i.m.	20 000 units/kg		24
Ampicillin sodium	s.c., i.m.	6–8		8
Dihydrostreptomycin sulphate	i.m.	10		12
Kanamycin sulphate	i.m.	6–8		12
Spectinomycin hydrochloride	i.m.	10		12
Erythromycin base (20%)	i.m.	10		12
Tylosin base (20%)	i.m.	12.5		12
Lincomycin hydrochloride monohydrate	i.m.	10		12
Trimethoprim/sulphadiazine	i.m.	8/40		24
Trimethoprim/sulphadoxine	i.m.	8/40		24
		Priming	*Maintenance*	
Oxytetracycline hydrochloride	i.m.	10	7.5	24
Sulphamethazine sodium	s.c., i.m.	110	55	24

doses (25 mg/kg) at 12-hour intervals would be required. An outbreak of *Salmonella dublin* infection in 5-week-old calves was successfully treated with spectinomycin. A priming dose (22 mg/kg), injected subcutaneously, was followed by oral administration of the drug at a total dose of 0.5 g for five days (Cook 1973). These calves had failed to respond to prior therapy with ampicillin, sulphamethazine, oxytetracycline and chloramphenicol.

Pigs

The applied aspect of chemotherapy in pigs is somewhat different from that in other species. This difference is related both to the system of management and to the functional anatomy of the pig. Parenteral dosage regimens for antimicrobial agents which might be used for the treatment of bacterial infections are given in Table 3.11. Since the intramuscular route of injection is used most commonly, the formulation of parenteral preparations is critical in determining absorption of drug substance from the injection site and the extent of tissue damage that may result. In pigs, treatment often consists of a single dose rather than a course of therapy, dose rates being indicated in Table 3.11. Pain and induration may occur following the intramuscular injecton of lincomycin. In addition, some tissue damage with scar tissue formation can result from sulphamethazine, oxytetracycline, erythromycin, and tylosin administration. Medication of the feed or the drinking water with antimicrobial agents may be used as a means of controlling various diseases in pigs. The drug concentrations which are added to the feed for this purpose are given in Table 3.12. Tylosin and sulphamethazine are often combined, in which case 100 g of each drug are mixed in a tonne of feed. Medication of the drinking water may be used, but this procedure is more wasteful than feed medication. Substances administered in the drinking water include tylosin, trimethoprim–sulphadiazine, lincomycin–spectinomycin, streptomycin, and sodium arsanilate. The pre-slaughter withdrawal time for sodium arsanilate is five days.

Table 3.12 Feed levels of antimicrobial agents used for disease control in pigs.

Drug	Amount in Feed (g/tonne)
Oxytetracycline	50–100
Chlortetracycline	50–100
Lincomycin–spectinomycin	40
Tylosin	100
Sulphamethazine	100
Neomycin sulphate	100
Furazolidone	50–100
Carbadox*	50
Virginiamycin	25

* Must be withdrawn 35 days prior to slaughter.

References

Alexander F. & Collett R. A. (1974) Some observations on the pharmacokinetics of trimethoprim in the horse. *Br. J. Pharmacol.* **52**, 142 p.

Angehrn P. & Then R. (1973) Investigations on the mode of action of the combination sulfamethoxazole/trimethoprim. *Chemotherapy* **19**, 1–10.

Atef M. & Nielsen P. (1975) Metabolism of sulphadiazine in goats. *Xenobiotica* **5**, 167–172.

Baggot J. D. (1977) *Principles of Drug Disposition in Domestic Animals: The Basis of Veterinary Clinical Pharmacology.* W. B. Saunders, Philadelphia.

Booth N. H. (1977) Drug and chemical residues in the edible tissues of animals. In *Veterinary Pharmacology and Therapeutics,* L. Meyer Jones, N. H. Booth and L. E. McDonald (eds.) 4th ed. Iowa State University Press, Ames, Iowa.

Boxenbaum H. G., Fellig J., Hanson L. J. *et al* (1977) Pharmacokinetics of sulphadimethoxine in cattle. *Res. Vet. Sci.* **23**, 24–28.

Cook B. (1973) Successful treatment of an outbreak of *Salmonella dublin* infection in calves using spectinomycin. *Vet. Rec.* **93**, 80.

Dalton R. G. (1968) Renal functional in neonatal calves: inulin, thiosulphate and paraaminohippuric acid clearance. *Br. Vet. J.* **124**, 498–502.

Davis L. E., Neff C. A., Baggot J. D. *et al* (1972) Pharmacokinetics of chloramphenicol in domesticated animals. *Am. J. Vet. Res.* **33**, 2259–2266.

Davitiyananda D. & Rasmussen F. (1974) Mammary and renal excretion of sulphadoxine and trimethoprim in cows. *Acta Vet. Scand.* **15**, 340–355.

Eberhart R. J., Watrous G. H., Hokanson J. F. *et al* (1963) Persistence of antibacterial agents in milk after intramammary treatment of clinical mastitis. *J. Am. Vet. Med. Assoc.* **143**, 390–394.

Gunnison J. B., Speck R. S., Jawetz E. *et al* (1951) Studies on antibiotic synergism and antagonism: The effect of sulfadiazine on the action of penicillin *in vitro* and *in vivo*. *Antibiotics & Chemotherapy* **1**, 259–266.

Hooke F. G. (1978) Antibiotics. In *The Therapeutic Jungle,* Proceedings No. 39. The Post-Graduate Committee in Veterinary Science, The University of Sydney, vol. **2**, pp. 813–897.

Huber W. G. (1977) Streptomycin, chloramphenicol and other antibacterial agents. In *Veterinary Pharmacology and Therapeutics,* L. Meyer Jones, N. H. Booth & L. E. McDonald (eds.) 4th ed. Iowa State University, Ames, Iowa.

Kaplan S. A., Weinfeld R. E. Cotler S. *et al* (1970) Pharmacokinetic profile of trimethoprim in dog and man. *J. Pharmac. Sci.* **59**, 358–363.

Miles C. P., Coleman V. R., Gunnison J. B. *et al* (1951) Antibiotic synergism requires the simultaneous presence of both members of a synergistic drug pair. *Proc. Soc. Exp. Biol. Med.* **78**, 738–741.

Nielsen P. (1973) Metabolism of sulphonamides in goats. *Acta. Vet. Scand.* **14**, 647–649.

Nielsen P. & Rasmussen F. (1975) Trimethoprim and sulphadoxine in swine: Half-lives, volume of distribution and tissue concentrations. *Zentral. für Vet.* (A), **22**, 564–571.

Nielsen P. & Rasmussen F. (1976a) Elimination of trimethoprim, sulphadoxine and their metabolites in goats. *Acta. Pharmacol. Toxicol.* **38**, 104–112.

Nielsen P. & Rasmussen F. (1976b) Influence of age on half-life of trimethoprim and sulphadoxine in goats. *Acta Pharmacol. Toxicol.* **38**, 113–119.

Nielsen P. & Rasmussen F. (1977) Half-life, apparent volume of distribution and protein-binding for some sulphonamides in cows. *Res. Vet. Sci.* **22**, 205–208.

Palmer G. H., Bywater R. J. & Francis M. E. (1977) Amoxycillin: Distribution and clinical efficacy in calves. *Vet. Rec.* **100**, 487–491.

Pilloud M. (1973) Pharmacokinetics, plasma protein binding and dosage of chloramphenicol in cattle and horses. *Res. Vet. Sci.* **15**, 231–238.

Rasmussen F. (1958) Mammary excretion of sulphonamides. *Acta Pharmacol. Toxicol.* **15,** 139–148.

Rasmussen F. (1959) Mammary excretion of benzylpenicillin, erythromycin, and penethamate hydroiodide. *Acta Pharmacol. Toxicol.* **16,** 194–200.

Rasmussen F. (1966a) *Studies on the Mammary Excretion and Absorption of Drugs.* Carl. Fr. Mortensen, Copenhagen.

Rasmussen F. (1966b) Mammary excretion of lincomycin in cows. *Acta Vet. Scand.* **7,** 97–98.

Rasmussen F. (1970) Renal and mammary excretion of trimethoprim in goats. *Vet. Rec.* **87,** 14–18.

Rasmussen F. & Hogh P. (1971) Irritating effect and concentrations at the injection site after intramuscular injection of antibiotic preparations in cows and pigs. *Nord. Vet. Med.* **23,** 593–605.

Rasmussen F. & Ladefoged O. (1974) Tissue damage at the injection site after intramuscular injection of drug preparations formulated by addition of polyvinylpyrrolidone. *Acta Vet. Scand.* **15,** 636–638.

Rasmussen F., Nielsen P. & Svendsen O. (1973) Tissue injuries, concentrations at the injection site and the concentrations in muscles, liver and kidney after intramuscular injection of injectable sulphadimidine 0.2 g/ml in pigs. *Nord. Vet. Med.* **25,** 256–261.

Rasmussen F. & Svendsen O. (1976) Tissue damage and concentration at the injection site after intramuscular injection of chemotherapeutics and vehicles in pigs. *Res. Vet. Sci.* **20,** 55–60.

Schipper I. A., Filipovs D., Ebeltoft H. *et al* (1971) Blood serum concentrations of various benzyl penicillins after their intramuscular administration to cattle. *J. Am. Vet. Med. Assoc.* **158,** 494–500.

Smith C. B., Dans P. E., Wilfert J. N. *et al* (1969) Use of gentamicin in combination with other antibiotics. *J. Infec. Dis.* **119,** 370–377.

Sonne M. & Jawetz E. (1969) Combined action of carbenicillin and gentamicin on *Pseudomonas aeruginosa in vitro. Appl. Microbiol.* **17,** 893–896.

Stowe C. M. & Sisodia C. S. (1963) The pharmacologic properties of sulfadimethoxine in dairy cattle. *Am. J. Vet. Res.* **24,** 525–535.

Theodorides V. J., DiCuollo C. J., Guarini J. R., *et al* (1968) Serum concentrations of chloramphenicol after intra-ruminal and intraabomasal administration in sheep. *Am. J. Vet. Res.* **29,** 643–645.

Weinstein E. (1975) Antimicrobial agents: General considerations. In *The Pharmacological Basis of Therapeutics,* Goodman L. S. & Gilman A. (eds.) 5th edn. pp. 1090–1112. Macmillan, London.

Whelton A., Schach von Wittenan M., Twomey T. M. *et al* (1974) Doxycycline pharmacokinetics in the absence of renal function. *Kidney Int.* **5,** 365–371.

Ziv G., Bogin E. & Sulman F. G. (1973a) Blood and milk levels of chloramphenicol in normal and mastitic cows and ewes after intramuscular administration of chloramphenicol and chloramphenicol sodium succinate. *Zentral. für Vet.* (A) **20,** 801–811.

Ziv G., Shani J. & Sulman F. G. (1973b) Pharmacokinetic evaluation of penicillin and cephalosporin derivatives in serum and milk of lactating cows and ewes. *Am. J. Vet. Res.* **34,** 1561–1565.

Ziv G. & Sulman F. G. (1973a) Serum and milk concentrations of spectinomycin and tylosin in cows and ewes. *Am. J. Vet. Res.* **34,** 329–333.

Ziv G & Sulman F G. (1973b) Penetration of lincomycin and clindamycin into milk in ewes. *Br. Vet. J.* **129,** 83–91.

Ziv G. & Sulman F. G. (1973b) Passage of polymyxins from serum into milk in ewes. *Am. J. Vet. Res.* **34,** 317–322.

Ziv G. & Sulman F. G. (1974a) Distribution of aminoglycoside antibiotics in blood and milk. *Res. Vet. Sci.* **17,** 68–74.

Ziv G. & Sulman F. G. (1974b) Analysis of pharmacokinetic properties of nine tetracycline analogues in dairy cows and ewes. *Am. J. Vet. Res.* **35,** 1197–1201.

4

The use of antibiotics in equine practice

S.W. RICKETTS & R. HOPES

The basic principles guiding the use of antibiotics are the same for all species (Short 1963, Alexander 1966, Brander 1966, Baggot 1977, English & Roberts 1979). Antibiotics are used to treat or to prevent infectious disease, usually of bacterial origin. Specific drugs are chosen depending on the sensitivity of the causal organism. The drug is used in therapeutic doses over a sufficient period of time to minimise the risk of producing reistant strains. Suitable guidelines for dosages and duration of therapy are usually provided by the drug companies concerned (Massam & Murray 1978). If the desired clinical result is not obtained after an adequate period of treatment, the drug used is changed to another to which the organism is also sensitive. The use of in-vitro antibiotic sensitivity tests may be criticised on theoretical grounds (Hinton 1976, Linton 1976) but, if properly performed (Mackintosh 1981), they are still the best guide that the clinician has available (Brander 1966).

It is not always possible to confirm the presence of a causal organism by laboratory techniques, and in these cases drugs are chosen depending on the organism or organisms likely to be involved. These may be deduced from past experience with the particular species and organ system involved. *Streptococcus zooepidemicus* (a beta-haemolytic Streptococcus) is a common cause of equine bacterial infection (Bazeley & Battle 1940, Bryans 1972) and is usually penicillin sensitive. Resistant strains do occur however and clinicians must be on their guard for this problem (Tobin 1978).

Veterinary surgeons should recognise the risks of antibiotic abuse and try to limit their use of these drugs (Randall 1969, Swann 1969, Roberts & English 1979). Sulphonamide (Bazeley 1940a) and potentiated sulphonamide drugs (Alexander & Collett 1975) may be conveniently used in equine practice, where appropriate, reserving antibiotics for use in specific circumstances.

Special considerations for the use of antibiotics in horses

Body weight

Total body weight varies from the Shetland pony to the Suffolk horse (Goodal 1965). Since dosages must be calculated on a body weight basis, large volumes of drugs may be needed in the larger types of horse, and this may cause problems with local reactions. For large volume intramuscular injections, doses should be divided and given into different sites.

Value

The value of different horses varies widely from those of sentimental value only to those worth millions of pounds; this may have a direct bearing on the veterinary surgeon's ability to use the antibiotic of choice.

Administration

The route and method of administration of an antibacterial drug is governed primarily by the site at which the desired response is needed. If local treatment is appropriate and the preparation used is readily absorbable at the site of action then this is usually ideal. For successful parenteral treatment, the chemical nature of the drug (e.g. its pH in solution) and binding characteristics govern its ability to be readily absorbed and transported via the bloodstream to the site of action (English & Roberts 1979). Horses vary widely in their response to interference by a veterinary surgeon and handlers vary widely in their ability to control their horses. Some situations may be potentially hazardous and the choice of antibiotic used and the route of administration may be governed by the risk of injury to the horse, handler and/or veterinary surgeon. Intravenous therapy is facilitated by the readily available jugular vein. There are several large muscle masses available for intramuscular injections but the gluteal area is preferred for its lower incidence of local reaction (Rossdale & Ricketts 1980). Oral therapy, with sulphonamide drugs in powder or paste form, is very useful in many cases. Most horses can be enticed to eat all but very bitter medicines in a warm, sweet mash. Oral drugs that are used to give systemic cover must, of course, be absorbed from the gastrointestinal tract giving adequate blood levels.

Many horses at livery, in training, or at stud, do not belong to those who look after them. Thus the practice of leaving antibiotic injections for follow-up treatment is often not acceptable. Apart from the undesirability of this practice on ethical grounds, the risk of legal action following accidents or reactions after injections by unqualified persons is very real. Suitable oral

                    Chapter 4

antibiotic preparations (e.g. sulphamezathine or potentiated sulphonamides) are thus a useful way of avoiding the costs of repeated veterinary attention.

Unwanted reactions and side-effects

The horse is renowned for its ability to react locally to injections of any kind (Rossdale & Ricketts 1980) and horse owners are equally renowned for their reactions to such occurrences. Intravenous injections are less likely to produce local reaction than intramuscular ones (Short 1963). With potentially irritant drugs (e.g. acidic solutions of oxytetracycline and tetracycline and alkaline solutions of the sodium salts of some sulphonamides) great care must be taken not to inject outside the vein or severe local reactions may occur (Gabel 1977). Even with non-irritant drugs, unwanted local reactions can occur if the horse is fractious or the handler is unable to control the horse in the correct manner, resulting in local trauma from the needle.

Unwanted systemic reactions may occur following antibiotic administration. Some horses appear to be allergic to penicillin (Walton 1980) and may show dramatic acute anaphylaxis with collapse or a generalised urticarial response (Ingham & Large 1969). The incidence of such hypersensitivity reactions is estimated to be less than 5% (Tobin 1978). The long term use of systemic antibiotics of any type may suppress the intestinal microflora and cause gastrointestinal upsets. The use of intravenous oxytetracycline has been particularly incriminated (Cook 1973, Baker & Leyland 1973, MacKellar *et al* 1973), and may be followed by acute diarrhoea which may become chronic and intractable. This same drug has been reported to be a possible trigger factor for some cases of acute salmonellosis in horses (Owen 1975). Roberts & English (1979) recommend that, wherever possible, oral antimicrobial therapy should not be used to treat gastrointestinal conditions in the horse. In addition to upsetting the normal intestinal flora, they point out that microbial fermentation in the large intestine may be disturbed and that fungal overgrowth may occur.

The long term local use of antibiotics at any site may cause problems of organ malfunction or infection with resistant bacteria or fungi (Alexander 1966). This is a particular problem with intestinal and genital therapy (Roberts & English 1979). The intestinal microflora is easily upset by medication, and diarrhoea and/or spasmodic or flatulent colic may follow. Prolonged antibiotic medication of the uterus may lead to fungal infections (Rossdale & Ricketts 1980).

Antibiotic medication of the penis of breeding stallions or the use of 'antiseptic' washes after coitus may cause problems with super-infection with *Klebsiella pneumoniae* and *Pseudomonas aeruginosa*. Some capsule types of *Klebsiella pneumoniae* are present in the normal microflora of the stallion's penis (Atherton 1975) but are kept to a low level by micro-ecological factors. Klebsiella organisms, being capsulated, resist antiseptics better than non-capsulated organisms and are frequently resistant to many antibiotics. The over-judicious use of genital antibiotics and antiseptics in the face of contagious equine metritis could contribute to the production of Klebsiella or Pseudonomas overgrowth. The normal microflora of the genitalia have been shown to inhibit the in-vitro growth of *Haemophilus equigentitalis* (Swerczek 1978b).

The use of systemic antibiotics in some horses may result in lethargy and inappetence. This may seriously upset schedules for racehorses in training and should be avoided if possible (Pascoe 1972). Trainers are not appreciative of this unwanted side-effect.

Contraindications

The main contraindications are the avoidance of penicillin in known allergically sensitive horses and the avoidance of drugs producing local reaction, e.g. the use by the intramuscular route to some sulphonamide and potentiated sulphonamide drugs and some long-acting penicillins (English 1958).

Rules of racing

If samples taken from a racehorse at a routine post-race 'dope' test are found to contain any substance, other than a 'normal' nutrient, that horse may be disqualified under the Rules of Racing (The Jockey Club 1978). This means that, if a horse needs antibiotic medication sufficiently close to a race that traces of the drug or its metabolites may be detectable in a test after the race, the trainer must be advised not to allow the horse to race. Unless essential, the use of any drug during the racing season should be avoided on these grounds.

Clearance times vary considerably from drug to drug and from horse to horse but guidelines have been given to practitioners by the Racecourse Security Services (Moss & Clarke 1977) and the British Equine Veterinary Association (Glendenning 1977). The use of procaine penicillin in racehorses should be particularly avoided, since procaine may sometimes be detected in post-race samples even after the eight-day withdrawal period recommended by the Royal College of Veterinary Surgeons (Tobin & Blake 1977, Roberts & English 1979).

The use of specific antibiotics

Penicillin appears to be the most popular antibiotic used in the horse.

However, it is often not appreciated that there is a very definite limit to the plasma concentrations achievable with this drug (English 1958, English 1965, Rollins *et al* 1972). Rapid renal clearance determines the maximal plasma concentration and little is gained by using dose rates higher than 25 000 IU benzylpenicillin/kg body weight. Nevertheless, some practitioners claim better clinical responses with higher doses and Tobin (1978) recommends that high doses should be used to assist the diffusion of penicillin into areas of difficult access by simple mass action. He points out that penicillin generally crosses cell membranes poorly and thus penetration into joint cavities, pleural and peritoneal cavities, and CSF may be limited. He suggests that 5×10^6 IU would be a conservative dose for an adult horse.

In man, probencid is used to reduce the rate of renal clearance of penicillin, giving higher plasma concentrations (Robinson 1964, Kampmann *et al* 1972). Limited trials with this drug (Allen *et al,* unpublished data), have shown no elevation of plasma penicillin concentrations in two pony mares.

Plasma penicillin concentrations are lower in the horse than in other species (English 1965). The fact that approximately 62% of benzylpenicillin is bound to plasma protein (Keen 1965) further reduces the amount of 'free' penicillin available. Long-acting penicillins (benethamine and benzathine) are not well absorbed by the horse and only low plasma concentrations are achieved after 24 hours (Glaxo 1975). Sodium benzylpenicillin will give a rapid high plasma concentration with maximal levels in 30 minutes. These drop rapidly to undetectable levels in a few hours. Procaine benzylpenicillin is absorbed from the site of injection over a 24 hour period.

To obtain optimal concentrations in the horse it has been suggested (English 1965) that crystalline (sodium) benzylpenicillin should be used to give a rapid plasma concentration peak, and this level should then be maintained by using procaine penicillin.

Chloramphenicol is now rarely used in equine medicine in the U.K. but in specific cases it must be remembered that its half-life in the horse is extremely short (English & Withy 1959, Pilloud 1973).

The use of antibiotics in specific conditions

Prophylaxis

In adult horses after surgery (Milne 1972), for injuries and wounds, where secondary bacterial infection is threatened, sulphonamides or penicillin–streptomycin combinations are useful. For foals during the adaptive period (Rossdale & Ricketts 1980), potentiated sulphonamides or penicillin–streptomycin combinations are useful and well tolerated.

On theoretical grounds, the use of potentiated sulphonamides is not likely to produce antibiotic-resistant strains (Barrett & Busby 1970). It has been demonstrated that the use of prophylactic antibiotic programmes for new born foals reduces the risk of neonatal infectious disease (Platt 1977).

Respiratory disease

Upper respiratory virus infections are a major cause of illness and disruption of training programmes in race and performance horses (Powell *et al* 1974, Rose *et al* 1974). At present, little can be done to treat viral infections (Scott 1971, Mumford & Rossdale 1980). Treatment consists of rest from exercise and, if possible, the improvement of ventilation, which may be a major contributing factor (Sainsbury 1981). The ventilation in many racing stables leaves a lot to be desired and the traditional husbandry of horses in training, in relation to stable clothing and the closure of windows usually makes matters worse. When there is a high rectal temperature and the horse is depressed and will not eat, antibacterial agents in the form of sulphonamide or penicillin–streptomycin combinations may be used to treat or guard against secondary bacterial infections. Acute or chronic bacterial pneumonia is rarely seen in adult horses in the UK.

Para-nasal sinusitis of bacterial origin usually presents a persistent unilateral nasal discharge (Baker 1972). Systemic antibacterial treatment alone is seldom effective but surgical exploration, local antibacterial irrigation, and expulsion of damaged molar teeth, if indicated, is usually successful. A differential diagnosis of para-nasal neoplasia (Leyland & Baker 1975) or mycosis (Greet 1981) and gutteral pouch mycosis (Cook 1968) must be borne in mind.

Acute bacterial pneumonia is sometimes seen in new born and older foals (Mahaffey 1962). Isolation of the causative organism should always be attempted and in this regard trans-tracheal washings are sometimes useful (Mansmann *et al* 1971, Bryans 1972, Beach 1981).

In cases from which a causative organism is isolated, the choice of antibiotic should be governed by in-vitro sensitivity tests. Mucolytic agents may help the action of antibiotics. In cases of *Cornybacterium equi* pneumonia in foals (Mahaffey 1962, Bain 1963, Rooney 1966, Linton & Gallagher 1969), treatment is seldom effective despite the use of large doses of antibiotics to which the organism is sensitive. This organism causes massive pulmonary damage with abscess formation.(Sippel *et al* 1968, Knight 1969). It is the cause of epidemics of respiratory disease in foals in some countries (Bain 1963). Smith & Robinson (1981) described an outbreak of *C. equi* pneumonia in five out of six foals of which four survived. The animal dying was the first to be affected and these authors emphasised that early diagnosis by trans-tracheal aspiration and appropriate treatment with penicillin and gentamicin was important. The organism was recovered from cobwebs in the stables and airborne infection was postulated.

Streptococcus equi causes acute upper respiratory lymphadenitis ('strangles') in non-immune foals, yearlings or adults (Bazeley 1940b, Bazeley 1942a, 1942b, Bazeley 1943, Mahaffey 1962, Woolcock 1975a). It may also cause a much milder disease which appears similar to other 'dirty noses' (Woolcock 1975b).

All cases of upper-resporatory infection in young horses should be screened by laboratory examinations for *Strep. equi* and positive cases should not be treated with penicillin unless this is necessary to save the horse's life. Penicillin acts by destroying the bacterial cell wall which may damage the organism's effectiveness as an antigen, thus compromising the host's antibody response. Penicillin also penetrates poorly into abscesses which may leave pockets of infection. Once treatment stops, abscesses often recur and may spread widely throughout the body ('bastard strangles') (Bryans 1972).

Gastrointestinal disease

Acute bacterial gastroenteritis is not commonly seen in adult horses in the UK. The incidence of salmonellosis throughout the world is sporadic (Gibbons 1980) and the reported incidence ranges from 1 to 27%. Gibbons (1980) and Wray *et al* (1981) both recorded a significant increase in disease and mortality caused by salmonellosis in horses during 1976. *Salmonella typhimirium* was the most common type isolated and drug sensitivity tests showed that most of the strains were resistant to streptomycin and sulphonamides, although resistance to other antibacterial drugs was low. Seventeen different patterns of antibiotic resistance were recorded but resistance to more than two antibiotics was uncommon. The majority of outbreaks occurred in teaching hospitals but a variety of 'stressful', predisposing factors have been suggested. These include transportation, change of environment, starvation and food deprivation, parturition and late pregnancy, over-work and over-training, early weaning and artificial rearing of foals, major surgery and anaesthesia, contamination of the environment, food and water, intercurrent disease and high parasitic burden (particularly Trichonema spp.) and anthelmintic treatment.

Antibacterial treatment directed towards eliminating Salmonella spp. from infected horses and symptomless carriers achieves questionable results (Jeffcott 1976). Smith (1981) suggests that treatment must include the correction of fluid and acid-base imbalances, minimising stress, the administration of intestinal absorbents and astringents, the administration of specific antimicrobial drugs to which the organism is sensitive in those cases where bacteriaemia is known to be present or its likelihood is high, as in foals. He recommends the use of chloramphenicol and potentiated sulphonamides. There is a poor response to antibiotic treatment in horses with severe intestinal damage. Bryans *et al* (1965) found furoxone to be helpful in the treatment of experimentally induced salmonellosis in foals. Smith (1981) states that there are no reports that the use of antimicrobial drugs in horses with salmonellosis prolongs the carrier state. He also recommends the use of corticosteroids and prostaglandin synthetase inhibitors (non-steroidal anti-inflammatory agents) to prevent shock and reduce discomfort. The use of oxytetracycline in horses should be avoided as this may precipitate acute diarrhoea and under some circumstances may convert a symptomless carrier into an acute case (Baker & Leyland 1973, Cook 1973, MacKellar *et al* 1973, Owen 1975).

Oral framycetin sulphate is sometimes useful in some cases of flatulent or fermentative colic, in which it is intended to reduce intestinal bacterial activity.

Individual cases or even outbreaks of enteritis in young foals are sometimes seen. A specific causal organism is seldom isolated, but some cases of rotavirus (Flewett *et al* 1975) or salmonella infections are seen (Mahaffey 1952). Unfortunately, we have no specific knowledge of pathogenic or potentially pathogenic serotypes of *E. coli* in the horse (Davies 1978).

In some cases of foal diarrhoea, an upset of the normal bacterial microflora may prolong symptoms after the infection, as such, has been removed. In these cases the oral administration of a proprietary *Lactobacillus acidophilus* culture (*Enpac*) is often beneficial. The majority of foals develop diarrhoea during the period of the mare's first post-partum oestrus as a result of a digestive upset associated with changes in milk composition (Johnston *et al* 1970). In some animals this 'physiological' upset may be sufficient to allow the development of a bacterial enteritis and some clinicians use oral framycetin sulphate prophylactically during the 'foal heat' period. Roberts & English (1979) recommend the use of systemic antibacterial treatment in cases of enteric disease and criticise the use of oral antibiotics for treatment and prophylaxis in foals. They warn of the danger of upsetting the intestinal bacterial flora and suggest that associated mucosal damage can lead to acquired lactase deficiency. They point out that that the 'primary lesion' in most neonatal septicaemia is usually some impairment of colostral transfer of immunity and suggest that treatment and prophylaxis should be directed towards that end. Well managed stud farms take all possible measures to maximise colostral immunoglobulin transfer and there is no doubt that the judicious use of oral antibacterial drugs can, on occasions, be far more successful than the use of parenteral antibacterials alone.

Genitourinary disease

Nephritis and cystitis in the adult horse are extremely rare. With modern methods of stud hygiene, neonatal nephritis caused by *Actinobacillus equuli* (Maguire 1958, Littlejohn 1959) is rarely seen.

Bacterial endometritis is a major problem for clinicians involved in reproductive practice (Peterson *et al* 1969, Woolcock 1980). Potentially pathogenic bacteria may be broadly classified into two types (Ricketts 1981): **1** those capable of causing venereal disease, e.g. *K. pneumoniae* capsule types 1 and 5 (Platt *et al* 1976), *Ps. aeruginosa* (Hughes *et al* 1966), and *H. equigenitalis* (Taylor *et al* 1978). **2** Those capable of invading genital tracts which are damaged or have defective local defence mechanisms, e.g. *Strep. zooepidemicus, E. coli,* Proteus spp. and *Staphylococcus aureus.* The isolation of these latter groups of organisms from the cervix of the mare during oestrus does not necessarily imply the presence of endometritis (Hughes 1980, Ricketts 1978, 1981) and further evidence from clinical examinations (Greenhof & Kenney 1975, Baker & Kenney 1980), cervical cytological examinations (Wingfield Digby 1978), and sometimes endometrial biopsy (Ricketts 1975a, 1975b, Kenney 1978) is needed before antibiotic treatment is instituted.

Water-soluble antibiotic preparations should only be used in the uterus of the mare, since non-therapeutic suspending agents in suspensions and pessaries may cause non-infectious endometritis in their own right (Mather *et al* 1979). The choice of antibiotic should be governed by in-vitro sensitivity tests and the results of previous clinical experience. *H. equigenitalis* is widely sensitive to most antibiotics except streptomycin (Taylor *et al* 1978) but benzylpenicillin or ampicillin has been recommended as the drug of choice (David *et al* 1977). Strains of *H. equigentitalis* sensitive to streptomycin have been reported from America (Swerczek 1978a). Some strains of *K. pneumoniae* and *Ps. aeruginosa* are relatively insensitive to antibiotics but gentamicin sulphate, polymixin B sulphate and neomycin sulphate seem to give the best results.

Hamm (1978) found that systemic treatment with gentamicin, at a dose rate of 4.4 mg/kg intravenously twice daily for up to 34 days, was necessary to treat *Ps. aeruginosa* and *K. pneumoniae* infections in stallions. Where these specific organisms are not involved, we have found that a water-soluble mixture of neomycin sulphate, polymixin B sulphate and nitrofurazone (*Vagifurin*) and sodium benzylpenicillin (*Crystapen*) is useful as a broad spectrum cover.

As in all instances, prevention and early diagnosis are of more value than the treatment of disease. Increasing knowledge of the importance and pathogenesis of endometrical disease in mares (Ricketts 1978) should lead to a reduction in the incidence of genital infectious disease in horses. A major help in this regard would be the controlled use of artificial insemination, in cases with specific veterinary indication (Rossdale 1978, Bowen 1978, Brook 1978, Anon 1978). In cases where a stallion was known to be infected or contaminated with potentially pathogenic organisms, then the use of semen extenders containing antibiotics might be useful in helping to treat the semen (Kenney *et al* 1975). Squires *et al* (1981) found that the maximum bactericidal effect on Klebsiella and Pseudomonas in raw or extended semen required incubation of the sample at 38°C for at least 15 minutes and thus the addition of the antibiotics to fresh skimmed milk extender was indicated. They suggest that the simplest treatment regimen for the control of susceptible strains of *K. pneumoniae* and *Ps. aeruginosa* is the addition of 1000 units of polymixin B sulphate per ml of extended semen.

Mastitis

Mastitis is uncommon in mares in comparison with some other species, but cases are sometimes seen in lactating or recently weaned mares and even in maiden fillies in training (Rossdale & Ricketts 1980).

Treatment of mares with local intramammary preparations is often difficult because of the small teat ducts and the animal's violent resentment. However, it should be attempted in conjunction with hot bathing of the udder, expression of secretions, and systemic antibiotic treatment.

Skin disease

In cases of bacterial dermatitis, the choice of antibiotic to be used should be based on in-vitro sensitivity tests. Although a normal skin commensal, *Staph. aureus* is capable of causing severe dermatitis (Fennel & Vass 1976).

Cases are often insensitive to penicillin. Sodium fusidate, used locally as an ointment, and cloxacillin, used systemically, have proved useful in such cases. *Dermatophilus congolensis* infection ('rain scald') is sometimes seen in exposed horses during wet weather (Thomsett 1979). In these cases, changes of management are usually of greater importance than the use of specific antibiotic drugs.

Griseofulvin has been used with success in dermatophyte infections (ringworm) (Georg & Kaplan 1957, Hiddleston 1970). Our experience is that the results obtained are not as good now as they were when the drug was first used and that greater success is achieved in *Trichophyton verucosum* infections than in *T. equinum* and *Microsporum equinum* infections. Natamycin (Oldenkamp 1979), used locally as an aqueous suspension containing 100 μg/ml natamycin, applied topically twice with an interval of four days, appears to give much better results in cases of *T. equinum* and *M. equinum* infection. Natamycin suspension can also be used to treat grooming brushes and stable clothing.

Infections of the limbs

Pus in the foot

If adequate drainage of the abscess is provided and a poultice is applied, antibiotic treatment is seldom necessary (Johnson & Bartels 1972). For cases of pyrexia and swelling of the limb, sulphonamide or penicillin–streptomycin combinations may be useful.

Cracked heels

This is sometimes a major problem in horses turned out in wet weather and under muddy conditions. The cause is usually damage to the skin by continual exposure to the mud and wet followed by infection with bacterial opportunists. Cases of *Dermatophilus congolensis* infection have been reported (Pascoe 1972). If the affected area is cleaned and dried and the horse is kept out of wet and muddy conditions, the infection usually clears rapidly. In cases that cannot be continually stabled, a mixture of liquid paraffin and sulphanilamide is antibacterial and protective.

Lymphangitis

The causal organism in these cases is seldom known, unless abscessation occurs, but *Strep. zooepidemicus* may be suspected in many cases. Intensive treatment with penicillin–streptomycin combinations should be augmented with the early use of anti-inflammatory drugs and forced exercise (Rossdale & Ricketts 1980).

Joint disease

Injuries may result in bacterial arthritis in adult horses. Wounds that definitely or possibly involve joints should always be treated with systemic antibiotics such as benzylpenicillin–streptomycin combinations. Septic arthritis ('joint ill') in foals (Van Pelt & Riley 1969), typically occurring at 3–6 weeks of age, is always potentially serious. Early diagnosis followed by intensive treatment is needed if chronic crippling disease is to be avoided. Both systemic and intra-articular antibiotic treatment is indicated. Specific bacterial organisms are seldom isolated from even the most purulent synovial fluid samples (Van Pelt 1969), but this may not necessarily mean that bacteria are not present.

We have isolated *Salmonella typhimurium* and *C. equi* from some cases, all of which have been intractable to treatment. In other cases, not involving these specific organisms, the use of 5% neomycin sulphate locally and combinations of penicillin and streptomycin systemically have produced recovery. In some cases, cephalosporin sulphate has been used both locally and systemically because of its known penetrating ability. Penetration of the antibiotics may be inhibited by vascular thrombosis in the local blood vessels (Van Pelt & Riley 1969). Some cases are associated with epiphyseal abscesses and these appear to have the worst prognosis (Rossdale & Ricketts 1980). Systemic antibiotic treatment should be maintained for at least ten days and the affected joint or joints should be drained of synovial fluid and injected with antibiotics every other day until the leycocyte count in the synovial fluid returns to within normal limits.

The early irrigation of the involved joint with large volumes of sterile saline solution may be beneficial (Norrie 1975). When using antibiotic preparations locally into a joint it must be remembered that some are irritant to joint surfaces: 5% neomycin sulphate is considered the drug of choice. There is some evidence to suggest that the early use of oral sodium salicylate in joint infections may protect hyaline cartilage against damage (Simmons & Chrisman 1965).

Meningitis

Meningitis has been seen in newborn foals and in some cases treatment with cephalosporin sulphate has been attempted, occasionally with apparently successful results.

Infections of eyes and ears

A proprietary ophthalmic preparation containing cloramphenicol is convenient for use in cases of eye infections caused by chloramphenicol-sensitive bacteria. Chloramphenicol is one of the few antibiotics which is capable of crossing the optic 'barrier' readily (Pilloud 1973)

Otitis is rarely seen in the horse, but some cases have been associated with otodectic mites. If treatment with an aural gammabenzene hexachloride preparation is not successful then secondary bacterial infection may have occurred and treatment with specific antibiotic drugs is indicated.

Chronic infections

The use of isoniazid, a hydrazide of isonicotinic acid, has been described in the horse (Roberts 1971). This is a relatively safe, effective and economical drug for long-term therapy in chronic infections. It has been used since 1953 and is well known as a treatment for human tuberculosis. Its mechanism of action is unknown. We have used the drug in horses with chronic pulmonary disease and chronic infections and abscesses in a variety of sites. In many cases, the clinical response to treatment appears to have been very satisfactory.

Immunostimulants

Lowe (1980) cited experimental work which suggests that levamisole (*Nemicide*) exerts an immunostimulant effect by restoring the number of T lymphocytes to normal when these are depleted. It also enhances the activity of these cells and, through them, enhances the activity of other immune mechanisms (phagocytosis, migration of phagocytes, haemotaxis, lymphokinase production, lymphocyte stimulation, lymphocyte and macrophage cytotoxicity). Lowe suggests a dose rate of 2.5 mg/kg by mouth on two consecutive days each week, usually for five weeks, in small animals. We have used this regimen in young foals with joint ill with possibly beneficial results. We have also used levamisole in the form of in-feed granules (*Nilverm*) at a dose rate of 5.5 mg/kg for cases of chronic upper respiratory disease in adult horses in training.

References

Alexander F. (1966) Some recent advances in veterinary chemotherapy. *Vet. Rec.* **78**, (Clinical Suppl. 1), I–IV.

Alexander F. & Collett R. A. (1975) Trimethoprim in the horse. *Equine Vet. J.* **7**, 203–6.

Anon (1978) Thoroughbred breeding and A. I. *Vet. Rec.* (Editorial) **102**, 537.

Atherton J. G. (1975) The identification of equine genital strains of Klebsiella and Enterobacter species. *Equine Vet. J.* **7**, 207–9.

Baggot J. D. (1977) Bioavailability and drug disposition in domestic animals (part II) *Vet. Rev.* XXIV **5**, 86–94.

Bain A. M. (1963) *Corynebacterium equi* infections in the equine. *Aust. Vet. J.* **39**, 116–21.

Baker G. J. (1972) Surgery of the head and neck. In *Equine Medicine and Surgery*, eds. Catcott E. S. and Smithcors J. F. American Veterinary Publications 752–91.

Baker J. R. & Kenney R. M. (1980) Systematic Approach the diagnosis of the infertile or subfertile mare. In *Current Therapy in Therogenology*.

Baker J. R. & Leyland A. (1973) Diarrhoea in the horse associated with stress and tetracycline therapy. *Vet. Rec.* **93**, 583–4.

Barrett M. & Bushby S. R. M. (1970) Trimethoprim and the sulphonamides. *Vet. Rec.* **87**, 43–51.

Bazeley P. L. (1940a) Sulphamilamide treatment of Streptococcal infections in horses. *Aust. Vet. J.* **16**, 187–93.

Bazeley P. L. (1940b) Studies with equine Streptococci, 2 Experimental immunity to *Strep. equi. Aust. Vet. J.* **16**, 243–59.

Bazeley P. L. (1942a) Studies with equine Streptococci, 3 Vaccination against strangles. *Aust. Vet. J.* **18**, 141–55.

Bazeley P. L. (1942b) Studies with equine Streptococci, 4 Cross immunity to *Strep. equi. Aust. Vet. J.* **18**, 189–94.

Bazeley P. L. (1943) Studies with equine Streptococci, 5 Some relations between virulence of *Strep. equi* and immune response in the host. *Aust. Vet. J.* **19**, 62–85.

Bazeley P. L. & Battle J. (1940) Studies with equine Streptocci 1. A survey of beta-haemolytic Streptococci in equine infections. *Aust. Vet. J.* **16**, 140–6.

Beach J. (1980) Technique of tracheo-aspiration in the horse. *Equine Vet. J.* **30**, 136–7.

Bowen J. M. (1978) CEM and AI. *Vet. Rec.* **102**, 349.

Brander G. C. (1966) The use of antibodies in the veterinary field. *Vet. Rec.* **79**, (Clinical Suppl. 4), IX–XI.

British Equine Veterinary Association (1976) Worming horses. B.E.V.A. Newsletter no. 4.

Brook D. (1978) CEM and AI. *Vet. Rec.* **102**, 561.

Bryans J. T. (1972) Bacterial and Spirochetal diseases. In *Equine Medicine and Surgery,* 2nd edn., eds. Catcott E. J. and Smithcors J. F. *American Veterinary Publications* 79–113.

Bryans J. T., Fallon E. H. & Shephard B. (1961) Equine Salmonellosis. *Cornell Vet.* 467–77.

Bryans J. T., Moore B. O. & Crow M. W. (1965) Safety and efficacy of furozone in the treatment of equine Salmonellosis. *Vet. Med. Small An. Clin.* **60**, 626–33.

Cook W. R. (1968) The clinical features of gutteral pouch mycosis in the horse *Vet. Rec.* **83**, 336–45.

Cook W. R. (1973) Diarrhoea in a horse associated with stress and tetracycline therapy. *Vet. Rec.* **93**, 15–16.

Davies M. E. (1978) Some studies on equine strains of *Escherichia coli. Equine Vet. J.* **10**, 115–21.

David J. S. E., Frank C. J. & Powell D. G. (1977) Contagious metritis 1977. *Vet. Rec.* **101**, 189–90.

English P. B. (1958) Penicillin blood levels in the horse with fortified benzathine. *Aust. Vet. J.* **34**, 82–8.

English P. B. (1965) The therapeutic use of penicillin: the relationship between dose rate and plasma concentration after parenteral administration of benzylpenicillin (penicillin G). *Vet. Rec.* **77**, 810–4.

English P. B. & Roberts M. C. (1979) Antimicrobial chemotherapy in the horse: I Pharmacological considerations. *J. Equine Med. Surg.* **3**, 259–68.

English P. B. & Withy D. (1959) Serum, urine and tissue levels of chloramphenicol in the horse. *Aust. Vet. J.* **35**, 187–93.

Fennell C. & Vass R. I. (1976) The treatment of equine skin infections using topical trichlora-carbanilide. *Equine Vet. J.* **8**, 42–5.

Flewett T. H., Bryden A. S. & Davies H. (1975) Virus diarrhoea in foals and other animals. *Vet. Rec.* **96**, 477.

Gabel A. A. (1977) Intravenous infections — complications and their prevention. *23rd Proc. Amer. Assoc. Equine Pract.* 28–9.

Georg L. K. & Kaplan W. (1957) Equine ringworm with special reference to *Trichophyton equinum. Amer. J. Vet. Res.* **18**, 798–810.

Gibbons D. F. (1980) Equine salmonellosis. A review. *Vet. Rec.* **106**, 356–9.

Glaxo (1975) Penicillin in horses. Glaxo Veterinary Research Newsletter.

Glendenning S. A. (1977) Anabolic steroids and drug abuse in the racehorse. *Vet. Rec.* **100**, 164.

Goodal D., Machin (1965) *Horses of the world.* Country Life Books.

Greenhof G. R. & Kenney R. M. (1975) Evaluation of reproductive stuatus of non-pregnant mares. *J. Amer. Vet. Med. Assoc.* **167**, 449–58.

Greet T. R. C. (1981) Nasal aspergillosis in three horses. *Vet. Rec.* **109**, 487–9.
Hamm D. H. (1978) Gentamicin therapy of genital tract infections in stallions. *J. Equine Med. Surg.* **2**, 243.
Hiddleston W. A. (1970) Antifungal activity of penicillin griseofulvin mycelium. *Vet. Rec.* **86**, 75–6.
Hinton M. (1976) Antibiotic sensitivity test data and advertising. *Vet. Rec.* **99**, 154.
Hughes J. P. (1980) Clinical examinations and abnormalities in the mare. In *Current Therapy in Theriogenology,* ed. Morrow D. A. p. 706–21. W. B. Saunders, Philadelphia.
Hughes J. P., Loy R. C., Asbury A. C. *et al* (1966) The occurrence of Pseudomonas in the reproductive tract of mares and its effect on fertility. *Cornell Vet.* **56**, 595–610.
Ingham B. & Large B. J. (1969) An introduction to allergy and its treatment. *Equine Vet. J.* **1**, 279–82.
Jeffcott L. B. (1976) Equine salmonellosis: some thoughts on epidemiology and treatment. *Vet. Drug* **6**, (12) 6–7.
Jockey Club (1978) *Rules of Racing.* Wetherby, Woolnough, Northants.
Johnson J. H. & Bartels J. E. (1972) Conditions of the forelimb. In *Equine Medicine and Surgery,* eds. Catcott E. S. & Smithcors J. F., *American Veterinary Publications,* p. 505–62.
Johnston R. H., Kamstra L. D. & Kohler P. H. (1970) Mare's milk composition as related to 'foal heat' scours. *J. Anim. Sci.* **31**, 549–53.
Kampmann J., Hansen J., Mølholm *et al* (1972) Effect of some drugs on penicillin half-life in blood. *Clin. Pharmacol. & Therap.* **13**, 516–19.
Keen P. M. (1965) The binding of three penicillins in the plasma of several mammalian species as studied by ultrafiltration at body temperature. *Br. J. Pharmacol.* **25**, 507–14.
Kenney R. M. Z. (1978) Cyclic and pathological changes of the mare endometrium as detected by biopsy, with a note on early embryonic death. *J. Amer. Vet. Med. Assoc.* **172**, 241–62.
Kenney R. M., Bergman R. V., Cooper W. L. *et al* (1975) Minimal contamination techniques for breeding mares: technique and preliminary findings. *Proc. 21st Ann. Conv. Amer. Assoc. Equine Pract.* 327.
Knight H. D. (1969) Corynebacterial infections in the horse: problems of prevention. *JAVMA* **155**, 446–52.
Leyland A. & Baker J. R. (1975) Lesions of the nasal and para-nasal sinuses of the horse causing dyspnea. *Br. Vet. J.* **131**, 334–44.
Linton A. H. (1976) The antibiotic sensitivity testing of pathogens commonly found in veterinary practice. *Vet. Rec.* **99**, 370–1.
Linton J. A. M. & Gallaher M. A. (1969) Suppurative bronochopneumonia in a foal associated with *Corynebacterium equi. Irish Vet. J.* **23**, 197–200.
Littlejohn A. (1959) Sleepy foal disease in Natal. *JSAVMA* **30**, (2) 143–7.
Lowe R. J. (1980) Levamisole as an immunostimulant. *Vet. Rec.* **106**, 390.
MacKellar J. C., Vaughan S. M., Smith R. J. G. *et al* (1973) Diarrhoea in the horse following tetracycline therapy. *Vet. Rec.* **93**, 593.
Mackintosh M. E. (1981) Bacteriological techniques in the diagnosis of equine genital infections. *Vet. Rec.* **108**, 52.
Maguire L. C. (1958) The role of *B. viscosum equi* in the causation of equine disease. *Vet. Rec.* **70**, 989–91.
Mahaffey L. W. (1952) Salmonella typhimurium in foals in Western Australia. *Aust. Vet. J.* **28**, 8.
Mahaffey L. W. (1962) Respiratory conditions in horses. *Vet. Rec.* **74**, 1295–314.
Mansmann R. A., Wheat J. D. & Jang S. S. (1971) Diagnostic usefulness of transtracheal aspiration in the horse. *Proc. 17th Amer. Assoc. Equine Pract.* 143–6.
Massam D. & Murray M. (1978) Compendium of data sheets for veterinary products. Pharmind Publications.
Mather E. C., Refsal K. P., Gustafsson B. K. *et al* (1979) The use of fibre-optic techniques in

clinical diagnosis and visual assessment of experimental intrauterine therapy on mares. *J. Reprod. Fert.* (Suppl.) **27**, 293.

Milne F. J. (1972) Equine abdominal surgery — in retrospect. *Equine Vet. J.* **4**, 175–81.

Moss M. A. & Clarke E. G. C. (1977) A review of drug 'clearance times' in racehorses. *Equine Vet. J.* **9**, 53–6.

Mumford J. A. & Rossdale P. D. (1980) Virus and its relationship to the 'poor performance' syndrome. *Equine Vet. J.* **12**, 3–9.

Norrie R. D. (1975) The treatment of joint disease by saline lavage. *Proc. 21st Amer. Assoc. Equine Pract.* 91.

Oldenkamp E. P. (1979) Treatment of ringworm in horses with natamycin. *Equine Vet. J.* **11**, 36–8.

Owen A. ap. R. (1975) Post stress diarrhoea in the horse. *Vet. Rec.* **96**, 267–70.

Pascoe R. R. (1972) Further observations on Dermatophilus infections in horses. *Aust. Vet. J.* **48**, 32–4.

Peterson F. B., McFeely R. A. & David J. S. E. (1969) Studies on the pathogenesis of endometritis in the mare. *Proc. 15th Amer. Assoc. Equine Pract.* 279–87.

Pilloud M. (1973) Pharmacokinetics, plasma, protein bindings and dosage of chloramphenicol in cattle and horses. *Res. Vet. Sci.* **15**, 231–8.

Platt H. (1977) Joint ill and other bacterial infections in thoroughbred studs. *Equine Vet. J.* **9**, 141–5.

Platt H., Atherton J. G. & Ørskov I. (1976) Klebsiella and enterobacter organisms isolated from horses. *J. Hyg. Camb.* **77**, 401–8.

Powell D. G., Burrows R. & Goodridge A. (1974) Respiratory viral infections among thoroughbred horses in training during 1972. *Equine Vet. J.* **6**, 19–24.

Randall C. J. (1969) The Swann Committee. *Vet. Rec.* **85**, 616–20.

Ricketts S. W. (1975a) Endometrial biopsy as a guide to diagnosis of endometrial pathology in the mare. *J. Reprod. Fert.* (Suppl.) **23**, 341–5.

Ricketts S. W. (1975b) The technique and clinical application of endometrial biopsy in the mare. *Equine Vet. J.* **7**, 102–8.

Ricketts S. W. (1978) Histological and histopathological studies of the endometrium of the mare. Fellowship thesis, Royal College of Veterinary Surgeons.

Ricketts S. W. (1981) Bacteriological examinations of the mare's cervix: techniques and interpretation of results. *Vet. Rec.* **108**, 46–51.

Roberts M. C. & English P. B. (1979) Antimicrobial chemotherapy in the horse, II The application of antimicrobial therapy. *J. Equine Med. Surg.* **3**, 308–15.

Roberts W. D. (1971) Isoniazid in equine therapy. *Proc. 17th Am. Assoc. Equine Pract.* 33–4.

Robinson O. P. W. (1964) The effect of probenecid in delaying the urinary excretion of the new penicillins derived from 6-amino-penicillanic acid. *Br. J. Clin. Pract.* **18**, 593–600.

Rollins L. D., Teske R. H., Condon R. J. *et al* (1972) Serum penicillin and dihydrostreptomycin concentrations in horses after intramuscular administration of selected preparations containing antibiotics. *J. Am. Vet. Med. Assoc.* **161**, 490–5.

Rooney J. R. (1966) Corynebacterial infection in foals. *Med. Vet. Pract.* **47**, 43–5.

Rose M. A., Rossdale P. D., Hopes R. *et al* (1974) Virus infection of horses at Newmarket 1972–73. *Vet. Rec.* **95**, 484–7.

Rossdale P. D. (1978) A.I. to keep control of CEM. *Vet. Rec.* **102**, 291.

Rossdale P. D. & Ricketts S. W. (1980) *Equine Stud Farm Medicine.* Bailliere Tindall, London.

Sainsbury D. W. B. (1981) Ventilation and environment in relation to equine respiratory disease. *Equine Vet. J.* **13**, 167–70.

Scott G. R. (1971) Guidelines for the control of equine viral infections. *Equine Vet. J.* **3**, 1–6.

Short G. V. (1963) Systemic antibacterials in equine practice. Proc. BEVA Conf., Manchester.

Simmons D. P. & Chrisman O. D. (1965) Salicylate inhibition of cartilage degeneration. *Artheritis & Rheumatism* **8**, 960–9.

Sippel W. L., Keahey E. E. & Bullard T. L. (1968) Corynebacterial infection in foals: etiology, pathogenesis and laboratory diagnosis *JAVMA* **153**, 1610–3.

Smith B. P. (1981) Equine salmonellosis: a contemporary view. *Equine Vet. J.* **13**, 147–51.

Smith B. P. & Robinson M. C. (1981) Studies of an outbreak of *Corynebacterium equi.* pneumonia in foals. *Equine Vet. J.* **13**, 223–8.

Squires E. L., McGlothlin D. E., Bowes R. A. *et al* (1981) Use of antibiotics in stallion semen for the control of *Klebsiella pneumoniae* and *Pseudomonas aeruginosa. J. Equine Vet. Sci.* **1**, 43–8.

Swann M. M. (1969) *Joint Committee on the use of antibiotics in animal husbandry and veterinary medicine.* HMSO, London.

Swerczek T. W. (1978a) Inhibition of the CEM organism by the normal flora of the reproductive tract. *Vet. Rec.* **103**, 125.

Swerczek T. W. (1978b) Contagious equine metritis in USA. *Vet. Rec.* **102**, 512–3.

Taylor C. E. D., Rosenthal R. O., Brown D. F. J. *et al* (1978) The causative organism of contagious equine metritis 1977 — proposal for a new species to be known as *Haemophilus equigenitalis. Equine Vet. J.* **10**, 136–44.

Thomsett L. R. (1979) Skin diseases of the horse. *Pract.* **1**, 15–26.

Tobin T. (1978) Pharmacology review: Haemotherapy in the horse — penicillins. *J. Equine Med. Surg.* **2**, 475–9.

Tobin T. & Blake J. W. (1977) Pharmacology of procaine in the horse: relationships between plasma and urinary concentrations of procaine. *J. Equine Med. Surg.* **1**, 188–94.

Van Pelt R. W. (1969) Idiopathic tenosynovitis in foals. *JAVMA* **155**, 510–7.

Van Pelt R. W. & Riley W. F. (1969) Clinicopathologic findings and therapy in spetic arthritis in foals. *JAVMA* **155**, 1467–80.

Walton G. S. (1968) Skin disease of domestic animals. I Skin manifestation of allergic response in domestic animals. *Vet. Rec.* **82**, 204–7.

Wingfield Digby N. J. (1978) The techniques and clinical application of endometrial cytology in mares. *Equine Vet. J.* **10**, 167–70.

Woolcock J. B. (1975a) Epidemiology of equine Streptococci. *Res. Vet. Sci.* **18**, 113–4.

Woolcock J. B. (1975b) Studies with atypical *Streptococcus equi. Res. Vet. Sci.* **19**, 115–9.

Woolcock J. B. (1980) Equine bacterial endometritis: diagnosis, interpretation and treatment. *Vet. Clin. N. Amer. Large Animal Pract.* **2**, 241–51.

Wray C., Sojka W. J. & Bell J. C. (1981) Salmonella infection in horses in England and Wales 1973–79. *Vet. Rec.* **109**, 398–401.

5

Pharmaceutical agents and the bovine udder

C.L. WRIGHT

Historical perspective

Antibiotics have been used extensively over the past 30 years in the control of bovine mastitis. Such was the optimism in antibiotic therapy that, in 1962, Edwards said of *Streptococcus agalactiae* that '. . . today this organism is relatively unimportant'. However, the disease is still spread worldwide and there is a high incidence of new infection. It could be said of all adult dairy bovines that they either have the infection, are developing the infection, or will become infected within the next lactation. Recent surveys reveal that mastitis due to streptococcal organisms, particularly *Streptococcus agalactiae,* is more prevalent and widely distributed than was previously thought (Greer & Pearson 1973). In Ireland, bulk tank surveys demonstrated a high infection rate (Pearson *et al* 1976) and clinical samples received from the south-west of Scotland revealed a high incidence of clinical mastitis due to *S. agalactiae* (Wright 1977). *Staphylococcus aureus* infection is also prevalent and, in recent years, the incidence of mastitis due to coliform organisms and other bacteria commonly found in the environment has become a source of concern (Howell 1972, Brander 1973, Pearson & Wright 1969, Marr 1978). Most mastitis of economic importance is caused by streptococcal, staphylococcal and coliform infection. Because of the wide range of response to infection, several approaches to therapy are required, but these cannot be relied upon entirely to solve the mastitis problem.

With the introduction of antibiotics shortly after World War II, and in particular the development of penicillins for the treatment of Gram-positive organisms, mastitis entered the therapeutic era. Unfortunately, the effectiveness of therapy has not been entirely beneficial and a false sense of security and reliance has developed concerning its role in mastitis control (Philpot 1969). Furthermore, the use of antibiotics in the treatment of mastitis has created problems for the milk processor and the consumer (Albright 1961). It must be said that antibiotics in milk supplies are largely the result of improper use of mastitis infusion preparations, or failure to conform to instructions on packaged preparations that the milk from treated quarters should be discarded. A review (Mercer *et al* 1976) of the various phases of development of anti-mastitis products made the point that the 'rediscovery' of effectiveness of treatment in non-lactating cows after a period of 22 years does not speak well for the logic and rationale used in selecting antibacterial agents for the treatment of bovine mastitis. Mastitis control is further complicated by the fact that the dairy farmer has a free choice of drugs used without a proper diagnosis or a good measure of clinical efficiency (Schalm & Ormsbee 1949), and these authors went on to state that major progress with therapy was treatment in the dry period.

The development of treatment of subclinical infections during the dry period has been extensively reviewed by Schultze (1975) as has therapy during lactation by Plommet & Le Louedec (1975). The optimism of previous years has been replaced by an awareness of the problems of the changing patterns of bacterial infections and the influence of differing methods of husbandry. Mastitis continues to constitute a national problem and continues unabated. As reported in France (Plommet & Le Louedec 1975), much of the blame for the continued prevalence of mastitis has been the lack of follow-up, poor hygiene, apathy and erratic use of therapeutic measures. In general, it is agreed by research workers firstly that control is intimately related to the milking process and that lactation and dry cow therapy are only part of the general approach to mastitis control, and secondly that the greatest success will follow procedures designed to prevent new infections rather than relying on direct treatment to eliminate established infections (Philpot 1969). Christie *et al* (1974), in a clinical study of the effect of dry cow treatment, examined data from the viewpoint of management skill and demonstrated that, with good management, a 13% greater return on treatment investment can be achieved compared with those farms with poor management.

One major difficulty is determining the efficiency of drug therapy and the prediction of the result of therapy. A large variation in response among herds and between cows within the herd, may be due to the type of organism involved, the location of infected sites, or the degree of udder induration (Ziv 1978), but these are only a few of the variable influences. Variation of the organism is largely uncontrolled; virulence, antibiotic resistance, and dose are difficult to measure in natural infections so that in any one individual, a variable response to antibiotic therapy may be attributed to yield, the stage of lactation, the extent of tissue damage, the number and location of infected foci, and also to the existing cell content of the milk. Ziv (1975) found a variation in the behaviour of various antibiotics in infected quarters compared with non-infected quarters in the same animal. With so many variable factors, it is not surprising that experimental results are inconsistent and equivocal.

Table 5.1   Common infecting organisms in bovine mastitis. (After Postle & Natzke 1974 & Bramley 1975.)

Staphylococcus aureus
Streptococcus agalactiae
Other Streptococci (including *Streptococcus uberis, Streptococcus dysgalactiae,* Enterococci, and Streptococci of group C and group G)
Coliform organisms (including *Corynebacterium pyogenes,* Serratia spp., Proteus spp., Pseudomonas spp., Pasteurella spp., Nocardia spp., Bacillus spp., and yeasts)
Coagulase-negative micrococci (consisting of the genera Staphylococcus and Micrococcus) and *Corynebacterium bovis*

The infecting organism

The two most common causal agents on a national scale are the Gram-positive *Staphylococcus aureus* and *Streptococcus agalactiae.* However, within individual herds a wide variety of Gram-positive and Gram-negative organisms, fungi and yeasts are capable of infecting cows and creating a herd mastitis problem in spite of sensible standards of hygiene and milking management. Most of these are opportunist invaders and remain localised. Infection with yeasts should always be suspected when there is a history of unsuccessful antibiotic treatment, but spontaneous cure is common. Postle & Natzke (1974) reporting on the efficacy of antibiotic treatment of subclinical infections used five main categories for recording (Table 5.1). Since 1974 a wide variety of additional organisms have been demonstrated as a possible cause of mastitis including Leptospira spp. (Ellis *et al* 1976), Bacillus spp. (Jones *et al* 1981), and Mycoplasma (Jasper 1974).

Antibiotic sensitivity

It has been said that drug abuse has led to the development of drug resistant strains of bacteria. In 1964, Dodd *et al* found 70% of *S. aureus* isolates from bovine milk were resistant to penicillin. House & Manley (1974) reported that 23% of their isolates were resistant to streptomycin. Le Louedec (1978), in a literature review, concluded that, whilst infection due to *Strep. agalactiae* are the most easy to cure, only 75% of infections due to *S. aureus* were cleared by cloxacillin and only slightly better results were achieved with a combination of ampicillin and cloxacillin. McDonald & Anderson (1981) investigating in-vivo antibiograms of 813 *S. aureus* isolates and coagulase-negative staphylococci isolates from milk samples obtained from cows in 24 herds, found that 90% were sensitive to 13 or more antimicrobial agents used in the field and concluded that an adequate selection of highly

Table 5.2. The bacterial sensitivity of *S. aureus* isolates from bovine milk tested using multidiscs.

Percentage of isolates resistant	
Penicillin	51
Nitrofurazone	40
Streptomycin	12
Tetracycline	12
Neomycin	4
Novobiocin	4
Erythromycin	2
Methicillin	0

effective antibiotic agents are available for intramammary staphylococcal infections. Figures obtained at Auchincruive using the Kirby–Bauer technique show 51% of isolates resistant to penicillin and 12% resistant to streptomycin. Multidiscs commonly used have been found to give inconsistent and inaccurate results. In any case, these bear little relation to clinical efficiency, and in-vitro results appear to be extremely optimistic. It would be more consistent to observe only the resistance pattern of a bacteria, not its sensitivity.

The antibiotic susceptibility patterns indicate that penicillin, streptomycin, nitrofurans and tetracyclines are not a good choice for therapy against *Staphylococcus aureus*. Beta-lactamase production is an important mechanism conferring resistance to penicillin by *S. aureus* and a range of Gram-negative bacteria. Only 9% of isolates were resistant to both penicillin and streptomycin (which was lower than expected) and, in addition, it was found that isolates resistant to either erythromycin or tetracycline were also resistant to nitrofurans and penicillin *in vitro*. This is in contrast to the findings of other workers (Jasper 1972, House & Manley 1974) and reflects the importance of local patterns of antibiotic usage. Cephalosporins, methicillin and cloxacillin act synergistically with penicillins blocking beta-lactamase *in vitro* but in-vivo results are less spectacular. The different response in some herds to cloxacillin therapy from the in-vitro sensitivity has been investigated using a mouse model (Anderson 1979).

There are few reports in the literature on bovine streptococcal antibiotic sensitivity other than a study of 455 streptococcal isolates from bovine intramammary infections (McDonald *et al* 1976). In this study 90% of the cultures were sensitive to carbenicillin, chloramphenicol, erythromycin and penicillin; neomycin and streptomycin were ineffective against *Streptococcus dysgalactiae, Streptococcus agalactiae* and *Streptococcus uberis* and mostly ineffective against *Enterococci* and *Streptococcus bovis*. This is con-

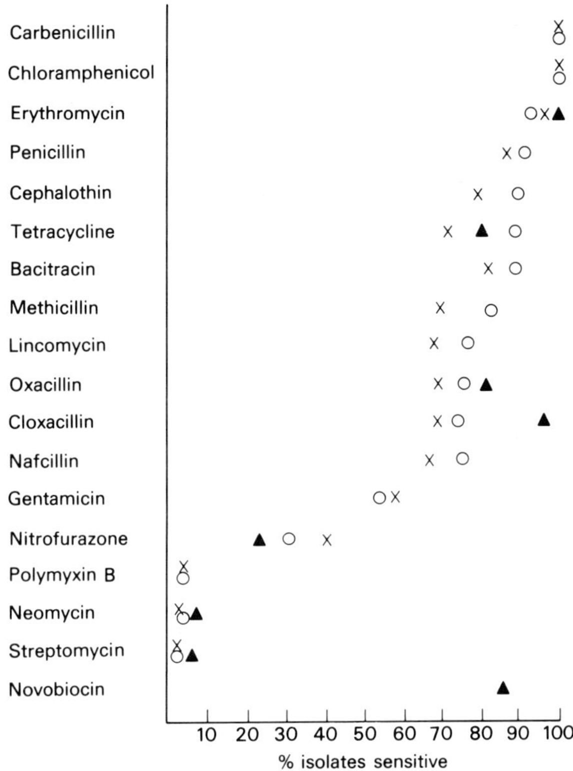

Fig. 5.1 In-vitro antimicrobial sensitivity of Streptococci. O= McDonald *et al* 1976, ▲ = West of Scotland Veterinary Division 1978, × = National Animal Diseases Centre.

sistent with our findings and with those of Davies (1961). The most recent survey of clinical mastitis in England and Wales reveals a high prevalence of cases due to *S. uberis* infection. We have found little success in the use of antibiotics for the complete control of this infection — an observation also made by Throop & Swanson (1958) and Misra & Marshall (1971), who found that most strains of *S. uberis* are penicillin-sensitive *in-vitro*, but treatment with penicillin usually does not cure. In our experience, a combination of penicillin with an aminoglycoside is commonly used to treat streptococcal infections and gives improved results. We have also found a marked decrease in sensitivity to tetracyclines and to novobiocin. Pearson (1976) has also reported strains of *S. agalactiae* growing in serum broth containing 0.2 IU/ml of penicillin. Enterococci which are quite resistant to most antibiotics but which rarely cause a herd mastitis problem, show the greatest sensitivity to chloramphenicol and to carbenicillin (McDonald *et al* 1976). Regardless of the in-vitro sensitivity, the final test must be in the in-vivo eradication of infection (McDonald *et al* 1976). In the first place, the causative organism should be sensitive to the drug chosen; however some of the most active drugs *in vitro* are poorly and unevenly distributed in the udder and are only absorbed to a limited extent (Ziv 1980b). Anderson (1979) suggested the response of lactating cattle with chronic staphylococcal mastitis to intramammary therapy with cloxacillin is sometimes disappointing despite the in-vitro sensitivity of the Staphylococci. Intramammary inoculation of cloxacillin also failed to cure experimental chronic disease in the mouse (Anderson 1979). Cloxacillin was significantly less active against intracellular Staphylococci than against those released from neutrophils by sonication, possibly because of their very low growth rate when inside cells (Craven & Anderson 1980a). These workers (1980b), using an in-vitro system, tested a range of antibiotics for possible intracellular action and found that only rifampicin showed intracellular killing; however, when used in intramammary therapy, rifampicin has been generally less effective than penicillin-based preparations.

In recent years the frequency of Gram-negative bacterial infection causing mastitis has increased. The main cause of these infections is *Escherichia coli* but infections by other genera such as Klebsiella spp, Citrobacter, Enterobacter, Proteus and Pseudomonas spp., may constitute a herd mastitis problem. Generally the infection is acute or per acute, and chronic

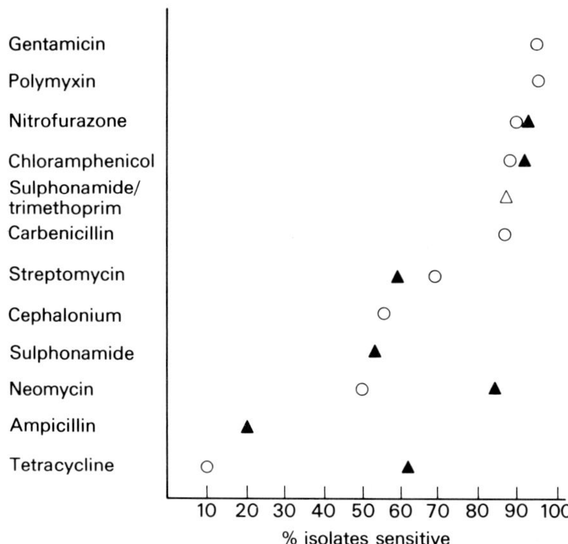

Fig. 5.2 In-vitro microbial sensitivity of *E. coli* isolates from cows with intramammary infection. ○ = McDonald *et al* 1976, ▲ = West of Scotland Veterinary Division 1978.

Table 5.3 Antibiotic activities.

Broad spectrum	Gram positive	Gram negative
Chloramphenicol	Penicillin G	Dihydrostreptomycin
Chlortetracycline	Cloxacillin	Framycetin
Oxytetracycline	Nafcillin	Neomycin
Sulphonamide/trimethoprim	Penethamate	Polymyxin
Ampicillin	Lincomycin	Streptomycin
Amoxycillin	Erythromycin	
Cephoxazole	Novobiocin	
	Tylosin	
	Oleandomycin	
	Spiramycin	
	Dapsone	

mastitis due to these infections is the exception rather than the rule, although persistent mammary excretion of *Pseudomonas aeruginosa* is not uncommon after infection. Hill *et al* (1979) demonstrated the excretion of *E. coli* for periods up to several weeks following experimental infection. McDonald *et al* (1977) found that when Gram-negative bacilli were ranked in order of decreasing antibiotic sensitivity, *E. coli* was the most sensitive followed by *Klebsiella pneumoniae* and Proteus spp.; Pseudomonas spp. were most resistant, showing 100% resistance to 13 of 17 antimicrobial agents tested. This agrees with the reports of other workers.

It is of interest that, of 78 isolates of *E. coli* obtained at Auchincruive, 50 were untypable using Weybridge reference strain antisera and the 28 typable isolates comprised 11 different serotypes. The wide variety of isolates and the preponderance of untypable strains is consistent with the findings of McDonald *et al* (1970) in America. Two of the serotypes isolated at Auchincruive proved to be chloramphenicol-resistant, and there is no evidence attributing this to the use of chloramphenicol in mastitis therapy.

It has been suggested previously (Philpot 1969, Uvarov 1971) that, in the absence of cultural information on the infecting organism, chemotherapeutic agents possessing a wide spectrum of antimicrobial activity should be selected. If we consider the in-vitro sensitivity pattern which is a most important consideration, then chloramphenicol would appear to be a logical choice. However, there is considerable argument about the use of this drug for the treatment of animals' disease (Report 1969), particularly where there is a high risk of antibiotic residues in the milk. Additionally, when given intramuscularly at normal dose rates (25 mg/ml), chloramphenicol does not achieve sufficient concentrations in the udder (Ziv 1980b). Several members of the cephalosporin group have been developed for intramammary use in lactating and non-lactating cows and are active against a wide range of Gram-negative and Gram-positive bacteria. Cephoxazole was reported to be of value in the treatment of coliform mastitis (Allenstein 1977) and, in combination with benzylpenicillin, bacteriologically efficient (Harris 1978). Cephalonium as an agent of prevention and treatment in the non-lactating bovine has been reported on, but the clinical trials show no advantage over other beta-lactam antibiotics. However, on the basis of sensitivity and evidence of synergism, there appears to be some merit in using such a combination of drugs.

Combination of antibiotics

Even though most intramammary infection is caused by Gram-positive bacteria, the ideal formulation for injection into the udder might be composed either of a single broad-spectrum antimicrobial or a mixture of two antimicrobial agents, one effective against Gram-positive, the other possibly against Gram-negative bacteria. If possible, synergistic antimicrobials should be used (McDonald *et al* 1977). Clinical studies in which synergy plays a demonstrable role in therapy are sparse. Whilst synergistic activity has been unequivocally demonstrated *in vitro;* efficacy *in vivo* may be limited. Combinations of sulphamethoxazole and trimethoprim have become increasingly important in the treatment of the toxic cow due to per acute mastitis, as a result of infection by a wide range of Gram-negative and Gram-positive bacteria. A number of other antibiotic combinations have been evaluated: penicillin and novobiocin (Hamdy *et al* 1975, Schultze & Mercer 1976), penicillin and cephoxazole (Boulton & Ross 1977), and ampicillin and cloxacillin in a wide variety of combinations (Postle & Natzke 1974), but mainly for use in the non-lactating udder. The combination of 10^6 IU penicillin plus 1g of dihydrostreptomycin is probably the most widely used and evaluated combination preparation for lactation therapy, but appears to have the limitations of all products in that the therapeutic response against *Staphylococcus aureus* is less than satisfactory, and this almost certainly reflects the pathogenesis of this organism (Anderson 1977).

Mixtures of antibiotics, especially for use in bovine mastitis, are increasing (Uvarov 1975); while many home mixed or improvised regimens continue to be used (Mercer *et al* 1976). In the USA in 1973 an interim policy allowing a maximum of four active ingredients was instituted to allow the development of efficacy data. Some substances such as papain and corticosteroids have had further restrictions imposed on them.

Role of corticosteroids

Two arguments have been used to support the use of corticosteroids in intramammary preparations, one is to prevent the inflammatory response when a mildly irritant product or base is used, and the other is to reduce the inflammatory response to the infecting organism, permitting penetration by the antibiotic.

Experimental studies by Mercer *et al* (1976) demonstrated that prednisolone was very rapidly absorbed from the normal udder and that absorption was reduced in the infected udder. Furthermore, corticosteroid treatment had little, if any, effect in altering the leucocyte response to experimental infection. It was considered that corticosteroids have a primary function of assisting in the detoxification process via their glucogenic effects. However, Swarbrick (1968) found that even large doses of corticosteroids failed to hasten the resolution of clinical mastitis. This finding was in line with other workers in Europe and he concluded that there was no justification for their inclusion. Carroll *et al* (1974) showed that massive doses of corticosteroids (flumethasone), either infused into mammary glands or given intramuscularly in cases of endotoxin-induced bovine mastitis, may have limited the swelling of treated quarters but otherwise failed to influence the course of infection. Several adverse effects of corticosteroids on leucocytes have been established, reducing phagocytosis, decreased diapedesis, and intraleucocyte killing of phagocytosed bacteria (Pappe *et al* 1981). The use of betamethasone parenterally in the treatment of per acute mastitis is widespread and is thought to be beneficial as a potent anti-inflammatory agent which may justify its inclusion in a treatment regimen for acute mastitis with systemic disturbances; however, there appears to be no clear cut demonstration of the beneficial effect (see also Chapter 20).

Lactational therapy

Intramammary and parenteral administration

The most common method of determining drug kinetics is by measuring the excretion rate of a particular drug in milk (Mercer 1976). However, several methods have been tried to estimate the levels of antibiotics in tissues. Examination of tissue homogenates and autoradiographic techniques can provide data on the kinetics of drug distribution throughout the normal or the infected udder. Frequent failures in treatment of acute mastitis may be due partly to poor or uneven distribution. The oedema and inflammatory debris in mastitis may prevent drug diffusion of locally infused antibiotic through the milk phase. Staphylococci in particular and other pathogens also are often tissue invasive and, in many cases, respond poorly to intramammary infusion although fully sensitive to the drug *in vitro*. Under these circumstances, parenteral treatment of acute mastitis is preferred as a major portion of the antibiotic is quickly removed by milking out when administered by the intramammary route. Parenteral therapy with antibiotic may produce a better distribution of drug through the udder and should be considered as an adjunct to local treatment in refractory or recurrent cases also.

In an excellent review of drug selection Ziv (1980b) states that oxytetracycline and chloramphenicol administered intramuscularly possess limited intramammary bioavailability properties and therefore should be administered intravenously at high dose rates. Effective passage of drug from the blood into the udder is best achieved with the macrolide antibiotics, but the antibacterial spectra of these drugs is limited to Gram-positive pathogens. Although macrolide and lincomycin have been used as seond-line antibiotics against Gram-positive bacteria (Burrows 1980), they may, under certain circumstances, be of particular value because of their propensity to achieve high tissue concentrations. The limited extent of penetration of the aminoglycoside antibiotics into milk can be related to their extremely poor solubility in non-polar solvents and their low oil-to-water partition coefficients (Ziv & Sulman 1974b). These authors suggest that inhibitory levels of aminoglycosides can only be maintained in milk for short periods, thus requiring frequent treatments with potential toxic effects.

The factors that influence the antibiotic absorption from the udder are related to the physicochemical properties of the drugs, in particular the degree of ionisation, lipid solubility, and protein binding. They indicate that absorption is by non-ionic diffusion — the rate of disappearance being independent of the dose but being influenced by the pH (Rasmussen 1966). These factors have been extensively studied by Ziv & Rasmussen (1975) and Ziv & Sulman (1974a).

Absorption from the udder can explain the reduction in antibiotic concentration, and the rate is governed by the drug's physical characteristics rather than its molecular configuration. The lipid solubility of undissociated drug—those with higher lipid:water coefficients are absorbed faster—is the rate-limiting factor with drugs which are highly ionised in milk. However, with less ionised drugs such as ampicillin and penethamate the rate-limiting factor becomes the dissociation constant (pKa) (Ziv 1975).

With some antibiotics, protein binding can influence the rate of absorption from the udder but most antibiotics are bound to milk proteins to some extent. Drugs with strong affinities to serum albumins are not necessarily highly bound by tissue proteins and, although binding diminishes antibiotic activity *in vitro,* it is not a measure of the in-vivo activity. Furthermore, the absorption rate will be rapid after the infusion of the drug due to saturation of binding sites, and thus the rate of absorption will decrease with increasing tissue affinity. Since extensively bound drugs cross biological membranes

Table 5.4   Binding of antibiotics to dry udder secretion and to udder tissue homogenates (Ziv *et al* 1976).

Antibiotics more than 50% bound to secretion
Cloxacillin
Novobiocin
Phenoxymethyl penicillin

Antibiotics more than 50% bound to tissue homogenates
Neomycin
Dihydrostreptomycin
Spiramycin
Polymyxin B

Antibiotics less than 50% bound to secretion and to udder tissue homogenates
Benzylpenicillin
Ampicillin
Cephaloridine (very slowly absorbed)
Erythromycin
Chloramphenicol

---

with difficulty, this reversible property tends to prolong the antibiotic retention in the udder.

In addition to udder tissue binding, the excretion of antibiotics from the udder is governed by the type of vehicle base. It is possible to prepare bases allowing quick, medium, and prolonged release rates of products from which the veterinarian can make an appropriate choice. In general, intramammary infusion with oil or ointment vehicles results in slower, less uniform and less complete distribution than with an aqueous vehicle, and the more irritant the vehicle the greater the excretion time (Schipper 1955). Many veterinary surgeons are returning to the use of antibiotic suspension in large volumes of sterile water to treat per acute mastitis, hoping to achieve greater distribution.

Antibiotic usage in dry cows

Dry cow therapy

Intramammary therapy at the end of lactation is considered to play an important part in controlling the relatively high rate of new infections occurring during the early part of the dry period. The udder secretions of cows in the dry period contain lactoferrins which are not conducive to the growth of Gram-negative organisms and new infection in the dry period is, therefore, generally with Gram-positive organisms. Several studies have

Table 5.5 Efficacy of antibiotic preparations in the non-lactating udder.

Preparation (source)	S. aureus		Streptococci other than S. agalactiae		Source of data
	Quarters infected (no.)	Quarters cleared (%)	Quarters infected (no.)	Quarters cleared (%)	
Benzathine cloxacillin 500 mg* (E. R. Squibb)	54	76	57	93	Postle & Natzke (1974)
Benzathine cloxacillin 500 mg* (Beecham–Massengill Pharmaceutical)	118	84	136	83	
Neomycin sulphate 500 mg (Upjohn Co)	81	62	139	75	
Procaine penicillin G 1 000 000 IU* (West Agro-Chemical)	38	47	98	86	
Procaine penicillin G 1 000 000 IU +dihydrostreptomycin sulphate 1 g*	713	87	1607	90	
Procaine penicillin G 5 000 000 IU +dihydrostreptomycin 500 mg*	53	55	98	86	
Procaine penicillin G 300 mg +Na-novobiocin 250 mg**	90	78	–	–	Uvarov (1971)
Procaine penicillin G 300 mg +Na-novobiocin 250 mg**	37	60	14	100	Brookbanks (1968)
Procaine penicillin G 300 mg +Na-novabiocin 250 mg** (Glaxo Laboratories)	114	64	35	100	Pearson & Wright (1969)
Procaine penicillin G 500 000 IU +Na-novobiocin 600 mg***	12	83	56	88	
Benzathine cloxacillin 500 mg (Beecham Animal Health UK)	160	83	114	96	Ziv et al (1981)
Sodium nafcillin 100 mg +procaine benzylpenicillin 300 mg +dihydrostreptomycin 100 mg (Gist Brocades, Holland)	277	84	174	90	
Cephalonium 250 mg (Glaxovet UK)	236	77	134	87	

* In 3% Al-monostearate and peanut oil, ** in 3% Al-monostearate and mineral oil, *** in 2% Al-monostearate and peanut oil.

been conducted in which the new infection rate in the dry period was measured. Neave *et al* (1950) found a 24% new infection rate; Ward & Schultz (1974) found that 9.5% of quarters became infected, principally with Streptococci, during the early part of the dry period, with an increased occurrence in the older cow. They reported that *Streptococcus uberis* was quite invasive in the early dry period, had a higher rate of occurrence in older cows, and that neomycin sulphate in an oil base reduced this infection rate. McDonald & Anderson (1981a), in one study of experimental infection, demonstrated that many new intramammary infections due to *S. uberis* may occur, especially during the last half of the non-lactating period. This must contribute to a variable response to dry cow therapy and to the recent observation of the high incidence of clinical cases due to *S. uberis* infection in post-parturient animals and in heifers before their first parturition (Cooper *et al* 1977).

The response and cure rate using dry cow therapy is extremely variable, ranging from 47% to 100% for primary pathogens isolated from natural infections. The cure rate is known to be directly related to the length of time the infection was in the udder; only 38% of infections of more than one year's duration responded to treatment in spite of massive doses of antibiotic (Schalm *et al* 1971). Since new infection in the dry period is principally with Gram-positive organisms, all antibiotics used should be active against Gram-positive organisms and the preparations usually also incorporate an antibiotic active against B-lactamase (penicillinase) producing *S. aureus* (e.g. cloxacillin, nafcillin, or a cephalosporin). Dry cow intramammary preparations generally also utilise methods for slowing the release of antibiotic from the infusion bolus such as formation of poorly soluble salts (e.g. procaine or benzathine penicillins) and incorporation in oily bases.

In a review of dry cow therapy (DCT), Shultze (1975) commented that the therapy of bovine mastitis, especially DCT, rests on a less than solid pharmacological basis. Ziv (1975) emphasised the special considerations to be taken into account in relating antibiotic concentrations in milk or dry cow secretions to the potential clinical efficiency in the udder. As a result of his studies of the pharmacokinetics of antibiotics, several general conclusions regarding the ideal antibiotic intended for mastitis therapy were derived and are summarised in Table 5.6.

Marr (1978) questioned the role of dry cow therapy in herds with low bulked milk cell counts and associated the rising incidence of 'coliform' mastitis herd problems with dry cow therapy. The unquestioned efficiency, however, of dry cow therapy in controlling udder infections with *Streptococcus agalactiae, Corynebacterium bovis,* non-coagulase producing Staphylococci, and recent infection with *Staphylococcus aureus* has much to recommend the practice. In a controlled experiment, Wright & Leaver

Table 5.6 Characteristics of an 'ideal' antibiotic for mastitis therapy.

Intramuscular injection
Low MIC against the majority of udder pathogens
High bioavailability from the i.m. injection site
Low degree of serum protein binding
Chemically, a weak base or otherwise highly non-ionised in serum
Sufficiently lipid-soluble
Having a long $t_{\frac{1}{2}}$ in the body

Intramammary infusion during lactation
Minimal irritability to the udder
Low MIC
Low degree of binding to milk and udder tissue proteins
Chemically, a weak base or otherwise highly non-ionised in milk
Sufficiently lipid-soluble
Short milk-withholding period required

Intramammary infusion during the dry period
Completely non-irritant to the udder. (Although mild udder irritation is tolerable, and perhaps desirable for antibiotics intended for therapy during lactation, this property can result in extensive damage to the udder in dry period therapy)
Low MIC with a preferred bactericidal mode of action to minimise chances of drug resistance developing when low levels of antibiotics are present in the udder in the latter part of the dry period
High degree of binding to dry udder secretions and udder tissue proteins
Chemically, a strong acid or a strong base
Highly hydrophilic properties
Large molecular weight
Stability of microbiological activity in dry udder secretions for at least 3 weeks

Table 5.7 The effect of dry cow therapy on the incidence of mastitis infections early in lactation 1979–80 (Wright & Leaver 1982).

Category	Control	Treated
Uninfected cows at drying off, uninfected at calving	43	51
Infected at drying off, uninfected at calving	5	25
Infected at drying off, infected at calving	18	7
New infections in the dry period	27	10
New infections post calving	14	24
Total incidence of infection	59	41

(1982) demonstrated no marked effect on the incidence of new udder infections post calving to coliform infections. In addition effective control of 'summer mastitis' was demonstrated and, in the untreated animal group, there was a steady increase in the prevalance of subclinical infection due to *Staphylococcus aureus*.

Prophylaxis of summer mastitis

This infection, which may be described as an acute necrotising mastitis in a non-lactating bovine, is most commonly associated with *Corynebacterium pyogenes, Streptococcus dysgalactiae* and *Peptococcus indolicus* alone or in combination. As early as the 1950s, prophylaxis using intramammary penicillin G had been carried out with success in cows and heifers (Pearson 1950, 1951). The use of long-acting, slowly absorbed intramammary preparations is to be recommended over the period from the end of June until the end of August. Experimental work has revealed the need for repeated infusion at four-week intervals where the incidence of summer mastitis is high. During the year of 1977, 216 cases of summer mastitis were examined; bacteria were recovered from 38 animals which had been treated with long-acting intramammary preparations and it was assumed that the antibiotic had been absorbed or was below inhibitory concentration. The repeated infusion is effective but adds to the cost involved, and it is unlikely that the use of existing antibiotic preparations will be regarded as a permanent solution to the problem of controlling summer mastitis.

Treatment of the acute case

The choice of therapy for per acute and acute cases of mastitis (normally occurring in lactating animals) is difficult. For economic reasons, many cases which do not involve systemic upset, will continue to be treated by intramammary therapy alone. In the absence of typing and sensitivity data for the organism, the choice of penicillin–aminoglycoside combinations are likely overall to be as efficacious as other treatments and are generally the most economic, both in cost of drug and in terms of withholding time for milk. When given by the intramammary route, absorption of both penicillin and aminoglycosides from the udder is poor and adequate concentrations are thereby maintained in the udder (Ziv 1975). However, previous experience on the particular farm or area and the clinical signs may suggest that this combination may be ineffective.

If Staphylococci are known to be involved, the inclusion of a penicillin or cephalosporin active against penicillinase-producing Staphylococci (e.g. nafcillin, cloxacillin, cephoxazole) would be advised. In the case of Mycoplasma spp. treatment appears to have a poor success rate. Jasper *et al* (1966) reported reasonable success using oxytetracycline and neomycin. The logical choice is either tetracycline or a macrolide — only these two groups having efficacy against Mycoplasma spp. Resistance to re-infection appears to be short-lived (Bennet & Jasper 1978).

Treatment of the per acute case

The per acute case of mastitis is characterised by high systemic temperature and treatment is of considerable urgency. In these cases parenteral therapy is essential and intramammary therapy, if used at all, should be with the same antibiotic. During per acute mastitis, repeated milking out is desirable and this also leads to loss of antibiotic when given intramammarily. Chloramphenicol, although active *in vitro,* does not penetrate the udder well and pharmacokinetic considerations argue against its use. The macrolides (tylosin, erythromycin) concentrate extremely well in the udder when given systemically but the narrow spectrum (Gram-positive) of this group may restrict their use in the per acute case. Tetracyclines should be given in large doses intravenously if suitable concentrations are to be achieved in the udder; high dosage is also recommended for sulphonamide–trimethoprim combinations (Ziv 1980b). MacDairmid (1978) argues that, for staphylococcal per acute mastitis, the order of choice of systemic therapy is tylosin (12.5–20 mg/kg every 24 hours); oxytetracycline (10 mg/kg i.v. every 12 hours) and sulphonamide–trimethoprim (48 mg/kg i.m. every 12 hours).

Because of its potential therapeutic effect in combatting the effects of endotoxins associated with Gram-negative infections, aspirin has been suggested as a part of the therapeutic regimen in coliform mastitis (Mercer & Teske 1977). Gingerich (1977) suggested that aspirin be given as part of a therapeutic regimen for mastitis and that 100 mg/kg given orally at 12-hour intervals is an appropriate dose. In addition, the in-vitro inactivation of endotoxin from *E. coli* strains by polymyxin B has been demonstrated (Ziv 1978) and products containing 100 mg of polymixin B appeared to be effective in reducing udder swelling and improving clinical conditions if administered in the early stages of acute bovine coliform mastitis (Ziv 1980).

Finally, the concomitant existence of other abnormalities — ketosis, post-parturient hypocalcaemia, metritis and acute digestive upset — must not be overlooked. In any case, the depression, dehydration and anorexia may be overcome by several pails of warm water containing half a gallon of molasses, 2–3 g of mineral supplement, and 40 g of acetylsalicylic acid in 500 ml of ethyl alcohol (Schipper 1967).

Conclusions

Throughout the literature reservations are expressed concerning the adequacies of antibiotic therapy in the control of mastitis. This would appear to be due to the lack of controlled efficacy trials, emphasis having been placed on the rapidity of elimination of the drug from the milk (Mercer 1976). The collection of data on the efficacy of mastitis treatment from naturally occurring infections in commercial herds is time consuming and expensive. Experimentally-induced infections, comparing different treatments, hold greater promise for the demonstration of efficacy. However, there is no doubt that antibiotic therapy has played a major role in the control of acute mammary infections in a changing agricultural scene. That the use of antibiotics for control of subclinical mastitis is only one part of any mastitis control scheme is generally recognised. The individual and management factors that determine how the mammary gland responds to invasion are still poorly understood, but the explanation of failure to respond to therapy would appear to lie in this area. Controlled studies are now being developed particularly with induced infection (Newbold 1974, Postle 1976, McDonald & Anderson 1981a). However, criteria for the diagnosis of intramammary infection still have to be agreed upon, but Griffith *et al* (1977) have developed a useful method of assessing the state of infection with predictable 99% accuracy for large field experiments. Postle (1976), using paired quarter samples, showed an error of 3% could be expected from a single sample. Together with these observations, Ziv (1975) has established certain criteria in relation to drug absorption, distribution and pharmacokinetics designed to rationalise the approach to developing intramammary formulations and a quicker evaluation of efficacy.

Armed with these techniques, newer drugs and formulations may result. The ultimate measure will be the clinical efficacy at farm level. Non-clinical mastitis should be treated preferably at the end of lactation. As for treatment of the acute case, more attention must be paid to those infections caused by Gram-negative organisms and the selection of broad spectrum antibiotics administered by the parenteral route. There is an urgent need for direction and rationalisation in this field.

References

Albright J. L., Tuckey S. L. & Woods G. T. (1961) Antibiotic in milk. *J. Dairy Sci.* **44,** 5, 779.

Allenstein L. C. (1977) A practitioner's approach to mastitis therapy. *J. Am. Vet. Med. Assoc.* **170,** 1199.

Anderson J. C. (1977) Experimental staphylococcal mastitis in the mouse: The indication of chronic mastitis and its response to antibiotic therapy. *J. Comp. Path.* **87,** 611.

Anderson J. C. (1979) Response to treatment of chronic mastitis induced in mice by strains of *Staphylococcus aureus* isolated from herds of different susceptibility to cloxacillin therapy. *Br. Vet. J.* **135,** 92.

Bennet R. H. & Jasper D. E. (1978) Factors associated with differentiations between cattle resistant and susceptible to intramammary challenge exposure to *Mycomplasma bovis*. *Am. J. Vet. Res.* **39,** 407.

Boughton E. (1979) *Mycoplasma bovis* mastitis. *Vet. Bull.* **49**, 377.

Boulton M. G. & Ross G. W. (1977) Resistance of cephaxazole–benzylpenicillin combinations to destruction by β lactamase associated with bovine mastitis. *J. Comp. Path.* **87**, 145.

Bramley A. J. (1975) Infection of the udder with coagulase negative micrococci and *Corynebacterium bovis*. *Proc. Semin. Mastitis Control IDF Bulletin Doc.* **85**, 327.

Brander G. C. (1973) Dairy herd environment and the control of mastitis. *Vet. Rec.* **92**, 501.

Burrows G. E. (1980) Pharmacokinetics of macrolides, lincomycins and spectinomycin. *J. Am. Vet. Med. Assoc.* **176**, 1072.

Carroll E. J., Lasmanis J., Jain N. C. *et al* (1974) Use of dimethyl sulphoxide–flumethazone combination for treatment of endotoxin-induced bovine mastitis. *Am. J. Vet. Res.* **35**, 6, 781.

Christie G. J., Keefe T. J. & Strom B. S. (1974) Cloxacillin and the dry cow. *Clin. VM/SAC* 1405.

Cooper M. G., Buddle B. M., Ashby M. G. (1977) Incidence of infection prior to first parturition. *Ann. Report Wallaceville, New Zealand, Anim. Res. Ctr. 1967—77.*

Craven N. & Anderson J. C. (1980a) The selection in vitro of antibiotics with activity against intracellular S. aureus. *J. Vet. Pharacol. Therap.* **3**, 221.

Craven N. & Anderson J. C. (1980b) Therapy of experimental staphylococcal mastitis in the mouse with cloxacillin and rifampicin, alone and in combination. *Res. Vet. Sci.* **31**, 295.

Davies E. M. (1961) Growing resistant to antibiotics. *Vet. Rec.* **73**, 17, 429.

Dodd F. H., Kingwill R. G., Neave F. K. *et al* (1964) *Staphylococcus aureus* recovered from infected quarters. NIRD Reports, 33.

Edwards S. J. (1962) Antibiotics in the treatment of mastitis. In *Antibiotics in Agriculture,* ed. M. Woodbine, Butterworth, London.

Ellis W. A., O'Brien J. J., Pearson J. K. L. *et al* (1976) Bovine leptospirosis:infection by the serogroup hebdomadis and mastitis. *Vet. Rec.* **99**, 368.

Gingerich D. A. (1977) Pharmacokinetics of drugs used systemically in mastitis therapy. *Proc. 10th Ann. Convent. Ann. Assoc. Bov. Pract.* p. 64.

Greer D. O. & Pearson J. K. L. (1973) *Streptococcus agalactiae* in dairy herds, its incidence and relationship to cell count and inhibitory substance levels on bulk milk. *Br. Vet. J.* **129**, 544.

Griffin T. K., Dodd F. H., Neave F. K. *et al* (1977) A method of diagnosing intramammary infection in dairy cows for large experiments. *J. Dairy Res.* **44**, 25.

Hamdy A. H., Olds W. L., Roberts B. J. (1975) Activity of penicillin and novobiocin against bovine mastitis pathogens. *Am. J. Vet. Res.* **36**, 259.

Harris A. M., Davies A. M., Marshall M. J. (1978) The treatment of clinical mastitis with cephoxazole and penicillin. *Vet. Rec.* **107**, 4.

Hill A. W., Shears A. L. & Hibbitt K. G. (1979) The survival of serum resistant *Escherichia coli* in the bovine mammary gland following experimental infection. *Res. Vet. Sci.* **26**, 32.

House J. A. & Manley M. (1974) Antibiotic sensitivity patterns of *Staphyloccus aureus* from bovine milk. *Cornell Vet.* **64**, 584.

Howell D. (1972) Survey on mastitis caused by environmental bacteria. *Vet. Rec.* **90**, 654.

Jasper D. E. (1972) Antimicrobial susceptibility of Staphylococci isolated from bovine mastitis. *Calf. Vet.*, (October).

Jasper D. E., Al-Aubaidi J. M. & Fabricant J. (1974) Epidemiologic observation on mycoplasma mastitis. *Cornell Vet.* **64**, 407.

Jasper D. E., Jasis N. C. & Brazil L. H. (1966) Clinical and laboratory observations on bovine mastitis due to Mycoplasma. *J. Am. Vet. Med. Assoc.* **148**, 1017.

Jones T. O. & Turnbull P. C. B. (1981) Bovine mastitis caused by *Bacillus cereus*. *Vet. Rec.* **108**, 271.

Le Louedec (1978) *Efficacité des Antibotiques contre le mammites bovines Staphylococcique et Streptococcique: Ann. Rech. Vet.* **9** (i), 63.

MacDairmid S. C. (1980) Antibacterial drugs used against mastitis in cattle by the systemic route. *N. Z. Vet. J.* **26**, 290.

McDonald T. J., McDonald J. S. & Rose D. L. (1970) Aerobic Gram-negative rods isolated from bovine udder infections. *Am. J. Vet. Res.* **31**, 1937.

McDonald J. S., McDonald T. J. & Stark D. R. (1976) Antibiograms of Streptococci isolated from bovine intramammary infections. *Am. J. Vet. Res.* **37**, 1185.

McDonald J. S., McDonald T. J. & Anderson A. J. (1977) Antimicrobial sensitivity of aerobic Gram-negative rods isolated from bovine udder infections. *Am. J. Vet. Res.* **38**, 10, 1503.

McDonald J. S. & Anderson A. J. (1981a) Experimental infection of bovine mammary glands with *S. uberis* during the non-lactating period. *Am. J. Vet. Res.* **42**, 3, 465.

McDonald J. S. & Anderson A. J. (1981b) Antibiotic sensitivity of *Staphylococcus aureus* and coagulase-negative Staphylococci isolated from infected mammary glands. *Cornell Vet.* **71**, 391.

Marr A. (1978) Bovine mastitis control : A need for appraisal? *Vet. Rec.* **102**, 132.

Mercer H. D., Geleta J. N., Schultz E. J. *et al* (1970) Milk out rates for antibiotics in intramammary infusion products used in the treatment of bovine mastitis: relationship of somatic cell counts, milk production level and drug vehicle. *Am. J. Vet. Res.* **31**, 9, 1549.

Mercer H. D., Geleta J. N., Baldwin R. A. *et al* (1976) Viewpoint of current concepts regarding accepted and tried products for control of bovine mastitis. *J. Am. Vet. Med. Assoc.* **169**, 10, 1104.

Mercer H. D. & Teske R. H. (1977) Special considerations for the development of drugs for acute clinical mastitis. *J. Am. Vet. Med. Assoc.* **170**, 1190.

Misra B. & Marshall R. T. (1972) *Streptococcus uberis* of bovine mastitis origin: isolation, characterisation and serology of two mucoid strains. *J. Dairy Sci.* **55**, 194.

Neave F. K., Dodd F. H. & Henriques E. (1950) Udder infections in the 'dry period'. *J. Dairy Res.* **17**, 37.

Newbould F. H. S. (1974) Antibiotic treatment of experimental *Staphylococcus aureus* infections of the bovine mammary gland. *Can. J. Comp. Med.* **38**, 411.

Paape M. J., Gwanzdauskas F. C., Guidry A. J. *et al* (1981) Concentrations of corticosteroids, leucocytes and immunoglobulins in blood and milk after administration of ACTH to lactating dairy cattle: Effect on phagocytosis of *Staphylococcus aureus* by polymorphonuclear leucocytes. *Am. J. Vet. Res.* **42**, 2081.

Pearson J. K. L. (1950) The use of penicillin in the prevention of C. pyrogenes infection of the non-lactating udder. *Vet. Rec.* **62**, 166.

Pearson J. K. L. (1951) Further experiments in the use of penicillin on C. pyrogenes infection of the non-lactating bovine udder. *Vet. Rec.* **63**, 215.

Pearson J. K. L. (1964) Antibiotics in slow and quick release bases. *Vet. Rec.* **76**, 409.

Pearson J. K. L. & Wright C. L. (1969) The place of dry cow therapy in mastitis control. *Vet. Rec.* **85**, 144.

Pearson J. K. L., Greer D. O. & Pollock D. A. (1976) *Streptococcus agalactiae* in the smaller herd. Its incidence in relationship to somatic cell counts. *Br. Vet. J.* **132**, 588.

Philpot W. N. (1969) Role of therapy in mastitis control. *J. Dairy Sci.* **52**, 708.

Plommet M. & Le Loudec C. (1975) The role of antibiotic therapy during lactation in the control of subclinical and clinical mastitis. I.D.F. Bulletin Document 85, Seminar on Mastitis Control, p. 265.

Postle D. S. & Natzke R. P. (1974) Efficacy of antibiotic treatment in the bovine udder as determined from field studies. *Vet. Med/SAC,* **69**, 1535.

Postle D. S. (1976) Observations on bacteriological isolate from pairs of quarter milk samples. *J. Am. Vet. Med. Assoc.* **168**, 220.

Radostits O. M. (1961) The clinical aspects of coliform mastitis in cattle. *Can. Vet. J.* **2**, 401.

Rasmussen F. (1966) *Studies on the mammary excretion and absorption of drugs.* Carl. F. Mortensen, Copenhagen.

Report (1969) *Joint Committee on Use of Antibiotics in Animal Husbandry and Veterinary Medicine.* HMSO, London.

Schalm O. W. & Ormsbee R. W. (1949) Effects of management and therapy on staphylococcic mammary infections. *J. Am. Vet. Med. Assoc.* **115**, 464.

Schalm O. W., Carrol E. J. & Jain N. C. (1971) *Bovine Mastitis.* Lea & Febiger, Philadelphia.

Schipper J. A. (1955) Comparison of vehicles in intramammary therapy of bovine mastitis. *Vet. Med.* **50**, 111.

Schipper I. A. (1967) Practical mastitis chemotherapy. *Vet. Med. Res.* **2/3**, 257.

Schultze W. D. (1975) Dry cow therapy : a review. *Proc. Nat. Mast. Council USA,* p. 41.

Schultze W. D. & Mercer H. D. (1976) Non lactating cow therapy using a formulation of penicillin and novobiocin. *Am. J. Vet. Res.* **37**, 1275.

Smith A., Neave F. K., Dodd F. H. *et al* (1966) Methods of reducing the incidence of udder infection in dry cows. *Vet. Rec.* **79**, 233.

Smith A., Neave F. K., Dodd F. H. *et al* (1967) The persistence of cloxacillin in mammary gland when infused immediately after the last milking of lactation. *J. Dairy Res.* **34**, 47.

Swarbrick O. (1968) Intramammary treatment of bovine mastitis. *Vet. Rec.* **82**, 1, 2.

Throop B. T. & Swanson E. W. (1958) A study of penicillin tolerance of some organisms infecting the bovine mammary gland. *J. Am. Vet. Med. Assoc.* **132**, 467.

Uvarov O. (1971) Drugs against mastitis. *Vet. Rec.* **88**, 674.

Uvarov O. (1975) *Review of Recent Trends in Veterinary Therapeutics. The Veterinary Annual,* 15th Issue. John Wright, Bristol.

Waldvogel F. A., Girard J. D. & Regamey C. (1975) Combinations of antibiotics in severe pneumonias due to Gram-negative bacilli. In *Clinical Use of Combinations of Antibiotics,* 90–108, ed. J. Klastersky. Hodder and Stoughton, London.

Ward G. E. & Schultz L. H. (1974) Incidence and control of mastitis during the dry period. *J. Dairy Sci.* **57**, 1341.

Watkins J. H., Buswell J. F. & Hutchinson I. (1975) The treatment of clinical mastitis with a combination of ampicillin and cloxacillin. *Vet. Rec.* **96**, 289.

Wright C. L. (1977) Annual Report. The West of Scotland Agricultural College, p. 112.

Wright C. L. & Leaver D. (1982) The Effect of Dry Cow Therapy on the Incidence of Mastitis Infection early in Lactation. (In press)

Ziv G. (1975) Pharmacokinetic concepts for systemic and intramammary antibiotic treatment in lactating and dry cows. *IDF Seminar on Mastitis Control, Doc.,* **85**, 314.

Ziv G. (1980a) Availability and usage of new antibacterial drugs in europe. *J. Am. Vet. Med. Assoc.* **176**, 1122.

Ziv G. (1980b) Drug selection and use in mastitis:systemic vs local therapy. *J. Am. Vet. Med. Assoc.* **176**, 1109.

Ziv G., Gordins S., Behcar G. *et al* (1976) Binding of antibiotics to dry udder secretion and to udder tissue homogenates. *Br. Vet. J.* **132**, 318.

Ziv G. & Rasmussen F. (1975) Distribution of labelled antibiotics in different components of milk following intramammary and intramuscular administration. *J. Dairy Sci.* **58**, 1637.

Ziv G., Storper M. & Saran A. (1981) Comparative efficacy of three antibiotic products for the treatment and prevention of subclinical mastitis during the dry period. *Vet. Q.* **3**, 74.

Ziv G. & Sulman F. G. (1974a) Absorption of antibiotic by the bovine udder. *J. Dairy Sci.* **58**, 1637.

Ziv G. & Sulman F. (1974b) Distribution of aminoglycoside antibiotic in blood and milk. *Res. Vet. Sci.* **17**, 68.

6

The addition of antibiotics to feedingstuffs

D.L. HUDD

Antibiotics occur in nature as the metabolites of certain moulds and bacteria. Their use in animal feeds evolved largely from the fermentation of vitamin B_{12}. In the 1940s, it was shown that liver extracts, fish meal, and cow manure contained a growth factor for chicks which was termed the animal protein factor (APF). It was then shown that this vitamin could replace the crude APF substance in promoting the growth of chicks (Ott *et al* 1948). Demand for B_{12}-rich supplements grew and, in 1949, it was noted that an APF supplement from chlortetracycline fermentation produced a growth response in chicks over and above that attributable to its B_{12} content (Stockstad *et al* 1949). Antibiotics themselves were subsequently found to enhance the health and growth of pigs, poultry, and other animals.

Since that time the use of antibiotics in feedingstuffs has increased in line with developments in intensive animal production. It is a convenient method for administering a pharmacologically active substance to large numbers of intensively raised animals to ensure that each receives an appropriate oral dose. Antibiotics are now commonly included in the feed of chickens, turkeys, pigs, veal calves, ruminating cattle, and fur-bearing animals.

The term 'antibiotic' has tended to become synonymous with 'antibacterial'. This is unfortunate because many antibiotics, as well as having direct effects at a cellular level on the host animal, also have activity against a variety of other living organisms including viruses, fungi, helminths, and protozoa. Their use in animal feeds reflects many of these properties. For growth promoting purposes they are included in the feed at low levels where they also improve the efficiency of feed utilsation. For therapeutic purposes they are used in feed usually at higher levels for their antibacterial, antifungal, anthelmintic, or antiprotozoal effects.

Impact of legislation on antibiotics in animal feeds

Smith (1977) recounted the events in the UK which led, in 1969, to the *Report of the Joint Committee on the Use of Antibiotics in Animal Husbandry and Veterinary Medicine,* commonly known as the Swann Report.

During the 1960s, the incidence of antibiotic resistance in bacteria pathogenic for farm animals increased to a point where it was complicating the treatment of disease. Although the therapeutic use of antibiotics was partly responsible, it was suggested that the feeding of antibiotics for growth promotion purposes was also contributory. This applied particularly in the case of the high incidence of penicillin- and tetracycline-resistant Staphylococci and tetracycline-resistant Clostridia and *Escherichia coli* in pigs and poultry.

The earlier discovery by Japanese workers of transmissible antibiotic resistance suggested that tetracycline-resistant *E. coli* from animals fed tetracyclines might constitute a reservoir of resistance potentially transmissible to pathogenic *E. coli* and Salmonellae affecting man. Anderson & Lewis (1965) reported a great increase in the incidence of antibiotic-resistant *Salmonella typhimurium,* especially in strains of phage type 29 considered to be of bovine origin. Originally sensitive to all antibiotics, this resistance, which was mainly transmissible, appeared first to streptomycin and tetracyclines and then to the sulphonamides and ampicillin. The use of antibiotics in calves for growth promotion purposes had not been permitted at that time so it was almost certainly their use for prevention and treatment of disease that led to the problem.

These observations and the implications of transmissible resistance were largely responsible for the UK government setting up the Swann Committee. Its report recommended amongst other things that antibiotics for nutritional use should be restricted to those which are of economic value to livestock production, have little or no application as therapeutic agents in man or animals, and which do not impair the efficacy of therapeutic antibiotics through the development of resistant organisms. Following the report, the tetracyclines and penicillin were prohibited from use as growth promoters in the UK and became available only on veterinary prescription. Also, tylosin, although it had not been implicated in resistance problems and is not used in human medicine, was prohibited from growth promotion use because it was used as a therapeutic agent in veterinary medicine. Zinc bacitracin was suggested as meeting the new requirements for a feed antibiotic.

In 1970, the Food and Drug Administration of the USA established a Task Force to examine the safety and effectiveness of antibiotics in animal feeds. A report was issued in 1972. Its proposals were to restrict penicillin and tetracyclines to prescription use only (Frazier & McNett 1978), but these have not been implemented.

In 1976, the tetracyclines and penicillin were also removed from the list of approved feed additives in EEC countries. Apart from their association with transmissible resistance, the tetracyclines had been implicated in leav-

Table 6.1 Permitted nutritional feed antibiotics in EEC (up to and including 37th commission directive, 8th June, 1981).

	Turkeys	Chickens for fattening	Layer replace-ments	Laying hens	Calves	Cattle for fattening	Swine	Lambs/ kids	Fur animals
Usual maximum age limit (weeks)	26		16		26		26	26	
Avoparcin		+					+		
Bacitracin (zinc)	+	+	+	+	+		+	+	+
Flavophospholipol	+	+	+	+	+	+	+		+
Lincomycin		+*	+*						
Mocimycin		+*					+*		
Monensin Sodium		+†				+			
Nosiheptide		+*					+*		
Spiramycin	+	+	+		+		+	+	+
Tylosin							+		
Virginiamycin	+	+	+		+		+		

*Annex II — free-sale or prescription only, at the discretion of the member state. †Anticoccidal use only.

ing tissue residues in the carcasses of meat animals (Brüggemann *et al* 1973). Certain macrolide antibiotics, including tylosin, are still approved for nutritional use in EEC countries.

Although the philosophy of the Swann Committee recommendations appeared to be sound, it has had little impact on the pattern of bacterial resistance in the UK. The amount of tetracycline-resistant *E. coli* in the pig population might have decreased slightly but the incidence of pigs excreting these organisms (100% in 1975) has not (Smith 1977). Tylosin continues to be an effective growth promoting antibiotic for pigs (Burckhardt 1976, Jones 1978). After 18 years of continual use in the USA, Europe, and elsewhere, there is no evidence that its use as a growth promoting antibiotic jeopardises the treatment of systemic diseases of animals. Thus, since 1972 there has been a movement in the UK, EEC, and USA towards a separation of those antibiotics selected for nutritional purposes and those selected for medicinal purposes. Those antibiotics currently listed in the Annexes of the EEC Feed Additive Directive 70/524 for growth promoting purposes are shown in Table 6.1.

Suggested features of antibotics for use as growth promoters

Suggestions of those features which would be desirable for antibiotics for growth promotion are given below. These are recommendations from the Swann Committee, EEC legislation, and independent workers.

Economic value in livestock production

Low levels of antibiotics for growth promotion are usually included in the feed of healthy growing animals to reduce production costs by enhancing growth and improving the efficiency of feed utilisation. An improvement in general health status may be concurrent in the flock or herd but control of disease is not the primary intention. Improvements in average daily gain and in feed conversion efficiency may be of the order of 3–4% in broiler chickens, 4–5% in pigs and veal calves, and 10% or more in ruminating cattle. Apart from reducing the time for animals to reach market weight, thus lowering overhead costs on buildings and labour, the effects of saving feed (which usually contributes 60–70% of the costs of raising meat animals) can be highly significant.

In 1976, in the UK alone, over 11 million tonnes of compounded feed were consumed by cattle, pigs, and poultry; in the EEC this figure exceeded 60 million tonnes (Williams 1977). EEC countries produce over 100 million pigs annually and a 5% reduction in feed consumed would represent a saving of 1 250 000 metric tonnes. Thus, cost effectiveness is most important in the selection of feed antibiotics and this is related both to the cost of the antibiotics themselves and to their efficacy in improving growth performance.

Lack of impairment of efficacy of therapeutic antibiotics

The Swann Committee Report states: 'The development of resistant strains of an organism is probably inevitable when a "feed" antibiotic is used but will be harmful only if the efficacy of a therapeutic antibiotic or antibiotics is thereby threatened. The development of organisms (which need not be pathogens) resistant to a "feed" antibiotic might impair the efficacy of a therapeutic antibiotic if:
a   the "feed" antibiotic were itself to be used in therapy, or
b   the "feed" antibiotic were to have cross-resistance with the therapeutic antibiotic, or
c   resistance to the "feed" antibiotic were to be part of a multiple resistance pattern transferable *en bloc* such that selection pressure imposed by the use of the "feed" antibiotic would favour the prevalence of multiple-resistant organisms.'

Some organisms may acquire resistance to antibiotics at the concentrations used in growth promotion. This will be of significance only if the organisms themselves are pathogens or if the resistance is transmissible *in vivo* to pathogens and there is cross-resistance with therapeutic antibiotics, resulting in a disease which may become more difficult to treat. Thus, the latter two criteria — transmissibility and cross-resistance — apply particularly to antibiotics which, at growth promoting levels, select for resistance, especially of the transmissible type in the Gram-negative *Enterobacteriaceae*. There is little basis for excluding from therapeutic use antibiotics which have no action against Gram-negative bacteria and which, at growth promoting levels, are poorly absorbed or not absorbed at all.

Residues in food products

EEC feed additive legislation (Council Directive 70/524, 1970) requires that antibiotics used at growth promoting levels should 'not harm the consumer by altering the characteristics of livestock products'. Thus, the use of growth promoting antibiotics should not leave 'unacceptable' traces of residue in meat, milk, or eggs destined for human consumption. An 'unacceptable' level of residue is that which exceeds an established tolerance for the compound. A tolerance can be described as the maximum safe residue or, in regulatory terms, as the maximum permitted residue (Hudd 1978).

The implementation of withdrawal periods to eliminate traces of residue from tissues may be difficult under commercial conditions and costly to monitor. However, some countries have adopted monitoring programmes and the detection of antibiotic residues can lead to rejection of carcasses and offal, with consequent loss to the livestock owner. If residues are known to be present following the growth promoting use of an antibiotic, questions as to their toxicological or microbiological safety arise. Thus, there is the tendency towards using those antibiotics for growth promoting purposes which are not or are very poorly absorbed from the alimentary tract. The molecular size of antibiotics may be of significance in this respect and absorption is certainly of importance in considering antibiotics to be given in feed for the treatment of systemic disease. Once absorbed, the main route of excretion of foreign compounds and their metabolites is through the kidney into the urine. However, it is known that some compounds are excreted partly or mainly through the liver and bile. Williams (1971) states that compounds of a molecular weight less than 300 tend to be excreted in the urine. With compounds of molecular weight of 300–500 a variation in the extent of their biliary excretion exists between species and these can be divided into three groups: good, moderate, and poor biliary excretors. Good biliary excretors include the chicken, where the minimum molecular weight for biliary excretion is in the region of 325 ± 50. The moderate biliary excretors include sheep, where the minimum may be in the region of 400. For the poor biliary excretors, which include rabbit and probably man, the minimum may be about 500. Studies of biliary excretion of compounds of molecular weights higher than 500 suggest that in all species these compounds are excreted to a great extent in the bile.

It is often stated for certain of the larger molecule antibiotics that virtually no absorption from the gastrointestinal tract occurs. This is usually based on the fact that no microbiological activity can be detected in the serum, urine, or in tissues. It may, however, not be true to conclude that no absorption occurs from the intestine. In the case of tylosin, for example, it is believed that growth promoting levels are well absorbed but rapidly eliminated by biliary excretion (Sieck 1978). It is noteworthy that, of the antibiotics used for growth promoting purposes, avoparcin, bacitracin and flavomycin all have popular molecular weights in excess of 1000 and there are no reports of residues appearing in tissues even when fed at high levels. The macrolide, tylosin (molecular weight 915) is used at low levels for growth promotion and can be used at higher levels for the treatment of systemic disease, but no residues (assay sensitivity 0.1 parts/10^6) appear in the tissues of pigs until a feed level of 550 parts/10^6 is exceeded (Kline 1970). On the other hand, the tetracyclines, with molecular weights of approximately 500, leave detectable residues when administered at growth promoting levels.

Colonisation of the gastrointestinal tract by pathogens

In the USA, following the report of the FDA Task Force on the use of antibiotics, Salmonella excretion studies have been required for antibiotics used at so-called 'sub-therapeutic' levels in the feed of pigs and poultry. In the UK, Smith (1977) stated ' . . .because chickens are an important source of food poisoning for human beings, it is apparent then that in assessing the suitability of an antibiotic for growth promotion use, account should be taken of its effect on Salmonella excretion. With this in mind it is suggested that consideration be given to enlarging the main recommendations of the Swann Report by stating that, apart from satisfying the criteria laid down, antibiotics used for growth promotion should also not favour the colonisation of the alimentary tract by Salmonellae.' Smith & Tucker (1975, 1978) investigated on a limited scale the effects of certain antibiotics on the colonisation and excretion of *Salmonella typhimurium* in chickens. They found increases of varying magnitude in chickens fed diets containing avoparcin, bacitracin, flavomycin, lincomycin, tylosin and virginiamycin. Monensin had no obvious effect on the Salmonella excretion pattern. These workers noted that they studied the effects of these additives only on one strain of Salmonella in one strain of chicken maintained under one method of management and it is conceivable that different results would be obtained under different conditions.

Antibiotics used for growth promoting purposes

Avoparcin

This is a glycopeptide antibiotic produced by the fermentation of a strain of *Streptomyces candidus:* molecular weight approximately 1500. It is used solely for growth promoting purposes and is not otherwise used in human or veterinary medicine. It is primarily active against Gram-positive bacteria and is inactive at levels up to 100 μg/ml against pathogenic Gram-negative bacteria.

In-vivo studies in chickens have shown that the use of avoparcin does not favour the selection of resistant Streptococci or Staphylococci and it is not cross-resistant with other therapeutic antibiotics tested (lincomycin, gentamicin, benzylpenicillin, cephalothin, chloramphenicol, streptomycin, vancomycin, minocycline and oxytetracycline (Walton 1978)).

Avoparcin is said to be virtually unabsorbed from the gastrointestinal tract and is rapidly eliminated as the unchanged antibiotic. In pigs, 100% of a single oral dose was recovered in the excreta within 48 hours. Of this, most was eliminated in the faeces with only a trace amount in the urine. Similar results were obtained in chickens. No detectable blood levels or residue appears in tissues from the feeding of avoparcin to broilers for 56 days or to pigs for 95 days at levels up to and including 100 parts/10^6 (assay sensitivity 0.1–0.5 parts/10^6). Limited studies have indicated that avoparcin may favour the colonisation and excretion of *Salmonella typhimurium* in chickens (Smith & Tucker 1978).

Zinc bacitracin

This is a polypeptide antibiotic produced by a strain of *Bacillus subtilis* originally isolated from a patient named Margaret Tracey; molecular weight 1488. It is used almost exclusively for growth promoting purposes although in the past it has had limited therapeutic use in human and veterinary medicine. It is active primarily against Gram-positive bacteria and it has not been widely associated with resistance development in either Gram-positive or -negative bacteria.

Walton (1977) reported on the effect of zinc bacitracin on *Escherichia coli* in animals receiving it in the feed. When these were grown on agar containing the antibiotic, structural lesions in the bacterial cell wall were revealed. When the treated cells were examined for susceptibility to therapeutic antibiotics it was shown that their minimum inhibitory concentrations (MICs) were reduced when compared with data obtained prior to zinc bacitracin treatment. No residues have been detected in chickens fed levels up to 1100 parts/10^6 in the feed for nine weeks (assay sensitivity 0.5–0.7

parts/10^6) or in pigs receiving 550 parts/10^6 for 106 days (Shor 1970, Kline 1970). In a Salmonella excretion study in chickens, bacitracin either did not influence or slightly increased the amount of *S. typhimurium* excreted (Smith & Tucker 1975).

Flavophospholipol (moenomycin, bambermycins, Flavomycin)

This is a phosphorus-containing glycolipid antibiotic produced by fermentation of a group of Streptomyces spp. comprising *S. bambergiensis, S. ghanaensis, S. geysirensis* and *S. ederensis;* molecular weight approximately 1700. It is used for growth promoting purposes and is not used in human or veterinary medicine. It is active mainly against Gram-positive bacteria.

Cross-resistance with flavophospholipol has not been detected in staphylococcal strains resistant to several antibiotics. In-vitro tests with Gram-negative bacteria show that some of these become sensitive to the antibiotic after acquiring R-factors, i.e. the MIC is lowered by R-factors to such an extent that the antibiotic (even in growth promoting doses) inhibits the ability of the bacteria to replicate. Some plasmids possessing R-factors are eliminated by the action of the antibiotic.

Young calves fed 10 mg/calf/day of flavophospholipol in the feed for 61 days showed lower mean percentages of faecal *E. coli* resistant to streptomycin and oxytetracycline than untreated controls. The percentage of *E. coli* exhibiting multiple resistance to three antibiotics was reduced from 23.9% to 10.4% and to two antibiotics from 18.9% to 11.4% (Dealey & Moeller 1977b).

Balance studies carried out in chickens and pigs have demonstrated that after oral administration flavophospholipol is almost completely eliminated as the intact molecule in the faeces. No measurable residues are found in the tissues or eggs of chickens fed the antibiotic for several months or in the carcasses of pigs and beef cattle after it had been given in the feed at many times the normal dosage.

In Salmonella excretion studies, chickens fed diets containing flavophospholipol excreted the organisms in larger amounts than the controls but results obtained tended to differ when the antibiotic was used on different occasions (Smith & Tucker 1975). However, in young calves, the feeding of flavophospholipol for eight weeks was found to reduce the duration and prevalence of Salmonella shedding and to significantly reduce the number of organisms resistant to streptomycin, ampicillin and oxytetracycline (Dealy & Moeller 1977a). Similar results have been reported in weaning pigs (Dealy & Moeller 1976).

Monensin sodium

This is an ionophorous polyether antibiotic produced by the fermentation of a strain of *Streptomyces cinnamonensis;* molecular weight 692. It has limited antibacterial activity and is used as an anticoccidial agent in broiler chickens, in which it is active against the six species of Eimeria, known to be pathogenic, and as a growth promoting antibiotic in ruminating cattle in which it produces beneficial changes in the production of ruminal volatile fatty acids (see below).

In in-vitro studies, various bacteria have been passaged 40 times in media containing sub-inhibitory concentrations of monensin and their sensitivity tested to other antibiotics commonly used in veterinary medicine. The bacteria included Staphylococci, Lactobacilli, Clostridia, *E. coli* and Bacteroides. It was concluded that these organisms, present in the enteric flora of ruminants and chickens, when exposed to monensin will not develop resistance to other antibiotics commonly used for the prevention and treatment of disease (ampicillin, chloramphenicol, chlortetracycline, erythromycin, lincomycin, neomycin, penicillin, spectinomycin, spiramycin, streptomycin, tylosin).

Studies in steers have shown that over 70% of monensin is excreted as the unchanged antibiotic in the faeces. In cattle receiving up to 500 mg/animal/day, no residues were detectable (assay sensitivity 0.05 parts/10^6) at zero time withdrawal. In chickens fed the recommended level for coccidiosis control, no residues are detectable after 24 hours' withdrawal.

In studies of Salmonella excretion, broiler chickens were experimentally infected with *Salmonella typhimurium*. No significant differences were observed either in the numbers of Salmonellae excreted or in the number of days of shedding between the treated and control chickens. Also Smith & Tucker (1978) found that monensin had no obvious effect on the Salmonella excretion pattern in chickens.

Macrolides and related antibiotics

Tylosin

This is a macrolide antibiotic produced by the fermentation of a strain of *Streptomyces fradiae* obtained from a soil sample from Thailand; molecular weight 915. This antibiotic was developed solely for use in animals and is not used in human medicine. As well as being an effective growth promoter in pigs, it is used in chickens, turkeys, cattle, and swine primarily for the control of respiratory infections. It is active mainly against Gram-positive bacteria and mycoplasmas while the Gram-negative Enterobacteriaceae show an inherent resistance to the antibiotic.

No detectable residues are found in the carcasses of pigs following the use of growth promoting levels of tylosin. Even following the feeding of 550 parts/10^6 tylosin in the ration for 105 days, no detectable residues are present at zero time withdrawal. When 1100 parts/10^6 is fed for 105 days, a residue is found in liver which is eliminated after 48 hours (assay sensitivity 0.22–0.33 parts/10^6) (Kline 1970).

Studies in pigs receiving tylosin in the presence of sulphadimidine have indicated that there is no effect on the duration of excretion of Salmonellae. From limited studies in chickens — although the antibiotic is not used for growth promotion purposes in this species — Smith & Tucker (1975, 1978) observed some increase in Salmonella excretion. However, Ridgway & Ryden (1966) reported that tylosin included in feed did not cause an increase in the carrier rate of chickens infected with *S. typhimurium*, indeed, at nine days post-infection there was a significant reduction both in mortality and in the carrier rate compared with controls.

Spiramycin

This is a macrolide antibiotic produced by the fermentation of a strain of *Streptomyces ambofaciens* obtained from a soil sample in northern France; molecular weight 842–898. It is used in human medicine, in veterinary medicine for the control of mycoplasmosis and the treatment of mastitis, and for growth promoting purposes. It is primarily active against Gram-positive bacteria and mycoplasmas.

Lincomycin

This is a lincosaminide antibiotic produced by the fermentation of *Streptomyces lincolnensis;* molecular weight 406. It was developed initially for use in human medicine and has similar antibacterial activity to erythromycin. It is also used for therapy in veterinary medicine and as a growth promoter in chickens.

When fed to chickens at 11 parts/10^6 for 24 days no residues were found at zero time withdrawal but a level of 110 parts/10^6 fed for nine weeks left residues in liver and kidney which remained for at least five days (Shor 1970). Pigs given lincomycin at 100 parts/10^6 in the feed require withdrawal period of six days, suggesting the presence of residues before that time (Anon 1978).

In chickens receiving lincomycin in the feed, *S. typhimurium* was found in higher concentrations in the faeces for longer periods of time than from chickens in the control groups (Smith & Tucker 1978). However, in pigs given feed containing 100 parts/10^6 lincomycin and exposed to a strain of *S. typhimurium*, the number of pigs which shed the organism in the faeces, the numbers of *S. typhimurium* in the faeces, and the length of time the organisms were shed were not affected when compared with results from unmedicated pigs (DeGeeter *et al* 1976).

Virginiamycin (Staphylomycine)

This is a mixture of two antibiotics produced by the fermentation of a strain of *Streptomyces virginiae* found in a soil sample from Belgium. Virginiamycin S is a polypeptide antibiotic and virginiamycin M is a macrocyclic lactone. Virginiamycin S is also known as a streptogramin type B antibiotic. The molecular weights are 823 and 525 (DeSomer & Dijck 1955, Cocito 1969). It has been used in human medicine for the treatment of staphylococcal infections and in veterinary medicine for the treatment of swine dysentery in pigs as well as for growth promoting purposes. It is primarily active against Gram-positive bacteria.

No detectable residues were found in the muscle tissue of chickens receiving a meal containing 100 parts/10^6 virginiamycin for four weeks (assay sensitivity 0.01 parts/10^6) or in muscle, liver, and abdominal fat of chickens fed 110 parts/10^6 for up to nine weeks.

In Salmonella excretion studies, the amount of *S. typhimurium* organisms excreted from chickens receiving virginiamycin was only slightly greater than that excreted by the groups fed antibiotic-free diets (Smith & Tucker 1975).

Resistance and cross-resistance to macrolide and related antibiotics

The Gram-negative enteric bacteria are naturally resistant to macrolide and related antibiotics (Vazquez 1975), probably because they do not penetrate the complex cell envelope of these organisms. Macrolide resistance in *Staphylococcus aureus* is often accompanied by cross-resistance to lincosamides (e.g. lincomycin) and streptogramin type B (e.g. virginiamycin S) antibiotics (Weisblum & Demohn 1969, Goldman & Heiss 1971).

The macrolide antibiotics used in human and animal medicine usually contain a 14- or 16-membered lactone ring (Vazquez 1975). The 14-membered ring macrolides include erythromycin and oleandomycin. The 16-membered ring macrolides include spiramycin and tylosin.

Staphylococcal resistance to macrolides and related antibiotics is generally of two major types: constitutive or inducible. In both forms resistance is due to ribosome modification by a specific methylase enzyme (Devriese 1976). The resistant strains have a decreased ability to bind the antibiotic(s) due to methylation of the ribosome. Differentiation between inducible and constitutive resistance in Staphylococci may be important when reviewing the growth promoting uses of macrolide and related antibiotics. Inducible resistance is a bacterial response to erythromycin and other 14-membered ring macrolides but not to the 16-membered ring macrolides. It can be produced by the presence of sub-inhibitory levels of antibiotic which appear to trigger the biosynthesis of the methylase enzyme. After induction of resistance, the inducibly resistant bacteria, in the presence of other macrolide or related antibiotics, can become fully resistant not only to the inducer but also to the other antibiotics (tylosin, spiramycin, lincomycin, and virginiamycin S).

In a population of *S. aureus,* organisms with constitutive resistance have the enzyme naturally present. A resistant population may appear in response to selection pressure from any of the macrolide or related antibiotics used at inhibitory levels. These bacteria will be resistant to macrolide and other related antibiotics. Devriese (1976) has noted that, although staphylococcal resistance to macrolides affects virginiamycin S, the strains remain susceptible to virginiamycin.

Most naturally occurring antibiotic resistance is determined by genes carried on plasmids and their presence in Staphylococci is well established (Lacey 1973). Transfer of the plasmids is mediated by bacteriophages in a process called transduction. It is unlikely that this method of transfer would transfer plasmids to organisms other than Staphylococci. Conjugal transfer of infectious resistance as in the Enterobacteriaceae has not been demonstrated in the Staphylococci. Conjugal transfer of plasmid-borne multiple resistance does occur in *Streptococcus faecalis* but has not been reported in other Streptococci. Silver *et al* (1977) followed the resistance pattern of faecal Streptococci in dogs fed virginiamycin in the diet at 50 parts/10^6. The main effect of the virginiamycin was to eliminate the more sensitive *Streptococcus bovis* and to replace it by *S. faecalis* some of which were resistant to virginiamycin and showed cross-resistance with erythromycin. This resistance was transferable to other strains of *S. faecalis* but these were replaced by the normal population soon after the cessation of treatment.

Mode of action of antibiotics in improving growth

Not all antibiotics with recognised antibacterial properties are effective in improving the growth performance of animals. Those that possess this action usually have a mainly gram-positive spectrum of activity but their chemical structures differ widely and cannot be related to their growth promoting potential (Hays 1964). Certain Gram-negative antibiotics (e.g. strepto-mycin) will enhance growth but others (e.g. neomycin) do not (Bunyan *et al* 1977). The growth promoting antibiotics do not exert a favourable influence in germ-free animals (Coates *et al* 1963).

Over the years three main theories have been advanced to explain the beneficial effects resulting from the feeding of antibiotics to animals. These are a metabolic effect, a disease control effect, and a nutrient-sparing effect.

Metabolic effect

Some of the antibiotics effective as growth promoters are readily absorbed into the bloodstream of the host animal. Others, as described above, are very poorly absorbed. Differences in absorption cannot readily be associated with the efficiency of antibiotics as growth promoters although they may have an influence on systemic infectious disease.

Disease control effect

It is often said that growth promotion benefits result solely from the control of pathogenic organisms capable of producing specific disease or non-specific detrimental effects resulting from toxin production. Many workers have noted a gut-thinning effect following antibiotic usage which is assumed to result from a reduction in bacterial toxin production, thus permitting improved absorption of dietary nutrients. Braude *et al* (1953) showed that improvements in growth performance due to the inclusion in feeds of antibiotics are inversely related to the performance level of untreated con-trol animals. The very wide range of performance data reviewed came from studies in both diseased and healthy pigs.

More recently Jones (1978) suggested that the standard practice of expressing improvements in growth rate and feed conversion efficiency as a percentage of the untreated control value may lead one to assume that, at certain levels of control performance, no effects can be obtained by the use of growth performance improvers. From a series of trials using the antibiotic tylosin at growth promoting levels in clinically healthy pigs under good commercial management conditions, he found that pigs were achieving a constant improvement of approximately 30 g/pig/day over a range of control gains from 417 to 683 g/pig/day. Thus, in this study it was only the *percen-tage* improvement in average daily gain that was inversely related to the control performance but the *absolute* improvement was constant. These results support the view that improvements in growth performance can be obtained in clincally healthy pigs kept under sanitary conditions. They also support the nutrient-sparing effect described below.

Nutrient-sparing effect

Germ-free animals grow better on the same ration than conventionally reared animals. Therefore, it is postulated that the presence of bacteria or certain bacteria in conventionally reared animals adversely influences the availability and absorption of nutrients. Recent studies have demonstrated that the use of antibiotics at growth promoting levels influences the metabolism of the enteric flora producing a nutrient-sparing effect which makes more of the dietary feed nutrients available for absorption by the host animal (Assche *et al* 1975a, 1975b, Vervaeke *et al* 1976, Henderickx *et al* 1976).

Henderickx *et al* (1976) describing the inter-relationship between the host animal and its enteric flora said: 'It is well known that a baby animal immediately after birth is invaded by micro-organisms from the mother and the environment. This disorderly mass of germs tries to organise itself; some strains are going to locate themselves in preferential sites of the intestinal tract with the consequence that an interaction between host and flora is established. This interaction can be positive, as was Pasteur's opinion that life without flora is impossible, or negative as proposed by Metchnikoff.' This group summarised the possible actions of the intestinal bacterial flora (Table 6.2). The ability of bacteria to synthesise vitamins is favourable whereas the production of toxins is unfavourable. In the metabolism of carbohydrates, the microbial digestion of cellulose to lactic acid and volatile fatty acids is advantageous because cellulose cannot otherwise be digested by the enzymes of the digestive juices. The same bacterial intervention for carbohydrates of the starch type constitutes a loss of energy. The microbial metabolism of proteins and fats may produce an unfavourable result because the end products may have either a toxic character or a reduced biological value.

The magnitude and type of bacterial metabolism in the intestine is dependent on the animal species, the age of the host, and the part of the intestinal tract involved. Thus, the interaction between enteric flora and host is of three types.

1 Competitive, as in carnivores, where the host uses different means to counteract the gut flora. These include a low gastric pH, active enzyme secretion, a large surface area for absorption, and rapid passage of intestinal contents which reduces the duration of contact between the bacteria and the substrate.

2 Cooperative, as in ruminants, where optimal conditions for the bacterial

Table 6.2 Possible actions of the intestinal flora. (After Henderickx *et al* 1976.)

1 Synthesis of vitamins

2 Production of toxins

3 Metabolism of carbohydrates

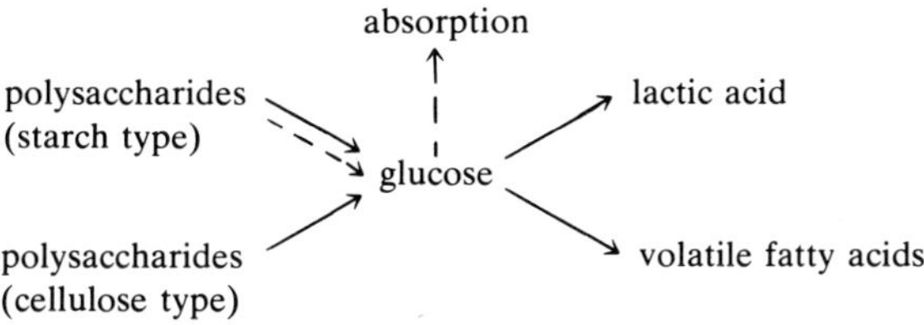

4 Metabolism of proteins

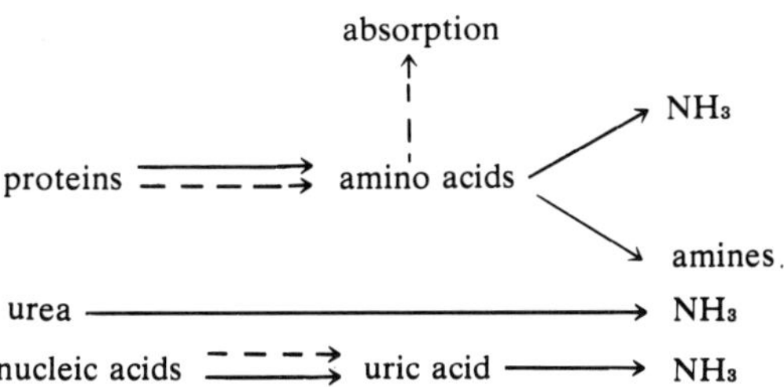

5 Metabolism of fats

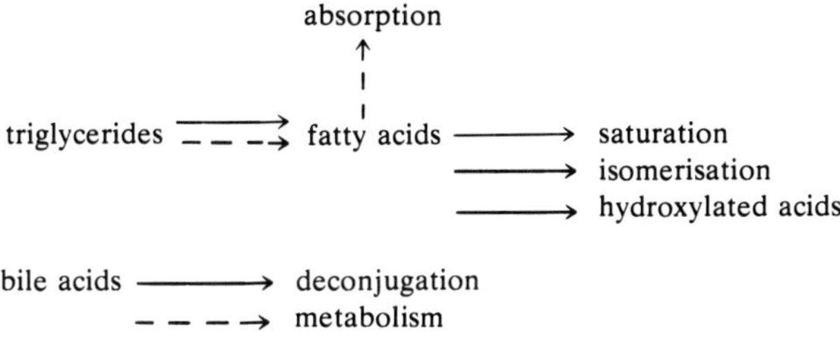

— —→ Normal metabolism,   ⟶ metabolism by the bacteria

flora are created by the host in providing large fermentation vessels, optimal pH, no secretion of enzymes and a slow evacuation of the contents.
3   Compromise, as in non-ruminating herbivores like the pig, where microbial action is competitive in the stomach and small intestine and cooperative in the caecum and the large intestine (Henderickx *et al* 1976).

Normal enteric flora of the early-weaned pig

In early-weaned piglets of five days of age, an analysis of the composition of

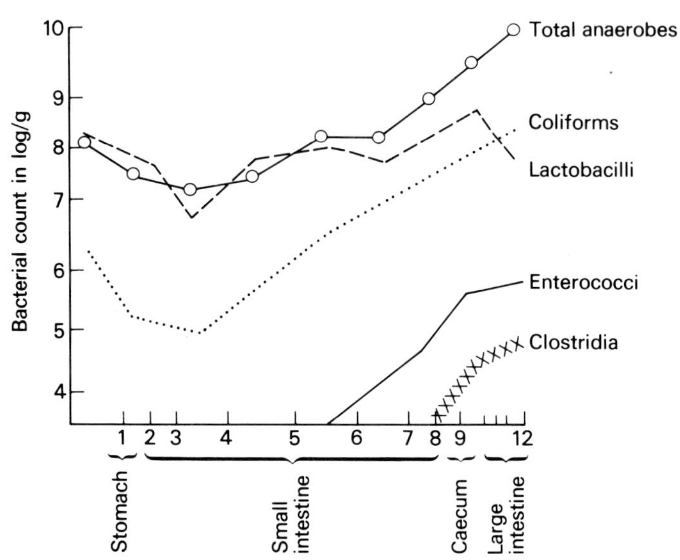

Fig. 6.1 Quantitative and topographical distribution of the gastrointestinal flora in early weaned piglets. (From Henderickx *et al* 1976.)

the enteric flora showed the presence of large numbers of Lactobacilli in the stomach and the small intestine (Fig. 6.1). Only small numbers of coliform bacteria were present in the stomach and the first part of the small intestine but, in the distal part, their numbers increased, reaching a maximum in the large intestine. Enterococci were present in the large intestine together with small numbers of Clostridia. A biochemical analysis of the microbial metabolites in such piglets indicated large amounts of lactic acid were present in the small intestine while volatile fatty acids and ammonia were present in high concentrations in the caecum and the large intestine.

Vervaeke *et al* (1976) studied the production rates of bacterial metabolites after incubation of stomach, ileal, and caecal contents of early-weaned piglets (Table 6.3). They found that bacterial activity in the stomach is low, the production of organic acids in the ileum is important, and the concentrations of volatile fatty acids and ammonia are markedly higher in the caecum than in the other segments, but that no lactic acid is produced in the caecum. They concluded that, if it is useful to inhibit bacterial action in the porcine gut, this has to occur in the small intestine. They also studied the effects of virginiamycin, flavophospholipol, and spiramycin on bacterial multiplication and metabolite production after the incubation of ileal contents from early-weaned piglets. They concluded that virginiamycin inhibits the multiplication of Streptococci and the production of lactic and volatile fatty acids. Flavophospholipol influences only the numbers of Streptococci and

Table 6.3 Production rate (μmol/ml) of bacterial metabolites after four hours incubation of stomach, ileal and caecal contents of early-weaned piglets. (Adapted from and reproduced with the permission of Vervaeke *et al* 1976.)

	Stomach	Ileum	Caecum
Lactic acid	+7.7	+74.5	−11.6
Volatile fatty acids	+5.8	+27.7	+64.3
Ammonia	+3.1	+ 8.4	+23.5

the production of lactic acid. Spiramycin influences the numbers of Streptococci and Lactobacilli and the production of organic acids.

From these experiments it was concluded that the influence of various feed additives on bacterial multiplication and metabolism is different. By analysis, it was demonstrated that a decrease in organic acid production results in a sparing of carbohydrates.

Continuous culture studies

To calculate the quantity of saved carbohydrate, a continuous culture technique has been used (Henderickx *et al* 1976). Intestinal contents are collected from a fistulated donor animal and are infused with a pump in a fermentation vessel kept under constant conditions. This is provided with an overflow so that the fermenting liquid is kept at a constant volume and, by adapting the pumping rate, a constant fermentation process is obtained. At certain locations of the intestinal tract there is both inflow and outflow — production of metabolites, absorption and secretion. With the continuous culture technique there is no absorption or secretion so that the difference between inflow and outflow is due entirely to metabolism.

The results indicated that the presence of virginiamycin on the continuous culture of ileal contents from piglets reduced the microbial fermentation of glucose leading to a calculated energy saving of 8.0 kcal/hour/100 g dry matter of intestinal contents. The use of spiramycin produced a calculated energy saving of 4.3 kcal/hour/100 g dry matter.

Antibiotic manipulation of rumen fermentation

The principal end products of rumen fermentation by cellulolytic and non-cellulolytic bacteria are microbial cells, volatile fatty acids (acetic, propionic, and butyric) and gases (carbon dioxide and methane). The volatile fatty acids are absorbed and utilised by the animal, while methane and carbon dioxide are lost by eructation (Fox 1977).

The decarboxylation of succinic acid produced by the cellulolytic bacteria on a roughage diet can account for approximately 75% of the rumen propionic acid production (Scheifinger & Wolin 1973). The carbon dioxide, hydrogen, and formic acid produced by these and other rumen bacteria are used by methanogenic bacteria to produce methane. Methane losses from the overall rumen fermentation represent an energy loss of approximately 8–10%. The production of propionic acid recovers considerably more energy in a form usable by the animal than the production of acetic or butyric acids. Approximately 70% of the energy requirement of the ruminant is supplied in the form of these three acids. Alterations in the proportions produced can have a considerable impact on the efficiency of the rumen fermentation as an energy supply source for the animal.

Since the early 1960s, attention has been focussed on the use of additives that will inhibit the production of methane thus diverting metabolic hydrogen into the production of other reduced end products of rumen fermentation, particularly propionic acid. The addition of hydrogen to in-vitro fermentation systems has been shown to increase the production of propionic acid — thus supporting the proposed inverse relationship between propionate and methane productions in the rumen (Nevel *et al* 1974). Many workers have shown that this effect can be achieved *in vitro* and *in vivo* by a wide variety of compounds but increases in propionate production have been variable. There is evidence that inhibition of methane production may result in increased losses in the form of gaseous hydrogen; and adaptation of the rumen microflora to certain inhibitors has also been suggested. The results in terms of improvements in growth performance have usually not been sufficient to justify the use of methane inhibitors in commercial animal production. However, the ionophore antibiotic monensin sodium has been shown to increase propionate production both *in vitro* and *in vivo* and this effect was maintained throughout a 148 day feeding trial (Richardson *et al* 1976). Numerous reports have appeared demonstrating the benefit of monensin on growth performance on a wide variety of rations. An improvement in feed conversion of approximtely 10% was obtained in confined beef cattle and an improvement in average daily gain was reported in pasture cattle (Raun *et al* 1976, Utley 1976, Potter *et al* 1976).

It has been shown that methane production is reduced when monensin is included in the ration but it appears that it is not acting as a direct methane inhibitor. Thornton *et al* (1976) used animals in metabolism cages to show a statistical reduction in methane produced by animals fed monensin. Also in-vitro fermentation studies indicate that methane production is decreased as the monensin level is increased. At the recommended use level, the rumen concentration of monensin is somewhere between 1 and 4 parts/10^6 on a weight/volume basis and, under these conditions, it reduces methane production by approximately 30%. Chalupa *et al* (1978) indicated that monensin did not increase hydrogen production, a trait common to all direct methane inhibitors. Studies by Romesser (1976) suggest that monensin is probably affecting a precursor of methane production such as the hydrogen availability to the methane-producing bacteria rather than having a direct effect upon the methanogenic bacteria themselves. When *Methanobacillus thermoautotrophicum* was grown in the presence of high concentrations of monensin, it has no effect on the ability of the organism to produce methane provided sufficient hydrogen and carbon dioxide were present. Nevel & Demeyer (1977) indicated that monensin appeared to interfere with formate, a hydrogen and carbon dioxide source for some methanogenic bacteria.

Since monensin produces benefits in cattle fed many types of rations, an effect on biochemical pathways common to both cellulolytic and non-cellulolytic rumen bacteria has been suggested (Fig. 6.2). The reductive tricarboxylic acid cycle found in both types of bacteria is a possible site as this uses reducing power in the form of (H^+) to produce succinic acid in the cellulolytic bacteria and propionic acid in some strains of non-cellulolytic bacteria; in addition it is involved in hydrogen and formate production by these organisms. A shift in the flow of this reducing power (H^+) from hydrogen or formate formation would result in increased reduced acid production.

The total numbers of rumen bacteria and protozoa appear to be unaffected by monensin (Dinius *et al* 1976, Richardson *et al* 1978) but there is

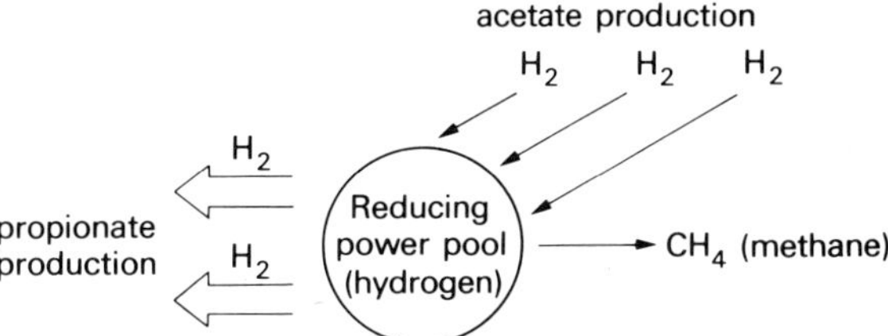

Fig. 6.2 Mode of action of monensin on rumen fermentation.

some indication (Short 1978) that a cellulolytic shift from Ruminococcus to Bacteroides occurs. Chen & Wolin (1978) indicate that high levels of monensin may favour certain species of rumen bacteria.

Summary of mode of action of growth promoting antibiotics

In monogastric animals, microbial action on dietary nutrients is in competition with the host animal. Each antibiotic has its own mode of action which may produce changes in the composition, topographical distribution, and metabolism of the enteric flora. In so doing the antibiotic can reduce the microbial fermentation of glucose and decrease the production of lactic acid, volatile fatty acids, and ammonia leading to a net energy gain by the animal. In healthy groups of animals raised under similar conditions, this may be seen to result in a constant improvement in average daily weight gain or efficiency of feed utilisation.

In ruminant animals, microbial action on dietary nutrients is cooperative. Without it, plant celluloses would not become available as energy sources to the host animal and non-protein nitrogen would not be assimilated into available amino acids. Antibiotics such as monensin sodium enhance the efficiency of microbial fermentation by increasing the production of propionic acid and reducing energy loss from the production of methane gas. The net energy gain to the animal may be observed as an increase in average daily weight gain in cattle at pasture and, most commonly, as an improvement in the efficiency of feed utilisation in confined cattle.

References

Anderson E. S. & Lewis M. J. (1965) Drug resistance and its transfer in *Salmonella typhimurium. Nature* **206**, 579.

Anon (1978) Product Notes (Lincomycin) *Vet. Rec.* **102**, 290.

Assche P. F. Van, DeMey L. E. & Descamps J. A. (1975a) *In vitro* study of the influence of Virginiamycin and Spiramycin on the composition and biochemical activities of the gastro-intestinal flora of piglets. I. Influence on the composition of the flora. *Zbl. Bakt. Hyg.* **231**, 153.

Assche P. F. Van, DeMey L. E. & Descamps J. A. (1975b) In vitro study of the influence of Virginiamycin and Spiramycin on the composition and biochemical activities of the gastro-intestinal flora of piglets. II. Influence on the biochemical activities of the micro-flora. *Zbl. Bakt. Hyg.* **231**, 163.

Braude R., Walker H. D. & Cunha T. J. (1953) The value of antibiotics in the nutrition of swine: A review. *Antibiot. & Chemoth.* **3**, 271.

Brüggemann J. von, Tiews J., Gropp J. *et al* (1973) The use of the Allgemeinen Hemmstofftest to detect tissue residues. *Tierphysiol. Tierernährg. Futtermittelkde.* **31**, 171.

Bunyan J., Jeffries L., Sayers J. R. *et al* (1977) Antimicrobial substances and chick growth promotion: The growth promoting activities of antimicrobial substances, including 52 used either in therapy or as dietary additives. *Poult. Sci.* **18,** 283.

Burchhardt I. (1976) Are antibiotic feed additives still effective in fattening pigs? *Deut. Geflugelwtsch. Schweinprod.* **12,** 273.

Chalupa W., Corbett W. & Brethour J. R. (1978) Manipulating rumen fermentation with monensin and amichloral. *Abstracts 70th Annual Meeting ASAS.*

Chen M. & Wolin M. J. (1978) Effect of monensin and lasalocid on the growth of rumen methane bacteria. *Proc. Annu. Meet. Am. Soc. Microbiol.*

Coates M. E., Fuller R., Harrison G. F. *et al* (1963) A comparison of the growth of chicks in the Gustafsson germ-free apparatus and in a conventional environment, with and without dietary supplements of penicillin. *Br. J. Nutr.* **17,** 141.

Cocito C. (1969) Metabolism of macromolecules in bacteria treated with virginiamycin. *J. Gen. Microbiol.* **57,** 179.

Council Directive concerning additives in feedingstuffs (70/524) (1970) *Offic. J. Europ. Commun.*

Dealy J. & Moeller M. W. (1976) Influence of Bambermycins on salmonella infection and antibiotic resistance in swine. *J. Anim. Sci.* **42,** 1331.

Dealy J. & Moeller M. W. (1977a) Influence of Bambermycins on salmonella infection and antibiotic resistance in calves. *J. Anim. Sci.* **44,** 734.

Dealy J. & Moeller M. W. (1977b) Effect of Bambermycins on Escherichia coli and antibiotic resistance in calves. *J. Anim. Sci.* **45,** 1239.

DeGeeter M. J., Stahl G. S. & Geng S. (1976) Effect of lincomycin on prevalence, duration and quantity of Salmonella typhimurium excreted by swine. *Am. J. Vet. Res.* **37,** 525.

DeSomer P. & Dijck P. van (1955) A preliminary report on antibiotic number 899, a Streptogramin-like substance. *Antibiot. & Chemoth.* **5,** 632.

Devriese L. A. (1976) In vitro susceptibility and resistance of animal staphyloccoci to macrolide antibiotics and related compounds. *Ann. Rech. Veter.* **7,** 65.

Dinius D. A., Simpson M. E. & Marsh P. B. (1976) Effect of monensin fed with forage on digestion and the ruminal ecosystem of steers. *J. An. Sci.* **42,** 229.

Fox B. P. (1977) The manipulation of rumen fermentation. *International Study week,* Gembloux, Belgium.

Frazier R. F. & McNett I. (1978) Antibiotics in feed-risk vs benefit. *Pig Am. Suppl.*

Goldmann S. F. & Heiss F. (1971) Resistance of Staphylococcus aureus to erythromycin, lincomycin and staphylomycin. *Z. Med. Mikrobiol. u. Immunol.* **156,** 168.

Hays V. W. (1964) *Antibiotics in Swine Rations.* Elanco Products Co., Indianapolis.

Henderickx H. K., Decuypere J. A. & Vervaeke I. J. (1976) The mode of action of some feed additives. *2nd Int. STAFAC Symp. Proc.,* Iowa.

Hudd D. L. (1978) Residue monitoring of food products of animal origin. *Br. Vet. J.* **134,** 243.

Jones P. W. (1978) The use of tylosin to improve the growth performance of clinically healthy pigs. *Proc. 5th Int. Pig Vet. Cong.* (Zagreb) Yugoslavia, Abstract K.B. 39.

Kline R. M. (1970) Antibiotic residue studies in edible swine tissues. In *Proceedings of the antibiotic presentations to the US Food and Drug Administration Task Force on the use of antibiotics in animal feeds,* pp. 290–308. The Animal Health Institute.

Lacey R. W. (1973) Genetic basis, epidemiology, and future significance of antibiotic resistance in staphylococcus aureus: A review. *J. Clin. Path.* **26,** 899.

Nevel C. J. Van, Prins R. A. & Demeyer D. I. (1974) The inverse relationship between methane and propionate in the rumen. *Z. Tierphysiol, Tierernahrg und Futtermittelkde* **33,** 121.

Nevel C. J. Van & Demeyer D. I. (1977) Effect of monensin on rumen metabolism in vitro. *Appl. Envir. Microb.* **34,** 251.

Ott W. H., Rickes E. L. & Wood T. R. (1948) Activity of crystalline vitamin B_{12} for chick growth. *J. Biol. Chem.* **174,** 1047.

Potter E. L., Cooley C. O., Richardson L. F. *et al* (1976) Effect of monensin on performance of cattle fed forage. *J. An. Sci.* **43**, 665.

Raun A. P., Cooley C. O., Potter E. L. *et al* (1976) Effect of monensin on feed efficiency of feedlot cattle. *J. An. Sci.* **43**, 670.

Report of the Joint Committee on the use of Antibiotics in Animal Husbandry and Veterinary Medicine (1969). HMSO, London.

Richardson L. F., Raun A. P., Potter E. L. *et al* (1976) Effect of monensin on rumen fermentation in vitro and in vivo. *J. An. Sci.* **43**, 657.

Richardson L. F., Potter E. L. & Cooley C. O. (1978) Effect of monensin on ruminal protozoa and volatile fatty acids. *Abstr. 11th Annu. Meet. ASAS MW Sect.*

Ridgway F. & Ryden R. (1966) Resistance studies of Salmonella typhimurium in chicks on a tylosin feed. *J. Comp. Path.* **76**, 23.

Scheifinger C. C. & Wolin M. J. (1973) Proprionate formation from cellulose and soluble sugars by combined cultures of Bacteriodes succinogenes and Selenomonas ruminantium. *Appl. Microb.* **26**, 789.

Shor A. L. (1970) Tissue residue levels in poultry products. In *Proceedings of the antibiotic presenations to the US Food and Drug Administration Task Force on the use of antibiotics in animal feeds,* pp. 95–115. The Animal Health Institute.

Short D. E. (1978) Rumen fermentation and nitrogen metabolism as affected by monensin. Thesis, University of Illinois.

Silver R. P., Leming B. & Cohen E. (1977) Effect of virginiamycin supplemented feed on plasmid determined erythromycin resistance in Group D streptococci. *Proc. 10th Int. Cong. Chemoth.* (Zurich). Abstract No. 127.

Smith H. W. (1977) Antibiotic resistance in bacteria and associated problems in farm animals before and after the 1969 Swann Report. In *Antibiotics and Antibiosis in Agriculture,* Woodbine M. (ed.), pp.344–356. Butterworths, London.

Smith H. W. & Tucker J. F. (1975) The effect of feeding diets containing permitted antibiotics on the faecal excretion of Salmonella typhimurium by experimentally infected chickens. *J. Hyg. Camb.* **75**, 293.

Smith H. W. & Tucker J. F. (1978) The effect of antimicrobial feed additives on the colonisation of the alimentary tract of chickens by Salmonella typhimurium. *J. Hyg. Camb.* **80**, 217.

Stockstad E. L. R., Jukes T. H., Pierce J. V. *et al* (1949) The multiple nature of the animal protein factor. *J. Biol. Chem.* **180**, 647.

Thornton J. H., Owens F. N., Lemenger R. P. *et al* (1976) Monensin and ruminal methane production. *J. An. Sci.* **43**, 336. (abstr.)

Utley P. R. (1976) Use of Rumensin in growing and finishing beef cattle — a review. *Proc. Georgia Nutr. Conf.*

Vazquez D. (1975) *Antibiotics III.* Mechanisms of action of Antimicrobial and Antitumour Agents, eds. J. W. Corcoran & F. E. Hahn. Springer-Verlag, New York.

Vervaeke I. J., Decuypere J. A., Henderickx H. K. *et al* (1976) Mode of action of some feed additives. *Proc. 4th Int. Pig Vet. Cong.* Iowa. Abstract AA4.

Walton J. R. (1977) A mechanism of growth promotion: non-lethal feed antibiotic induced, cell wall lesions in enteric bacteria. In *Antibiotics and Antibiosis in Agriculture,* pp. 259–264. Woodbine M. (ed.) Butterworths, London.

Walton J. R. (1978) The effect of dietary avoparcin on the antibiotic resistance patterns of enteric and pharyngeal bacteria isolated from broiler chickens. *Zbl. Vet. Med. B.* **25**, 290–300.

Weisblum B. & Demohn V. (1969) Erythromycin — inducible resistance in staphylococcus aureus: Survey of antibiotic classes involved. *J. Bacteriol.* **98**, 447.

Williams D. R. (1977) Feed Additives — whose responsibility? *Br. Vet. Assoc. Annu. Cong.* (Swansea).

Williams R. T. (1971) Species variations in drug biotransformations. In *Fundamentals of drug metabolism and drug disposition,* eds. B. N. LaDu, H. E. Mandel & E. L. Way, pp. 187–205. Williams & Wilkins, Baltimore.

7

Antibiotic resistance in veterinary practice

A.H. LINTON

Without question antibiotics have become established as one of the most useful tools in the hands of the veterinary surgeon. As therapeutic agents they have proved highly beneficial in the relief of suffering and in saving life. Their use in prophylaxis, and, under restricted conditions, for growth promotion, has played a significant role, both economically and epidemiologically in controlling infectious disease and in contributing to the ever growing demands for animal proteins.

These benefits have not been without certain disadvantages, some of which are listed in Table 7.1. A number have already been referred to by other authors in this book (Chapters 3, 4, 5, & 6) but, as therapeutic agents, the most important single factor which decides the success or failure of an antibiotic in the treatment of an infectious disease is the sensitivity of the causal agent to the antibiotic of choice.

Each micro-organism by virtue of its biological nature exhibits differences in susceptibility to the same antibacterial agent (Table 7.2). The Gram-positive bacteria are usually susceptible to a range of antibiotics which have little activity against Gram-negative bacteria, and vice versa. The broad spectrum antibiotics, on the other hand, have the unique property of being effective against both Gram-positive and Gram-negative species. Apart from the range of susceptibility of bacteria, some species readily acquire resistance to antibiotics to which they are normally sensitive and acquisition can be demonstrated both *in vitro* and *in vivo*.

Table 7.1 Problems associated with the use of antibiotics.

Toxicity to animals undergoing treatment
Hypersensitive reactions
Inhibition of normal flora
Superinfection by antibiotic resistant or insusceptible micro-organisms
Antibiotic resistance (acquired) by bacteria
Prolonged excretion of enteric pathogens
Antibiotic residues in animal products (meat, milk)
Inhibition of starter bacteria in the dairy industry by antibiotics in milk

---

Table 7.2 The antibiotic sensitivity/resistance patterns of common veterinary organisms (Linton 1982).

	Erythromycin	Novobiocin	Bacitracin	Benzylpenicillin	Methicillin (celbenin)	Cloxacillin (orbenin)	Cephaloridine	Carbenicillin (pyopen)	Ampicillin (penbritin)	Tetracycline	Chloramphenicol	Neomycin	Gentamicin	Streptomycin	Polymixin	Griseofulvin	Nystatin	Amphoteracin
Gram-positive bacteria																		
*Staphylococcus aureus**	+	+	+	+	+	+	+	+	+	+	+	+	+	+				
*Staphylococcus aureus** (penicillinase producers)	+	+	+	−	+	+	+	−	−	+	+	+	+	+	−	−	−	−
Streptococcus spp (Lancefield types A B C G)	+	+	+	+	+	+	+	+	+	+	+	−	−	−	−	−	−	−
Streptococcus faecalis	(+)	−	(+)	(+)	(+)	(+)	(+)	−	+	+	+	−	−	−	−	−	−	−
Gram-negative bacteria																		
Pasteurella multocida	+	+	−	+	+	+	+	+	+	+	+	+	+	−	+	−	−	−
*Haemophilus influenzae**	(+)	+	−	−	(+)	−	(+)	+	+	+	+	+	+	+	+	−	−	−
*Escherichia coli**	−	−	−	−	−	−	+	+	+	+	+	+	+	+	(+)	−	−	−
Salmonella spp*	−	−	−	−	−	−	+	+	+	+	+	+	+	+	+	−	−	−
*Pseudomonas aeruginosa**	−	−	−	−	−	−	−	+	−	−	−	−	+	−	+	−	−	−
Rickettsiae	−	−	−	−	−	−	−	−	−	+	+	−	−	−	−	−	−	−
Lymphogranuloma group	−	−	−	−	−	−	−	−	−	+	+	−	−	−	−	−	−	−
Fungi																		
Candida albicans	−	−	−	−	−	−	−	−	−	−	−	−	−	−	−	−	+	+
Dermatophytes	−	−	−	−	−	−	−	−	−	−	−	−	−	−	−	+	−	−
Viruses**	−	−	−	−	−	−	−	−	−	−	−	−	−	−	−	−	−	−
c: bactericidal s: bacteriostatic	s	s	c	c	c	c	c	c	c	s	s	c	c	c	c	s	s	s

*These species may acquire resistance by the transfer of R plasmids; the choice of antibiotic for therapy must be determined by sensitivity testing.
**Viruses are unaffected by the various antibiotics in clinical use. The considerable variety of antibiotics which affect DNA and RNA synthesis, and are capable of inhibiting virus replication in vitro (e.g. actinomycin, ribavirin), are far too toxic for normal clinical use so chemotherapeutics are employed. Sensitivity alone does not necessarily indicate the drug of choice for therapy; pharmacological properties must also be taken into consideration.
+: sensitive, (+): less sensitive or different strains give different levels of sensitivity, −: resistant.

Chapter 7

The incidence of antibiotic resistance *in vivo* is directly related to the intensity of antibiotic usage for whatever purpose and the route by which the antibiotic is administered. For instance, it is well established that antibiotics administered by the oral route in any (even sub-lethal) dosage have a profound effect on the gut flora both in its composition and in the selection of antibiotic-resistant strains. With the ever increasing use of antibiotics, the incidence and range of antibiotic resistance has steadily increased and it is doubtful that the process has yet reached equilibrium. This has created concern that the usefulness of antibiotics in the treatment of disease will decline with time.

Antibiotics and the emergence of bacterial resistance

If the main deleterious effect of antibiotic use is the emergence of resistant populations, it is important to discuss how these arise. Antibacterial agents do not cause bacteria to become resistant; their use selects resistant populations where resistant bacteria are already present. But where do these resistant bacteria come from? Surveys of culture collections made before the antibiotic era have revealed that genes coding for antibiotic resistance to various agents were already present (Richmond 1965). These resistance genes were not obvious until antibiotics became available but, once they did, the few bacteria carrying them were selected at the expense of sensitive strains and emerged to become dominant in microbial populations.

A number of questions may assist in clarifying the problem. How did resistance genes arise in the first place? Are new resistance genes being developed with time? What are the main mechanisms for the emergence of antibiotic resistance in sensitive populations? These questions will be considered below.

How did resistance genes arise prior to the antibiotic era?

At the moment we have no clear answer to this question. One theory is that they evolved from genes coding for different cellular functions but which were capable of stepwise modification by mutation (Gale *et al* 1981, Pollock 1967). Many resistances are due to enzyme inactivation of antibiotics. Thus chloramphenicol is inactivated by an acetylating enzyme (chloramphenicol acetyltransferase which uses acetyl-coenzme A as a co-factor). This may have evolved from some other enzyme which also used the co-factor. Analogous origins have been proposed for the enzymes which inactivate β-lactams and aminoglycosides (Richmond 1980).

Are new resistance genes being developed with time?

Without doubt, genes coding for resistance are evolving all the time. In some cases it is a matter of enzyme induction which occurs when the bacteria are exposed to an antibiotic. The genes coding for these antibiotic-destroying enzymes are already present but an ever increasing capacity to produce the enzyme is induced by exposure to the antibiotic. Induction of penicillinase in staphylococci during penicillin therapy is one example.

Many genetic resistance determinants (R determinants) are sited on relatively small pieces of extrachromosomal DNA (R plasmid) which can be lost or gained by a bacterium (see below) without loss of viability. Many of these genes can in turn change their position on DNA molecules by a process of transposition whereby a defined piece of the DNA moves from one DNA molecule to another. Thus by this process the genetic content is undergoing continuing evolution and new combinations of genes are likely to appear in the future.

What are the main mechanisms for the emergence of antibiotic resistance in erstwhile sensitive populations?

The situation is aggravated by the fact that R plasmids in one bacterium may be transferred to sensitive ones by several mechanisms; they include transformation, transduction, and conjugation.

Transformation. This is a method of transfer by which free DNA is transferred from one cell to another. If the DNA codes for antibiotic resistance, the recipient cell becomes instantly resistant. Transformation occurs rarely in nature, but can be demonstrated readily in the laboratory.

Transduction. This involves a bacterial virus (bacteriophage or phage) which carries the DNA from one bacterium to another. The phage replicates in an antibiotic-resistant bacterium. During the stage of phage maturation, when the new phage DNA is assembled within new phage coats, by chance the new phage particle may pick up a small piece of bacterial DNA instead of phage DNA. This is carried by the phage to a sensitive bacterium and the DNA coding for resistance is released into the sensitive cell during the process of phage infection. Transduction is especially important for the transfer of resistance genes between staphylococci and has been shown to occur *in vivo*.

Conjugation (sexual mating). This occurs in many Gram-negative bacteria, including Enterobacteriaceae, *Pseudomonas* spp., *Vibrio* spp., etc. The resistant donor bacterium synthesises a surface structure (sex pilus) which can attach to a receptor site on a sensitive (recipient) bacterium. The DNA coding for resistance (often called an R plasmid) is then transferred from the donor cell into the recipient cell. The mechanism is referred to as conjugal transfer and involves a form of DNA replication which results in a copy of the R plasmid being transferred into the recipient cell. Once the recipient cell has acquired the plasmid DNA it, in turn, becomes a donor cell. The whole process of plasmid transfer and conversion of the recipient into a donor takes about an hour, although the actual DNA transfer occupies less than 10 minutes. Because recipients can become donors, the spread of resistance genes through a population can occur rapidly.

R plasmids may code for resistance to one or many antibiotics and the R plasmid may be transferred in part or whole. The range of resistance acquired by the recipient cell depends, therefore, on the number of R determinants transferred.

Transfer by conjugation occurs not only between bacteria of the same species, e.g. between *Escherichia coli,* but also between species of different genera of Gram-negative bacteria, e.g. between *E. coli* and *Salmonella* spp. or *Shigella* spp. Since transfer can occur between non-pathogens and pathogens, the reservoir of R plasmids in non-pathogenic micro-organisms is of great importance in clinical medicine.

How does the use of antibiotics influence the resistance?

It must be re-emphasised that, apart from processes involving enzyme induction, antibiotics *per se* do not create antibiotic resistance or, indeed, affect the transfer frequencies of R plasmids. What they do is to inhibit the sensitive members of a population and select the resistant ones. Overall, therefore, the use of antibiotics for whatever purpose in animals, agriculture and man, selects an ever widening range of resistant bacteria which is arising particularly by gene transfer. Transfer is rarely demonstrated in the gut of normal animals not receiving antibiotics; the converse, however, is invariably true.

The use of one antibiotic will obviously select strains of bacteria resistant to that particular agent. If, however, the resistant bacteria carry R plasmids coding for a number of R determinants, the same antibiotic will select strains resistant to all.

There is little evidence that fundamentally new mechanisms of resistance are appearing at any great frequency — rather resistant strains, consequent upon adaptation and mixing of resistance genes by transfer and transposition, are on the increase and the position is aggravated by the increase in antibiotic usage.

The incidence of antibiotic resistance in domestic animals

As already emphasised, antibiotic resistance arises by selection consequent upon the use of antibiotics. The incidence of antibiotic resistance in domestic animals will be considered without prejudice to the purpose for which the antibiotic was used, i.e. therapy, prophylaxis, or growth promotion. Since the incidence of antibiotic resistance in animal pathogens differs quite markedly from that experienced in members of the indigenous flora, especially of the mouth and gut, they are considered separately.

Acquired antibiotic resistance in animal pathogens

Acquired resistance is not uniformly experienced in all groups of animal pathogens. The bovine mastitis streptococci, for example, are as sensitive to benzylpenicillin today as they were when this antibiotic was first introduced to clinical use. Consequently widespread use of the proprietary intra-mammary preparation, *Streptopen* (a mixture of streptomycin and benzyl-penicillin), has reduced the incidence of the penicillin-sensitive mastitis streptococci which have been replaced by penicillin-resistant staphylococci and naturally insusceptible *Escherichia coli*.

Acquired resistance is found mainly in two groups of organisms: *Staphylococcus aureus* and the enteric Gram-negative bacilli. Soon after penicillin was used in the intramammary treatment of bovine mastitis, penicillin-resistant strains of *St. aureus* began to appear. Invariably these strains produced large amounts of the enzyme penicillinase (β-lactamase) which split the active penicillin molecule at the β-lactam bridge, thereby rendering the drug ineffective. By 1961, 70% of all isolates were penicillin resistant (Pearson 1977) and this level has been maintained to date.

The other group of pathogenic micro-organisms, the salmonellae, in which antibiotic resistance is a very real problem has demonstrated an uneven incidence of antibiotic resistance. Despite the ever-increasing oral use of antibiotics in animal husbandry and veterinary medicine, relatively few Salmonella serotypes in the UK have shown resistance to thera-peutically useful antibiotics (Table 7.3). A large proportion have been resistant to sulphonamide and streptomycin — neither of which are indi-cated in treatment — but relatively few have been found to be resistant to broad spectrum antibiotics. Where problems of multi-resistance have arisen this has occurred almost exclusively in a relatively small number of phage types of one serotype, *Salmonella typhimurium*. In the 1960s, an outbreak occurred in calves which was caused by phage type 29 (Anderson 1968).

Table 7.3 The percentage of all salmonella isolates, submitted to the Central Veterinary Laboratory, resistant to individual drugs. (From Linton 1981.)

	Su	S	T	C	N	A	F	Trm
1971	55	81	1	<1	<1	4	2	0
1972	34	91	3	1	4	1	<1	0
1973	66	76	5	<1	1	<1	1	0
1974	64	48	5	<1	1	<1	<1	0
1975	77	39	3	<1	1	<1	1	<1
1976	75	65	5	<1	1	1	1	<1
1977	49	46	9	6	1	1	1	<1
1978	66	54	18	12	6	7	1	1
1979	56	54	16	11	7	8	2	5

Su	Sulphonamide (50 μg)	A Ampicillin (10 μg)
S	Streptomycin (10 μg)	F Furazolidone (15 μg)
T	Tetracycline (10 μg)	Trm Trimethoprim/sulphamethoxazole (25 μg)
C	Chloramphenicol (10 μg)	(Data 1% and above rounded up to the nearest %)
N	Neomycin (10 μg)	

Initially the strain was sensitive to most available antibiotics but the range of resistances increased with time as more antibiotics were used for prophylaxis and therapy. The outbreak came to an end in 1968–69.

More recently a series of phage types of *S. typhimurium* (types 193, 204, 204C, etc.) — each derived from a parent phage type (type 49) by R plasmid transfer (Threlfall *et al* 1978, 1980, Rowe *et al* 1979) — have caused serious outbreaks in calves with subsequent spread to man. These strains carry between four and seven R determinants including resistance to sulphonamides, streptomycin, tetracycline, chloramphenicol, ampicillin, kanamycin/neomycin, and trimethoprim.

Since outbreaks in animals by multi-resistant strains of salmonella have been relatively few it must be deduced that other factors, in addition to the selective pressure of antibiotics, must be important. The circumstances which encourage the genetic events by which resistance is transferred to salmonellae must be rare. However, once a multi-resistant strain has arisen what started as a rare event can explode into a countrywide epidemic by the movement of infected calves — a practice very common in the calf industry (Linton 1981).

Acquired antibiotic resistance in the normal flora

The composition of the normal gut flora of domestic animals is highly complex and varies from species to species and with age. It is not surprising, therefore, that the incidence of antibiotic resistance also varies between animal species and between different bacterial species which make up the complex flora. The most work has been done studying *E. coli* in the regular meat animals.

Animals kept at pasture and the older ruminant in which the rumenal flora has developed, carry relatively few antibiotic-resistant strains of *E. coli* (Linton 1977). This is due, in part, to the fact that the specialised rumenal flora displaces the conventional flora of the younger animal and consequently the numbers of *E. coli* are relatively small. Also, animals at pasture are rarely treated with antibiotics and certainly receive none as growth additives. In contrast, housed animals, especially those managed intensively, often receive oral antibiotics as growth promoters and therapeutically to control scours, etc. Even low levels of antibiotics, as used for growth promotion, select resistant strains. Consequently antibiotic-resistant *E. coli* are prevalent in the gut flora of calves, pigs, and poultry (Fig. 7.1) and this is particularly the case with animals reared intensively, such as veal calves (Linton *et al* 1981). Strains of *E. coli* resistant to seven or eight antibiotics are regularly encountered.

The widespread use of oral antibiotics in domestic animals over many years, and the transfer of R plasmids between members of the gut flora, has resulted in many multi-resistant O serotypes of *E. coli* being regularly present. These have become established in the stable gut flora and persist long after the antibiotic pressure has been withdrawn. Because they are good colonisers of particular animal species, these antibiotic-resistant strains are found frequently even in animals not being given antibiotics.

The importance of antibiotic-resistant bacteria

A knowledge of the natural susceptibility or insusceptibility of various animal pathogens (see Table 7.2) enables the clinician to select the best antibiotic for treatment. Infection by a species which is able to acquire resistance genes presents an unpredictable problem and, apart from clinical experience of likely events, the only rational approach is to determine the sensitivity/resistance spectrum of the causal agent and select the best antibiotic based on that information.

Acquired antibiotic resistance in animal infections is most commonly experienced in *Staphylococcus aureus, Pseudomonas aeruginosa* and salmonellae. Infections by multi-resistant *Salmonella typhimurium,* for instance, may cause fatal septicaemia, particularly in calves, and are virtually untreatable by antibiotics. They also reach man by cross-infection (see Fig. 7.1). In man, most infections with antibiotic-resistant strains of salmonellae, are neither more nor less important than infections by sensitive ones, since

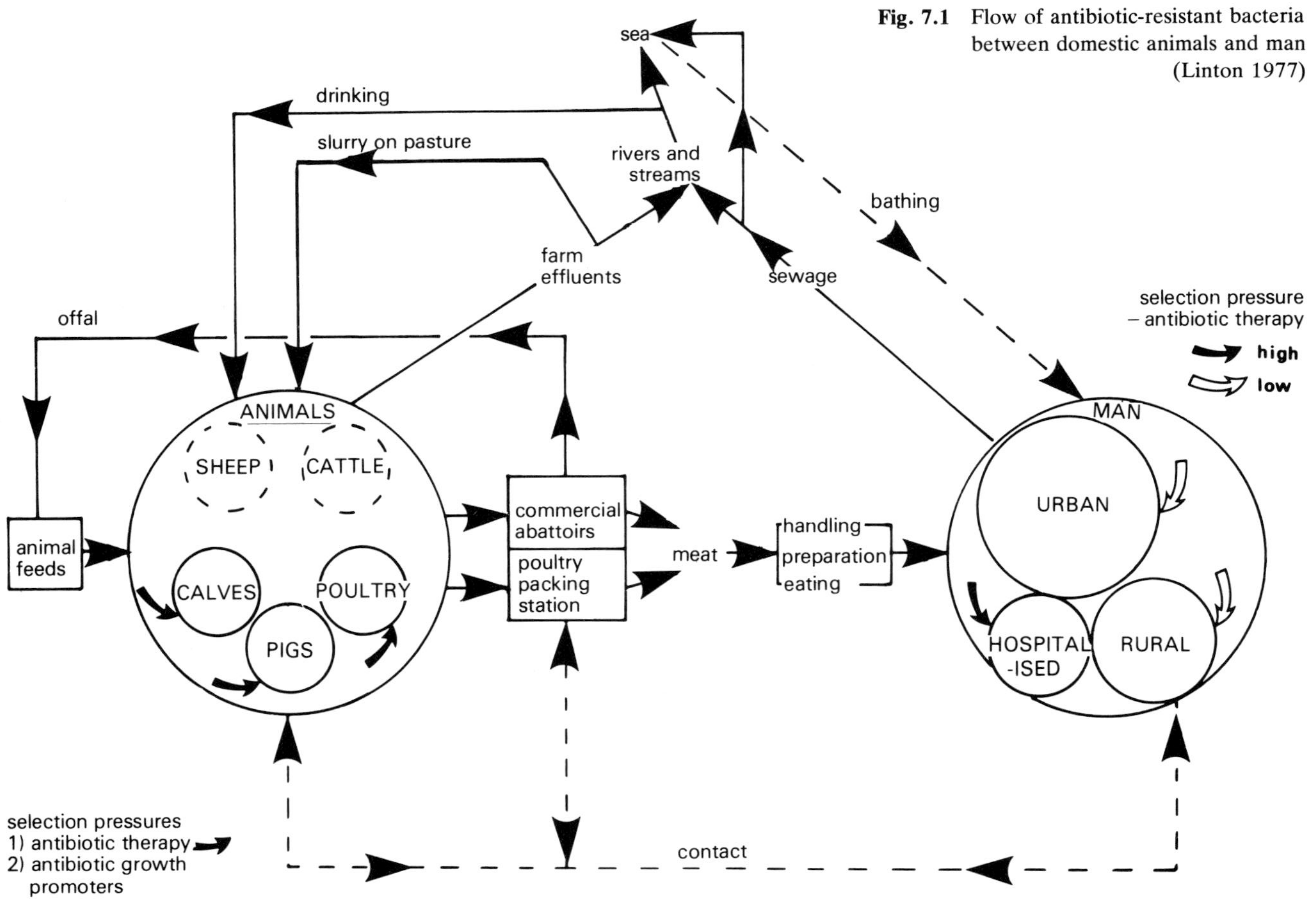

Fig. 7.1 Flow of antibiotic-resistant bacteria between domestic animals and man (Linton 1977)

antibiotics are rarely indicated for treatment. In a few cases, however, particularly infections in the very young or elderly, salmonellae can cause fatal meningitis or septicaemias.

The significance of antibiotic-resistant *E. coli* is less clear. Infections by *E. coli* in animals, such as coliform mastitis, are usually caused by antibiotic-sensitive strains derived from the cows' gut flora (Linton *et al* 1979). Resistant strains of animal origin are likely to be of greatest importance as a rich reservoir of R plasmids both for animal pathogens and, indirectly, for man. There is suggestive evidence that the *S. typhimurium* responsible for the outbreak in the calf industry which began in 1977 derived their R plasmids from non-pathogenic gut organisms (Linton *et al* 1981).

Carcasses of animals at slaughter are frequently contaminated by antibiotic-resistant *E. coli* from the gut flora (Linton 1977, Linton *et al* 1977a, Linton *et al* 1977c). These pass along the food chain (Fig. 7.1) and eventually colonise man (Linton *et al* 1977b). There is no evidence that these strains cause disease episodes in man, such as urinary tract infections, but they are a potential source of R plasmids for the indigenous gut flora of man and may be transferred to human pathogens. R plasmids regularly found in *E. coli* have now been demonstrated in *Haemophilus influenzae* (Saunders *et al* 1978) and gonococci (Elwell *et al* 1977, Sox *et al* 1979).

Guidelines for the appropriate use of antibiotics

As pointed out earlier, antibiotic resistance arises as a consequence of the use of antibiotics. The use of these agents in animals and man is certainly excessive; they are too often used where, on rational grounds, they are not indicated, or the wrong agent is used, or they are given for too long a period, or at too high a dose. There is need, therefore, for a more prudent use of these agents both in the human and veterinary fields. Only by so doing will the rate of increase of antibiotic resistance be limited.

Objectives for antibiotic use

The first of these is the successful treatment of infection in the patient, but treating one patient may increase the risk to others of acquiring an infection with resistant organisms. To minimise this risk:

1   The antibiotic used should be one to which the infecting organism has been shown to be sensitive, or, if this is not practicable, to which the putative infecting organism can be expected to be sensitive.
2   It should have as narrow a spectrum of activity as possible.
3   It should be given in dosage adequate to effect cure.
4   It should be used for the least possible time.

5 It should be given where possible by routes other than the oral route, which has a profound effect on the gut flora.

The therapeutic use of antibiotics

The decision to administer an antibiotic is the responsibility of the veterinary surgeon who has the animal under his care. In good clinical practice the correct use of antibiotics for treatment depends on accurate clinical diagnosis supported, whenever possible, by laboratory evidence of the nature of the infecting organism and its susceptibility to antibiotics. In many cases, however, it is necessary to begin treatment before the causative organism has been isolated and in others it may not be possible to obtain laboratory evidence of its identity. In these circumstances 'best-choice' treatment of severe infections must be based on experience and on a knowledge of the current antibiotic susceptibility of the more likely causes of the infection. It must be stressed, however, that a good laboratory service can do much to improve the quality of antibiotic prescribing. Reporting of results must be as rapid as possible to provide the veterinary surgeon with sound information as early as possible in the course of treatment.

Large numbers of preparations containing mixtures of antibiotics increase the risk of antibiotic resistance arising. Apart from certain well established fixed-ratio combinations such as streptopen and co-trimoxazole, these preparations should be discouraged.

The prophylactic use of antibiotics

The prophylactic use of antibiotics is frequently practised to safeguard intensively reared animals against potential infection. However, this should not be used routinely in the absence of proven infection and is no substitute for good hygiene in animal-rearing establishments.

Antibiotics should be used prophylactically only when there is good evidence that the treatment will significantly reduce the frequency of infection. With few exceptions it will be successful in situations in which the risk of infection is short lived and where the antibiotic is given before the infecting organism has gained a foothold in the animal.

The use of antibiotics for growth promotion (see Chapter 6)

Following the recommendations of the Swann Committee (Anon 1969), the use of therapeutically important antibiotics for growth promotion has been banned in the UK except under veterinary prescription. The ban has not been altogether successful (Linton 1981) but it was introduced in the belief that many antibiotic growth promoters select for resistant bacteria. Other non-therapeutic antibiotics and non-antibiotic products are available and their use should be encouraged to avoid the complications arising from the use of therapeutically important antibiotics.

It must be emphasised, however, that banning the use of therapeutic antibiotics for growth promotion is likely to have limited effect unless there is a significant reduction in their administration to animals (and man) for other purposes.

References

Anderson E. S. (1968) Drug resistance in *Salmonella typhimurium* and its implications. *Br. Med. J.* **3**, 333–339.

Anon (1969) *Swann Report. Report of the Joint Committee on the use of antibiotics in Animal Husbandry and Veterinary Medicine.* HMSO, London

Elwell L. P., Roberts M., Mayer L. W. *et al* (1977) Plasmid-mediated β-lactamase production in *N. gonorrhoeae. Antimicrob. Agents & Chemoth.* **11**, 528–533.

Gale E. F., Cundliffe E., Reynolds P. E. *et al* (1981) *The Molecular Basis of Antibiotic Action,* 2nd edn. John Wiley, New York.

Linton A. H. (1977) Antibiotic resistance — the present situation reviewed. *Vet. Rec.* **100**, 354–360.

Linton A. H. (1981) Has Swann failed? *Vet. Rec.* **108**, 328–331.

Linton A. H., Handley B., Osborne A. D. *et al* (1977a) Contamination of pig carcasses at two abattoirs by *Escherichia coli* with special reference to O-serotypes and antibiotic resistance. *J. Appl. Bacteriol.* **42**, 89–110.

Linton A. H., Howe K., Bennett P. M. *et al* (1977b) The colonization of the human gut by antibiotic resistant *Escherichia coli* from chickens. *J. Appl. Bacteriol.* **43**, 465–69.

Linton A. H., Howe K., Hartley C. L. *et al* (1977c) Antibiotic resistance among *Escherichia coli* O-serotypes from the gut and carcasses of commercially slaughtered broiler chickens: a potential public health hazard. *J. Appl. Bacteriol.* **42**, 365–378.

Linton A. H., Howe K., Sojka W. J. *et al* (1979) A note on the range of *Escherichia coli* O-serotypes causing clinical bovine mastitis and their antibiotic resistance spectra. *J. Appl. Bacteriol.* **46**, 585–590.

Linton A. H., Timoney J. F. & Hinton A. H. (1981) The ecology of chloramphenicol resistance in *Salmonella typhimurium* phage type 204 and *Escherichia coli* in calves with endemic salmonella infection. *J. Appl. Bacteriol.* **50**, 115–129.

Pearson J. K. L. (1977) Intramammary therapy: its achievement and limitations. In *Antibiotics and Antibiosis in Agriculture,* ed. M. Woodbine. Butterworths, London.

Pollock M. R. (1967) The function and evolution of penicillinase: a problem of biochemical evolution. *Br. Med. J.* **4**, 71–77.

Richmond M. H. (1965) Wild-type variants of exo-penicillinase from *Staphylococcus aureus. Biochem. J.* **94**, 584–593.

Richmond M. H. (1980) *The Evolution of Antibiotic Resistance.* E. R. Squibb Lectures on the Chemistry of Microbial Products. The Squibb Institute for Medical Research, Princeton.

Rowe B., Threlfall E. J., Ward L. R. *et al* (1979) International spread of multiresistant strains of *Salmonella typhimurium* phage types 204 and 193 from Britain to Europe. *Vet. Rec.* **105**, 468–469.

Saunders J. R., Elwell L. P., Falkow S. *et al* (1978) β-lacatamases and R-plasmids of

Haemophilus influenzae. Scand. J. Infect. Dis. (Suppl.) **13,** 16–122.
Sox T. E., Mohammed W. & Sparling P. F. (1979) Transformation-derived *Neisseria gonorrhoeae* plasmids with altered structure and function. *J. Bacteriol.* **138,** 510–518.
Threlfall E. J., Ward L. R., Ashley A. S. *et al* (1980) Plasmid-encoded trimethoprim resistance in multiresistant epidemic *Salmonella typhimurium* types 204 and 193 in Britain. *Br. Med. J.* **280,** 1210–1211.
Threlfall E. J., Ward L. R. & Rowe B. (1978) Epidemic spread of *Salmonella typhimurium* phage type 204 in bovine animals in Britain. *Vet. Rec.* **103,** 438–440.

PART 3
IMMUNOLOGY AND PARASITOLOGY

8

Basic immunology and vaccination

R. BOMFORD

This chapter is not intended to cover all of the vast field of contemporary immunology. For this, the reader is referred to the many excellent textbooks now available (see p. 158). Rather, it is intended to focus attention on those aspects of classical and contemporary immunology, particularly the mechanisms of resistance to infection which are most relevant to large animal vaccination.

Humoral and cell-mediated immunity

When an animal is exposed to foreign material that can be recognised by the immune system (an antigen) two types of immune response are possible.

Humoral immunity results from the appearance of circulating immunoglobulins (antibodies) capable of attaching to the antigen. Alternatively immune lymphocytes may be generated carrying cell-surface receptors which enable them to recognise the antigen and mediate a variety of immunological reactions (such as the tuberculin reaction or graft rejection). This type of immunity is called cell-mediated and can only be transferred from animal to animal by injections of immune cells and not by serum. As will be explained more fully below, humoral and cell-mediated immunity are attributable to different populations of cells and are responsible for resistance to different types of infection. Some of their more important characteristics are summarised in Table 8.1. Humoral and cell-mediated immunity are not mutually exclusive and may coexist in the same animal.

Active and passive immunity

Active immunity is a general term for the state of humoral or cell-mediated immunity that is established as a result of the stimulation of an animal's immune system by an antigen. Passive immunity is acquired by an animal following the transfer of immune serum or cells from an immune donor.

Table 8.1 Humoral and cell-mediated immunity.

Humoral immunity	Cell-mediated immunity
Mediated by antibody (immunoglobin)	Mediated by cells (immune lymphocytes, sometimes cooperating with macrophages)
Transferred between animals by antibody (e.g. tetanus antitoxin, lamb dysentery antiserum)	Transferred between animals only by cells, not by antibody
Confers resistance to extracellular viruses, bacteria and bacterial toxins	Confers resistance to intracellular viruses and bacteria (e.g. Mycobacteria, Brucella)

Vaccination is expected to elicit active immunity of a type which will confer immunity to infection. For this to occur, three conditions must be fulfilled.

1 The vaccine must contain the right antigen. Organisms frequently possess antigens which generate a strong immune response, without conferring any protective immunity.

2 The antigen must be injected in a form that will stimulate the maximum immune response. When a vaccine is prepared from killed organisms, or part of an organism such as a toxin, materials called adjuvants (to be discussed below), which render the antigens more capable of provoking an immune response, are usually added. Vaccines consisting of living attenuated organisms generally do not require an adjuvant.

3 The immune system of the animal must be capable of responding to the antigen. In practice this means that the animal should preferably not be very young, when the immune system may be immature, or either old or sick, both these latter states being associated with a diminished responsiveness of the immune system.

Successful vaccination provides long-lived immunity over months or years. This is sometimes the result of chronic stimulation of the immune system by persisting antigen or of immunological memory (p. 150).

In the veterinary field, passive immunity is provided to animals by injections of antiserum preparations such as tetanus antitoxin or lamb dysentery antiserum. The advantage of passive immunity is that it is instantaneously effective, there being no lag period while the host immune response develops, as after vaccination. It also provides protection in animals whose own immune system is immature or impaired. The major drawback is that protection is short-lived. Homologous antisera (from the same species as the recipient) have a half-life of about three weeks, as a result of destruction by the normal processes of catabolism of serum proteins. Heterologous sera, from a different species, disappear from the circulation abruptly about two weeks after injection because the host begins to make antibodies against them. The antigen–antibody complexes which are formed can cause a potentially dangerous pathological reaction called serum sickness, an example of the general phenomenon of hypersensitivity (p. 157).

Passive immunisation occurs naturally when antibodies are transferred from the mother to the foetus via the placenta, or to the newborn in the colostrum. This phenomenon can be exploited to provide protection of the newborn by vaccinating the mother. Thus sows may be vaccinated with *E. coli* antigens to provide piglets with resistance against the enteritis caused by this bacterium.

The cellular basis of antibody production

Antibodies are protein molecules, composed of four polypeptide chains — two light and two heavy — joined together by disulphide bridges into a Y shape (Fig. 8.1). The two sites capable of binding to antigens are located at the ends of the prongs of the Y. An antibody molecule can therefore bind to two antigenic sites simultaneously. This can cause cross-linking of molecules of antigen, seen as immunoprecipitation of soluble antigens or haemagglutination of red cells.

The other end of the antibody molecule, at the base of the Y, is known as the Fc region, because, in certain types of antibodies, it contains a receptor

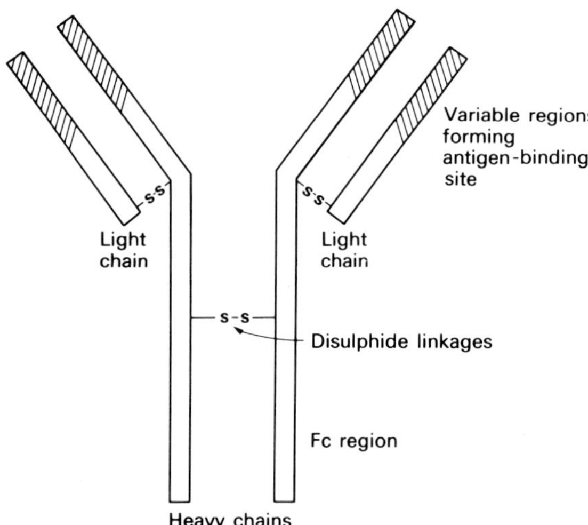

Fig. 8.1　Y-shaped arrangement of polypeptide chains in antibodies.

capable of binding serum components known as complement. The receptor
becomes able to interact with complement only after the antibody has
combined with antigen. Complement is involved in the destruction of
micro-organisms and cells to which antibody has become attached. Its
nature and function will be discussed more fully on p. 152.

The recognition of an antigen by an antibody requires molecular com-
plementarity between the antigenic determinant and the antigen-binding
site on the antibody (the 'lock and key' analogy). An animal has the capability for making approximately a million different antibody molecules. The
specificity of the antigen-binding site is controlled by the amino acid sequence of the polypeptide chains in that part of the molecule; thus the ends of
the light and heavy chains which form the site vary widely in their sequences
between different antibodies. This section of the chain is known as the
variable region. The other ends of the chains, the constant regions, are
uniform in amino acid sequence.

One question that has greatly puzzled immunologists is that, given that
there are about a million different antibody molecules, each with specific
amino acid sequence in the variable regions, are there correspondingly a
million separate genes in the genome providing the necessary genetic information? This question has now been partially answered. The genes coding
for the constant and variable regions are on the same chromosome, but in
embryo cells the two genes are separated from each other by a stretch of
DNA about 1000 base pairs long. There are one or a few copies of the
constant region gene, but many copies of the variable region gene. During
development of the cell the constant region gene becomes more closely
coupled up to one of the variable region genes, which will code for the
specificity of the antibody the cell will eventually make. Even though each
cell contains many variable region genes, it is generally believed that there
are still not enough to code for the entire range of antibody molecules. This
difficulty is overcome if it is assumed that precursors of antibody-forming
cells can carry different sets of variable region genes. The favoured hypothesis for the origin of this variation is that crossing-over occurs between the
multiple copies of the variable region genes during the development, creating new DNA base sequences not present in the germ line.

Antibodies are synthesised by differentiated lymphocytes called plasma
cells. The precursors of plasma cells carry immunoglobulin (antibody)
molecules of a single specificity in their cell membranes. These cell surface
immunoglobulins function as receptors, to which antigen can combine,
provided that it will fit into the antigen-recognising region of the immunoglobulin.

For some antigens which consist of a series of repeated identical antigenic determinants (e.g. some bacterial polysaccharides like dextrans or

levans, or single proteins such as collagen), the binding of antigen is sufficient to trigger the plasma cell precursor to differentiate into a plasma cell which will secrete antibody. However, for the majority of antigens it is now clear that the participation of a second type of lymphocyte is required for antibody production. This cell does not itself synthesise antibody but, after combining with antigen through a cell surface receptor (the chemical nature of which is still not fully understood, but which is certainly not entirely immunoglobulin), it produces soluble factors which stimulate or 'help' the plasma cell precursor to initiate antibody synthesis. The antibody-producing lymphocyte has come to be known as 'B' lymphocyte and the second cell as a 'helper T or T_H' cell. One model for the interaction between B and T_H cells is shown in Fig. 8.2.

Fig. 8.2 is a simplification, in that it is now certain that macrophages are involved in the initiation of the immune response. T lymphocytes are particularly responsive to antigen associated with histocompatibility antigen on the macrophage surface membrane.

The two categories of lymphocytes received the designation T and B because of their different migration patterns in the body. All lymphocytes originate from stem cells in the bone marrow. Those that are destined to synthesise antibody migrate, in birds, to a lymphoid organ called the bursa of Fabricus and then on to the lymph nodes and spleen. Passage through the bursa is essential to acquire the capacity for antibody formation; hence the designation B cells. The mammalian equivalent of the bursa has not been

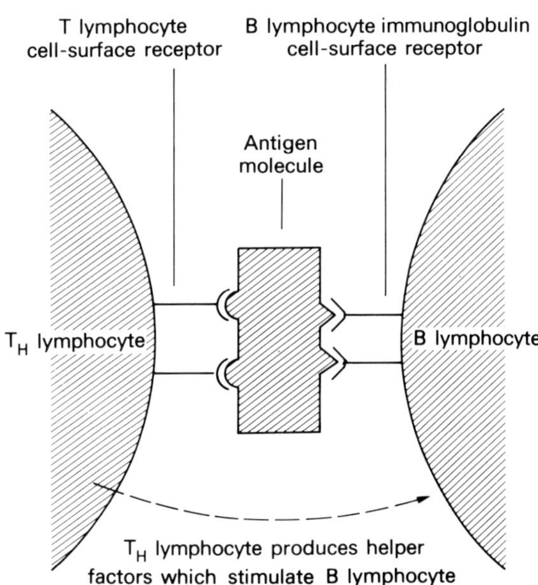

Fig. 8.2 A model for the interaction between T_H and B lymphocytes.

Table 8.2 Origin of T and B lymphocytes.

	Site of production of precursors from stem cells	Site of differentiation to T or B cells	Site of immunological function
B cells	Bone marrow	Avian bursa of Fabricius, mammalian bursal equivalent	Lymph nodes, spleen, etc.
T cells	Bone marrow	Thymus gland	Lymph nodes, spleen, etc.

identified with certainty, although the favoured candidate is the foetal liver. Future T cells must pass through the thymus gland on their way from the bone marrow to the peripheral lymphoid organs. The migration patterns of T_H and B cells are shown in Table 8.2.

Immunological memory

Not all of the B cells which come into contact with antigen go on to produce antibody. Some of them are stimulated to divide to produce more cells which are capable of recognising antigen, but which differentiate into plasma cells only after a second encounter with antigen. These cells are known as memory cells, and are responsible for the well known phenomenon of the secondary immune response; or the increased antibody production after a second exposure to antigen. It has also been established that there are T_H memory cells.

Clearly, memory cells might play a very important role in vaccination. The vaccine may confer protection by eliciting the formation of antibody (which will be immediately available if infection strikes) or alternatively by generating memory cells, which are relatively long-lived — lifespans of up to four months having been recorded in the mouse. When repeated vaccinations are administered, the best response is obtained by allowing an interval of weeks or months between injections. This may be explicable in terms of a need to allow the full complement of memory cells to develop before the animal is re-exposed to antigen.

Immunological adjuvants

As mentioned previously, most veterinary vaccines which are made from killed microbial material contain an adjuvant. Some examples are listed in Table 8.3. The most commonly used adjuvants are the gels of aluminium

Table 8.3 Immunological adjuvants used in large animal vaccines.

Adjuvant	Chemical composition	Used in
Aluminium salts	Aluminium hydroxide gel Aluminium phosphate gel Alum	Sheep Clostridium vaccine Sheep and pig Pasteurella vaccine Swine Erysipelas vaccine Tetanus vaccine
Oil emulsions (Freund's adjuvant)	Mineral oil and emulsifying agent	Louping ill vaccine Sheep foot rot vaccine
Saponin	Mixture of glycosides of triterpenoids	Foot-and-mouth disease vaccine

salts, and water-in-oil emulsions made with mineral oil. Both of these materials improve the immune response by holding the antigen at the site of injection so that it is slowly made available to the immune system, and not immediately degraded or excreted. Aluminium gels bind antigens electrostatically and, in the oily emulsions, the antigen is enclosed in the water droplets in the oil.

It is likely that adjuvants not only form an antigen deposit but also interact with the immune system. The most probable cellular site of action of adjuvants is the macrophage. There is evidence that macrophages which have been exposed to adjuvants are more effective at presenting antigen to lymphocytes and triggering an immune response.

Antibody and resistance to infection

Antibodies differ among themselves according to the antigen they can recognise, but can also be divided into classes with respect to the structure of their heavy chains. The different classes of antibody play distinct roles in resistance to infection. Table 8.4 summarises the properties of the major classes of antibody.

After subcutaneous or intramuscular vaccination the first antibody to appear in the blood will usually be IgM followed by IgG. Both these classes of antibody are able to neutralise bacterial toxins and viruses. Virus neutralisation occurs by coating of the virus cell-surface receptors, which are needed for attachment to and penetration of host cells. Bacteria or viruses which are covered by IgM or IgG antibodies become more susceptible to phagocytosis by macrophages. Antibodies which promote phagocytosis are given the general title of opsonising antibodies.

IgA antibodies are found mostly in the sero-mucous secretions (saliva,

Table 8.4 Location and function of major classes of immunoglobulin.

Designation	Location	Function
IgM	Blood	First immunoglobulin to be produced after infection. Neutralisation and opsonisation viruses and bacteria
IgG	Blood and extravascular fluids	Neutralisation viruses and bacterial toxins. Opsonisation
IgA	Seromucous secretions	Immunity on external epithelial surfaces
IgE	Blood, and fixed to mast cells and basophils	High levels produced by parasite infection. Responsible for atopic allergy (e.g. hay fever and asthma)

tears, nasal fluids, colostrum, secretions of lung and gastrointestinal tract), where they form a first line of defence against invading micro-organisms. IgA antibody is formed locally at the site of infection by plasma cells in the relevant epithelium. This means that the conventional routes of vaccination — subcutaneous or intramuscular — may not be very effective against infections which are controlled by local IgA. One large animal vaccine which is believed to act through the IgA response is that against infectious bovine rhinitis virus, and this is administered intranasally.

IgE antibodies possess a molecular configuration which enables them to attach to mast cells and, when antigen is bound by IgE, the mast cell is triggered to degranulate. Histamine and other pharmacologically active agents are thereby released. This is the cause of such undesirable allergic reactions as hay fever and asthma. These reactions are called anaphylaxis, and are discussed more fully below. Very high levels of IgE antibody are sometimes found in animals suffering from nematode infections, but there is still controversy as to whether this antibody plays a protective role.

Complement

After a virus or a bacterium has been coated by antibody, the Fc region of the attached antibody becomes able to combine with complement. This is called complement fixation. The term 'complement' describes a group of nine serum proteins, designated C1 to C9. The first component of complement to react with antigen–antibody complexes is C1, followed by the rest in the order C4, 2, 3, 5, 6, 7, 8. 9. The whole process can be envisaged as a sequence or cascade of enzymatic reactions, each step catalysing the next. The components of complement which are known to be important in resis-

Table 8.5 Categories of T lymphocytes.

Category	Name	Function
Helper	T_H	Stimulates B cells to antibody formation
Killer	T_C	Cytotoxicity — kills foreign and virus-infected cells
Delayed-type hypersensitivity	T_{DH}	Releases factors which stimulate macrophages to enhanced bactericidal activity (e.g. Brucella immunity)
Suppressor	T_S	Inhibits function of B and other T lymphocytes

tance to infection are C3, C5, C8 and C9.

C3 is broken down during complement fixation into two pieces, C3a and C3b. Macrophages have a cell-surface receptor for C3b, which facilitates the phagocytosis of particles carrying bound C3b. C5 suffers a similar degradation into C5a and C5b. C5a is chemotactic for polymorphonuclear leucocytes. Fixed C8 and C9 between them generate a phospholipase activity which damages cell membranes. This contributes to the destruction of enveloped viruses and Gram-negative bacteria. The latter are rendered more susceptible to the enzyme lysozyme which is present in the lysosomal vesicles of polymorphs and macrophages.

The cellular basis of cell-mediated immunity

It is now clear that the lymphocytes which are involved in cell-mediated immunity are T cells, although they are distinct from the T_H cells which take part in antibody production. A summary of the presently-recognised categories of T cells is presented in Table 8.5.

Cell-mediated immunity and resistance to infection

T_C cells

T_C cells (the subscript c stands for cytotoxic) are able to attach to foreign cells by cell-surface receptors and to lyse them by a mechanism that is not yet fully understood. The first function which was ascribed to T_C cells was the destruction of grafts of foreign tissue (homograft rejection), since T_C cells are very efficient at recognising foreign transplantation (histocompatibility) antigens. However, it is obvious that invasion by foreign tissue is not a naturally occurring hazard (except during pregnancy, an immunologically interesting situation, where special mechanisms must have been evolved to avoid rejection of the foetus), and T_C cells were suspected to have some role other than frustrating the efforts of transplantation surgeons. It has recently

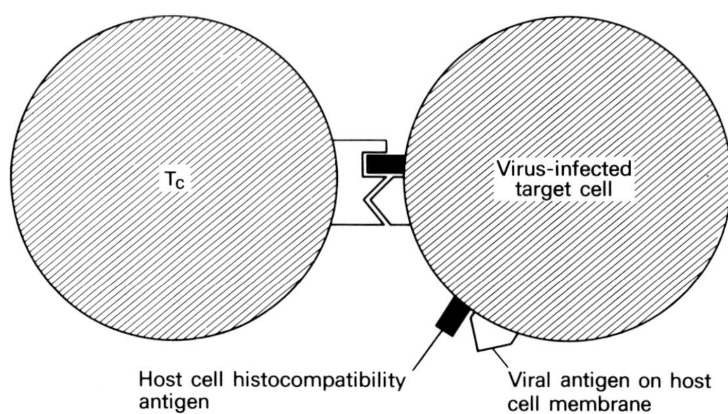

Fig. 8.3   Interaction between T killer cell and target host cell, and a result of which the latter is lysed.

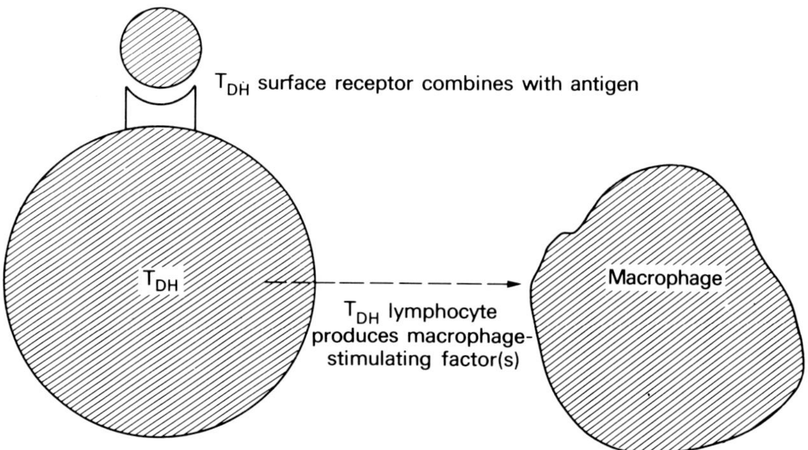

Fig. 8.4   Interaction between T_{DH} and macrophage, as a result of which the macrophage bactericidal capacity is enhanced.

been discovered that T_C cells can lyse virus-infected cells; in order to do this they must recognise some part of the target cell histocompatability antigen as well as viral antigen on the cell surface (Fig. 8.3).

T_{DH} cells

When T_{DH} cells recognise antigen through their cell-surface receptors they are stimulated to release soluble factors which control the physiology of macrophages (Fig. 8.4). As in the case of T_H cells, T_{DH} cells are responsive to antigen presented on the surface of macrophages. The best known of the factors released by T_{DH} cells is called MIF, or macrophage migrating inhibition factor. This slows down the movement of macrophages and so probably helps to localise them at the site of infection. Another factor, MAF (macrophage activation factor) increases the ability of macrophages to kill bacteria.

T_{DH} cells received their $_{DH}$ because they are responsible for the reaction of delayed-type hypersensitivity. A classical example of this is the tuberculin reaction, e.g. in guinea pigs — a reddening of the skin appearing 24 hours after the intradermal injection of material from the tubercule bacillus into infected animals. The delayed-type hypersensitivity reaction is the product of the recognition of antigen by T_{DH} cells, followed by the immigration, retention, and activation of macrophages.

T_{DH} cells provide protective immunity against bacteria which grow in macrophages, such as Mycobacteria, Listeria or Brucella. Animals infected with parasites frequently display delayed-type hypersensitivity to parasite antigens, although the precise role, if any, of these reactions in resistance to parasitic infection has yet to be clarified.

A number of large animal vaccines are thought to act through cell-mediated immunity, largely because protection is not correlated with antibody. The type of cell-mediated immunity is unknown, although it may be inferred that, for the viruses (e.g. orf or sheep pustular dermatitis), T_C cells are likely to be involved, and for the bacteria (anthrax, Brucella ,Salmonella) T_{DH} cells. It is interesting that most of these vacccines contain living organisms (although some Brucella vaccines use only killed bacteria). In contrast, the many viral (e.g. foot-and-mouth disease and louping ill) and bacterial (e.g. Clostridium, Erysipelas, *Fusiformis nodosus,* tetanus) vaccines known to protect through IgM or IgG antibodies are prepared from killed organisms or toxins. It may be that cell-mediated immunity is most readily evoked by living organisms capable of infecting host cells and changing their surface antigens so they are recognised as foreign by T_C or T_{DH} cells.

T_S cells

Several different types of T_S (suppressor) cells are now recognised which inhibit the functions of other categories of T or B cells. Their role is to exert feedback control over immune responses to foreign antigens, and they may also be important in preventing auto-immune reactions against the body's own constituents. As yet there is no known example of T_S cells interfering with vaccination, although this is clearly a theoretical possibility. The factors which control the triggering of T_S cells rather than other types of lymphocytes are beginning to be understood. For instance, in the case of some antigens, the intravenous injection of large doses of antigen will selectively elicit the appearance of T_S cells specifically capable of switching off the immune response to that antigen. Clearly, vaccines should be constituted and administered in such a way as to minimise the stimulation of T_S cells.

Macrophages

Some of the functions of the macrophage have already been alluded to in passing, but since the importance of this cell in the immune system is gaining increasing recognition, they will be described in more detail. Macrophages originate from precursors in the bone marrow, and are liberated into the bloodstream as relatively immature cells — monocytes. These migrate from the bloodstream to sites of inflammation, and also settle down to form the fixed population of macrophages in various organs, e.g. the Kupffer cells of the liver.

A role for macrophages in the initiation of the immune response has been adduced from the results of experiments *in vitro*. Mouse spleen cell suspensions incubated with an antigen such as sheep red blood cells will generate cells secreting antibody against the red blood cells. This does not happen if the macrophages are selectively removed from the spleen cell population prior to incubation with antigen. Separation of the macrophages is accomplished by allowing them to adhere to the culture vessel, and removing the non-adherent lymphocytes; or by the addition of iron particles which are phagocytosed by the macrophages, allowing them to be dragged to the bottom of the culture vessel with a magnet.

The details of the interactions between antigen, macrophages, and lymphocytes at the outset of the immune response have not yet been established. An early idea was that macrophages concentrate antigen on their cell surfaces, so that lymphocytes can be more effectively triggered. It is now suspected that more complicated processes occur. An important recent discovery is that, for the generation of T_H cells *in vitro,* the macrophages and lymphocytes in the culture must be syngeneic (i.e. from the same strain of mouse, and therefore carrying the same histocompatability antigens). It is now believed that the receptors T_H cells can only recognise antigens if they become intimately associated with host histocompatability antigens, and that this happens on macrophage surfaces.

The major role of the macrophage in the control of infection is exercised through phagocytosis. Materials coated by antibody are much more readily phagocytosed, because there are receptors on the macrophage membrane for the Fc region of IgG molecules, and also, as mentioned above, for C3b. The phagocytosed particles find themselves in cytoplasmic vesicles (phagosomes), which fuse with lysosomes to form phagolysosomes. The contents of the phagosomes are thus exposed to the enzymes (e.g. lysozyme) contained in the lysosomes. Gram-negative bacteria whose membrane has been damaged by complement are more susceptible to enzymatic attack.

It is now recognised that macrophages are major secretory cells. They release materials which are important for resistance to infection (C3 and interferon), a large number of enzymes (e.g. collagenase and esterase) which may play a role in chronic inflammation, pharmacologically-active agents (prostaglandins), and molecules which affect other cells involved in the immune response (e.g. colony stimulating factor, which promotes the formation of macrophages and granulocytes in the bone marrow, and lymphocyte activation factor, which improves the response of T lymphocytes to antigen). The phagocytic and secretory functions of macrophages can be enhanced by exposure to antigen–antibody complexes, and also to factors secreted by T lymphocytes. Such macrophages are referred to as activated. Thus the effector role of macrophages is stimulated by an ongoing humoral or cellular immune response.

Hypersensitivity reactions

The term 'hypersensitivity' is used to encompass all the pathological reactions that may follow the introduction of antigen into an animal that is already immune. Three types of hypersensitivity which are liable to cause anaphylaxis and complications during vaccination or serum therapy have already been mentioned. Their properties are summarised in Table 8.6.

If, in response to a previous immunisation, an animal has mounted an IgE response, there will be a danger of anaphylaxis after subsequent vaccination. When the injection is subcutaneous and antigen does not escape from the site of injection, the reaction will be confined to a local wheal and

Table 8.6 Classification of hypersensitivity reactions.

Time of appearance	Designation	Mediator
Immediate	Anaphylaxis	IgE on mast cells
	Complex-mediated	
	Arthus reaction	IgG-antigen complexes formed at site of injection of antigen into an immune animal
	Serum sickness	IgG-antigen complexes formed during clearance of a large quantity of antigen from the circulation
Delayed	Delayed-type hypersensitivity	T_{DH} cells

flare. However, if antigen reaches the circulation and combines with IgE on mast cells in sites such as the lungs or bronchi, the consequent histamine release will cause violent contraction of smooth muscle fibres. Signs of distress such as salivation or increased respiratory rate will appear. An intramuscular or subcutaneous injection of adrenaline should be given which modulates the release of histamine in the lung, and causes bronchodilation by a direct action, thus alleviating the respiratory distress by two mechanisms.

The injection of antigen into an animal in which IgG antibodies are circulating can cause complex-mediated hypersensitivity. After subcutaneous injection, antigen–antibody complexes in antibody excess can be deposited locally causing, amongst other things, histamine release and the attraction of neutrophil polymorphs. This is a consequence of complement fixation by the antigen–antibody complex. Split C5 is responsible for triggering histamine release from mast cells. The complexes also interact with the blood-clotting mechanism, leading to aggregation of platelets, which also contain histamine. The subsequent oedematous and necrotic reaction is called the Arthus reaction. Serum sickness results when large quantities of antigen reach the circulation. Antigen–antibody complexes in antigen excess can be formed. These are small, soluble, and not quickly cleared. They also trigger histamine release from mast cells, leucocytes, and platelets.

There is a considerable danger of serum sickness after treatment with heterologous antisera, and adrenaline should be available in case the signs (similar to those of anaphylaxis) appear. If it is suspected that the animal is already immune to the antiserum, for instance if multiple doses have already been given, an antihistamine drug may be injected 15–30 minutes before the antiserum.

References

Lachmann P. J. & Peters D. K. eds. (1982) *Clinical Aspects of Immunology,* 4th edn. Blackwell Scientific Publications, Oxford.
Herbert W. J. (1980) *Veterinary Immunology.* Blackwell Scientific Publications, Oxford.
Humphrey J. H. & White R. G. (1970) *Immunology for Students of Medicine,* 3rd edn. Blackwell Scientific Publications, Oxford.
Roitt I. (1980) *Essential Immunology,* 4th edn. Blackwell Scientific Publications, Oxford.
Tizard I. R. (1977) *An Introduction to Veterinary Immunology.* W. B. Saunders, Philadelphia.

9

Clinical immunology — immunisation

J. SCARNELL

The principles underlying the induction of increased resistance to infectious diseases by means of immunisation has been discussed in Chapter 8. This chapter will illustrate the practical implementation of these principles. While it may be too much to expect that perfect immunisation schedules can be evolved, great benefit must surely result from a better understanding of how current knowledge has been derived and how best this may now be applied. To this end the control of three diseases in large animal practice will be discussed: tetanus in the horse, salmonellosis caused by *Salmonella dublin* in the calf, and *Escherichia coli* diarrhoea in the unweaned pig.

Immunological responses are complex and among the determinants involved are:

1   the species of animal and its stage of development
2   the dose and particular presentation of the antigens
3   the concentration and type of adjuvant used.

In addition there is much individual variation. For these reasons specific recommendations can only be taken to apply to a specified product.

Prophylaxis of tetanus in the horse

The control of tetanus involves humoral antitoxic immunity to bacterial exotoxins. These antitoxins serve to neutralise the specific toxins which are produced at the site of localised proliferation of the organism before they are absorbed and reach susceptible cells.

Because tetanus has such characteristic signs, the disease has long been recognised and one of the earliest references in the horse was about 300 BC by Aristotle. It is not possible to define the precise economic importance of tetanus in the horse in the UK, since there are no returns of the total horse population and the disease is not notifiable. Its significance, however, is not measured only by its economic importance. Some infectious diseases have long been associated with intense public as well as scientific interest. Tetanus has this reputation. Also in some areas, the risk of infection is recognised to be particularly high, especially in the newborn foal.

No progress in the control of tetanus could be made until the essential features of its aetiology were recognised and the causative organism isolated. Almost immediately following this achievement, one of the most important advances in bacteriology was made: the discovery that experimental animals could be stimulated to produce antibodies against the organisms and thereby cease to be susceptible. In order that antitoxin could be obtained in considerable quantities, at first horses were immunised using iodised toxin. Antitoxin was later produced on a very large scale during the 1914–18 war from horses which were inoculated with toxin–antitoxin mixtures. Detoxification by formol and the antigenicity of the toxoids thus produced were then investigated and brought into field use for horses, especially from 1930 onwards when alum precipitation was discovered to enhance its antigenic value. However, marked local reactions were sometimes reported, particularly in thoroughbreds, and this led to investigations of other adjuvants such as aluminium hydroxide (Chodnik *et al* 1959). There is still a slight risk of reactions following the use of such vaccines and, although the incidence is low, the implications can be serious especially for valuable bloodstock and racehorses in training. Further purified fractions have therefore been introduced in order to develop a more suitable vaccine (Kerry *et al* 1976).

There are thus two main methods of inducing protection against tetanus — antitoxin for passive immunisation and toxoids for active immunisation. Active immunisation is the better method. Assessments from sales figures of tetanus prophylactics of the number of horses inoculated have several limitations: tetanus antitoxin is also used in other domesticated animals, the dosages for prophylaxis and treatment are very different, and it is not known how much toxoid has been used in primary courses and how much for repeat injections. The indications, however, are that active immunisation should be more generally applied.

The horse is the most susceptible of domesticated species to tetanus toxin on a body weight basis (Smith 1954); furthermore, unlike some cows and sheep, horses do not develop natural active immunity to tetanus and circulating antibodies do not arise naturally in them. The only evidence of such a response is seen in a few horses which show evidence of feeble potentiation when a primary dose of toxoid is injected. To ensure optimum protection, strict attention to the vaccination schedule is thus required. The following approach to tetanus prophylaxis will consider in particular the pregnant mare, the foal, and the necessity for repeat inoculations.

Prophylaxis in pregnant mares

The main aim is to achieve peak antitoxin concentrations in the colostrum,

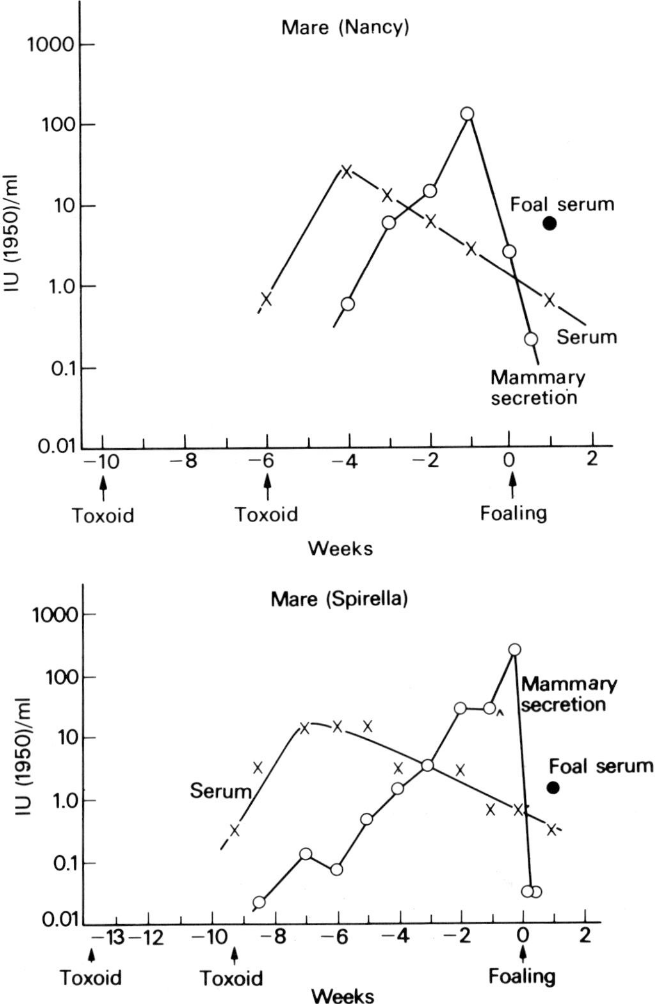

Figs. 9.1a & b   Tetanus antitoxin titres for two mares. × = serum, ○ = mammary secretion, ● = foal serum.

since the foal is essentially agammaglobulinaemic before birth. Absorption of gammaglobulin is greatest soon after birth and ceases completely after 24 hours or so (Jeffcott 1971). In addition, Jeffcott (1974) measured the serum and colostrum protein patterns in mares before and after foaling and showed that, after parturition, the levels of protein and *Clostridium perfringens* (*welchii*) type A antibody fell rapidly, even in the colostrum of hyper-immune mares. Tetanus antitoxin follows a similar pattern as shown in Figs. 9.1a and 9.1b.

The exact process by which the mammary gland selectively concentrates immune proteins into colostrum is not known. Even in the cow — to which most publications refer — the mechanisms are not understood, but it has been suggested that changes in the circulating concentrations of oestrogen and progesterone in the last 4–6 weeks of pregnancy are involved. The aim, therefore, should be to achieve peak concentrations in the serum throughout this period and this can be achieved by completing the primary course, or injecting a booster dose, between one and two months before foaling (Liefman 1981). If too short or too long an interval is allowed, the duration of transferred protection to the foal will be shortened. Foals expected early in the season tend to be carried longer than those due later and variations in the length of pregnancy up to two weeks on each side of the anticipated date can occur.

Prophylaxis in the foal

The foal from the non-immune mare

There has been a tendency to accept that the newborn do not respond to a given antigenic stimulus (e.g. Burnett 1962) and clearly a knowledge of the age by which immunological competence develops in the foal is required. The typical response which has been obtained to inoculation of a foal from a non-immune mare with an adsorbed tetanus toxoid is illustrated in Figs. 9.2a and 9.2b. These foals were inoculated at 1 and 5 weeks and at 5 and 9 weeks of age, respectively. There was a good response in both animals with no evidence of either immunological immaturity or tolerance.

If vaccine is suitably administered, the foal newly born to a non-immune mare can apparently produce a response which is little different from that in a foal inoculated later in life. Inevitably though there will be a delay in this response during which cases of *tetanus neonatorum* might arise. Rossdale & Scarnell (1961) reported that, on certain studs in the Newmarket area, the incidence of tetanus was sometimes as high as 2%. On such studs, tetanus antitoxin in single or repeated doses generally appeared to protect, but there were certain limitations. Thus, a case of hyperacute tetanus had been reported within three days of birth and several cases had occurred at 2–3 weeks of age within three days of a dose of 1500 IU antitoxin.

The foal from the immune mare

Possible interference with response to vaccines by maternally transferred antibodies has long been recognised: e.g. in children to poliomyelitis and

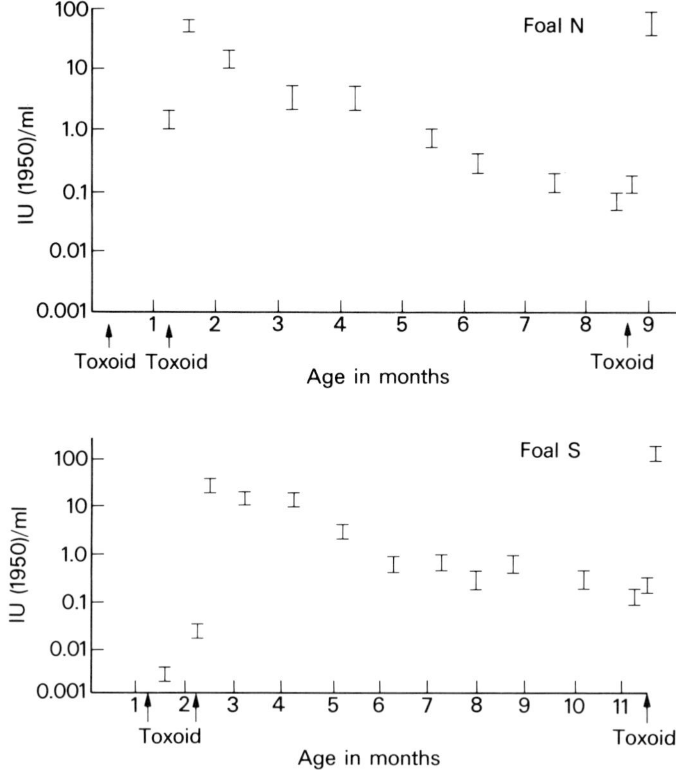

Figs. 9.2a & b   Tetanus antitoxin titres for two foals.

diphtheria, in calves to rinderpest, in lambs to *Cl. perfringens (welchii)* type D, in puppies to distemper, and in foals to African Horse Sickness vaccines. While, with living vaccines, multiplication is required to produce an active response, adsorbed preparations of tetanus toxoid in simultaneous active and passive immunisation have been used satisfactorily in man.

The influence of mineral carriers on the response was emphasised by Fulthorpe (1965). Rossdale & Scarnell (1961) and Kerry *et al* (1976) have recorded residual antitoxin titres in foals up to six months of age which had been suckled by vaccinated dams. A typical example of the interference by maternally transferred antibody to the response to tetanus vaccine is shown in Fig. 9.2c, but there was an excellent response to a third injection of toxoid which indicated that adequate sensitisation is possible during the period of passive protection. It is suggested therefore that a suitable compromise is achieved by delaying inoculation of the foal until it is four months of age.

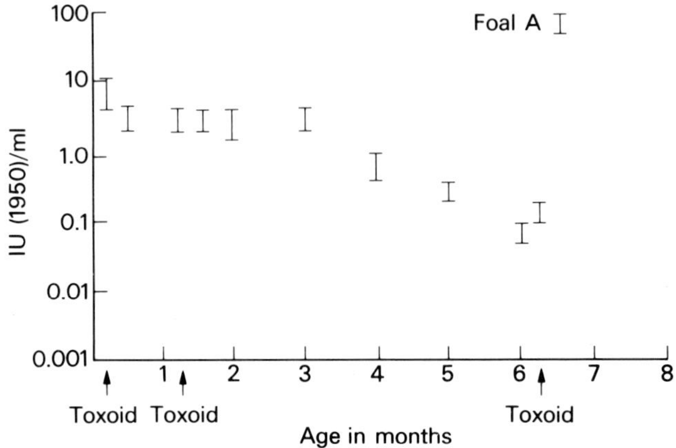

Fig. 9.2c Tetanus antitoxin titres for a third foal.

Table 9.1 Tetanus antitoxin titres in ponies* (Scarnell 1974).

| | Initial Course | | | ca five-year booster | | |
	Pre-1st	Pre-2nd	1 month post-inoculation	Pre-inoculation	Post-inoculation 7 days	21 days
Steady Aim	ND†	1.0–2.0	10–20	0.1–0.5	10–20	50–100
Nancy	ND	0.5–1.0	4–10	0.02–0.05	50–100	50–100
Daisy	ND	1.0–2.0	5–10	0.1–0.2	200–500	200
Hilda	ND	2.0–5.0	25–50	0.02–0.05	100–200	100–200
Spirella	ND	0.2–0.5	10–20	<0.01	50–100	50–100
Nicola	ND	1.0–2.0	10–20	0.5–1.0	10–20	20–50
Stella	ND	1.0–2.0	10–20	0.05–0.1	20	10–20
Bebe	ND	1.0–2.0	20–50	0.2–0.5	100–200	50–100
Suna	ND	0.02–0.04	10–20	0.2–0.5	10–20	20–50
Morgan	ND	2.0–4.0	4–10	0.02–0.05	10–20	20–50
Anthea	ND	0.5–1.0	10–20	0.1–0.5	50–100	100–200
Gareth	ND	0.02–0.04	0.5–1.0	0.05	5–10	10–20

*In IU (1950)/ml serum, †ND = None detectable.

Persistence of protection and rapidity of recall

This has been studied (Scarnell 1974) in a group of cross-bred pony mares first immunised with two doses of an aluminium adsorbed tetanus toxoid. The concentrations of antitoxin in repeated samples of sera were determined. Five years later, after several foalings, those mares which were still available were re-inoculated with an aluminium phosphate adsorbed tetanus toxoid. The responses were determined and the results are shown in Table 9.1 where it may be seen that, within five years of the initial course, the concentration of circulating antitoxin may fall to a very low level but that, after repeat inoculation, recall is rapid and even higher concentrations of antitoxin are then attained.

It is suggested, therefore, that immunised brood mares should be re-inoculated between 1 and 2 months before foaling; their foals should be actively immunised with a primary course of two doses starting at about four months of age; the dose should be repeated after one year and then at approximately three-yearly intervals.

Salmonellosis in calves due to *Salmonella dublin*

The precise mechanisms of immunity against Salmonella infections are not fully understood. Both cellular and humoral factors play a part. Cell-mediated immunity appears to predominate and to act via macrophages which have been activated by immune lymphocytes. Challenge bacteria are thus killed before they reach, and multiply in, the reticuloendothelial system. Only active immunisation is, therefore, likely to be of value. The agglutinating somatic and flagellar antibodies which are so useful in identification and classification do not appear to be involved.

Live vaccines that protected chickens against *S. gallinarum* were developed by Smith (1956), who then studied several variants of *S. dublin* (Smith 1965). Preliminary experiments with these were carried out in mice, but variations in their virulence and immunogenicity for the calf precluded direct application. The results in a group of Channel Island calves inoculated with various preparations and challenged orally with a fully virulent strain of *S. dublin* are shown in Table 9.2. They indicate the limitations of antiserum, even when homologous and prepared from hyperimmunised animals, but

Table 9.2 The immunising ability of live vaccines and antisera against *S. dublin* infection in calves.

Immunising agent	No. of Calves used	Cumulative mortality on the following days after challenge						No. of survivors
		2	3	4	5	6	7	
Antiserum (M*) (450 ml)	5	1	2	4	4	4	5	0
Vaccine 17A	8	0	2	6	6	6	8	0
Vaccine 9S	7	0	0	0	2	4	4	3
Vaccine 51	5	0	0	0	0	1	1	4
Vaccine 51 + 9S	2	0	0	0	0	0	0	2
Controls	14	4	10	13	13	13	14	0

*Prepared in calves against live *S. dublin* and given 2 hours before challenge (Smith 1965).

Table 9.3   The incidence of clinical *S. dublin* infection in vaccinated calves in an intensive beef unit (Smith 1965).

Vaccine	No. of calves vaccinated	No. developing infection in relation to vaccination	
		within 1 week	after 1 week
51	312	5	3
9S	312	2	9
Dead coagulase-negative Staphylococcus	312	5	35

Table 9.4   *S. dublin*: problem herds in demonstration trial (Scarnell 1968).

Reference	Inoculated died/total	Controls died/total
Herd 19	2/15	11/21
Herd 31	2/31	5/30

justified further examination of the vaccine strain which came to be known as HWS 51. This was carried out in barley-beef type calves of which ten were vaccinated with HWS 51 and ten were maintained as controls. After oral challenge with virulent *S. dublin* three weeks after vaccination, six of the unvaccinated calves died. All the vaccinated calves survived. The vaccine was then tested in an intensive rearing unit where *S. dublin* was known to be endemic. Calves were randomised sequentially on arrival into three groups and the results are shown in Table 9.3 (Smith 1965).

Throughout this work, 24-hour broth cultures were used for vaccination but such preparations are not suitable for wide scale use. A freeze-dried preparation was therefore made which proved to be stable for at least two years when stored at 2–8°C. The results of experimental challenge in calves agreed with those obtained in the previous work, and the product was assessed in the field against natural challenge. Of 513 vaccinated calves, 155 developed clinical signs of *S. dublin* infection (30.5%) compared with 104 of 188 unvaccinated animals (55.3%). On some of the farms not all the clinical assessments were evaluated bacteriologically, but the results show a statistically highly significant benefit to the inoculated calves ($\chi^2 = 37.22$; $p = < 0.001$). During this trial, the ranges of protection which might subsequently be expected were as shown in Table 9.4 in two adequately controlled groups.

The protection achieved by this vaccine strain was only partial. Clinical signs were not prevented on challenge. Calves could be ill, sometimes very ill, but, in contrast with control, uninoculated calves, recovery was much more rapid and mortality markedly reduced.

Field use of this strain as a vaccine has shown that some anaphylactoid reactions can be expected, although no cases developed in the preliminary work. The signs of this reaction resemble those of anaphylaxis, but no specific prior sensitisation has been recognised. In the calf, it is associated with acute respiratory distress and collapse. The mediators released in cattle have not been investigated, but it would seem logical to suppose that they are the same as those involved in other hypersensitivity type reactions. The subject has been discussed by Burka & Scarnell (1978), who suggest that treatment with aspirin and meclofenamate would appear to be indicated, in addition to the prompt subcutaneous injection of adrenaline. Another possible problem is that of inoculation of calves which have already been exposed to infection. In man, the use of *S. typhi* vaccines late in the incubation period may induce so-called 'provocation typhoid'. Similarly, some Salmonella vaccines increase the frequency of fatal bacteraemia in mice which are already infected. The identification of precipitating factors in investigation is difficult but there have been two incidents associated with prior *S. typhimurium* infection in which this problem might have been involved. Many calves must have been infected by the time of vaccination, and a few calves recognised to be excreting *S. dublin* and/or *S. typhimurium* have been experimentally inoculated but with no adverse reaction.

Protection afforded by this vaccine is not related to antibody response to somatic and flagellar antigens. Calves inoculated with HWS 51 do not produce 'O' antibodies. They do produce 'H' antibodies, but in many species these have long been known not to protect. The evidence that immunity in man is cell-mediated is that protection against typhoid in WHO vaccine field trials was not correlated with antibody titres; in calves, serum from immune donors did not protect against *S. dublin*; and, while calves immunised with a rough *S. dublin* vaccine did not have 'O' antibodies, they displayed delayed hypersensitivity reactions to *S. dublin* extracts.

The existence of cross-protection between several different Salmonella serotypes also suggests that neither 'H' nor 'O' antigens are involved in the protective response. Most investigations into heterotypic challenge have been done in laboratory animals (e.g. Smith & Halls 1966) but the results reported by Rankin and his colleagues (1967), shown in Table 9.5, indicate that vaccination of calves against *S. dublin* may protect against *S. typhimurium* to some extent. Clearly, further investigations are required.

There is also the problem of susceptibility of some live vaccines to inactivation *in vivo* by antibiotics or other antibacterial drugs. The subject is very complex but, in general, simultaneous administration may reduce the immune response. One oral preparation containing trimethoprim and

Table 9.5   The protection afforded by *S. dublin* 51 vaccine to calves experimentally challenged with *S. typhimurium*. (From Rankin *et al* 1967.) $p = 0.02$.

Group	Dead	Alive	Totals
Non-vaccinated	16	8	24
Vaccinated	7	17	24

sulphadiazine has been tested for compatability. Inoculation three days after completion of the course, or medication seven days after inoculation, had no marked effect on vaccine response as measured by subsequent resistance to artificial oral challenge. It is therefore suggested that the vaccine should be used on the farm of origin of calves one week before transportation but, where this is not practicable, that vaccine should be given at the collecting centre or as soon as possible after arrival at the rearing farm. It must also be emphasised that it is imperative that good husbandry and hygiene should be practised. Vaccines and drugs are not a substitute for these measures.

Immunisation against *E. coli* diarrhoea in the unweaned piglet

The rational immunoprophylaxis of enteric *E. coli* disease of the newborn pig has now become possible through research into the mechanisms of enteropathogenicity of the serotypes involved in this increasingly common problem. It utilises the transfer of various anti-adhesive and bactericidal antibodies in the colostrum and milk of actively immunised sows. These antibodies prevent adhesion and proliferation of the relevant entero-pathogenic serotypes and the associated enterotoxic interference with intestinal mucosal metabolism.

Pathogenesis

E. coli is, of course, a normal inhabitant of the large intestine, but disease is characterised by colonisation of the anterior small intestine with entero-pathogenic strains of particular serotypes which are able to multiply freely there (Sojka 1965). Numbers of *E. coli* in the small intestine as much as 5000-fold higher than normal are commonly found in clinically affected pigs. Arbuckle (1970) showed that many of these strains adhere to the gut wall and Smith & Linggood (1971) used genetic engineering techniques to identify the factors responsible for adherence in the newborn. They were the K88 capsular antigens. Jones & Rutter (1972) then demonstrated that these antigens were associated with pathogenicity. K88 positive strains caused high piglet mortality but a laboratory prepared mutant without K88 did not adhere to the gut wall and caused only low levels of mortality. They suggested that the K88 antigens functioned as adhesives *in vivo,* prevented the removal of these strains by gut peristalsis and permitted the multiplication and build-up of organisms in the proximal small intestine. The hypothesis has been substantiated by others including Jones & Rutter (1974) and Nagy *et al* (1976). The stages of *E. coli* disease are believed to be as follows:

1 exposure to pathogen
2 adhesion to the upper small intestine
3 production and release of toxins affecting water and electrolyte balance
4 diarrhoea, dehydration, death.

With improved serological typing procedures it has been determined that most of the pathogenic strains isolated from diarrhoea in newborn pigs in the UK possess these K88 antigens (Sojka 1971) (Table 9.6). In Ireland, from the Abbotstown laboratory, Sweeny (1975) has reported that 96.7% of his isolates were K88 positive.

Conventional *E. coli* vaccines were deficient in K88 antigens and an experimental vaccine rich in K88 antigens was therefore prepared and examined in gilts for efficiency to confer passive protection to their piglets against experimental challenge (Nagy *et al* 1978). Four serotypes of *E. coli* were used in the product, and strains selected for their ability to produce K88 antigens in aerated cultures as follows:

08:K87 (B), K88 ab (L)
0138:K81 (B), K88 ac (L)
0141:K85 ab (B), K88 ab (L)
0149:K91 (B), K88 ac (L)
Purified antigens K88 ab, K88 ac.

Table 9.6 *E. coli* infection in pigs

Weybridge number	International serotype	Disease associated
G7	08:K87(B), K88ab(L)	Pre-weaning scour
G1253	0147:K89(B), K88ac(L)	Pre-weaning scour
G205	08:K87(B), K88ac(L)	Pre-weaning scour
E68I	0141:K85ab(B), K88ab(L)	Pre-weaning scour
G491	0138:K81(B), K88ac(L)	Pre-weaning scour
Abbotstown	0149;K91(B), K88ac(L)	Pre-weaning scour
E145	0141:K85ac(B)	Oedema
E68II	0141:K85ab(B)	Oedema
E57	0138:K81(B)	Oedema
E4	0139:K82(B)	Oedema

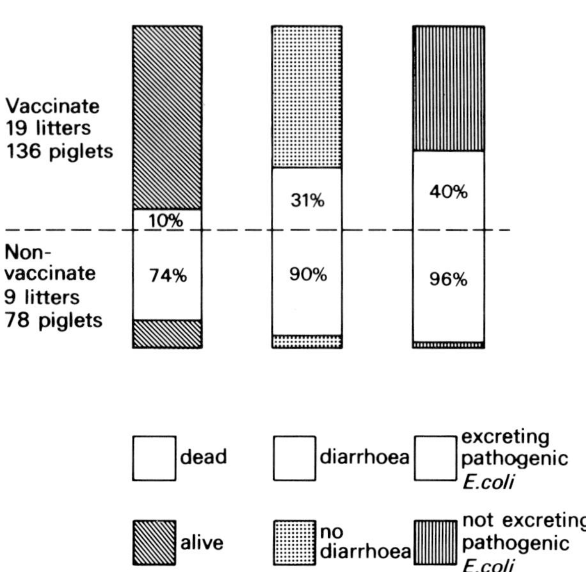

Fig. 9.3 Mortality, diarrhoea and excretion data in vaccinated and control groups after laboratory challenge with *E. coli* 0149.

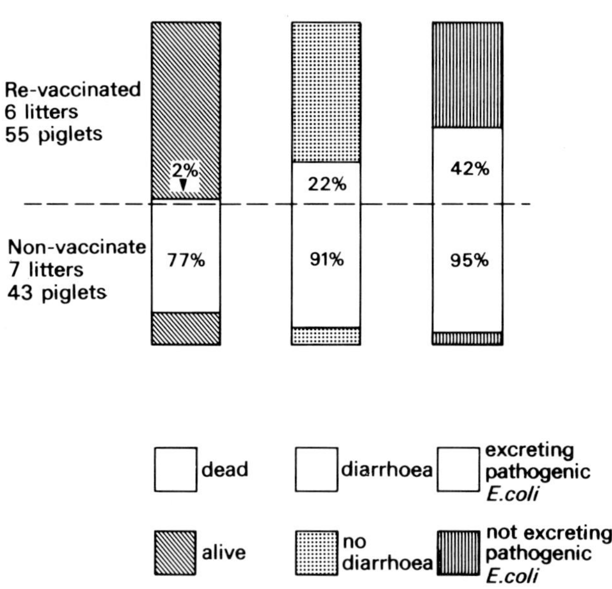

Fig. 9.4 Mortality, diarrhoea and excretion data in re-vaccinated and control groups after laboratory challenge with *E. coli* 0149.

After inactivation and the addition of alhydrogel as adjuvant, gilts were inoculated 6–8 weeks and again two weeks before farrowing. Piglets were challenged orally with 10 000 million organisms (many times greater than might be expected from natural exposure) of an Abbotstown strain of *E. coli* — 0149:K91 (B), K88 ac (L). Observations were made daily on mortality, diarrhoea, and excretion until death or cessation of excretion of the challenge strain. The results, compared with those from litters of control unvaccinated gilts, are shown in Fig. 9.3. Single doses were repeated in their subsequent pregnancies and the results in these litters are shown in Fig. 9.4.

Field trials

Field trials were therefore organised in the UK, on farms where *E. coli* was reported to be endemic, to compare the incidence of *E. coli* disease in new born piglets from vaccinated dams with that in piglets from dams inoculated with a placebo product (Scarnell 1978). The 25 farms included in the trials varied from small mixed farms to specialised pig units, some of them being highly automated and housing up to 2000 breeding sows. Husbandry varied from the traditional straw bed to modern crate farrowing on partially slatted concrete floors. Quality of hygiene and management varied greatly. Sows and gilts were numbered and divided into two groups, one to receive the coded vaccine, the other the coded placebo. Efforts were made to achieve an equal distribution between the groups as regards age, number of previous farrowings, previous health record, type of husbandry, and housing. Inoculation proceeded sequentially so that the numbers in one group did not greatly exceed those in the other. A total of 599 pregnant sows were inoculated, 301 with the vaccine and 298 with the placebo.

The number of piglets observed in the trials was about 6000. They were inspected daily for at least three weeks after birth. Whenever diarrhoea occurred in either group, rectal swabs were obtained from one or more piglets in the litter concerned, placed in Stuart's transport medium, and dispatched for bacteriological examination. After swabs had been taken, the farmer was free to use therapy to minimise economic loss. At post-mortem examination of piglets suspected of dying from *E. coli* infection, swabs were taken from the stomach, duodenum, ileum and large intestine. Farmers were supplied with specially designed record sheets and made daily recordings of litter data covering births, clinical illness, diarrhoea, deaths, specimens taken, and treatment given.

Swabs were examined by culture on blood agar plates. All *E. coli* isolates were tested by slide agglutination against a range of antisera covering the pathogenic *E. coli* shown in Table 9.6. All *E. coli* isolates, whether or not haemolytic or serotypable, were examined *in vivo* for enterotoxic properties

Table 9.7 UK field trial data.

	Vaccine	Placebo	
Scour days per piglet born alive	0.3	0.6	
Percentage of litters in which diarrhoea occurred	35.7	45.5	$p<0.019$
Percentage of sampled litters in which *E. coli* were serotyped	5.8	26.6	$p<0.001$
Percentage of sampled litters in which enterotoxic *E. coli* were found	10.0	25.6	$p<0.012$
Percentage of death/total live births	10.5	11.6	$p<0.162$

by the intestinal loop technique (Smith & Halls 1967). This consists of the inoculation of cultures into ligated segments of the small intestine of anaesthetised piglets, and comparing the visible reactions induced 24 hours later with those of control segments. A confirmed challenge was recognised on eleven of the 25 farms. The results in the two groups on these 11 farms in terms of diarrhoea, *E. coli* serotypes identified, and enterotoxic properties demonstrated, may be summarised as shown in Table 9.7.

The differences in the incidence of diarrhoea week by week between the two groups were very highly significant. In week one, there was a 54.3% reduction in scour days, $p<0.001$; in week two a 43.9% reduction, $p<0.001$; and in week three a 52.5% reduction, $p<0.001$ (Fisher's exact probability test). During the three-week period of observation, vaccination thus resulted in the following reductions: 22% in the incidence of diarrhoea; 50% in the number of scour days; 78% in the number of *E. coli* serotypes isolated, and 61% in the number of enterotoxic *E. coli* found. Controlled trials in other countries demonstrated further benefits, including increased weight gain at weaning (Nielsen & Wittenburg 1979).

Conclusion

This account of the development of effective methods of protection against the diseases associated with infection by *Cl. tetani, S. dublin,* and *E. coli* has summarised various aspects of applied immunoprophylaxis and illustrated three different immunological mechanisms — anti-toxic, cell-mediated and humoral antibacterial.

Bibliography

Parish H. J. & Cannon D. A. (1962) *Antisera, Toxoids, Vaccines and Tuberculins in Prophylaxis and Treatment,* 4th edn. E. & S. Livingstone, Edinburgh.

Stableforth A. W. & Galloway I. A. (1959) *Infectious Diseases of Animals.* Butterworths, London.
Topley and Wilson's Principles of Bacteriology, Virology and Immunity, 6th edn. (1975). Edward Arnold, London.

References

Tetanus

Burnett F. M. (1962) *The Integrity of the Body,* p. 79. Oxford University Press.
Chodnik K. S., Watson A. R. A. & Hepple J. R. (1959) *Vet. Rec.* **71,** 904.
Fulthorpe A. J. (1965) *J. Hyg.* (Camb.) **63,** 243.
Jeffcott L. B. (1971) *Perinatal Studies in Equidae with Special Reference to Passive Transfer of Immunity.* PhD thesis, University of London.
Jeffcott L. B. (1974) *J. Comp. Path.* **84,** 93.
Kerry J. B., Thomson R. O., Epps H. B. G. *et al* (1976) *Dierg. Tijds.* **45,** 333.
Liefman C. E. (1981) *Aust. Vet. J.* **57,** 57.
Rossdale P. D. & Scarnell J. (1961) *Vet. Rec.* **73,** 184.
Scarnell J. (1974) *Vet. Rec.* **95,** 62.
Smith L. D. S. (1954) *Introduction to the Pathogenic Anaerobes,* p. 98. University of Chicago Press.

Salmonellosis

Burka J. F. & Scarnell J. (1978) *Vet. Rec.* **102,** 483.
Rankin J. D., Taylor R. J. & Newman G. (1967) *Vet. Rec.* **80,** 720.
Smith H. W. (1956) *J. Hyg.* (Camb.) **54,** 419.
Smith H. W. (1965) *J. Hyg.* (Camb.) **63,** 117.
Smith H. W. & Halls Sheila, (1966) *J. Hyg.* (Camb.) **64,** 637.

E. coli

Arbuckle J. B. R. (1970) *J. Med. Microbiol.* **3,** 333
Jones G. W. & Rutter J. M. (1972) *Infect. Immun.* **6,** 918.
Jones G. W. & Rutter J. M. (1974) *Amer. J. Clin. Nutrit.* **27,** 1441.
Nagy L. K., Bhogal B. S. & Mackenzie T. (1976) *Res. Vet. Sci.* **21,** 303.
Nagy L. K., Walker P. D., Bhogal B. S. *et al* (1978) *Res. Vet. Sci.* **24,** 39.
Nielsen A. F. & Wittenburg J. (1979) *Vet. Tids.* **62,** 419.
Scarnell J. (1978) *Proc. Int. Pig. Vet. Soc.* (Zagreb).
Smith H. W. & Halls S. (1967) *J. Path. Bact.* **93,** 499.
Smith H. W. & Linggood M. A. (1971) *J. Med. Microbiol.* **4,** 467.
Sojka W. J. (1965) *E. coli* in domestic animals. *Rev. Ser. 7. Commw. Bur. Anim. Hlth.* Farnham Royal, Bucks.
Sojka W. J. (1971) *Vet. Bull.* **41,** 509.
Sweeney E. J. (1975) *Irish Vet. J.* **29,** 127.

10

Modern anthelmintics for farm animals

J. ARMOUR

For ease of presentation, the modern anthelmintics currently available for the internal parasites of farm animals will be considered on a host species basis, namely cattle, small ruminants, and pigs. Since comprehensive and authoritative reviews on this subject were published by Gibson (1975) Kelly *et al* (1976) and Frimmer & Lammler (1977), only the agents developed since 1975 and those reviewed by the above authors and still widely used in practice will be discussed in this chapter. It is also proposed, where appropriate, to indicate how anthelmintics may be used prophylactically as well as curatively. Since many of the appropriate references are listed in the above reviews only limited references will be used in the current text. Where further details of the mode of action of anthelmintics are required, the reader is referred to Van den Bossche (1976) and Rew (1978).

Cattle

Gastrointestinal nematodes

The common gastrointestinal nematodes of cattle are: *Ostertagia ostertagi,* Haemonchus spp. and *Trichostrongylus axei* in the abomasum; *Cooperia oncophora, Nematodirus helvetianus, Bunostomum phlebotumum* and *Strongyloides papillosus* (in young calves) in the small intestine; and *Oesophagostomum radiatum* in the large intestine. In certain tropical and subtropical areas, *Toxocara* (Neoascaris) *vitulorum* is also prevalent in the small intestine of calves. At one time specific anthelmintics were prescribed for individual parasites, but modern anthelmintics have a wide spectrum of activity although the degree of this activity may vary according to the species of helminth involved, route of administration, and dosage rate.

Wide spectrum anthelmintics

The wide spectrum anthelmintics currently available for cattle, originate mainly from five chemical groupings; benzimidazoles, tetramisoles, pyrantel, organophosphates, and avermectins.

1   The *benzimidazoles* are characterised by a very wide spectrum of activity and low mammalian toxicity. They bind strongly to nematode tubulin, a protein necessary for the formation and viability of microtubules and this occurs principally in absorptive intestinal cells, resulting in a complete absence of microtubules in the intestinal cells of the nematode within 24 hours of treatment. The inability of the intestinal cells to absorb nutrients causes a reduction in glycogen and the parasites are effectively starved. From this mode of action it is clear that benzimidazole efficiency increases as the length of exposure of the nematode to a threshold level of the drug increases. Repeated administration of divided doses to prolong exposure and administration by the oral route may therefore enhance drug activity and benzimidazoles given orally are particularly effective in ruminants in which prolonged passage through the rumen and hence a reduced rate of absorption leads to a continued exposure of the parasite to the drug (see also Chapter 1). For similar reasons, the most effective benzimidazoles are the less soluble compounds such as fenbendazole, oxfendazole and albendazole, which remain in solid form precipitates within the gut lumen for longer periods of time. When a benzimidazole drug passes directly to the abomasum following oral administration, the time for passage through the gastrointestinal tract is reduced and efficiency is correspondingly decreased. Eight of the benzimidazoles which have been synthesised are now available for clinical use, namely thiabendazole, cambendazole, mebendazole, oxibendazole, flubendazole, fenbendazole, oxfendazole and albendazole. These compounds are generally of very low toxicity in mammalian hosts, and it has proved virtually impossible to find a median lethal dose (LD_{50}) for some of them, such as thiabendazole and fenbendazole. Four compounds are known to be teratogenic: parbendazole, cambendazole, oxfendazole and albendazole; these should not be used in early pregnancy at greater than therapeutic dose rates. In some countries idiosyncratic reactions to cambendazole have necessitated its withdrawal.

Pro-benzimidazoles. The drug febantel is closely related to the benzimidazoles and, since it converts in the host to both fenbendazole and oxfendazole, it has been included in Table 10.2. Thiophanate does not fall into any of the chemical groupings outlined above but is classified in the allophanate group which is similar in chemical composition to the benzimidazoles; indeed thiophanate converts to a benzimidazole structure in the host. For this reason details of its efficacy are included in Table 10.2.

Anthelmintic efficiency has been graded as shown in Table 10.1. Details of benzimidazole drugs, including route of administration, anthelmintic efficiency against the common gut nematodes of cattle, withdrawal period (based on UK data) and special information are given in Table 10.2. Anthelmintic efficiency against adult and developing larval stages of the

Table 10.1   Key to anthelmintic efficiency.

A	>90%
B	75–90%
C	50–75%
D	<50%
U	Insufficient evidence

common gastrointestinal nematodes is high, but only the less soluble compounds which promote the maintenance of a threshold level of drug for a few days are effective against arrested larval stages and lungworms.

2 *Tetramisole* is a racemic mixture of D- and L-forms. The L-form — levamisole — is more potent and less toxic than dexamisole and is the compound generally used, although tetramisole is still marketed in some countries. Levamisole can be given subcutaneously or orally and is also effective by topical application — the so-called 'pour-on' technique. It acts as a ganglion stimulant of nematode nerves leading to neuromuscular paralysis of the parasites. In contrast to the benzimidazoles the peak concentration of levamisole is more important since excretion is very rapid, with more than 90% excreted in 24 hours. Mammalian toxicity is greater than with the benzimidazoles although, in normal usage, toxic effects are seldom seen. The effects are similar to those on the nematodes and ganglion stimulation is manifested by muscle tremors, salivation, bradycardia, respiratory embarrassment and constriction of the pupils. In low doses administered daily or every two days, levamisole is also used as an immunostimulant

Anthelmintic details regarding levamisole are given in Table 10.3 from which it can be seen that activity against developing larvae and adult forms of gut nematodes is high; the drug is also effective against lungworms including arrested larvae of this species (Oakley 1981).

3 *Pyrantel tartrate* and its methyl analog, *morantel tartrate,* are wide spectrum anthelmintics given by the oral route and with very high efficiency against adult stages of gut nematodes, particularly those species which dwell in the lumen. Activity is less against immature forms, especially those found in the mucosa, and negligible against arrested larvae or lungworms. Pyrantel is a depolarising muscle relaxant in nematodes (and to a lesser extent in the host) and produces paralysis of the parasites. Toxicity in the host is rare unless the normal dosage rate is exceeded by at least five times. The anthelmintic details are given in Table 10.3. Morantel tartrate is combined with a specific lungworm anthelmintic, diethylcarbamazine citrate, to provide action against both gut and lung nematodes.

Recently, a sustained release bolus containing morantel tartrate has been developed for use in cattle (Jones 1981) and in some countries this is

Table 10.2 Benzimidazoles and pro-benzimidazoles used against common bovine gastrointestinal nematodes.

Drug (formulation)	Efficiency			Withdrawal period (days)		Ovicidal	Comments and other activity
	adults	larvae	arrested larvae	meat	milk		
Thiabendazole (drench, paste, in-feed)	A	B	Nil	Nil	Nil	Yes	Use at >100 mg/kg
Fenbendazole (drench, in-feed)	A	A	A/B	14	3	Yes	Lungworms and cestodes
Albendazole (drench)	A	A	A/B	14	Not used	Yes	Lungworms, cestodes and fluke (1.3 × normal dose)
Oxfendazole (drench)	A	A	A/B	14	Not used	Yes	Lungworms and cestodes
Febantel (drench)	A	A	A/B	14	Not used	Yes	For arrested larvae use at >10 mg/kg
Thiophanate (drench, in-feed)	A	A	B	7	3	Yes	Double dose in severe infections

Note. Parbendazole, oxibendazole and cambendazole are also available in some countries and are active against adult and developing larvae of gastrointestinal nematodes. Cambendazole also has activity against lungworms and cestodes.

Table 10.3 Non-benzimidazoles used against bovine gastrointestinal nematodes.

Drug (formulation)	Efficiency			Withdrawal period (days)		Ovicidal	Comments and other activity
	adults	larvae	arrested larvae	meat	milk		
Levamisole (s.c. drench, in food or drink, dermal)	A	A	D	3	1	No	Lungworms. Toxic signs may appear × 3
Morantel tartrate (drench) (sustained-release bolus)	A	B	D	14	Zero	No	Combined with diethylcarbamazine citrate for lungworms. Bolus releases drug over 90 days and prevents larval intake over this period.
Ivermectin (s.c.)	A	A	A	21	Not used	No	Lungworms and several ecto-parasites

Note. Tetramisole is not included since it is largely replaced by levamisole. The organophosphates, trichlorfon, coumaphos and crufomate are used as in-feed anthelmintics and in some countries as pour-on agents.

the only formulation of morantel now available. This bolus is of sufficient weight to prevent its regurgitation and it settles in the reticulum/rumen following administration with a special dosing gun. The bolus is designed to provide the continuous release of morantel for 90 days after administration. During this period it will prevent the development of ingested larvae of gastrointestinal nematodes and, to a lesser extent (60 days), of lungworm larvae.

4 In cattle several *organophosphates* are widely used as anthelmintics including trichlorphon, coumaphos and crufomate. By the oral, topical or, in some instances, parenteral route they all have a good activity against the adult stages of common gut nematodes but not against the immature stages, including arrested larvae. The organophosphates inhibit cholinesterase both in nematodes and host. This inhibition results in accumulation of acetyl-choline at nerve endings leading to stimulation initially and then paralysis of nerve transmission. These anthelmintics have a relatively narrow safety margin which depends upon differential sensitivity of mammalian and nematode cholinesterase. Toxic signs include excessive salivation, purging and myosis. Response to prompt treatment with atropine sulphate is usually good, although large doses of atropine must be given. Anthelmintic details of these compounds are referred to in Table 10.3.

5 Recently a new family of antiparasitic agents, the *avermectins* have been discovered. The avermectins are produced as a fermentation metabolite of the actinomycete, *Streptomyces avermitilis*. Studies with the natural Ba component, a macrocyclic lactone, have shown it to be a broad spectrum anthelmintic in various host species (Egerton *et al* 1979). A chemically modified derivative, ivermectin, has been commercially developed for use in cattle and sheep.

The avermectins act against nematodes by blocking nervous transmission. The basic principle of this is that the action of the neurotransmitter GABA (gamma amino butyric acid) is potentiated, resulting in a rapid abolition of the inhibitory post-synaptic potential and a slower disappearance of the excitatory post-synaptic potential.

Specific treatments for arrested larvae

The majority of studies on the efficiency of anthelmintics against nematode larvae arrested in their development have been undertaken in areas where the abomasal parasite *O. ostertagi* predominates. The arrested larvae of this species are important since, depending on the numbers present, they can cause clinical disease or production loss due to the pathological changes induced in the abomasum following resumption of their development. Until comparatively recently, none of the anthelmintics available were effective against arrested larvae and several authors assumed that this inefficiency was due to the low metabolic rate of the arrested larvae preventing uptake and metabolism of the anthelmintic. However, Australian workers (Prichard *et al* 1978) have shown that the efficiency against arrested larvae is influenced more by the length of exposure of the nematode to effective levels of the anthelmintic. Therefore, some of the newer and less soluble benzimidazoles have proved to be effective as indicated in Table 10.2. Some variation in the activity of these agents has also been recorded by various workers including the present author, and it seems likely that one reason for this is related to the interaction between the routes taken by the administered compound. Thus, if the drug bypasses the rumen and goes directly to the omasum or abomasum (this can happen in up to 50% of cases according to McEwan & Oakley 1978), the period of exposure is reduced. In contrast, when the drug reaches the abomasum via the rumen, the rate of metabolism is reduced and the period of exposure of the nematode to the critical level of drug is prolonged. At normal dosage rates the less soluble benzimidazoles (fenbendazole, oxfendazole and albendazole) are the most effective against arrested larvae. Good activity against arrested *O. ostertagi* larvae has also been recorded with the closely related drugs, febantel and thiophanate, albeit at rates higher than that recommended or given in divided doses over five days. Recently ivermectin has been shown to be highly effective against arrested larvae and, since this drug is given by injection, the problem of rumen bypass is obviated (Armour *et al* 1980).

Toxocara vitulorum

Successful treatment of this ascarid can be achieved by using one of the piperazine compounds; although these are not available as ruminant preparations, the use of one of the horse or pig preparations should achieve the same results. Alternatively, one of the benzimidazoles with good activity against ascarids (e.g. cambendazole or morantel) could be tried.

Drug resistance

Resistance to thiabendazole and the other benzimidazoles has been recorded mainly from geographical areas where Haemonchus spp. predominate and the numbers of annual treatments are more numerous than in temperate zones such as Western Europe. This resistance or 'tolerance' as it is frequently labelled is sometimes incomplete and may be overcome by using higher dosage rates. Disturbingly, cross-tolerance has been reported between different benzimidazoles and even to chemically distinct drugs such as morantel tartrate and levamisole (Le Jambre 1978). Most of these reports refer to the nematode species of sheep, but some involve cattle nematodes.

In Europe, reports of anthelmintic tolerance are scarce other than in special circumstances such as an experimental regimen where continual dosing has selected resistant strains of nematodes. Nevertheless, many of the current control measures for gastrointestinal parasitism could be conducive to the selection of drug tolerant strains of nematodes. These measures recommend that cattle be moved to clean grazing after treatment; such a manoeuvre could lead to the latter grazing being contaminated solely with eggs from worm burdens surviving after treatment and theoretically less susceptible to the anthelmintic employed. The work of Le Jambre and his colleagues indicates that nematodes have sufficient genetic variation to develop resistance to several different anthelmintics at rates at least equal to that which develops to a single drug. On this basis it is probably better policy to alternate the anthelmintics used on a farm provided that the alternation occurs between different generations or populations of worms and that the alternative drugs are from a different chemical group.

Route of administration

As can be seen from Tables 10.2 and 10.3, most cattle anthelmintics are available as different preparations and administration is therefore possible by various routes. The effective therapeutic dose is best guaranteed when the drug is administered as a drench, paste, or by injection. Administration in feed or drinking water (Downey & O'Shea 1977) may be labour saving but has several disadvantages. Unless the cattle feed or drink individually there is no guarantee that a therapeutic dose will be obtained by each animal and subtherapeutic doses may promote the development of drug tolerance. Also, since depression of appetite is a common consequence of internal parasitism, the quantity of anthelmintic consumed may be sup-optimal. Where topical preparations of anthelmintics have been used, the activity obtained, while good, has been generally less than that achieved following oral or parenteral administration. Unless a strong economic or management case can be made for in-feed or topical application of cattle anthelmintics, the traditional route is to be preferred, particularly when the agents are being used therapeutically, rather than prophylactically. In the latter context the field performance of the morantel sustained-release device will be observed with interest.

Treatment of lactating cows

There is considerable debate at present on the role of gastrointestinal parasitism in limiting milk production in dairy cows. Positive evidence on increased milk yields following therapy with anthelmintics (notably thiabendazole) has come from various countries (Bliss & Todd 1974; Van Adrichem & Shaw 1977), although whether the improved yields can be ascribed wholly to the anthelmintic effect of the drugs or some other action, is not clear. While lactating cattle sometimes display an increased nematode faecal egg count, similar to the post-parturient effect seen in parasitised ewes, this increase is seldom of a great magnitude or duration. Nevertheless, it does indicate an increase in numbers of adult worms probably recruited from larvae which were arrested until the endocrinological or immuno-logical effects of parturition induced their maturation. If agents such as thiabendazole which are not active against arrested larvae in cattle are to be effective, they must therefore be given during lactation and not prior to calving. In contrast, some of the agents such as fenbendazole which are effective against arrested larvae, could be given prior to calving. Govern-ment regulations preclude the sale of milk for some days from cows treated with these newer drugs and so their use will be confined, appropriately, to late pregnancy or calving since colostrum has to be discarded. Thiaben-dazole, morantel tartrate including the bolus, the rapidly metabolised organophosphates and levamisole have minimal or no restriction placed on their use in the UK and they remain the agents of choice for use in lactating cows suspected of harbouring burdens of adult gastrointestinal nematodes.

Prophylactic use of anthelmintics

Advances in our knowledge about the epidemiology of gastrointestinal parasites of cattle have been considerable in the past decade, and efficient prophylactic control programmes have evolved incorporating a combination of drug therapy and management procedures. These systems are based on the knowledge that, in many geographical zones, the numbers of third stage (L_3) infective larvae of gastrointestinal nematodes fluctuate seasonally. For example, in temperate countries in the northern hemisphere, the L_3 over-winter on herbage and soil and infect cattle grazing in early spring; by late spring the overwintered L_3 succumb and from mid-July onwards are replaced by fresh L_3 which develop from eggs deposited by the calves infected in spring from the overwintered L_3; many L_3 ingested during autumn become arrested in development. Clearly, in these zones anthel-mintics are best applied at three points:

1   At three and six weeks after beginning spring grazing to reduce pasture contamination.

2   In mid-July prior to the seasonal increase and preferably accompanied by a move to 'clean' grazing, i.e. not utilised by cattle in that year. Where such a move is not possible, treatment should be continued at monthly intervals until housing.

3   At housing, with ivermectin or one of the benzimidazoles effective

against arrested larvae which are known to accumulate during autumn.

Based on local epidemiology, similar systems involving the prophylactic use of anthelmintics have been developed in temperate areas of the southern hemisphere (Anderson 1971) and in arid tropical countries. Information is lacking, however, on the possible use of similar prophylaxis in the humid tropics, where it seems likely that the seasonal fluctuations in numbers of L_3 will be less marked.

Lungworms

Several compounds are now available for the treatment of cattle infected with lungworm *Dictyocaulus viviparus*. The clinical disease caused by this parasite can be divided into three different phases: 1 the pre-patent disease due to blockage of the small bronchi and bronchioles by the eosinophil exudate produced in response to the developing larvae migrating up the bronchi, 2 the patent disease caused by reactions to the adult parasite in the main bronchi and a primary pneumonia resulting from the reaction around aspirated eggs produced by these adults, and 3 the post-patent disease in which few, if any, lungworms are present and which is due to widespread alveolar epithelialisation of unknown origin. Successful removal of both pre-patent and patent infections can be achieved by the benzimidazoles, fenbendazole, oxfendazole and albendazole and ivermectin. There have been good results against larval and adult *D. viviparus* with levamisole. Occasionally adverse reactions occur following treatment of heavy infections.

In Europe, seasonal arrested development during autumn by *D. viviparus* similar to that described for Ostertagia spp., is now recognised as an important feature of the epidemiology of this parasite since maturation of the arrested larvae (at the 5th larval stage) in spring results in pasture contamination. Fenbendazole has been tested against larvae and it has a reported efficiency of approximately 75% at the normal dose level for cattle, i.e. 7.5 mg/kg bodyweight (Inderbitzen & Eckert 1978). Levamisole is also reported as being effective against arrested lungworm larvae (Oakley 1981). Data on these compounds are given in Table 10.4. A lungworm-specific drug, diethylcarbamazine citrate, is still used for the treatment of pre-patent husk because of its high activity against the larval stages responsible for pre-patent husk. This drug is a piperazine derivative and causes paralysis of the lungworms due to a hyperpolarisation of the muscle cell membranes in the parasites. Administration is usually by intramuscular injection on each of three successive days, although the two latter doses may be given orally; it is relatively non-toxic. Diethylcarbamazine citrate is also marketed in combination with morantel tartrate and only a single treatment using this product is recommended.

Table 10.4 Anthelmintics against the cattle lungworm *Dictyocaulus viviparus*.

Drug	Formulation	Efficiency		Comments
		adults	larvae	
Diethylcarbamazine citrate	Injection or oral	B/C	A	Repeat treatment on 3 successive days
Levamisole	s.c. injection Oral	A	A	(Table 10.3)
Cambendazole	Oral	B	B	In severe infestations repeat treatment in 2 weeks
Fenbendazole	Oral	A	A	(Table 10.2)
Albendazole	Oral	A	A	(Table 10.2)
Oxfendazole	Oral	A	A	(Table 10.2)
Ivermectin	s.c. injection	A	A	(Table 10.3)

Note. Only fenbendazole and levamisole have so far been shown to be effective against arrested *D. viviparus*.

Prophylaxis against D. viviparus

Unlike the gut nematodes, the ecology of the free-living stages of *D. viviparus* is much less predictable and hence tactical seasonal treatments are generally unreliable as a method of prophylaxis. Since a lungworm vaccine is available for preventing parasitic bronchitis, it is better to reserve anthelmintics for treating sporadic outbreaks of the disease and use the vaccine on farms where the disease is endemic.

Liver fluke

Fascioliasis in cattle, unlike in sheep, is usually a chronic debilitating disease produced by the haematophagous activities of the adult liver fluke, *Fasciola hepatica (F. gigantica* in many tropical countries), in the main bile ducts. Subacute fascioliasis has also been reported where a mixture of young flukes in the parenchyma and adults in the bile ducts cause a syndrome in which both impaired liver function and anaemia occur (Eckert *et al* 1977). The acute syndrome with sudden death rarely occurs and then only in young calves. Fasciolicides for use in cattle should therefore be highly efficient against the adult stages in the bile ducts and several drugs with good activity are available. Although some of these fasciolicides are also efficient against parenchymal stages in sheep, this activity is less marked in cattle where the fibrous nature of the reaction to young migrating flukes (particularly if they are retarded or arrested in development) appears to protect the parasite by limiting the transport and uptake of the anthelmintic.

Fasciolicides for cattle

On a world-wide basis, five compounds are mainly used for the treatment of bovine fascioliasis: hexachlorophene, oxyclozanide, niclofolan, nitroxynil, and rafoxanide.

Hexachlorophene is a chlorinated hydrocarbon with a very good activity against adult flukes but disappointing efficiency against parenchymal stages at the recommended dosage rate. It has rather a narrow therapeutic index, hence toxic reactions characterised by nervous excitability and impairment of vision have been reported.

Oxyclozanide is similar in activity to hexachlorophene against adult flukes and, at the normal dosage rate, is not particularly effective against young migrating flukes. It is less toxic than hexachlorophene, although transient scouring and reduced milk yields have been reported following its use. However, in many countries it is the only agent which can be used in lactating cattle without restrictions on the sale of milk.

Niclofolan, like oxyclozanide, is highly effective against adult flukes at a dose rate of 3 mg/kg but requires much higher doses to remove immature stages. Toxicity occurs at four times the recommended dosage rate. Two other related compounds, bromophenophos and brotianide, have a similar efficiency to niclofolan and are also used in some European countries; another, closantel, will soon be available.

Nitroxynil possesses some advantage in that, apart from rafoxanide, it is the only injectable anthelmintic among fasciolicides currently in vogue. It possesses an excellent activity against adult flukes and some activity against the later parenchymal stages, i.e. flukes of more than six weeks. On occasions a slight local reaction is seen at the site of injection and a yellow staining of the skin due to nitroxynil may also occur. The maximum tolerated dose is 3–4 times the recommended dosage rate and toxicity under normal usage is rare. Nitroxynil increases the metabolic rate of the treated animal and toxic reactions can be recognised by a rise in body temperature and increased respiratory rate.

The above drugs have a similar mode of action in that they selectively uncouple phosphorylation reactions in liver flukes and so interfere with ATP production. Nitroxynil also provokes a toxic irreversible paralysis of flukes and it is not clear if the anthelmintic effect is obtained due to this property or the uncoupling effect.

Rafoxanide belongs to the salicylanilide chemical group and by the oral or subcutaneous route is a highly effective anthelmintic against adult flukes and the later parenchymal stages. Like the previously mentioned compounds it also acts by interfering with ATP production. It is well tolerated and toxic effects are rare except for occasional inappetence. It should not be

Table 10.5 Anthelmintics against *Fasciola hepatica* in cattle.

Drug (formulation)	Adult flukes	Immature flukes	Withdrawal period (days) meat	milk	Comment
Oxyclozanide (drench, in-feed)	A	C/D	14	Zero	Increased dose rate may cause side-effects
Rafoxanide (drench, injection)	A	B/C	28	Not used	Very safe
Nitroxynil (injection)	A	B/C	30	Not used	–
Albendazole (drench)	A	D	14	Not used	1.3 × dose rate used for nematodes.
Niclofolan (drench)	A	C/D	14	Zero	Increased dose rate needed to remove immatures may cause side-effects

Note. Bromophenophos, a drug with similar activity to niclofolan, is used in some European countries. Another, closantel, is under development. A benzimidazole ('Fasinex') is also under development which has very good activity against bile duct and parenchymal stages.

given to cattle producing milk for human consumption.

Recently, the benzimidazole, albendazole has been shown to have a good activity against flukes at twice the dosage rate recommended for roundworm therapy. Oxfendazole and fenbendazole have also shown good activity against adult flukes in preliminary, and as yet unpublished, trials, albeit at high dosage rates (Corba Pers. Commun.) Another new benzimidazole has been described by Boray (1982) and is currently under development. It has a very high activity against bile duct and parenchymal stages of liver fluke in cattle. Relevant details of these fasciolicides are given in Table 10.5.

Prophylaxis with fasciolicides

The anthelmintics currently available are effective only against the bile duct stages of fluke in cattle and clearance of parenchymal stages is minimal; as a result *F. hepatica* eggs usually re-appear in the faeces of treated animals within a few weeks of treatment. Therefore, a prophylactic programme designed to prevent the appearance of fluke eggs in the faeces and prevent infection of the snail intermediate host would require an impractical number of annual treatments. In practice, one or two annual treatments are given, mainly to young cattle at times when adult fluke burdens are known to accrue. In Europe this occurs during the winter and early spring and the recommended times for treatment are December and April in endemic areas or a single treatment in January or February, where burdens are expected to be lighter.

There is insufficient evidence on the significance of fluke infections in older cattle or lactating dairy cows. Nevertheless, there are data, particularly from western Europe, that strongly indicate production losses due to fluke in dairy cows and a production benefit from treatment during early lactation. This benefit is reflected in increased yields and improved milk quality (Koopman 1969, Hörchner *et al* 1970, Black & Froyd 1974). With the current restrictions on the use of available fasciolicides, oxyclozanide and niclofolan (in certain countries) are the only compounds to be used in lactating animals without a requirement for the discarding of milk.

Dicrocoelium dendriticum and *Paramphistomum* spp.

See pp. 192–194.

Cestodes

Moniezia species do occur in cattle, particularly calves, but they are not generally considered worthy of treatment. Nevertheless, three anthelmintic groups are available which are highly effective against these species. These are niclosamide, some benzimidazoles (cambendazole, fenbendazole, oxfendazole, and albendazole) and praziquantel. Since the problem is considered to be a minor one, the use of one of these benzimidazoles in a roundworm control programme should ensure control of Moniezia spp.

Combined anthelmintics for roundworms and flukes

It has been the custom for many years for pharmaceutical companies possessing a good roundworm anthelmintic and a good fasciolicide to develop a formulation in which these two agents were combined. In some of these formulations it was difficult to combine the two constituents at their respective optimal dosage rates, and hence suboptimal dosing took place. The advent of the benzimidazole, albendazole, with its unique activity against all helminth groups may have erased the problem of stability between different chemical groups, but this author has long considered that the combined drenches were unnecessary for cattle since, in many countries, the different helminthiases occur at different seasons, and therefore treatment with a combined anthelmintic which included a roundworm agent and a fasciolicide was unnecessary and indeed wasteful. Combinations of effective roundworm anthelmintics and fasciolicides available include thiabendazole–rafoxanide, levamisole–oxyclozanide, and thiophanate–brotianide.

Sheep and goats

Gastrointestinal nematodes

The common gastrointestinal nematodes of sheep include *H. contortus,* Ostertagia spp., and *T. axei* in the abomasum; Trichostrongylus spp., Nematodirus spp. (including *N. battus*). *Cooperia curticei, Strongyloides papillosus* and *Bunostomum trigonocephalum* in the small intestine; *Chabertia ovina,* Trichuris spp., and Oesophagostomum spp., in the large bowel. In temperate countries, the most important of these are *N. battus* in lambs and Ostertagia spp. and Trichostrongylus spp. in lambs and older sheep particularly during late pregnancy and lactation. In tropical and subtropical zones, *Haemonchus contortus* and *Oesophagostomum columbianum* are of particular importance. Treatment of sheep with a drug specific in its action against a particular nematode is now rare, with the exception of *N. battus*. Unlike cattle, sheep usually harbour a variety of gut nematodes; hence the advent of the wide spectrum anthelmintics has been a particular boon.

Wide spectrum anthelmintics

The anthelmintics available and widely used against sheep gastrointestinal nematodes are given in Tables 10.6 and 10.7. The range of anthelmintics is broadly similar to that used in cattle and most of the agents possess a high efficiency against the relatively wide range of nematodes found in sheep and goats. Several drugs which were ineffective against arrested larval stages in cattle have a good activity against generically related species in sheep; this is probably a reflection of the greater availability of drug due to the fact that the depth of the gastrointestinal mucosa in sheep is less then in cattle and therefore access to mucosal-dwelling larval stages is enhanced. Indeed, many of the larval stages of sheep parasites are to be found in the lumen of the gastrointestinal tract whereas, in cattle, contact with the mucosa is more intimate. An obvious exception to this is the large intestinal nodular worm *O. columbianum* where the larval stages are enclosed in a distinct nodule.

Low-level medication

World-wide epidemiological studies have shown that the increase in nematode faecal egg counts of adult female sheep and goats which occurs during the peri-parturient period (the so-called spring, post-parturient, or pei-parturient rise — PPR) is primarily responsible for the contamination of grazing areas from which susceptible lambs or kids become infected with gastrointestinal nematodes. The period of the PPR can extend from four weeks prior to parturition until 8–10 weeks after, with a peak at 4–6 weeks

Table 10.6 Benzimidazoles used against gastrointestinal nematodes of sheep and goats.

Drug (formulation)	Efficiency			Withdrawal period (days)		Ovicidal	Comments
	adults	larvae	arrested larvae	meat	milk		
Thiabendazole (drench, in-feed)	A	A/C	A/C	Nil	Zero*	Yes	Increase dose × 2 for *N. battus* and arrested larvae
Mebendazole (drench)	A	A/C	U	7	Not known	Yes	–
Oxibendazole	A	A/C	U	4	3	Yes	–
Cambendazole (paste)	A	A/B	U	28	Not used	Yes	Not from 1 week prior to service until 4th week of pregnancy Tapeworms and lungworms
Fenbendazole oxfendazole (drench, in-feed)	A	A	A	14	3	Yes	Lungworms and tapeworms
Albendazole (drench)	A	A	A	10	Not used	Yes	Lungworms, tapeworms, adult fluke (increased dose rate, *see* Table 10.9)
Thiophanate (drench, in-feed, feed blocks)	A	A/B	A/B	7	3	Yes	Available in feed blocks
Febantel	A	A/B	A/B	7	Zero	Yes	–

*Not used in lactating animals when milk is used for cheese production.

Table 10.7 Non-benzimidazoles used against gastrointestinal nematodes of sheep and goats.

Drug (formulation)	Efficiency			Withdrawal period (days)		Ovicidal	Comments and other activity
	adults	larvae	arrested larvae	meat	milk		
Levamisole (s.c. in-feed)	A	A/B	A/B	3	1	No	Lungworms
Morantel tartrate (drench)	A	B	U	14	Zero	No	Marketed combined with diethylcarbamazine citrate
Ivermectin (oral)	A	A	A	21	Not known	No	Lungworms

post-parturition. For complete control of the PPR which involves nematodes with a minimum pre-patent period in the host of about three weeks, at least three and possibly four anthelmintic treatments would be required over the twelve week period when nematode egg output is increased; this is often impractical and also costly. Where flocks are given supplementary feed it is possible to incorporate anthelmintic daily in the feed but this is only practical in intensive management systems. In less intensive situations an alternative to in-feed administration of an anthelmintic is to incorporate the drug in a feed block primarily used to supply essential energy or minerals. Neither of these systems guarantees daily uptake of the required amount of drug and apart from inefficient control could predispose to the development of anthelmintic tolerance.

A more attractive approach is the recent development reported from Australia in which anthelmintic is administered orally in a capsule containing a matrix of sterylamine ethoxylate and drug; the capsule localises in the rumen and steadily releases the anthelmintic over a critical period such as the peri-parturient phase (Anderson & Laby 1977). Although this development is still in the early stage it appears the most practical method of low-level medication. The drugs used in daily low-level programmes are those with ovicidal properties such as the benzimidazoles (thiabendazole, fenbendazole, oxfendazole, and albendazole) plus the related drugs thiophanate and febantel.

Lungworms

Sheep and goats harbour several species of lungworms, including *Dictyocaulus filaria*, *Muellerius capillarus*, *Protostrongylus rufescens*, and *Cystocaulus ocreatus*. Of these, *D. filaria* is considered to be the most pathogenic and this lungworm is a major problem in sheep flocks in several Mediterranean and Middle East countries. Although vaccination with an

Table 10.8 Anthelmintics against lungworms of sheep and goats.

Drug (formulation)	*Dictyocaulus filaria* adults	*Dictyocaulus filaria* larvae	*Muellerius capillarus*	*Protostrongylus refescens*	*Cystocaulus ocreatus*
Diethylcarbamazine citrate (injection, drench)	A/B	A			
Levamisole (s.c. injection)	A	A			
Some benzimidazoles — thiabendazole, fenbendazole, oxfendazole, cambendazole, albendazole, (drench, paste, in-feed)	A	A	Few significant results available as yet except that fenbendazole is very effective against *P. rufescens* and *C. ocreatus*		
Thiophanate (drench, in-feed)	A/B	A/B			
Ivermectin (drench, s.c.)	A	A	Not yet known		
Febantel (drench)	A	A	A	A	

X-irradiated larval vaccine is used to control *D. filaria* in some areas where the parasite is endemic, many flock-owners still rely on anthelmintics. In addition drugs such as levamisole, the new benzimidazoles (fenbendazole, oxfendazole and albendazole) the pro-benzimidazoles, thiophanate and febantel, and the avermectins should all prove beneficial. While the efficiency of these drugs (see Table 10.8) is high against adult and larval *D. filaria*, less is known about their effect against the smaller lungworms, though fenbendazole is known to be highly effective against naturally occurring *O. ocreatus* and *P. rufescens* (Eslami & Anwar 1976). Because of the complicated life-cycles of the small lungworms, material for experimental infections is difficult to obtain — hence the scarcity of data on the efficiency of anthelmintics against these species.

Liver fluke

Liver fluke infections in sheep (and probably in goats) are recognised as causing three clinical syndromes, namely acute, subacute, and chronic fascioliasis. The acute disease is due to haemorrhage and large scale disruption of liver parenchyma by young *F. hepatica* migrating through the parenchyma within six weeks of infection; the subacute disease is partly due to the same pathogenic process and partly to the anaemia caused by the haematophagic activity of the adult flukes in the bile duct. The chronic disease is due to the anaemia produced by adult flukes present in the bile ducts for several weeks, i.e. from twelve weeks post infection onwards.

Boray *et al* (1967) reviewed the drugs available for the treatment of immature and mature fluke infections in sheep. The anthelmintics currently used for these different clinical phases of fascioliasis are given in Table 10.9. Several drugs are effective in chronic fascioliasis, but only four — diamphenethide, nitroxynil, rafoxanide, and brotianide — are highly effective at marketed dose levels against the parenchymal stages of the liver fluke and therefore can be recommended for treating the subacute and acute diseases. Brotianide is a compound used principally in sheep and is closely related to clioxanide, a drug which was formerly used for the treatment of fascioliasis but has largely been supplanted by the four drugs mentioned above. It is closely related to rafoxanide (being a thiosalicylanilide) and acts in a similar manner by interfering with production of ATP. At a dose rate of 7.5 mg/kg it is highly effective against parenchymal stages and adult flukes and has a good safety margin. In treatments of severe acute fascioliasis the aromatic amine diamphenethide, which is available only for use in sheep, has proved outstanding against young flukes in the liver parenchyma and as a result the clinical response is dramatic. The high efficacy of diamphenethide is due to the deacetylated metabolite formed locally in the liver of sheep and this is responsible for the activity against the liver parenchymal stages.

Of the other drugs, also available for cattle, rafoxanide is probably the most widely used since nitroxynil is unpopular with some sheep owners due to the fleece staining with yellow dye which can occur at the site of injection. As in cattle, oxyclozanide is the only drug permitted for use where sheep and goats are milked, unless the milk or byproducts are discarded.

As mentioned above (p. 186) two drugs, namely closantel and a new benzimidazole (Boray 1982) are under development. Both are effective by injection or orally and closantel promises to control flukes down to six weeks old and the benzimidazole those down to one or two weeks old.

Dicrocoelium dendriticum

Very few drugs are consistently effective against the small liver fluke, *D. dendriticum*. Thiabendazole at a dose rate of 200–300 mg/kg body weight (i.e. 5–6 times the level for roundworms) is highly effective against the adult stages. Cambendazole has proved to be efficient at dose rates of 30 and 40 mg/kg against the adult stages (Sibalic *et al* 1971), while another benzimidazole, fenbendazole had an efficiency of 90% at high dosage rates, either in a single oral dose of 150 mg/kg or five repeated doses of 25 mg/kg. Recently, Eckert and his colleagues (Pers. Commun.) have shown that the

Table 10.9 Anthelmintics used against *Fasciola hepatica* in sheep and goats.

Drug (formulation)	Adult* flukes	4–8 week** old flukes	1–4 week*** old flukes	Withdrawal period (days)		Comments and other activity
				meat	milk	
Oxyclozanide (drench, in-feed)	A	C	D	14	Nil	Very safe; efficiency increases at higher dose rate. Tapeworms
Rafoxanide (drench)	A	A/B	D	28	Not used	Very safe; *Haemonchus* and *Oestrus ovis*
Nitroxynil (s.c. injection)	A	A/B	D	30	Not used	
Brotianide (drench, in-feed)	A	A/B	D	21	Not used	Increase dose rate for acute disease
Diamphenethide (drench)	A/B	A	A	7	Not used	Outstanding drug against very young flukes
Albendazole (drench)	B	C	D	14	Not used	1.5 × dose rate for nematodes. Not in 1st month of pregnancy

* chronic, ** sub-acute, *** acute fascioliasis.

Closantel and Fasinex are under development. Closantel is very effective against adults and 6–8-week-old flukes. Fasinex has an activity similar to diamphenethide.

cestocidal drug, praziquantel, was highly effective against adult stages in sheep. Further studies are required to evaluate these compounds and the other new benzimidazoles against *D. dentriticum* in cattle.

Paramphistomum spp.

The cestocidal drug, niclosamide, is probably the best drug available for the treatment of paramphistomiasis; at 50 mg/kg body weight several authors have reported high efficiency against the immature stages in the small intestine and the adult in the forestomachs. Oxyclozanide is also effective against the intestinal stages of these trematodes. More recently, Corba *et al* (1976) have reported that the fasciolicide, brotianide, has a high efficiency against the mature paramphistomes in the rumen and possibly the juvenile flukes in the small intestine. Current work at the same institute indicates that fenbendazole at 15 mg/kg is highly effective against adult and immature paramphistomes.

Combined products for nematodes and liver fluke

The indiscriminate use of a combined drench for the treatment of gastro-intestinal nematodiasis and fascioliasis can be wasteful. As mentioned above (p.187), the optimal times for treating the different helminthiases do not usually coincide, at least in Europe and North America, and unless the local epidemiology indicates a common seasonal cycle of infection with both classes of helminth, the use of combined drenches should be discouraged.

Cestodes

Tapeworms of the genera Moniezia, Thysanosoma, Avitellina and Stilesia have been reported as causing disease in sheep and goats in various parts of the world. For many years copper sulphate and lead or tin arsenates — all relatively cheap products — have been used for the treatment of tapeworms in sheep, and the arsenates have proved particularly effective against species of all four genera. In the more developed areas of the world the advent of the less toxic, but highly effective niclosamide, has resulted in this drug being used on farms with a tapeworm (moniezia) problem in lambs; it is also effective against *Thysanosoma actinoides.* Recently, the drug praziquantel has been developed and this is currently the most potent and one of the safest cestode drugs available. It also possesses the rare attribute of activity against both adult and larval cestodes. In ruminants it is highly effective against Moniezia spp., *Avitellina centripunctata,* and *Stilesia globipunctata* at 2.5–15.0 ml/kg. It is, however, rather costly and this may limit its use in large animals. Fortunately, in most countries, tapeworms are considered a minor and occasional problem, and treatment with a specific drug is unnecessary. In these situations the wide spectrum roundworm anthelmintics with accompanying action against Moniezia spp. are likely to be used; these include cambendazole, oxfendazole, fenbendazole and albendazole.

The prophylactic use of anthelmintics for sheep

The seasonal fluctuations in the free-living and infective stages of sheep helminths are now well documented from many areas of the world and anthelmintic treatments should be applied accordingly. For example, as mentioned previously, consideration should be given to controlling the peri-parturient rise in nematode faecal egg counts either by low-level medication or preferably by treating the ewes and moving them to worm-free grazing. Heavy infections in lambs occur most frequently during the post-weaning period and, where worm-free grazing is not available for this period, then regular anthelmintic therapy is advisable.

Liver fluke infections are also known to occur seasonally, and treatment should be applied accordingly. In western Europe, pasture infections with metacercariae (the infective stage) increase in early autumn. Therefore treatment with an anthelmintic effective against the young liver flukes, e.g. (diamphenethide, rafoxanide, nitroxynil) should be given from autumn onwards; in contrast, most fluke populations found in sheep at the end of the winter are adults and therefore one of the many drugs effective against adult flukes is required. With the excellent compounds now available, the best (and often most expensive) should be employed at the most critical times and local epidemiological knowledge sought to provide this information.

Pigs

Helminths of pigs

The common helminths of pigs are *Hyostrongylus rubidus* in the stomach, *Ascaris suum* and *Strongyloides ransomi* in the small intestine, and Trichuris spp. and Oesophagostomum spp. in the large intestine. Where pigs are kept at pasture (a decreasing number in developed countries), *Ascarops strongylina* and *Physocephalus sexulatus* occur in the stomach, *Macracanthorhynchus hirudinaceus* in the small intestine, Metastrongylus spp. in the lungs, *Fasciola hepatica* in the liver, and *Stephanurus dentatus* in the kidney. All of the latter parasites require an intermediate host, hence their prevalence in pigs at pasture.

Anthelmintic usage

Under modern pig husbandry systems, clinical parasitism is rarely seen and the main effects of helminths are as 'production-inhibitors' e.g. poor milk yield of sows, reduced weight of litters, reduced growth of piglets and poor food conversion ratios. Anthelmintics are widely used to alleviate reduced productivity due to the common helminths and it is the drugs used in this context that will be discussed. Some reference will be made to treatment of specific parasites found in grazing pigs, particularly in less developed countries.

The routine administration of anthelmintics to pigs is almost entirely in feed, although some treatments are given to individual pigs thought to be heavily parasitised. The in-feed formulation is usually either a powder, pellets, or granules and palatability of the product is important. As with all in-feed drugs, the main problem is to ensure adequate uptake of medicated feed in *ad libitum* feeding systems. In some countries continuous low-level medication is practised in an attempt to ensure an adequate uptake, but the efficiency of this type of therapy is not as well documented as the single in-feed treatment.

The anthelmintics available and most widely used are given in Table 10.10. Piperazine salts have a relatively narrow spectrum of activity in pigs and have not been included except in combination with other drugs, since their use other than in combination is decreasing. Unlike the ruminant anthelmintics there are, as yet, no compounds for pigs which are virtually 100% effective against the larval and adult stages of the common helminths. Thus, although preliminary work with the avermectins looks promising, diagnosis of the problem species involved is usually still necessary.

Where routine therapy is practised it is usual to carry out a programme which includes regular treatment of the sow as well as the growing stock. As in ruminants, the sow displays a marked increase in nematode faecal egg count during the peri-parturient period, and this is indirectly responsible for most of the infections found in the growing pigs. A popular worm-control treatment programme is as follows:

Sows. Prior to entering the farrowing house and possibly at weaning.
Weaners. On purchase or movement to the fattening house — usually about 8–12 weeks of age.
Fatteners. Eight weeks after entering fattening house.
Boars. Every six months.

Where *Strongyloides ransomi* is a problem, young unweaned piglets may be given specific treatment. It is best to use an anthelmintic with a high therapeutic index such as thiabendazole for this purpose. For treatment of lungworm infections or where Macrocanthorhynchus is present, levamisole

Table 10.10 Anthelmintics for nematodes in pigs (in-feed unless stated).

Drug	*Ascaris suum* adults/larvae	*Hyostrongylus rubidus* adults/larvae	*Oesophagostomum* spp. adults/larvae	*Trichuris suis* adults/larvae	Comments
Thiabendazole	D/D	A/C	A/C	D/D	No withdrawal; ovicidal
Parbendazole	A/D	A/D	A/D	B/U	16 days withdrawal, ovicidal
Cambendazole	A/B	A/C	A/C	D/D	14 days withdrawal, not sows for 5 weeks after service
Fenbendazole Flubendazole	A/B	A/A	A/B	A/D	14 days withdrawal, ovicidal, also active vs. *Metastrongylus*
Tetramisole	A/B	A/C	A/C	B/B	7 days withdrawal, ovicidal, also active vs. *Metastrongylus*
Dichlorvos	A/D	A/D	A/D	A/A	No withdrawal
Morantel	A/B	A/C	A/C	D/D	14 days withdrawal
Febantel	A/C	A/C	A/C	A/D	Increased dose rate vs. *Trichuris*. 7 days withdrawal
Thiophanate	A/C	A/B	A/B	A/B	7 days withdrawal; ovicidal

Note. Several drugs combined with piperazine to remove Ascaris e.g. thiabendazole. For treatment of clinical parasitism injectable levamisole is recommended. Oxyfendazole and ivermectin with efficacy similar to fenbendazole will be available shortly.

by injection has proved particularly useful. Successful treatment of Ascarops or Physocephalus spp. has been reported with trichlorfon and sodium fluoride, both drugs which are now less frequently used in pigs.

Finally, arrested larval development is known to occur frequently in certain pig nematode life-cycles (*H. rubidus* and Oesophagostomum spp.) and this should be considered when choosing an anthelmintic. Evidence is lacking about efficiency against arrested larval stages in pigs but recourse to the drugs effective against these stages in ruminants (e.g. one of the latest benzimidazoles or the avermectins) may alleviate the problem.

Where pigs are kept at pasture the same principles for the control of roundworms apply as with ruminants, i.e. pigs should be dosed and move to other grazing at a time when pasture levels of infective larvae are known to be declining. This principle will not control *A. suum* since the egg containing the infective stage of this parasite remains viable for several years. If Metastrongylus lungworms are a problem, then tetramisole or fenbendazole should be used.

Acknowledgements

The author wishes to acknowledge the assistance given by Dr James Bogan in the preparation of this paper.

References

Adrichem P. W. M. van & Shaw J. C. (1977) Effects of gastrointestinal nematodiasis on the productivity of monozygous twin cattle. II Growth performance and Milk Production. *J. Anim. Sci.* **45**, 423–429.

Anderson N. (1971) Ostertagiasis in beef cattle. *Victoria Vet. Proc.* **30**, 36–38.

Anderson N. & Laby R. (1977) A New Concept in Anthelmintic Use. *Proc. 8th Congr. Wld. Assoc. Vet. Parasit.* (Sydney) p. 4.

Armour J., Bairden K. & Preston J. M. (1980) A study of the anthelmintic efficiency of ivermectin against naturally occurring bovine gastrointestinal nematodes. *Vet. Rec.* **107**, 226–227.

Bliss D. H. & Todd A. C. (1974) Milk production by Wisconsin dairy cattle after deworming with thiabendazole. *Vet. Med./Small An. Clin.* **69**, 638–640.

Boray J. C., Happich F. A. & Andrews J. C. (1967) Comparative therapeutic tests on sheep infected with mature and immature fluke. *Vet. Rec.* **80**, 218–224.

Boray J. C. (1982) The anthelmintic activity of fasinex in sheep and cattle. *Vet. Rec.* In Press.

Bossche H. Van den (1976) In *Biochemistry of Parasites and Host-Parasite Relationships* 553–573. North Holland, Amsterdam.

Corba J., Pacenovsky J. & Krupner I. (1976) Study on the efficacy of Brotianide (Dirian). *Vet. Med. Res.* **2**, 181–189.

Downey N. G. & O'Shea J. (1977) Calf parasite control by means of low-level anthelmintic administered via the drinking water. *Vet. Rec.* **100**, 265–266.

Eckert J., Keller H., Hosh J. *et al* (1977) Subacute fascioliasis in cattle. *Schwiez Arch. Tierheith* **119**, 135–148.

Egerton J. R., Ostlind D. A., Blair L. S. *et al* (1979) Avermectins, new family of potent anthelmintics; efficacy of the B_{1a} component. *Antimicrob. Agents Chemother.* **15**, 372–378.

Eslami A. H. & Anwar (1976) Activity of fenbendazole against lungworms in naturally infected sheep. *Vet. Rec.* **99**, 129–130.

Frimmer M. & Lammler G. (1977) *Pharmacology and Toxicology,* pp. 75–106. F. R. Schattauer Verlag, New York.

Hörchner F., Hennings R., Verspohl F. *et al* (1970) MediKamentelle BeKämpfung der Fasciolose der Rinder im LandKreis SteinFurt II Ergebnisse nach der 3-Jahrigen BehandlungsaKtion. *Berl. Munch. Tierarztil. Wschr.* **83**, 21–26.

Gibson T. E. (1975) *Veterinary Anthelmintic Medication,* 3rd ed. Tech. Comm. No. 33. Commonwealth Institute of Helminthology, St. Albans.

Inderbitzen F. & Eckert J. (1978) Die Werkung von Fenbendazole (Panacur) gegen gehemunte Stadien von *Dictyocaulus viviparus* und *Ostertagia ostertagi* bei Kalbern. *Berl. Munch. Tierart. Wacht.* **91**, 395–399.

Jones R. M. (1981) A morantel sustained release bolus for the control of parasitic gastroenteritis in cattle. *Vet. Parasitol.* **8**, 237–251.

Kelly J. D., Gordon H. McL. & Whitlock H. V. (1976) Anthelmintics for sheep: historical perspectives, classification/usage, problem areas and future prospects. *N. S. W. Vet. Proc.* **12**, 18–31.

Koopman J. J. (1969) Observations about the control of fascioliasis in cattle. *Tijdschr. Diergeneesk.* **94**, 1046–1053.

Le Jambre I. F. (1978) Anthelmintic resistance in gastrointestinal nematodes of sheep. In *The Epidemiology and Control of Gastrointestinal Parasites of Sheep in Australia,* Donald A. D., Southcott W. H. and Dineen J. K. (eds.) CSIRO, Melbourne.

McEwan A. D. & Oakley G. A. (1978) Anthelmintics and closure of the oesophageal groove in cattle. *Vet. Rec.* **102**, 314–315.

Oakley G. A. (1981) Efficacy of levamisole against inhibited Dictyocaulus viviparus infection in cattle. *Res. Vet. Sci.* **30**, 127–128.

Prichard R. K., Donald A. D., Dash K. M. *et al* (1978) Factors involved in the relative anthelmintic tolerance of arrested larvae of *Ostertagia ostertagi*. *Vet. Rec.* **102**, 382.

Rew R. S. (1978) Mode of action of common anthelmintics. *J. Vet. Pharmacol. Therap.* **1**, 183–198.

Ross J. G. (1970) The economics of *Fasciola hepatica* infections in cattle. *Br. Vet. J.* **126**, 13–15.

Sibalic S., Lepojen Olga & Miklijan S. (1971) The efficiency of cambendazole against *Dicrocoelium dendriticum*. *Vet. Glasn.* **25**, 835–839.

Sibalic S., CvetKovic Lja., Lepojev Olga *et al* (1975) A study of the effect of cambendazole on *Ascaris suum* migrating larvae in artificially infected piglets. *Proc. 2nd Europ. Multicoll. Parasitol.* (Trogir) p. 107.

11

Anthelmintics for use in equine practice

J. DUNCAN

Horses, ponies and donkeys are hosts to a large variety of parasites, and it is well nigh impossible to find any grazing animal which is not harbouring a number of species at any particular time. The common internal parasites of British horses are shown in Table 11.1. The most common stomach parasites of the horse are undoubtedly stomach 'bots', the larval stages of horse bot flies (Gastrophilus spp). In the small intestine there are three common parasites: *Parascaris equorum* and *Strongyloides westeri* are most frequently found in young animals and the tapeworm *Anoplocephala perfoliata* is found in horses of all ages.

It is in the large intestine that numerous strongylid worms are to be found and these are divided, mainly on a size basis, into large (i.e. over 1.5 cm) and small (i.e. under 1.5 cm) strongyles. There are only two large strongyles common in Britain, *Strongylus vulgaris* and *Strongylus edentatus,* but the small strongyles consist of approximately 30 species which are commonly referred to as Trichonema spp. Also in the large intestine, mainly the colon, is found the horse pinworm *Oxyuris equi.*

A brief description of the life-cycles and pathogenic significance of these parasites and the influence of the host and the environment on their development is given prior to the discussion of control measures based on drug treatment.

Table 11.1 Common internal parasites of the horse.

Predilection site	Parasite	Common name
Stomach	Gasterophilus spp.	Bots
Small intestine	*Parascaris equorum*	Roundworm
	Strongyloides westeri	Threadworm
Ileum/caecum	*Anoplocephala perfoliata*	Tapeworm
Caecum/colon	*Strongylus vulgaris*	Large strongyles
	Strongylus edentatus	
	Trichonema spp.	Small strongyles
Colon	*Oxyuris equi*	Pinworm

Gasterophilus spp.

Infection with horse bots is common, as shown by the frequent finding of larvae in the stomach at post-mortem examination and by the presence of fly eggs on the hairs of many horses during the late summer and autumn. Bot flies have only one generation per year. The flies are active during July–September and eggs are laid during this period. After hatching, the larvae migrate to the stomach and develop there for 9–10 months. When mature, the following June, they are passed out in faeces to pupate and develop to the adult stage.

The pathogenic significance of bot larvae in the stomach is controversial. There are a few reports from Australia and the USA (Rainey 1948, Rooney 1964) incriminating bots as the cause of gastric disorders, but large numbers of these parasites can be found in horses which have shown no signs of gastrointestinal upset: their pathogenicity therefore remains obscure. However, the adult flies themselves cause a great deal of annoyance during the process of egg-laying and any measures which will reduce fly populations can only be beneficial. From the life-cycle it is obvious that removal of the bots after they have accumulated in the stomach during the late autumn and winter will effectively break the life-cycle.

Strongyloides westeri

In very young foals from two weeks to four months infection with the threadworm *Strongyloides westeri* is common. The life-cycle is as follows (Lyons *et al* 1973). Foals are commonly infected by larvae in their dam's milk and these develop into adult female worms in the small intestine, only the female of this species being parasitic. Infections may also occur by skin penetration of infective larvae. Eggs which are produced by these female worms are found in the faeces of foals by the second week of life and in severe infections diarrhoea may occur between 2 and 4 weeks of age. This parasite has another unusual feature in that it may have one or several free-living cycles before again producing third stage infective larvae. Although attempts have been made to treat mares in order to kill tissue-dwelling larvae and thus reduce infection of their foals, this has proved difficult and the main approach is to treat the scouring foal with an anthelmintic effective against *S. westeri.*

Parascaris equorum

The second common parasite of foals is the large roundworm *Parascaris equorum* and recent experimental studies have provided information on the life-cycle and pathogenesis of this parasite (Lyons *et al* 1976, Clayton &

Duncan 1978, Nicholls *et al* 1978). Adult male and female worms live in the small intestine of foals and young horses and the females produce sticky, round, thick-shelled eggs which become infective in 3–4 weeks. These larvated eggs are resistant to adverse environmental factors and may remain on pastures and in stables for several years. After ingestion, the eggshells are digested and the larvae migrate via the liver, lungs, and trachea to the small intestine where they mature and begin producing eggs approximately three months after infection. During their migration through the lungs, *P. equorum* larvae may produce a mild respiratory illness evidenced by coughing and a mucoid or mucopurulent nasal discharge, but they exert their main effect on their return to the small intestine where they cause unthriftness and in some cases emaciation and death. Because of the resistance of the egg, control is achieved by anthelmintic treatments to remove adult parasites from young foals and thus reduce the numbers of infective eggs available for foals of either the same or succeeding generations.

Anoplocephala perfoliata

The only tapeworm of horses in the UK is *Anoplocephala perfoliata* which is 4–5 cm long, white in colour and found in the ileum, around the ileo-caecal valve, and in the caecum. Typical eggs, each containing a hexacanth embryo, are released from mature proglottids and are passed in the faeces. These are ingested by forage mites, the intermediate host, in which the larval cystereroid develops. Ingestion of infected mites allows the adult tapeworm to develop in the small intestine of the horse. As in bot infection, the pathogenic significance of tapeworms is not well understood and only rarely is specific treatment called for.

Strongylid spp.

Heavy mixed infections with strongyles are common in equine animals of all ages. The pre-parasitic phase of the life-cycle is similar in all species. Adult worms live in the large intestine and typical thin-shelled, oval eggs are passed in the faeces. Under optimum conditions these eggs develop to infective third stage larvae on pasture in approximately two weeks.

After ingestion, in the case of the large strongyles there is an extensive larval migratory phase within the tissues of the host before the parasites reach maturity. *S. vulgaris* larvae travel to the cranial mesenteric artery and *S. edentatus* to the liver and parietal peritoneum in the region of the flanks before returning to the large intestine — the total time taken for this migration being approximately six months (*S. vulgaris*) and eleven months (*S. edentatus*), respectively. The small strongyles, on the other hand, spend some time developing in the large intestinal mucosa before reaching maturity in the lumen and the pre-patent periods range from 6 to 12 weeks.

This group of parasites is probably the most pathogenic of the equine helminths and anaemia, unthriftiness, and death are not uncommon in heavy strongyle infections. There is apparently little acquired immunity and horses of all ages may be infected either from overwintered third stage infective larvae (L$_3$) on pasture or from L$_3$ which accumulate on pasture from eggs passed in the faeces of untreated horses during the grazing season. Pasture larval levels may, however, be reduced to low levels by regular treatment of all grazing animals between April and October.

Oxyuris equi

Infection with adult pinworms is extremely common and, in the dorsal colon, the large white, female parasites reach a length of 10 cm while the males are about 1 cm in length. The female migrates to the anus to lay masses of ovoid, operculate eggs which are flattened on one side, on the perineal skin; thus eggs are rarely found in faecal samples. The infective third larval stage develops within the eggs in 4–5 days either on the skin, on the ground, or on contaminated objects and hatches after ingestion. The L$_3$ develops to the L$_4$ in the colonic mucosa before returning to the lumen to become adult — the whole cycle taking about five months.

O. equi is considered to be a non-pathogenic scavenger but the process of egg laying by the female parasites causes perineal irritation and tail rubbing. Control of oxyuriasis is achieved during routine strongyle control since virtually all the drugs active against strongyles are active against pinworms.

Anthelmintics

An ideal equine anthelmintic should possess the following qualities:
1 The drug should be efficient against all stages of the parasite
2 The preparation should be either non-toxic to the host or have a wide margin of safety
3 The drug should be easily administered
4 The cost of the treatment must be reasonable.

It is now appropriate to consider the drugs currently available in the UK (Table 11.2) and see to what extent they meet these criteria. Prior to the introduction of thiabendazole in 1962, the principal equine anthelmintics available were piperazine and phenothiazine. Neither of these drugs possessed 'broad-spectrum' anthelmintic activity but piperazine is still used as an efficient treatment for *P. equorum* infection. Benzimidazole anthelmintics,

Table 11.2 Formulation and dosage of anthelmintics for equine use.

Active principle	Trade name (UK)	Presentation	Recommended dose rate
Piperazine citrate	Citrazine	Powder	200 mg/kg
Thiabendazole	Equizole	Powder	44–50 mg/kg
	Thibenzole	In-feed pellets, pony paste	(88–100 mg/kg for *P. equorum*)
Mebendazole	Equivurm	Granules	5–10 mg/kg
	Telmin	Paste	
Fenbendazole	Panacur	Granules, suspension	7.5 mg/kg
Oxfendazole	Synanthic	Granules	10 mg/kg
	Systamex	Paste	
Febantel	Bayverm	Paste	6 mg/kg
Oxibendazole	Equitac	Paste	10 mg/kg
Pyrantel embonate	Strongid P.	Granules, paste	19 mg/kg
Dichlorvos	Astrobot	Resin pellets	8.3 g/500 lbs
Metriphonate	Neguvon	Paste	35 mg/kg

Table 11.3 Efficiency of anthelmintics against the common internal equine parasites.

	P. equorum	Strongyloides	Large strongyles	Small strongyles	*O. equi*	'Bots'
Piperazine	+	−	−	+	+	−
Thiabendazole	±	+	+	+	+	−
Mebendazole	+	−	+	+	+	−
Fenbendazole	+	+	+	+	+	−
Oxfendazole	+	+	+	+	+	−
Febantel	+	ND	+	+	+	−
Oxibendazole	+	+	+	+	+	−
Pyrantel embonate	+	−	+	+	+	−
Dichlorvos	+	ND	+	+	+	+
Metriphonate	+	ND	−	−	+	+

Key. + Highly effective; ± poorly effective; − not effective; ND no data available.

other than thiabendazole, available as equine preparations, are mebendazole, fenbendazole, oxfendazole, oxibendazole and the pro-benzimidazole febantel. The other major equine anthelmintics are pyrantel embolate and the organophosphorus compounds, dichlorvos and metriphonate.

Table 11.3 summarises the efficiency of these drugs against the adult stages of the major equine parasites. Unfortunately, much of the trial work carried out with these drugs made no assessment of their activity against developing larval stages in the tissues of the host, and it is only recently that there has been an attempt to assess such activity. However, from the table it is apparent that most of the drugs in current use have a broad spectrum of activity against adult gastrointestinal nematodes. Exceptions are piperazine, which has poor activity against large strongyles, and thiabendazole which has to be used at double the normal dose rate for reasonable activity against *P. equorum*.

Some of these compounds have not been tested against *Strongyloides westeri* infection in foals (e.g. dichlorvos) but activity against this parasite has been demonstrated in the case of thiabendazole, fenbendazole and oxfendazole. The only drugs with high activity against developing bot larvae in the stomach are dichlorvos and metriphonate.

Activity of anthelmintics against tissue-dwelling larval stages

Only a few of the major equine anthelmintics have been tested for activity against tissue-dwelling larval stages, although most have been shown to have some activity against larvae present in the lumen of the intestine. Fenbendazole and oxfendazole have been shown to have a significant effect against Trichonema spp. larvae in the mucosa of the large intestine and some effect against migrating large strongyles at increased dose rates (Duncan *et al* 1977). This could provide a basis for an increased interval between treatments.

Prophylactic use of anthelmintics

Although control measures on different horse establishments will vary according to conditions, in general *all* animals should be regularly treated with a broad spectrum anthelmintic at 4–6 week intervals in order to reduce parasite populations both in the animals and in the environment.

Good management is also important in reducing the level of parasitism including stable hygiene, pasture rotation, the retention of the least contaminated paddocks for nursing mares and their foals, treatment and isolation of new arrivals, and mixed grazing with other non-equine species.

Anthelmintic resistance

There are few reports of resistance to equine anthelmintics. Strains of horse strongyles resistant to thiabendazole were first reported from North America in 1965 (Drudge & Lyons 1965) after this drug had been the sole drug used, over a period of 3–4 years, in a group of brood mares. It was found, however, that the addition of piperazine to the thiabendazole overcame this resistance. In the UK in 1974 there was also evidence of acquired resistance of some small strongyles to thiabendazole and mebendazole on stud farms where the former drug had been used extensively

Table 11.4 General properties of equine anthelmintics.

Drug	Action	Presentation	Palatability	Dose rate/ activity	Toxicity
Piperazine	Causes a flaccid paralysis in nematodes	The only salt available for horses; marketed as a powder for administration via stomach tube or in feed	Usually well accepted	200–220 mg/kg. Activity limited mainly to *P. equorum* and small strongyle species	Low
Benzimidazole anthelmintics					
Thiabendazole	Interfere with absorption of nutrients by parasites' intestinal cells which effectively starves them	Powder or paste for oral administration	Medicated feeds sometimes refused but paste overcomes this problem	Broad spectrum including Strongyloides infection at 44–50 mg/kg but *P. equorum* needs 88–100 mg/kg	Very low
Mebendazole	As thiabendazole	Granules for in-feed medication or paste for oral administration using dosing syringe	Usually well accepted in feed but may be given by stomach tube or easily as paste	Broad spectrum at 5–10 mg/kg excluding Strongyloides	Non toxic at up to 40 times the normal dose rate
Fenbendazole	As thiabendazole	Granules for in-feed administration and paste or 10% suspension for oral administration	Well accepted in food and easily given as paste or suspension	Broad spectrum at 7.5 mg/kg. Strongyloides infection in foals may need up to 50 mg/kg	Extremely safe, apparently impossible to overdose
Oxfendazole	As thiabendazole	Granules for in-feed administration	Well accepted	Broad spectrum at 10 mg/kg	Very low

Drug	Mode of action	Formulation	Acceptability	Spectrum	Safety
Febantel		Paste	Well accepted	Broad spectrum at 6 mg/kg excluding Strongyloides	Very low
Oxibendazole		Paste	Well accepted	Broad spectrum at 10 mg/kg. 15 mg/kg for Strongyloides	Very low
Pyrantel embonate	A nematode muscle relaxant which produces worm paralysis	Granules and paste in a dosing syringe	Usually well accepted in feed and easily given as paste	Broad spectrum against adult GI parasites at 19 mg/kg	Safe up to 20 times recommended dose rate
Dichlorvos	An organophosphorus compound which acts as a cholinesterase inhibitor resulting in excess acetyl choline at nerve endings and leading to initial stimulation then paralysis of parasites	A resin pellet formulation for in-feed administration which allows slow release of the active principle on passage through the gut	Not always accepted in feed	Broad spectrum against helminths and bots at 33–43 mg/kg	Exercise care in pregnant animals and in those suffering from other conditions or being treated with other drugs having cholinesterase-inhibiting activity. Pellets appearing in the faeces are toxic for fowl and wild birds.
Metriphonate	As for dichlorvos	Paste	Administer carefully, can cause local irritation	Activity limited to *P. equorum, O. equi* and bots at 35 mg/kg	As for dichlorvos

(Round *et al* 1974). At the same time in the USA it was shown that mebendazole was ineffective against strongyles which were resistant to thiabendazole. Recently there have been further reports from Australia and Canada of cross-resistance of small strongyles to several benzimidazoles (Barger & Lisle 1979, Slocombe & Cote 1977). There is no evidence of resistance to piperazine, pyrantel, or dichlorvos, which are chemically unrelated to the benzimidazole group compounds and it is obvious therefore that treatments with these unrelated drugs should be substituted at intervals in a benzimidazole-based programme.

Other parasite infections and their treatment

Lungworm infection

Very little work has been carried out on *Dictyocaulus arnfieldi* infection of horses and donkeys and the pathogenesis, epidemiology, and therapy of this infection are not well understood. Successful treatment of confirmed cases has been reported using 100 ml diethylcarbamazine citrate daily for three days in drinking water and by dosing with thiabendazole at 440 mg/kg on two occasions with one day's interval between treatments. In Germany, levamisole, at 5 mg/kg given intramuscularly on two occasions with a 3–4 week interval, has been used in the treatment of lungworm infection in donkeys, but this drug is not particularly suited for horses as it has a narrower safety margin than in cattle and sheep and it is poorly active against strongyle infections. Fenbendazole, at a dose rate of 30 mg/kg, is recommended for the treatment of lungworm in horses and mebendazole paste, at a dose rate of 15–20 mg/kg/day for four days, has been shown to be 75–100% effective in a critical trial in donkeys (Clayton & Neave 1979).

Fluke and tapeworm infection

Although eggs of *F. hepatica* can be found frequently in horse faecal samples, treatment, like that for tapeworm, is rarely called for. There are reports, however, of rafoxanide and oxyclozanide being used successfully in the horse and niclosamide has been shown to be effective against *Anoplocephala perfoliata* infection.

References

Barger I. A. & Lisle K. A. (1979) Benzimidazole resistance in small strongyles of horses. *Aust. Vet. J.* **55,** 594–5.

Clayton H. M. & Duncan J. L. (1978) Clinical signs associated with *Parascaris equorum* infection in worm-free pony foals and yearlings. *Vet. Parasitol.* **4,** 69–78.

Clayton H. M. & Neave R. M. S. (1979) Efficacy of mebendazole against *Dictyocaulus arnfieldi* in the donkey. *Vet. Rec.* **105,** 571–2.

Drudge J. H. & Lyons E. T. (1965) Newer developments in helminth control and *Strongylus vulgaris* research. *Proc. Am. Assoc. Equine Practit.* 11th Annual Convention, pp. 381–9.

Duncan J. L., Macbeth D. G., Best J. M. J. *et al* (1977) The efficacy of fenbendazole in the control of immature strongyle infections in ponies. *Equine Vet. J.* **9,** 146–9.

Fletcher R. B. (1960) *Dictyocaulus arnfieldi* infestation in horses. *Vet. Rec.* **72,** 1171.

Lyons E. T., Drudge J. H. & Tolliver S. C. (1973) On the life cycle of *Strongyloides westeri* in the equine. *J. Parasitol.* **59,** 780–7.

Lyons E. T., Drudge J. H. & Tolliver S. C. (1976) Studies on the development and chemotherapy of larvae of *Parascaris equorum* (Nematoda: Ascaridoidea) in experimentally and naturally infected foals. *J. Parasitol.* **62,** 453–9.

Nicholls J. M., Clayton H. M., Pirie H. M. *et al* (1978) A pathological study of the lungs of foals infected experimentally with *Parascaris equorum. J. Comp. Pathol.* **88,** 261–74.

Rainey J. W. (1948) Equine mortality due to Gasterophilus larvae (stomach bots). *Aust. Vet. J.* **24,** 116–19.

Rooney J. R. (1964) Gastric ulceration in foals. *Vet. Pathol.* **11,** 497–503.

Round M. C., Simpson D. J., Haselden C. S. *et al* (1974) Horse strongyles' tolerance to anthelmintics. *Vet. Rec.* **95,** 517–18.

Slocombe J. O. D. & Cote J. F. (1977) Small strongyles of horses with cross resistance to benzimidazole anthelmintics and susceptibility to unrelated compounds. *Can. Vet. J.* **18,** 212–16.

PART 4
REPRODUCTION

12

Pharmacological treatment of reproductive disorders in the mare

W. EDWARD ALLEN

Several groups of substances are extensively employed to control various aspects of reproductive function in mares. In addition, there are a number of other agents which may be used in specific circumstances to increase fertility. The aim of this chapter is to review the literature concerning these various preparations and to indicate their modes of action and the clinical situations in which they may be employed. The basic changes which occur during a normal oestrous cycle in the mare are summarised in Fig. 12.1.

Prostaglandins

The use of prostaglandin (PG)F$_{2\alpha}$ and its synthetic analogues for the regulation of luteal activity in the mare has increased steadily since it was first

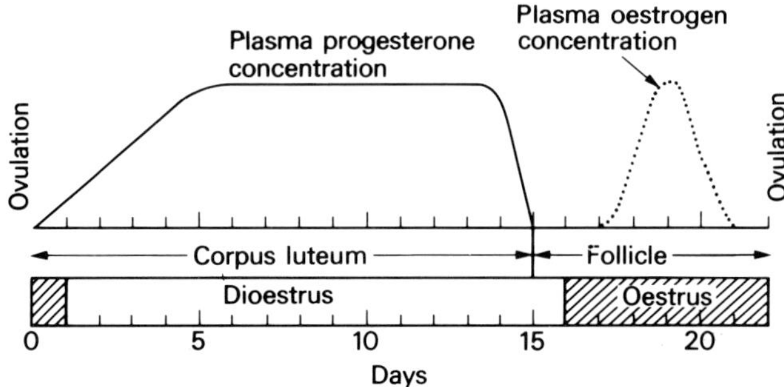

Fig. 12.1 Diagrammatic representation of the main behavioural, hormonal, and ovarian changes during an average (21 day) oestrous cycle in the mare. Note that oestrus usually ends 1–2 days after ovulation; that the corpus luteum begins to regress 14 days after ovulation, i.e. 2–3 days before the next heat in a 21 day cycle; and that the oestrous cycle length is very variable, i.e. 19 days upwards. Variations (except in 'prolonged dioestrus') are due to the time taken for follicles to mature; the luteal phase is relatively constant at 14–16 days. Ovulation can occur 30 days after the first day of oestrus. The longest cycles occur in spring.

213

shown that a subcutaneous injection of $PGF_{2\alpha}$ on day six of dioestrus caused a rapid return to oestrus (Douglas & Ginther 1972). This was confirmed by Allen & Rowson (1973) who used sythetic prostaglandin analogue and demonstrated that its luteolytic properties were responsible for the rapid return to heat. Since then considerable data have been accumulated on the efficacy of PG as a luteolytic agent in mares and, as a consequence, the administration of $PGF_{2\alpha}$ or its synthetic analogues has replaced the traditional method of causing luteolysis by irrigating the mare's uterus with saline.

During the first five days of its life (i.e. about the first four days of dioestrus) the developing corpus luteum (CL) is refractory to the effects of PG (Douglas & Ginther 1973, Allen & Rowson 1973). In the normal cyclical mare the CL begins to regress on the 14th day after ovulation, so that the use of exogenous PG after this time will only augment natural luteolysis. Treatment between days 5 and 14, and at times when there is abnormal persistence of luteal function, is followed by a rapid decline in peripheral blood concentrations of progesterone and a return to oestrus in 2–5 days (Douglas & Ginther 1972, Allen & Rowson 1973, Noden *et al* 1973, Hughes 1975), with ovulation 7–12 days after treatment. Some mares thus treated however, will ovulate without showing signs of heat (Kenney *et al* 1975). The induced oestrus may be of normal length (Douglas & Ginther 1975b) or slightly longer than usual (Burns *et al* 1979). Blood luteinising hormone (LH) concentrations are similar to those in normal periods of oestrus (Noden *et al* 1973, Oxender 1974, Noden *et al* 1974), as are concentrations of oestradiol, oestrone and androstenedione (Noden *et al* 1975). Prostaglandin administration has no effect on the length of dioestrus or oestrus in the post-treatment cycle (Douglas & Ginther 1972). Various routes of administration (subcutaneous, intramuscular, and intrauterine) have been investigated by several workers (Allen & Rowson 1973, Oxender 1974, Douglas & Ginther 1974a, 1974b, 1975a) and no differences in efficacy were found.

The minimal effective luteolytic dose of $PGF_{2\alpha}$ (free acid equivalent) has been estimated to be between $6\mu g/kg$ (Douglas & Ginther 1975a) and $9 \mu g/kg$ (Oxender *et al* 1975). Similar studies have been carried out on synthetic analogues of $PGF_{2\alpha}$ (Allen *et al* 1974). Doses of PG which do not cause complete luteolysis will produce a temporary reduction in luteal function as judged by circulating blood progesterone concentrations (Thompson & Witherspoon 1974, Allen *et al* 1974, Lamond *et al* 1975, Kiefer 1979). However, some workers, using a particular synthetic analogue, have apparently stimulated oestrus in mares which had non-luteal concentrations of progesterone in peripheral blood before treatment (Thompson & Witherspoon 1974, Lamond *et al* 1975, Tolksdorff *et al*

1976). This was not confirmed by Kenney *et al* (1975).

The local administration of PG either into the uterus or directly into the CL did not improve the luteolytic efficacy of the drug (Douglas & Ginther 1974b, 1975a) from which the authors concluded that PG may have, at least in part, a central effect on the hypothalamus or pituitary. They further showed (Douglas *et al* 1974) that the absence of a uterus did not significantly affect the luteolytic efficacy of PG, although, following later experiments which involved a comparison of luteolysis after administration of PG into either the carotid or the uterine artery, they considered the primary site of PG-induced luteolysis to be at the ovarian rather than at the pituitary–hypothalamic level. More recently it has been shown that $PGF_{2\alpha}$ is the natural luteolysin in mares (Douglas & Ginther 1976a, Neely *et al* 1979, Vernon 1979). The uterus responds differently to $PGF_{2\alpha}$ (tham salt) than to oxytocin (Capraro *et al* 1976).

In field studies, only 73–74% of PG-treated mares subsequently showed oestrus (Berwyn-Jones & Irvine 1974, Shepherd *et al* 1976); the reasons for the apparent failures are discussed later (p. 217). Conception rates following the induction of oestrus with PG are, however, generally thought to be acceptable (Witherspoon *et al* 1975, Noden 1975, Hughes 1975, Kenney *et al* 1975, Loy & Sharma 1976).

The immediate side-effects of overdosing with $PGF_{2\alpha}$ and its analogues have been well documented (Allen *et al* 1974, Goynings *et al* 1975, Miller *et al* 1976, Nelson 1976) and comprise sweating, hyperglycaemia, locomotor incoordination, hyperthermia, dyspnoea and hypergastromotility (Goynings *et al* 1977). These latter authors concluded that the largest non-toxic dose of $PGF_{2\alpha}$ is 0.53 mg/kg/day. Tolksdorff *et al* (1976) observed no side-effects in foals which were suckling mares that had been treated with PG, and Miller & Lauderdale (1976) could find no adverse effect of repeated doses of PG on fertility; although Spincemaille *et al* (1975) noted that repeated administration of PG resulted in udder development. More detailed studies (Douglas & Ginther 1976b) showed that, although daily injections of PG did not inhibit oestrus and normal follicular growth, heat terminated without ovulation and the follicle regressed. Subsequent heats were ovulatory.

Practical applications of PG in mares

The luteolytic property of PG is used widely in mares to control reproductive function in the following situations.

To shorten dioestrus

In cases where the mare was not covered during the previous oestrus either because of management difficulties (e.g. non-availability of stallion, ovulation occurring more rapidly than expected, results of bacteriological swabs awaited, etc.) or due to anticipated double ovulation. PG administration after day eight of the cycle may not be followed by appreciable shortening of the interovulatory period (Hughes & Loy 1978).

In mares with endometritis. Spincemaille *et al* (1975) reported that three spaced injections of PG in a mare with an endometritis caused by pseudomonas infection resulted in ovulation occurring three times within 25 days, and spontaneous resolution of the infection. Allen & Hadley (1973) and Newcombe & Allen (unpublished observations) have shown that mares with endometritis usually have shortened luteal activity, this being an apparently natural 'cleansing' mechanism. However, the use of PG may be of value in such circumstances and requires further investigation.

After foal heat. The use of this heat for covering mares has long been controversial. Its advantages are mainly that it is easy to detect due to its regular occurrence, and some mares thereafter do not show spontaneous oestrus (i.e. enter a 'lactational anoestrus'). However, some mares still have a post-partum endometritis at this heat, especially if uterine involution is slow, and a higher number of early foetal deaths have been recorded after conception at this heat as compared with others (Merkt 1966, 1968).

Several authors have obtained good conception rates when luteolysis has been induced after the foal heat ovulation (Witherspoon *et al* 1975, Tolksdorff *et al* 1976, Cornwell 1977), and Kreider *et al* (1975) and Tolksdorff *et al* (1976) have found such conceptions to be less likely to end in foetal death than natural foal heat conceptions. Burns *et al* (1979), however, did not increase conception rates by using this method. Data presented by Allen & Rossdale (1973) and Allen & Cooper (1975) suggest that most cases of 'lactational anoestrus' are associated with the persistence of luteal function.

Possibly to facilitate ease of detection of oestrus in individual mares which are kept out of contact with other horses, and where veterinary advice on the mare's reproductive status is not available. Two injections of PG at 14-day intervals, at a time of the year when the mare could reasonably be assumed to have started cyclical activity, would in most cases ensure that the mare was in heat 4–5 days after the second injection.

PG will not intensify oestrous behaviour in mares which are prone to having silent heats. However, a knowledge of when the mare should be in heat after PG administration may allow more rigorous methods of oestrus detection to be employed, with a consequently better chance of recognising behavioural changes in the 'shy' mare.

To shorten persistent luteal function (prolonged dioestrus)

The suggestion that some mares do not show cyclical activity during the breeding season due to a retained CL (Cameron 1942, Lieux 1966) was confirmed by Hughes *et al* (1972) who showed that this syndrome could occur spontaneously and was not influenced by season. The efficacy of PG in terminating such prolonged luteal function (prolonged dioestrus) has been demonstrated by Allen & Rossdale (1973) and Loy & Sharma (1976). The latter authors recorded that, although 59 of 60 mares treated in prolonged dioestrus subsequently ovulated in 2–15 days, only 46 of these mares showed oestrus. It is not uncommon to find one or more large follicles in the ovaries of mares in prolonged dioestrus, although one ovary still contains a functional CL. Regression of this CL (due to PG administration) may at one extreme be followed by the rapid ovulation of existing follicles in two or three days and the mare may not show any signs of oestrus. Conversely, all follicles which are palpable at the time of luteolysis may become atretic and newly developed follicles will ovulate at the end of the induced oestrus (Loy *et al* 1979). The fate of follicles which are present at the time of luteolysis may be governed by their age, with only the youngest follicles ovulating rapidly. More rarely follicles may ovulate during a period of prolonged dioestrus. Should PG be administered in this situation, before the young CL is five days old, then only the mature CL will regress and treatment will seem to have failed. The young CL should then regress after its usual 14 day lifespan.

To interrupt pregnancy

Two situations may arise in which it is desirable to curtail an established or probable pregnancy.

After inadvertent mating, or after accidental mating with the wrong stallion. PG administered after the sixth day following ovulation will induce luteolysis and a return to oestrus. Unless the mare is being examined regularly to pinpoint the time of ovulation, luteolytic therapy should be given ten days after the termination of oestrus. This will allow for any discrepancy between ovulation (or ovulations) and the end of heat.

After the diagnosis of twin pregnancy. Mares can rarely carry two foetuses successfully to term and it is thus desirable, should twin conception be confirmed, to abolish the pregnancy. However, for two reasons it is necessary to make a diagnosis and to institute treatment before 36 days after the first conception. Firstly, because although PG has been shown to be effectively luteolytic on days 27 (Allen 1977) and 32 (Kooistra & Ginther 1976) of gestation, only 7 of 15 mares given luteolytic doses of PG between days 40 and 120 aborted (Douglas & Ginther 1973) and 13 ponies at 80–300 days of pregnancy required on average 3.7 twelve-hourly injections of PG until abortion occurred (Douglas & Ginther 1974a). Secondly, Allen & Cooper (1975) reported that thoroughbred mares which are producing pregnant mare serum gonadotrophin (PMSG) will not return to oestrus despite low levels of progesterone in the peripheral circulation; these mares have small inactive ovaries. Conversely, in ponies (Allen 1973, Allen 1978a) which are producing PMSG, luteolysis is followed by oestrus which is anovulatory. Follicles appear to become distended with blood with the consequent formation of active corpora haemorrhagica (Allen 1977) and oestrous activity ceases as progesterone concentrations rise. Several such anovulatory cycles may occur. Thus in both thoroughbreds and ponies interruption of pregnancy after establishment of the endometrial cups cannot be followed by a further pregnancy until the cups regress spontaneously.

Mares in which spontaneous embryonic death occurs before the 36th day of pregnancy enter a luteal-dominated phase with persistence of the CL verum. This condition is similar clinically to prolonged dioestrus, although uterine tone (a feature of pregnancy) is usually more marked. The associated luteal activity can be curtailed with PG (Kooistra & Ginther 1976).

To synchronise oestrus and ovulation

Although at present there are few clinical indications for the synchronisation of ovulation in mares, two methods involving the use of prostaglandins have been suggested. Palmer & Joussett (1975a, 1975b) showed that a double sequence of PG and human chorionic gonadotrophin (hCG) injections during the breeding season would stimulate 75% of treated mares to ovulate during a 4-day interval. Holtan *et al* (1977) have suggested a method employing PG, hCG and progesterone. Modifications of these systems have been used by many workers with varying degrees of success (Hyland & Bristol 1979, Luque *et al* 1979, Voss *et al* 1979, Martin *et al* 1980, Scheffrahn *et al* 1980, Loy *et al* 1981).

In most of the clinical situations described above, luteolysis was traditionally achieved by the infusion of saline into the mare's uterus. However, as such procedures are cumbersome and may be dangerous to the operator, and since some mares contracted an endometritis as a result of such treatment, the use of PG has become widespread for inducing luteolysis in mares. A recent statistical analysis has shown that PG treatment is more effective than uterine infusion in the induction of fertile oestrus (Lieux 1980). It is still the duty of the clinician to ensure that PG is only employed in situations which warrant its use, and that it is not administered inadvertently to pregnant mares. The use of PG for inducing parturition in mares is considered later.

Human chorionic gonadotrophin (hCG)

This hormone is obtained from the urine of pregnant primates. It is biologically similar to the pituitary gonadotrophin, luteinising hormone (LH), and is used in many species to stimulate or accelerate the process of ovulation. Pure preparations of the pituitary hormones LH and FSH (follicle stimulating hormone) are very expensive and are not generally available for clinical use.

In the mare, ovulation usually occurs about 24 hours before the end of oestrus; in fact oestrus terminates as a consequence of ovulation. There is no fixed relationship between the first day of heat and the day of ovulation, but this interval tends to be shortest in the summer months. For highest fertility, service should occur within the 48 hours which precede ovulation, although conception will occur to some stallions when the period between service and ovulation is longer; some post-ovulation services are also fertile (Allen 1981). In order to ensure the optimal relationship between service and ovulation, it is common practice for hCG to be administered at the time of mating because this will stimulate most mares with a developing follicle to ovulate within the subsequent 48 hours (Mirskaya & Petropavlovsky 1938, Day 1939, 1940, Davison 1947). Further controlled experiments (Loy & Hughes 1966, Sullivan *et al* 1973, Voss *et al* 1974) confirmed these findings and showed that the induction of ovulation with hCG did not cause a reduction in conception rate. Although Loy & Hughes (1966) found that daily doses of 2000 or 3000 international units (IU) of hCG administered intramuscularly for 16 days did not interfere with the subsequent induction of ovulation, evidence has been presented (Sullivan *et al* 1973) that continued use of a single dose of hCG (2000 IU) in three successive oestrous periods resulted in an increased interval between the first day of heat and the day of ovulation at the third oestrus when compared with control animals. Saltiel & Camberos (1979) have also urged caution in the routine use of hCG in mares. However Roser *et al* (1979) found that, although repeated hCG injections in twelve mares stimulated anti-hCG antibody formation in five of them, ovulatory refractoriness did not develop in any of the mares, and the hCG antibodies did not cross-react with equine LH *in vitro*. Four of the five antibody-producing mares conceived to service at one oestrus, but only two produced foals at term (Roser *et al* 1980).

Interesting data have been presented on the possible mode of action of hCG in mares by Shilova *et al* (1976). A dose of 2500 IU hCG given intravenously caused a marked increase in urinary oestrogen (mainly oestrone) over the following 24 hours, and the authors suggest that this further stimulates endogenous luteinising hormone (LH) release by the hypophysis. Webel *et al* (1970) noted that there was accelerated maturation of the ovum in hCG-treated mares. Shilova *et al* (1976) also found that doses of 1500–6000 IU hCG given intravenously stimulated ovulation but that the time of ovulation did not depend on the dose. However, the higher doses (4500–6000 IU) were followed by reduced conception rates. After the administration of 6000 IU hCG, the increase in urinary oestrogen was mainly due to increased excetion of 17 β-oestradiol which the authors suggest may accelerate the passage of the ovum zygote down the fallopian tube. Tsukada *et al* (1975) have used hCG in oil in combination with pregnant mare serum gonadotrophin (PMSG) to induce oestrus in apparently anoestrous mares. The use of hCG in pregnant mares (before the 40th day of gestation) should be avoided as this may cause embryonic or foetal death (Allen 1974, 1975), especially if the dose is repeated.

Practical application of hCG in mares

The practical situations in which hCG (2000–3000 IU) may be used to stimulate ovulation are:
1 When oestrus is prolonged.
2 When a stallion is heavily booked and the number of services per heat must be minimised.
3 When a mare is visiting, or being visited by, a stallion and only one service is feasible.

The use of hCG to stimulate ovulation in mares which are thought to be unlikely to ovulate otherwise at the end of oestrus is unfounded. After the first ovulation in the spring, the vast majority of mares ovulate at the end of each ensuing oestrus. The similarity between a follicle and an early corpus haemorrhagicum on palpation *per rectum* often causes a clinician to erroneously assume that a mare which has gone out of season has not ovulated.

Gonadotropin releasing hormone (GnRH)

Luteinising hormone releasing hormone (LHRH) or luteinising hormone releasing factor (LHRF) is a decapeptide produced in the hypothalamus. It is carried in a local portal blood system to the anterior pituitary gland, where it stimulates the release of follicle stimulating hormone (FSH) and luteinising hormone (LH). The GnRH available at present is synthesised chemically, and a more potent analogue has recently become available.

The use of GnRH in mares was first recorded by Arbeiter (1973) who gave a single dose of 500 μg or five daily doses of 100 μg to anoestrous mares. This caused enlargement of the ovaries in all mares, and the growth of follicles up to 4cm diameter in over half of them; no ovulations occurred. Heinze & Klug (1975), however, found no evidence of follicular activity in anoestrous mares after a single injection of 1–4 mg GnRH. During normal oestrus a single dose of 1 mg GnRH on day 2 did not hasten ovulation (Downey *et al* 1974), nor did doses of 1–5 mg given 96 hours after PG-induced luteolysis (Noden & Oxender 1976). Ovulation did occur more quickly, however, when mares were given 2 mg GnRH daily from day 2 of oestrus (Downey *et al* 1974) or a single dose of 2 mg on day 3 (Kreider *et al* 1976), although this latter treatment had a detrimental effect on conception. Twenty out of 30 mares with developing or persistent follicles ovulated in 12–96 hours after administration of 1–4 mg GnRH intramuscularly (Heinze & Klug 1975).

Synthetic GnRH did not stimulate follicular growth in anoestrous pony mares (Allen & Alexeev 1980), but did cause increased FSH and LH release in pony foals and ovarectomised pony mares (Wesson *et al* 1980). There is also evidence that it hastens ovulation during oestrus (Ersklbiljic *et al* 1980), and it is now being used more commonly in oestrous synchronisation systems.

Transient increases in serum LH occurred after single injections of 400 μg GnRH during oestrus and anoestrus (Ginther & Wentworth 1974, Garcia & Ginther 1975), although the latter authors showed that a sustained rise in serum LH could be achieved by the continuous intravenous infusion of 2.37 μg/kg at a rate of 10 μg/100 kg/hour, and that pretreatment with 17β-oestradiol (5 mg), 24 hours before GnRH, potentiated its LH-releasing effect. The transient influence of single doses of GnRH on serum LH concentrations has been confirmed (Evans & Irvine 1975, Noden & Oxender 1976). Evans & Irvine (1975) have also shown that 1 mg GnRH in anoestrous mares caused a 400% increase in serum FSH concentration in 12 hours. They concluded that there is probably only a single gonadotrophin releasing hormone in the mare and that the differential release of LH and FSH in mares could result from a changing pituitary responsiveness to a constant GnRH input (Evans *et al* 1980). These authors have described a technique for inducing fertile ovulations in mares in late anoestrus by giving GnRH (0.4–1.4 mg/day for 3–5 days intramuscularly) at 10 day intervals, and at the same time stimulating the normal cyclic luteal phase with exogenous proesterone. Results were less promising in deep anoestrus. (Evans & Irvine 1976, 1977, 1979).

Pregnant mare serum gonadotrophin

Pregnant mare serum gonadotrophin (PMSG) is produced in the pregnant mare by the endometrial cups, and high concentrations of the hormone are found in the mare's blood between the 40th and 120th days of gestation. This period of pregnancy is also characterised by massive ovarian activity for which the PMSG is probably partially, but not wholly, responsible.

Despite various claims as to the efficacy of PMSG in inducing follicular growth and oestrus in non-pregnant mares (Cameron 1942, Naumenkov 1968, Mazurczak *et al* 1968, Maraspin & Stewart 1977), it is generally believed that this hormone is incapable of influencing ovarian function (Day 1940, Loy & Swan 1966) when administered to acyclical mares at conventional dose rates (i.e. up to 6000 IU/mare).

Progestogens

Progesterone in non-pregnant mares

Loy & Swan (1966) first described the use of progesterone in mares to suppress oestrus, particularly the foal heat. Daily doses of 100 mg intramuscularly in oil were necessary, although this did not always inhibit follicular growth and, on withdrawal of treatment (Loy *et al* 1967), some of these follicles ovulated whilst others regressed and were replaced by new follicles. This is similar to the situation which exists in prolonged dioestrus. Goncharov (1973) gave a single intramuscular dose of 500 mg progesterone to 18 mares which had not shown heat by 21 days *post partum*. Treatment was followed by heat in 5–17 days with a conception rate of 56%. In studies on the synchronisation of oestrus in ponies, Holtan *et al* (1974) gave mares 50 mg progesterone/day starting at various stages of the cycle. This resulted in some degree of synchronisation, and this study confirmed the findings of others (Loy & Swan 1966, Palmer 1976) that, to suppress ovulation, treatment had to be started in dioestrus. However, Van Niekerk *et al* (1973) gave daily intramuscular injections of 100 mg progesterone in oil for 7 days to mares in prolonged oestrus in spring, which terminated oestrus and also reduced follicular growth. After withdrawal of treatment oestrus began again within three days, was of normal duration (7–8 days), and ended in ovulation with a conception rate of 75–80%. The authors concluded that progesterone blocked the release of pituitary gonadotrophin with a subsequent build up until the termination of treatment.

In further synchronisation experiments (Holtan & Ginther 1975, Holtan *et al* 1977) it was shown that a 10 day course of 75 mg progesterone daily in pony mares, with injections of $PGF_{2\alpha}$ on day 7, and 2000 IU hCG on day 15 after commencement resulted in acceptable conception rates. Evans & Irvine (1976, 1977) found that injections of 150 mg progesterone in oil daily for 11 days to anoestrous mares resulted in peripheral blood levels of the hormone similar to those of the normal luteal phase of the cycle, although daily injections of progesterone in aqueous solution (at the same dose rate) did not achieve physiological levels in the circulation until day 21 (Ganjam *et al* 1975). These authors also concluded that there are no specific progesterone binding proteins in mares. The administration of 100 mg progesterone/day blocks the LH rise which usually follows the injection of oestradiol (Garcia & Ginther 1976) and, if carried on for at least three weeks, stimulates an increase in uterine tone which is similar to that of early pregnancy (Holtan *et al* 1979). A slow-release preparation (crystaline progesterone in propylene glycol) caused plasma progesterone concentrations to be raised above 1 ng/ml for 7–11 days after doses of 1–2 g (Hawkins 1979, Hawkins *et al* 1979).

Progesterone in pregnant mares

It has been common practice to administer exogenous progesterone to pregnant mares which have suffered pregnancy failure in previous years (Hammond 1944, Day 1957, DuPlessis 1964, Doganeli 1969, Goncharov 1972). Either 100–300 mg progesterone is implanted as subcutaneous pellets or 250–500 mg progesterone in oil is given every 10–30 days (Ganjam *et al* 1975). There is some scepticism as to the efficacy of such treatments (Short 1965, McGee 1969, Ganjam *et al* 1975, Hawkins *et al* 1979) because, firstly there is no evidence that pregnancy fails in mares as a primary result of insufficient ovarian or placental progestogen production, and secondly the doses of progesterone commonly employed could not produce physiological concentrations in the blood. In an attempt to maintain pregnancies in mares in which luteolysis was induced on the 27th day after conception, Allen (1977) found that 150 mg in oil on alternate days was not consistently effective. However, mares given 100 mg progesterone/day after ovariectomy on day 25 of gestation remained pregnant for as long as treatment continued (Holtan *et al* 1979). Furthermore, 100 mg pellets of progesterone are only absorbed at a rate of 0.31–0.41 mg/day (Allen 1976, 1982), and one mare implanted with 4 × 100 mg pellets returned to heat after pregnancy failure and conceived again despite the continued presence of the pellets. Implanting a total of 2 g pelleted progesterone in anoestrous pony mares did not raise plasma concentrations above 1 ng/ml (Allen 1982). Injections of 250 mg progesterone in oil during the sixth month of pregnancy caused an increase in plasma progesterone concentrations for 48 hours (Dinger & McCall 1981). It is possible that the use of exogenous progesterone may be beneficial to equine pregnancy in a way which is as yet not understood.

Synthetic progestogens

Several synthetic progestogens have been used experimentally in mares in attempts to temporarily inhibit pituitary gonadotrophic function and thus synchronise oestrus. In the majority of trials, however, these substances have not inhibited oestrus but have in fact stimulated follicular growth and ovulation (Table 12.1). Acceptable conception rates at such induced ovulations have been achieved in some of these trials. The mode of action of progestogens in this context is unclear.

Allyl trenbolone is a progestogen which does inhibit oestrus and this has recently become available for use in mares. Webel (1975) reported that daily oral dosage of this drug at rates of 0.176–0.44 mg/kg was effective. Similar inhibitory effects on oestrous behaviour have been found in subsequent trials (Table 12.1) Higher doses of allyl trenbolone are required to block ovulation than those required to block oestrus (Palmer 1979). The drug has been shown to have no adverse effect on fertility (Squires *et al* 1979b, Palmer 1979, Heesemann *et al* 1980, Turner *et al* 1981).

One of the major practical uses of this progestogen would appear to be in the management of the irregular oestrous cycles which occur commonly at the beginning of the breeding season. Treated mares have been shown to undergo their first ovulation significantly in advance of control mares (Squires *et al* 1979). Attempts to induce oestrus and ovulation in mares in deep winter anoestrus by progestogen treatment and subsequent withdrawal have generally been unsuccessful (Squires *et al* 1979a, Allen *et al* 1980).

Nittschelm & Van der Horst (1977) have shown that 10 mg chlormadinone acetate daily caused an increase in blood progesterone concentrations from below 1 ng/ml to 4–6 ng/ml. This occurred in intact and ovariectomised mares, but not ovaro-hysterectomised mares, from which the authors concluded that the uterus produced the progesterone which they detected.

The use of progestogens in mares with evidence of suspected early foetal resorption (Günzel & Merkt 1979) or in those given PG in early gestation (Stolla & Leidl 1979) have not proved successful in maintaining pregnancy.

Oestrogens

Natural and synthetic oestrogens are rarely used in stud work despite several claims as to their efficacy in various conditions (Arbeiter 1971). The situations in which the use of oestrogens have been advocated are the following.

Table 12.1 Effect of progestogens in mares.

Progestogen	Dose and route of administration	Reproductive state of mares	Result	Author
Norethisterone oenanthate (SV2)	3 mg/kg i.m. one dose	Acyclic and 'Nymphomaniac'	Good	Jochle & Merkt 1964 Merkt 1965
6-α Methyl-17α-acetoxy progesterone (MAP)	425–1782 mg/ day orally	Cycling and early spring	Not consistent	Loy & Swan 1966
Melengoestrol acetate (MGA)	10–20 mg/day i.m.	Cycling	Not consistent	Loy & Swan 1966
MAP	100 mg/day i.m.	Post-partum	No delay of foal heat	Loy & Swan 1966
Chlormadinone acetate (CAP)	125 mg i.m. one dose	–	Ovulation in 6–18 days	Mahler 1968
CAP	5 mg/day orally	Anoestrus	Oestrus in 8–24 days, 44% conception	Zerobin 1969
MGA	0.5–1.0 mg/day orally	Cycling?	Prolonged oestrus and persistent follicles	Bowen 1969
CAP	80–150 mg i.m. one dose, or 5 mg/day orally	Acyclic	Oestrus in 4–34 days	Arbeiter 1971
CAP	40–60 mg/day orally	Ovarian subfunction	Hastened oestrus, 65% conception	Hoppe *et al* 1972

Table continued overleaf

Table 12.1 continued

Progestogen	Dose and route of administration	Reproductive state of mares	Result	Author
CAP	50–80 mg/day orally	Ovarian dysfunction	Temporary blockage of pituitary gonadotrophin activity	Baier *et al* 1972
17-Hydroxyprogesterone n-Caproate	20–40 mg i.m. one dose	–	Stimulated follicular growth	McCall 1972 McCall & Sorensen 1972
MAP	150–200 mg i.m. one dose	Anoestrus	Oestrus and ovulation in 6–26 days, 50% conception	Metteuzzi 1972
CAP	40–60 mg/day orally	Anoestrus	Oestrus and ovulation, 78% conception compared with 33% controls	Hoppe *et al* 1974
CAP	50 mg i.m. then 10 mg/day orally	Anoestrus	Oestrus in 7–8 days, 45% conception	Arbeiter & Jochle 1975
Allyl trenbolone	0.022–0.176 mg/kg/day orally	Oestrus	Inhibition of oestrus, over 80% back in heat 9 days after withdrawal	Webel 1975

Allyl trenbolone	0.044 mg/kg orally for 12 days	Anoestrus	No effect	Squires *et al* 1979b and
		Prolonged oestrus (seasonal)	Cessation of oestrus in 3 days. Short, ovulatory oestrus after treatment	Heesemann *et al* 1980
		Oestrus	Oestrus but not ovulation, suppressed	Squires *et al* 1979b
Allyl trenbolone	20 mg/Shetland pony/day for 10 days orally	Anoestrus	No effect	
		Early seasonal ovarian activity	Synchronised oestrus	
	1.0, 0.5 or 0.25 mg intravaginally for 20 days	Cycling	Higher dose inhibited ovulation and synchronised oestrus. Lowest dose inhibited oestrus but not ovulation	Palmer 1979
Allyl trenbolone	30 mg orally/day/ thoroughbred for 10–15 days	Anoestrus	No response	
		Shallow anoestrus Long oestrus Lactational anoestrus	Oestrus within 8 and ovulation within 18 days	Allen *et al* 1980
Allyl trenbolone	0.044 mg/kg orally for 15 days	Small follicles during early breeding season	Reduced size of largest follicles. Hastened subsequent ovulation	Turner *et al* 1981

To induce abortion

It has been suggested that a dose of 40 mg stilboestrol given intramuscularly should be repeated after 48 hours and again 3–4 days later (Anon 1950). However, manual dilatation of the cervix and rupture of the chorio-allantoic membrane will produce a more rapid result. Stilboestrol is also recommended for relaxing the cervix prior to induction of parturition.

To induce oestrus

Burkhardt (1954) considered the injection of 8–10 mg stilboestrol worthwhile, although such induced heats are often sterile (DuPlessis 1964). Doses of 5–15 mg are more likely to induce oestrus when follicles are present (Burkhardt 1947, Day 1957), but this is still unreliable and larger doses (20–50 mg) usually inhibit follicular growth and depress pituitary function (Burkhardt 1947). Oestradiol (5–10 mg) or diethylstilboestrol (15–25 mg) cause slight ovarian stimulation in lactational anoestrus (Baier *et al* 1972).

Nishikawa *et al* (1952) gave mares 2–10 mg stilboestrol per day for between 10 and 20 days, starting 7–8 days after ovulation. This suppressed follicular growth and the next ovulation occurred on average 66 days after the one before treatment. Stallion-like behaviour also occurred, but had usually disappeared by the time of the first post-treatment ovulation. In nearly 50% of cases, this first ovulation was not accompanied by oestrous behaviour. Treated mares came into heat in the autumn and had fertile heats through the winter. A single dose of 20 mg stilboestrol at various stages of the cycle (Allen 1976) did not appear to depress pituitary function but was associated with an increased incidence of silent heats and prolonged dioestrus and also stimulated stallion-like behaviour. The administration of 10 mg oestradiol per day to mares increased the inter-ovulatory interval by suppressing follicle development and ovulation (Woodley *et al* 1979, Burns & Douglas 1981); luteolysis was not affected.

As a treatment for ovarian dysfunction

Arbeiter (1971) suggested the use of hexoestrol (5–25 mg) or oestradiol benzoate (5–15 mg) in cases of ovarian dysfunction. Azzie (1975) implanted 500 mg oestradiol benzoate in these mares in the winter for 3–4 weeks. He calculated that 3–4 mg were absorbed daily. Treated mares were in oestrus for 10–14 days but the ovaries then became hard and small and mares showed male-like behaviour and improved in body condition. Removal of the implant was followed by an oestrus of good fertility, possibly due to a rebound phenomenon.

As a treatment for persistent endometritis

Both Day (1944, 1957) and Azzie (1975) recommended the use of implants (1 g stilboestrol of 500 mg oestradiol benzoate), and Deubler (1952) suggested the intravaginal deposition of 100 mg stilboestrol in oil as an adjunct for treating persistent endometritis and pyometra in mares.

As a pregnancy diagnosis

Nishikawa (1955) reported that 3 mg stilboestrol given 13–16 days post ovulation induced signs of oestrus in mares in which the corpus luteum had regressed. These signs merged with the subsequent normal oestrus. They noted no harmful effects, and Reddy & Khan (1976) found this method to be 90% accurate when used on days 16 and 17 after the last service. However, the method does not distinguish between pregnancy and prolonged dioestrus.

To stimulate pituitary-LH release

Pattison (1975) has shown that 2–4 mg 17 β-oestradiol or oestradiol benzoate caused a surge of LH secretion in 12 hours. This effect was blocked by the administration of progesterone (Pattison 1975, Garcia 1977). As expected, oestradiol-17β (0.5 μg) also augmented the effect of GnRH on LH release and, if the course of GnRH was delayed until after oestradiol treatment (1.5 mg/day for 3 days) had finished, the LH response was almost identical to the prolonged peri-ovulatory LH surge of the normal mare (Vivrette & Irvine 1979).

To prevent abortion

In an experiment involving 576 pregnant mares, Nishikawa (1959) gave low doses of stilboestrol (2–10 mg) repeatedly over a two month period beginning at about five months of gestation. This resulted in a lower abortion rate in treated mares (3.3%) than in controls (12.7%).

Induction of parturition

Oxytocin

Reports by Purvis (1972) and Britton (1972) on the use of oxytocin for the induction of parturition in the mare have stimulated much interest in this technique over recent years. Purvis (1972) suggested a single intramuscular dose of oxytocin (120 IU/450 kg) if the cervix was relaxed, but recommended the use of oestradiol (3 mg/450 kg) or stilboestrol (30 mg/450 kg) 12 hours before induction to dilate the cervix in cases where this had not already occurred spontaneously. Hillman (1975) and Hillman & Ganjam (1979) also obtained good results with this method, although Klug & Lepel (1974), using oxytocin alone, encountered some cases of retained placenta. Rossdale & Jeffcott (1975) and Jeffcott & Rossdale (1977) gave oxytocin intravenously as a continuous infusion (0.09 IU/kg) and considered pretreatment with stilboestrol to be unnecessary; as a result, second stage labour was more stressful than usual. More recently, however, Pashen (1980) induced normal parturitions using small (2.5–10 IU) single intravenous injections of oxytocin. The major prerequisites suggested for induction by this method are adequate gestation length, the presence of milk or milk-like secretion in the udder, and relaxation of the cervix. In the author's experience the first of these requirements must be assessed in the context of known gestation lengths for the breed of horse involved and more particularly for the time of year. Pregnancies which terminate in February and March are considerably longer than those ending in September. Udder development in pony mares is not essential, and lactation in such mares appears to be stimulated after induction by nuzzling of a mature foal; indeed Britton (1972) suggested induction after nine months as a method of obtaining foster mothers. Ensuring adequate relaxation of the cervix is a humanitarian requirement. The initial dose of oxytocin appears to stimulate a transient period of discomfort after 10–15 minutes, which soon subsidies. This seems to 'trigger off' the normal parturition process which then begins some time later and usually proceeds uneventfully.

Vanderplassche *et al* (1971) have suggested the use of 60 IU oxytocin as an intravenous infusion in 1–2 litres of saline administered over two hours for the treatment of retained placenta, and Asbury (1972) gives a routine dose of 80–100 IU oxytocin to all mares 1½ hours after foaling to help separation of the allantochorion.

Glucocorticosteroids

Repeated small doses (Campbell 1971, Drost 1972) or occasional large doses (Burns 1973) of dexamethasone do not seem to affect the length of gestation. However Alm *et al* (1974) found that large daily doses (100 mg) of dexamethasone in late gestation (days 321–324) did shorten the length of pregnancy with the production of weak, though healthy, foals. No improvement was obtained when combinations of dexamethasone, progesterone, oestradiol and $PGF_{2\alpha}$ were used (Alm *et al* 1975). Rossdale & Jeffcott (1975) encountered dystocia in both of two mares after dexamethasone induction.

Prostaglandins

Preliminary reports (Rossdale *et al* 1976, Jeffcott & Rossdale 1977) on the use of synthetic PG to induce parturition are encouraging and suggest that such inductions, although not as rapid as those following oxytocin injection, may be less trouble. Exogenous PG (Rossdale *et al* 1979) and oxytocin (Pashen 1980) appear to stimulate release of endogenous PG, as judged by measurement of PG metabolite in peripheral blood.

Christiansen (1975) and Van Niekerk & Morganthal (1976) have reported the use of various combinations of glucocorticoids, oestrogens, oxytocin and PG, and it may well be some time before the best method of induction becomes apparent. Despite the criteria which have been suggested for consideration before induction of parturition in mares is attempted, and despite the parameters measured to compare the success or failure of various methods, one pertinent feature which has not been evaluated is the temperament of the mare. It is generally held that mares have some control over the onset of second stage labour, and that this can be postponed to some extent if the mare is upset by constant surveillance or other disturbances. The way in which environmental conditions may influence the course of an induced foaling requires consideration.

Antibiotic treatment of endometritis

There is little firm experimental evidence on which to base a rational approach to the treatment of equine endometritis, so that most treatment regimens are based on clinical impressions of efficacy. Once the antibiotic of choice has been selected, the main dilemma is whether the drug should be placed directly into the uterus or administered by other routes. The advantages of intrauterine therapy are:
1 A high concentration of antibiotic is initially achieved in the infected organ, and antibiotic could be present in therapeutic concentrations in any inflammatory exudate.
2 Absorption of the antibiotic into the circulation should ensure continued return of the drug to the endometrium for a period of time.

The advantages of other parenteral routes of administration, i.e. intramuscular or intravenous are:
1 Ease of administration, especially if dosing is required two or three times daily, although indwelling uterine catheters may to some extent overcome this problem (Kourtum 1969, Bredin 1976, Threlfall 1980).
2 The introduction of other bacteria (e.g. from the vestibule) into the uterus during manipulation is avoided.
3 Any local toxic effect of the antibiotic on the endometrium is avoided.

If the intrauterine route is adopted, then one must consider how often, and for how long, antibiotic should be administered. In addition, what dose rate, and in what volume, should be employed? It is thought that large volumes of liquid will completely fill the uterine lumen, although unless there is pus present this lumen is only potential and should easily be filled by small volumes. On the other hand, the pressure created by large volumes of fluid may physically aid diffusion of antibiotic into the endometrium or endometrial glands. There appears to be little danger of fluid entering the Fallopian tubes, as increased pressure in the equine uterus tends to compress the papilla at the utero-tubal junction, thus closing the ostium. However, it is probable that more antibiotic is lost due to refluxing *per vaginum* when large volumes are used.

This subject has been reviewed by Davis & Abbitt (1977) who are critical of the unnecessary use of antibiotics in general, and appear to favour the intrauterine route of administration over other parenteral routes when such therapy is essential. Use of the intrauterine route is also supported by Morrow *et al* (1972), Ellsworth (1972), Northway (1973), Bredin (1976), Conboy (1978), and Threlfall (1980). The recommendations of these authors vary between an infusion volume of 25 ml minimum and $500\mu l$ maximum (antibiotic suspended in saline), and between administration at once or twice weekly intervals (Northway 1973) and daily administrations either for 20 days at very high dose rates (Ellsworth 1972) or three times daily for five days (Threlfall 1980). The addition of proteolytic enzymes to antibiotic solutions for infusion has been suggested by Huval (1969).

In mares in which discharge was present after service it was found that intrauterine antibiotic therapy could be carried on until the 3rd day post-ovulation with no deleterious effect on fertility (Newcombe & Allen 1973), although in a controlled experiment Wearly *et al* (1972) found no advantage in the routine post-breeding use of antibiotics in 'problem' mares.

A recent investigation (Arbeiter *et al* 1976) into the endometrial concentration of antibiotic achieved after the intravenous or intramuscular administration of sodium benzylpenicillin and ampicillin showed that both intramuscular and intravenous administration of sodium benzylpenicillin was followed by concentrations in the endometrium which were 20–80% lower than those in serum. Intravenous ampicillin however achieved endometrial values 10–50% higher than serum concentrations; therapy should be repeated every 4–8 hours. Subsequently the fate of intrauterine sodium benzylpenicillin has been studied (Allen 1978b, Allen & Clarke 1978). In order to maintain therapeutic blood concentrations, administration is necessary every five hours. Experimentally-induced inflammation of the endometrium with Lugol's iodine caused a four-fold increase in absorption but did not achieve the serum concentrations which followed intramuscular administration. Mechanical irritation of the uterus by biopsy sampling increased the rate at which the endometrium took up penicillin after intramuscular injection (Allen & Ayliffe 1981). It was also found that penicillin solution was retained in the uterus more fully when the volume was small and when air was expelled from the vagina after administration to prevent straining. Oxytetracycline is absorbed from the equine uterus, but at a very slow rate (Lock *et al* 1980).

The bacteria which most commonly cause endometritis in mares are β-haemolytic Streptococci, *Escherichia coli* and *Staphylococcus aureus*. These organisms are opportunist pathogens and are normal inhabitants of the vestibule and perineum. Klebsiella spp., *Haemophilus equigenitalis,* and *Pseudomonas aeruginosa* are specific venereal pathogens and their isolation should be followed by appropriate control measures to prevent spread of infection. Antibiotics should be chosen after sensitivity testing, but it is often desirable to commence therapy before results are available in which case a broad spectrum drug should be chosen. In the USA gentamicin is the most commonly used antibiotic (Conboy 1978), but its efficacy has been doubted (Threlfall 1980) and it is costly. Penicillin and streptomycin, or ampicillin are probably the drugs of choice, unless sensitivity tests indicate otherwise. Oxytetracycline is not commonly used (Conboy 1978) and is often not effective (Threlfall 1980). Klebsiella spp. are usually sensitive to chloramphenicol and neomycin and Pseudomonas spp. are usually sensitive to gentamicin and polymixin B, although a reduction in fertility after the intrauterine use of neomycin and polymixin B has been reported (Wearly *et al* 1972). *Haemophilus equigenitalis* is sensitive to most antibiotics except (the common strain) streptomycin. After isolation of venereal pathogens it is important for the vestibular area, especially the clitoris, to be effectively treated to eliminate the carrier state.

Miscellaneous

Clomiphen, which promotes secretion of anterior pituitary gonadotrophins, has been used with apparent success in acyclical mares (Moberg 1972, Robinson 1977) at a dose of 100 mg/day for five days. High doses may, however, cause strong oestrous behaviour with no ovulation (Moberg 1972). An antiserum to an equine pituitary fraction has been shown to block ovulation and cause degeneration of apparently pre-ovulatory follicles (Pineda & Ginther 1972); in addition, when administered during dioestrus, it causes demise of the CL (Pineda *et al* 1972, 1973, Douglas *et al* 1974, 1975) which suggests that the pituitary normally releases a luteotrophic substance. Equine pituitary fractions have been used to induce

Table 12.2 Agents most commonly used in veterinary practice to control reproductive function in mares.

Pharmacological agent	Indications for use
Prostaglandin	To curtail luteal function in: 1 Normal cycles (including after foal heat) 2 Prolonged dioestrus 3 Twin or unwanted pregnancies (before day 36) 4 Persistent luteal function after early embryonic death 5 To induce parturition
Human chorionic gonadotrophin	To accelerate ovulation: 1 In prolonged oestrus 2 To reduce the length of oestrus
Progesterone	To maintain pregnancy
Oestrogens	To relax cervix before oxytocin induction of parturition
Oxytocin	1 To induce parturition 2 To aid expulsion of foetal membranes
Antibiotics	To treat endometritis. Suggest that: 1 Parenteral dose 2 Administered intrauterinely in small volumes 3 Daily until up to three days after ovulation, or longer at other times
Allyl trenbolone (progestogen)	To inhibit oestrus and synchronise ovulation

ovulation and multiple ovulation in anoestrous mares (Douglas *et al* 1974, Lapin *et al* 1975), and multiple ovulation in cycling mares (Douglas *et al* 1974, 1975), and ovulation in mares with persistent follicles (Tsukada *et al* 1975). In mares in which early twin pregnancies have been diagnosed, it is common for one conceptus to be destroyed by manual crushing *per rectum*, in the hope that the other will survive. However, this procedure often causes termination of the pregnancy, possibly due to PG release from the traumatised uterus. It has been suggested (Pascoe 1979) that simultaneous oral treatment with meclofenamic acid (an antiprostaglandin) may be useful in preserving such pregnancies.

In conclusion, Table 12.2 list the pharmacological agents discussed above which are most commonly used in veterinary practice to control reproductive function in mares, and shows the main indications for their use.

Acknowledgements

The author is indebted to Miss J. Jones and Miss B. Robertson for typing the manuscript.

References

Allen W. E. (1973) A clincal and endocrinological study of reproduction in the mare. PhD thesis, University of London.

Allen W. E. (1974) Administration of human chorionic gonadotrophin (HCG) to pony mares. *Vet. Rec.* **94**, 505.

Allen W. E. (1975) Pregnancy failure induced by human chorionic gonadotrophin in pony mares. *Vet. Rec.* **96**, 88–90.

Allen W. E. (1976) The pregnancy protecting effect of progesterone against human chorionic gonadotrophin challenge in mares. *Irish Vet. J.* **30**, 23–7.

Allen W. E. (1977) Effect of prostaglandin analogue on progesterone-treated pony mares during early pregnancy. *Equine Vet. J.* **9**, 92–5.

Allen W. E. (1978a) Some observations on pseudopregnancy in mares. *Br. Vet. J.* **134**, 263–9.

Allen W. E. (1978b) Plasma concentrations of sodium benzyl penicillin after intrauterine infusion in pony mares. *Equine Vet. J.* **10**, 171–3.

Allen W. E. (1981) Fertility in pony mares after post-ovulation service. *Equine Vet. J.* **13 (2)**, 134–5.

Allen W. E. (1982) The effect of implanted progesterone pellets on plasma progestagen concentrations in anoestrus pony mares. *Equine Vet. J.* **14**, (3), 244–6.

Allen W. E. & Alexeev M. (1980) Failure of an analogue of gonodatrophin releasing hormone (HOE-766) to stimulate follicular growth in anoestrous pony mares. *Equine Vet. J.* **12 (1)**, 27–8.

Allen W. E. & Ayliffe T. R. (1981) The effect of repeated biopsy sampling on endometrial concentrations of sodium benzylpenicillin following intramuscular injection in pony mares. *Res. Vet. Sci.* **31**, 281–3.

Allen W. E. & Clarke A. R. (1978) Absorption of sodium benzyl penicillin from the equine uterus after local Lugol's iodine, compared with absorption after intramuscular injection. *Equine Vet. J.* **10**, 174–5.

Allen W. E. & Hadley J. C. (1973) Peripheral blood levels of progesterone in pony mares during the oestrous cycle and early pregnancy. *Vet. Rec.* **93**, 77.

Allen W. R. & Cooper M. J. (1975) The use of synthetic analogues of prostaglandins for inducing luteolysis in mares. *Ann. Biol. Anim. Bioch. Biophys.* **15**, 461–9.

Allen W. R. & Rossdale P. D. (1973) A preliminary study upon the use of prostaglandins for inducing oestrus in non-cycling thoroughbred mares. *Equine Vet. J.* **5**, 137–40.

Allen W. R. & Rowson L. E. A. (1973) Control of the mare's oestrous cycle by prostaglandins. *J. Reprod. Fert.* **33**, 539–43.

Allen W. R., Stewart F., Cooper M. J. *et al* (1974) Further studies on the use of synthetic prosaglandin analogues for inducing luteolysis in mares. *Equine Vet J.* **6**, 31–5.

Allen W. R., Urwin V., Simpson D. J. *et al* (1980) Preliminary studies on the use of an oral progestagen to induce oestrus and ovulation in seasonally anoestrous thoroughbred mares. *Equine Vet. J.* **12**, 141–5.

Alm C. C., Sullivan J. J. & First N. L. (1974) Induction of premature parturition by parenteral administration of Dexamethasone in the mare. *JAVMA* **165**, 721–2.

Alm C. C., Sullivan J. J. & First N. L. (1975) Effect of dexamethasone, progesterone, oestrogen and $PGF_{2\alpha}$ on gestation length in normal and ovariectomised mares. *J. Reprod. Fert.* (Suppl. 23) 637–40.

Anon (1950) Artificially induced abortion. *JAVMA* **116**, 32–3.

Arbeiter K. (1971) Therapeutische Steroid hormon — Anwending beim pferd. *Wein. Tieřarztil. Mschr.* **58**, 328–32.

Arbeiter K. (1973) Report on the use of LH releasing hormone in the horse. *Zuchthygiene* **8**, 182.

Arbeiter K., Awad-Maselmeh M., Kopschitz M. M. *et al* (1976) Uterusgewebespiegel-und

Blutserumspiegelbestimmungen bei der Stute nach parenteraler verabreichung von Penicillin und Ampicillin. *Wein. Tierärztl. Mschr.* **63**, 298–304.

Arbeiter K. & Jochle W. (1975) A progestagen (Chlormadinone Acetate — CAP) for cycle control and infertility treatment in the mare. *Ann. Biol. Anim. Bioch. Biophys.* **15**, 385–6.

Ashbury A. C. (1972) Management of the foaling mare. *Proc. 18th Conv. Am. Assoc. Equine Pract.* 487–90.

Azzie M. A. J. (1975) Some clinical observations on the effect of an implant of oestradiol benzoate in brood mares. *J. Reprod. Fert.* (Suppl.) **23**, 303–6.

Baier W., Berchtold M. & Brummer H. (1972) Erfahrungen über die Behandlung von Zyklusstörungen bei der Stute. *Wein Tieräztl. Mschr.* **59**, 13–15.

Berwyn-Jones M. D. & Irvine C. H. G. (1974) Induction of luteolysis and oestrus in mares with a synthetic prostaglandin analogue (ICI 81008). *N.Z. Vet. J.* **22**, 107–10.

Bowen J. M. (1969) An induced cystic ovarian condition in the mare. *6th Int. Congr. Anim. Reprod. & AI, Paris 1968.* 1559–61.

Bredin K. J. (1976) Off-season treatment of endometritis in thoroughbred mares with ampicillin. *Irish Vet. J.* **30**, 100–2.

Britton J. W. (1972) In Purvis 1972.

Burkhardt J. (1947) Anoestrus in the mare and its treatment with oestrogen. *Vet. Rec.* **59**, 341.

Burkhardt J. (1954) Treatment of anoestrus in the mare by uterine irrigation. *Vet. Rec.* **66**, 375–6.

Burns P. J. & Douglas R. H. (1981) Effects of daily administration of estradiol-17β on follicular growth, ovulation and plasma hormones in mares. *Biol. Reprod.* **24**, 1026–31.

Burns S. J. (1973) Clinical safety of dexamethasone in mares during pregnancy. *Equine Vet. J.* **5**, 91–3.

Burns S. J., Irvine C. H. G. & Amoss M. S. (1979) Fertility of prostaglandin-induced oestrous compared to normal post-partum oestrous. *J. Reprod. Fert.* (Suppl.) **27**, 245–50.

Cameron H. S. (1942) Clinical observations on the use of equine gonadotrophin in the mare and cow. *JAVMA* **100**, 60.

Campbell D. L. (1971) Corticosteroids in first trimester pregnant mares. *S. West Vet.* **24**, 103–5.

Capraro D. L., Vernon M. W., Abrams R. M. *et al* (1976) Effects of oxytocin and $PGF_{2\alpha}$ on mare uterine motility. *J. Anim. Sci.* **43**, 277.

Christiansen J. (1975) Inducktion of føodsel hos hoppe. *Dansk Vet. Tidsskr.* **58**, 784–6.

Conboy H. S. (1978) Diagnosis and therapy of equine endometritis. *Proc. 24th Ann. Conv. Am. Assoc. Equine Pract.* 165–71.

Cornwell J. C. (1977) Endocrine status of the periparturient mare and induction of oestrous after foal heat with prostaglandin $F_{2\alpha}$. *Diss. Abstr. Int.* **37B**, 5453.

Davis L. E. & Abbit B. (1977) Clinical pharmacology of antibacterial drugs in the uterus of the mare. *JAVMA* **170**, 204–7.

Davison W. F. (1947) The control of ovulation in the mare with reference to insemination with stored sperm. *J. Agric. Sci.* **37**, 287–90.

Day F. T. (1939) Ovulation and the descent of the ovum in the fallopian tube of the mare after treatment with gonadotrophic hormones. *J. Agric. Sci.* **29**. 459.

Day F. T. (1940) Clinical and experimental observations on reproduction in the mare. *J. Agric. Sci.* **30**, 244.

Day F. T. (1944) Discussion in Hammond 1944.

Day F. T. (1957) The veterinary clinician's approach to breeding problems in mares. *Vet. Rec.* **69**, 1258–67.

Deubler M. J. (1952) Observations of the routine use of cervical cultures in mares. *Vet. Med.* **47**, 182–4.

Dinger J. E. & McCall J. P. (1981) Plasma progestagen levels in pregnant mares following administration of exogenous progesterone. *Theriogenology* **15**, 405–14.

Doganeli M. Z. (1969) Successful evisel and corluton treatment of a mare which had aborted the two previous pregnancies. *Vet. Fak. Derg. Ankera. Univ.* 48–9.

Douglas R. H., Garcia M. C. & Ginther O.J. (1974) Effect of equine pituitary antiserum and PGF$_{2\alpha}$ in hysterectomised mares. *J. Anim. Sci.* **39**, 989.

Douglas R. H., Garcia M. C. & Ginther O. J. (1975) Luteolysis with prostaglandin F$_{2\alpha}$ or an antiserum against an equine pituitary fraction in hysterectomized mares. *Am. J. Vet. Res.* **36**, 1793–5.

Douglas R. H. & Ginther O. J. (1972) Effect of prostaglandin F$_{2\alpha}$ on length of dioestrous in mares. *Prostaglandins* **2**, 265–8.

Douglas R. H. & Ginther O. J. (1973) Effect of prostaglandin F$_{2\alpha}$ in ewes and pony mares. *J. Anim. Sci.* **37**, 308.

Douglas R. H. & Ginther O. J. (1974a) Effect of PGF$_{2\alpha}$ on oestrous cycle and pregnancy in mares. *J. Anim. Sci.* **39**, 205.

Douglas R. H. & Ginther O. J. (1974b) Route of PGF$_{2\alpha}$ injection and luteolysis in mares. *J. Anim. Sci.* **39**, 206.

Douglas R. H. & Ginther O. J. (1975a) Route of prostaglandin F$_{2\alpha}$ injection and luteolysis in mares. *Proc. Soc. Exp. Biol. Med.* **148**, 263–9.

Douglas R. H. & Ginther O. J. (1975b) Effects of prostaglandin F$_{2\alpha}$ on oestrous cycle or corpus luteum in mares and gilts. *J. Anim. Sci.* **40**, 518–22.

Douglas R. H. & Ginther O. J. (1976a) Concentration of prostaglandin F$_{2\alpha}$ in uterine venous plasma of anaesthetised mares during the oestrous cycle and early pregnancy. *Prostaglandins* **11**, 251–60.

Douglas R. H. & Ginther O. J. (1976b) Effects of repeated daily injections of prostaglandin F$_{2\alpha}$ on ovaries in mares. *Prostaglandins* **12**, 881–94.

Douglas R. H., Nuti L. & Ginther O. J. (1974) Induction of ovulation and multiple ovulation in seasonally-anovulatory mares with equine pituitary fractions. *Theriogenology* **2**, 133–42.

Downey B. R., Irvine D. S., Parker W. G. *et al* (1974) Estrus and ovulation time in GnRH treated mares. *J. Anim. Sci.* **39**, 206.

Drost M. (1972) Failure to induce parturition in pony mares with dexamethasone. *JAVMA* **160**, 321–2.

DuPlessis J. L. (1964) Some observations and data in thoroughbred breeding. *J. S. Afr. Vet. Med. Assoc.* **35**, 215–21.

Ellsworth K. S. (1972) A practical approach to the treatment of endometritis. *Proc. 18th Ann. Conv. Am. Assoc. Equine Pract.* 487–90.

Ersklbiljic M., Varadin M. & Borjanovic S. (1980) Induction of ovulation in cows and mares by application of LH/FSH-releasing hormone. *9th Int. Congr. Anim. Reprod. A.I.* **3**, 92.

Evans M. J. & Irvine C. H. G. (1975) Release of equine FSH and LH following GnRH administration. *N.Z. Med. J.* **82**, 239.

Evans M. J. & Irvine C. H. G. (1976) Induction of oestrous and ovulation in the anoestrous mare with exogenous gonadotrophin releasing hormone. *8th Int. Congr. Anim. Reprod. & A.I., Crackow* Vol. III, 463–6.

Evans M. J. & Irvine C. H. G. (1977) Induction of follicular development, maturation and ovulation by gonadotrophin releasing hormone administration to acyclic mares. *Biol. Reprod.* **16**, 452–62.

Evans M. J. & Irvine C. H. G. (1979) Induction of follicular development and ovulation in seasonally acyclic mares using gonadotrophin releasing hormones and progesterone. *J. Reprod. Fert.* (Suppl.) **27**, 113–21.

Evans M. J., Irvine C. H. G. & Turner J. E. (1980) Daily GnRH administration during the mare's oestrous cycle: differential release of LH and FSH. *J. Anim. Sci.* **51**, (Suppl) 276.

Ganjam V. K., Kenney R. M. & Flickuger R. (1975) Effect of exogenous progesterone on its endogenous levels. Biological half-life of and lack of progesterone bindings in mares. *J. Reprod. Fert.* (Suppl.) **23**, 183–8.

Garcia M. C. (1977) Regulation of luteinising hormone secretion in the mare. *Diss Abstr. Int.* **37B**, 5552.

Garcia M. & Ginther O. J. (1975) Plasma luteinising hormone concentration in mares treated with gonadotrophin-releasing hormone and estradiol. *Am. J. Vet. Res.* **36**, 1581–4.

Garcia M. C. & Ginther O. J. (1976) LH control by estradiol and progesterone in mares. *J. Anim. Sci.* **43**, 285.

Ginther O. J. & Wentworth B. C. (1974) Effect of a synthetic gonadotrophin-releasing hormone on plasma concentrations of luteinising hormone in ponies. *Am. J. Vet. Res.* **35**, 79–81.

Goncharov V. (1972) Progesterone and pregnancy in mares. *Konevod. Konnyi. Sport* No. 9, 32.

Goncharov V. (1973) Stimulation of oestrous with progesterone. *Konevod. Konnyi. Sport* No. 7, 31–2.

Goynings L. S., Lauderdale J. W. & Geng S. (1975) Quoted by Lauderdale & Miller 1975.

Goynings L. S., Lauderdale J. W., Geng S. *et al* (1977) Pharmacologic and toxicologic study of prostaglandin $F_{2\alpha}$ in mares. *Am. J. Vet. Res.* **38**, 1445–52.

Günzel A. R. & Merkt H. (1979) Oestrous and fertility following progestagen treatment of mares showing clinical evidence of early pregnancy failure. *J. Reprod. Fert.* (Suppl.) **27**, 453–5.

Hammond J. (1944) Principles affecting the reproductive function. *Vet. Rec.* **56**, 41–6.

Hawkins D. L. (1979) Injectable progesterone therapy in the mare. *Proc. 25th Ann. Conv. Am. Assoc. Equine Pract.* 123–9.

Hawkins D. L., Neely D. P. & Stabenfeld G. H. (1979) Plasma progesterone concentrations derived from the administration of exogenous progesterone to ovariectomised mares. *J. Reprod. Fert.* (Suppl.) **27**, 211–6.

Heesemann C. P., Squires E. L., Webel S. K. *et al* (1980) The effect of ovarian activity and allyl trenbolone on the oestrous cycle and fertility of mares. *J. Anim. Sci.* **51**, (Suppl.) 284.

Heinze H. & Klug E. (1975) The use of GnRH for controlling the oestrous cycle of the mare. *J. Reprod. Fert.* (Suppl.) **23**, 275–7.

Hillman R. B. (1975) Induction of parturition in mares. *J. Reprod. Fert.* (Suppl.) **23**, 641–4.

Hillman R. B. & Ganjam V. (1979) Hormonal changes in the mare and foal associated with oxytocin induction of parturition. *J. Reprod. Fert.* (Suppl.) **27**, 541–6.

Holtan D. W., Douglas R. H. & Ginther O. J. (1974) Ovulation control in mares with Progesterone or $PGF_{2\alpha}$. *J. Anim. Sci.* **39**, 211.

Holtan D. W., Douglas R. H. & Ginther O. J. (1977) Estrus, ovulation and conception following synchronisation with progesterone, prostaglandin $F_{2\alpha}$ and human chorionic gonadotrophin in pony mares. *J. Anim. Sci.* **44**, 431–7.

Holtan D. W. & Ginther O. J. (1975) Pregnancy rate after progesterone — $PGF_{2\alpha}$ — HCG in mares. *J. Anim. Sci.* **41**, 359.

Holtan D. W., Squires E. L., Lapin D. R. *et al* (1979) Effect of ovariectomy on pregnancy in mares. *J. Reprod. Fert.* (Suppl.) **27**, 457–63.

Hoppe R., Bienkowski J. & Lipczynski A. (1972) Treatment of non-cycling mares by oral application of Chlormadinone Acetate. *7th Int. Congr. Anim. Reprod. A.I., Munich.* Summaries p. 124.

Hoppe R., Bienkowski J. & Lipczynski A. (1974) The treatment of non-cycling mares by oral application of chlormadinone acetate (CAP). *Theriogenology* **2**, 1–9.

Hughes J. P. (1975) Quoted by Lauderdale & Miller 1975.

Hughes J. P. & Loy R. G. (1978) Variation in ovulatory response associated with the use of prostaglandins to manipulate the lifespan of the normal diestrus corpus luteum or the prolonged corpus luteum of the mare. *Proc. 24th Ann. Conv. Am. Assoc. Equine Pract.* 173–5.

Hughes J. P., Stabenfeldt G. H. & Evans J. W. (1972) Clinical and endocrine aspects of the oestrous cycle of the mare. *Proc. 18th Ann. Conv. Am. Assoc. Equine Pract.* 199–248.

Huval L. J. (1969) The use of proteolytic enzymes in the treatment of uterine infections in mares. *Proc. 15th Ann. Conv. Am. Assoc. Equine Pract.* 334.

Hyland J. H. & Bristol F. (1979) Synchronisation of oestrous and timed insemination of mares. *J. Reprod. Fert.* (Suppl.) **27**, 251–5.

Jeffcott L. B. & Rossdale P. D. (1977) A critical review of current methods for induction of parturition in the mare. *Equine Vet. J.* **9**, 208–15.

Jochle W. & Merkt H. (1964) Behandling von Azyklic and Nymphomanie bei Stuten mit einem Depot-Gestagen. *Dtsch. Tierärztl. Wschr.* **71**, 201–2.

Kenney R. M., Ganjam V. K., Cooper W. L. *et al* (1975) Use of PG Tham salt in mares in clinical anoestrous. *J. Reprod. Fert.* (Suppl.) **23**, 247–50.

Keifer B. L., Roser J. F., Evans J. W. *et al* (1979) Progesterone patterns observed with multiple injections of a $PGF_{2\alpha}$ analogue in the cyclic mare. *J. Reprod. Fert.* (Suppl.) **27**, 237–44.

Klug E. & Lepel J. D. (1974) Uber die Mögliehkeit der Geburtsein — leitung beim Pferd mit Oxytocin. *Dtsch. Tierärztl. Wschr.* **81**, 349–52.

Kooistra L. H. & Ginther O. J. (1976) Termination of pseudopregnancy by administration of prostaglandin $F_{2\alpha}$ and termination of early pregnancy by administration of prostaglandin $F_{2\alpha}$ or colchicine or by removal of embryo in mares. *Am. J. Vet. Res.* **37**, 35–9.

Kortum W. (1969) An indwelling uterine infuser for cattle and horses. *JAVMA* **155**, 1942–5.

Kreider J. L., Cornwell J. C., Bercovitz A. B. *et al* (1975) Induction of oestrous in mares after foal heat with $PGF_{2\alpha}$. *J. Anim. Sci.* **41**, 363.

Kreider J. L., Cornwell J. C. & Godke R. A. (1976) Effect of GnRH on oestrous, ovulation and fertility in the mare. *J. Anim. Sci.* **42**, 263–4.

Lamond D. R., Buell J. R. & Stevenson W. S. (1975) Efficacy of a prostaglandin analogue in reproduction in the anoestrous mare. *Theriogenology* **3**, 77–86.

Lapin D. R., Douglas R. H., Nuti L. C. *et al* (1975) Induction of ovulation in anoestrous mares. *J. Anim. Sci.* **41**, 365.

Lauderdale J. W. & Miller P. A. (1975) Regulation of reproduction in mares with prostaglandins. *Proc. 21st Ann. Conv. Am. Assoc. Equine. Pract.* 235–44.

Lieux P. (1966) Abnormal cervix conditions and their relationship to infertility. *Proc. 12th Ann. Conv. Am. Assoc. Equine Pract.* 133–44.

Lieux P. (1980) Prostaglandin injection versus saline douche as a luteolytic agent. *Proc. 26th Ann. Conv. Am. Assoc. Equine Pract.* 133–4.

Lock T., Bevill R., Memon M. *et al* (1980) Absorption of oxytetracycline following intrauterine treatment in mares. *9th Int. Congr. Anim. Reprod. A.I.* **3**, 195.

Loy R. G., Buell J. R., Stevenson W. *et al* (1979) Sources of variation in response intervals after prostaglandin treatment in mares with functional corpora lutea. *J. Reprod. Fert.* (Suppl.) **27**, 229–35.

Loy R. G. & Hughes J. P. (1966) The effects of human chorionic gonadotrophin on ovulation, length of oestrous and fertility in the mare. *Corn. Vet.* **56**, 41–50

Loy R. G., Hughes J. P., Richards P. *et al* (1967) Effects of progesterone on reproductive functions in post-partum mares. *J. Anim. Sci.* **26**, 947.

Loy R. G., Pemstein R., O'Canna D. *et al* (1981) Control of ovulation in cycling mares with ovarian steroids and prostaglandin. *Theriogenology* **15**, 191–200.

Loy R. G. & Sharma O. P. (1976) Effects of prostaglandin on non-cyclic mares. *J. Anim. Sci.* **43**, 294.

Loy R. G. & Swan S. M. (1966) Effects of exogenous progestagens on reproductive phenomena in mares. *J. Anim. Sci.* **25**, 821–6.

Luque E. H., Rivera O. E. & Montes G. S. (1979) Induction of synchronised ovulation in mares injected with prostaglandins and extra hypophyseal gonadotrophins. *Rev. Med. Vet.* (Buenos Aires) **60 (3)**, 158–63.

Mahler R. (1968) Quoted by Hoppe *et al* 1974.

Maraspin L. & Stewart M. (1977) The usefulness of prostaglandin $F_{2\alpha}$ and pregnant mare serum in controlling the oestrous cycle in the thoroughbred mare. *Anat. Rec.* **187**, 644.

Martin J. C., Klug E. & Brede D. (1980) Synchronisation of oestrous cycle in the mare. *9th Int. Congr. Anim. Reprod. A.I. Madrid* **3**, 91.

Matteuzzi A. (1972) Contributo alla Conoscenza e alla Terapia Dell'anestro Nella Cevalla. *Nuova. Vet.* **48**, 168–74.

Mazurczak J., Ganowicz M. & Topa K. (1968) Control of the oestrous cycle in half-bred mares during the breeding season. *Med. Wet.* **24**, 539–41.

McCall J. P. (1972) Progesterone treatment of anovultory mares. *Diss. Abstr. Int.* **33B**, 1256–7.

McCall J. P. & Sorensen A. M. (1972) Progesterone treatment of anovulatory mares. *J. Anim. Sci.* **35**, 248.

McGee W. R. (1969) A practical program to reduce the incidence of embryonic and perinatal mortality. *Proc. 15th Ann. Conv. Am. Assoc. Equine Pract.* 141–50.

Merkt H. (1965) Erfahrungen mit einem konzeptionsverhütenden Steroid in der Behandling der Azyklie bei Grosstieren. *Dtsch. Tierärztil. Wschr.* **72**, 76–80.

Merkt H. (1966) Foal heat and embryonic resorption. *Zuchthygiene* **1**, 102–108.

Merkt H. (1968) Embryonic mortality and twin pregnancy in the horse. *Münch. Tierärztl. Wschr.* **81**, 369–70.

Miller P. A. & Lauderdale J. W. (1976) Mare fertility after repeated $PGF_{2\alpha}$ injections. *J. Anim. Sci.* **43**, 297.

Miller P. A., Lauderdale J. W. & Geng S. (1976) Effects of various doses of Prostin F2 Alpha on oestrous cycles, rectal temperature, sweating, heart rate and respiration rate in mares. *J. Anim. Sci.* **42**, 901–11.

Mirskaya L. M. & Petropavlovsky V. V. (1938) Reduction of the normal duration of heat in the mare by aid of Prolan. *Corn. Vet.* **28**, 58–61.

Moberg R. (1972) Uber die Verwendung von Clomiphen in der Behandling der anovulatorischen Brunst bei der Stute. *7th Int. Congr. Anim. Reprod. A.I. Munich* Summaries 126.

Morrow G. L., Jackson R. S. & Teiter S. M. (1972) Gentamicin therapy for endometritis in the mare. *Proc. 18th Ann. Conv. Am. Assoc. Equine Pract.* 411–16.

Naumenkov A. (1968) The use of PMS in horse breeding. *Konevod. Konnyi. Sport* **3**, 23.

Neely D. P., Kindahl H., Stabenfeldt G. H. *et al* (1979) Prostaglandin release patterns in the mare; physiological, pathophysiological, and therapeutic responses. *J. Reprod. Fert.* (Suppl.) **27**, 181–9.

Nelson A. M. R. (1976) The therapeutic activity, post-treatment fertility and safety of prostaglandin $F_{2\alpha}$-Tham salt in clinically anoestrous mares: A review. *Equine Vet. J.* **8**, 75–7.

Newcombe J. R. & Allen W. E. (1977) Some aspects of the susceptibility of the mare to uterine infection and the effect of endometritis on reproductive function. *Proc. Colloques de la Société Nationale pour l'étude de la Sterilité et de la Fécondité*, pp. 289–303 Masson.

Nishikawa Y. (1959) *Studies on Reproduction in Horses.* Japanese Racing Association, Tokyo.

Nishikawa Y., Harada N. & Sugie T. (1952) Studies on the effect of continuous injections of stilboestrol on the functions of ovaries in mares. *2nd Int. Congr. Physiol. Pathol. Anim. Reprod. A.I. (Copenhagen)* **1**, 173–9.

Nishikawa Y., Sugie T. & Kuroda N. (1955) Studies on the determination of corpus luteum stage and the early diagnosis of pregnancy by the injection of Oestrogen. *Bull. Natn. Inst. Agric. Sci. G.* **10**, 147–64.

Nitschelm D. & Van Der Horst C. J. G. (1977) The influence of chlormadinone acetate treatment on the concentration of some steroids in the blood, on the ovarian activity, and on the sexual behaviour of the mare. *Tijdschr. Diergeneesk* **102**, 805–16.

Noden P. A. (1975) Oestrus, ovulation and changes in some hormones during the oestrous cycle of mares and after Prostaglandin $F_{2\alpha}$ *Diss. Abstr. Int.* **36B**, 2648–9.

Noden P. A. & Oxender W. D. (1976) LH and ovulation after GnRH in mares. *J. Anim. Sci.* **42**, 1360.

Noden P. A., Oxender W. D. & Hafs H. D. (1973) LH after $PGF_{2\alpha}$ in mares. *J. Anim. Sci.* **37**, 323.

Noden P. A., Oxender W. D. & Hafs H. D. (1974) Estrus, ovulation, progesterone and luteinising hormone after prostaglandin $F_{2\alpha}$ in mares. *Proc. Soc. Exp. Biol. Med.* **145**, 145–50.

Noden P. A., Oxender W. D. & Hafs H. D. (1975) Estradiol, estrone and androestendione after prostaglandin $F_{2\alpha}$ ($PGF_{2\alpha}$) in mares. *Fed. Proc.* **34**, 316.

Northway R. B. (1973) A treatment regimen for equine cervicitis and metritis. *Vet. Med. Small Anim. Clin.* **68,** 269–70.

Oxender W. D. (1974) Prostaglandin $F_{2\alpha}$ control of ovulation in cows and mares. *Proc. 5th Tech. Conf. A.I. Reprod. (Chicago)* 36–40.

Oxender W. D., Noden P. A., Bolenbaugh D. L. *et al* (1975) Control of oestrous with prostaglandin $F_{2\alpha}$ in mares: minimal effective dose and stage of oestrous cycle. *Am. J. Vet. Res.* **36,** 1145–7.

Palmer E. & Joussett B. (1975a) Synchronisation of oestrous and ovulation in the mare with a two PG-HCG sequences treatment. *Ann. Biol. Anim. Bioch. Biophys.* **15,** 471–80.

Palmer E. & Joussett B. (1975b) Synchronisation of oestrous in mares with a PG analogue and HCG. *J. Reprod. Fert.* (Suppl.) **23,** 269–74.

Palmer E. (1976) Different techniques for synchronisation of ovulation in the mare. *8th Int. Congr. Anim. Reprod. A.I. (Crackow)* **III,** 495–9.

Palmer E. (1979) Reproductive management of mares without detection of oestrous. *J. Reprod. Fert.* (Suppl.) **27,** 263–70.

Pascoe R. R. (1979) A possible new treatment for twin pregnancy in the mare. *Equine Vet. J.* **11 (1),** 64–5.

Pashen R. L. (1980) Low doses of oxytocin can induce foaling at term. *Equine Vet. J.* **12 (2),** 85–7.

Pattison M. L. (1975) Hormonal control of the equine reproductive cycle: Temporal relationship of luteinising hormone and estradiol as studied by radioimmunoassay. *Diss. Abstr. Int.* **35B,** 4276–7.

Pineda M. H., Garcia M. C. & Ginther O. J. (1973) Effect of antiserum against an equine pituitary fraction on corpus luteum and follicles in mares during dioestrous. *Am. J. Vet. Res.* **34,** 181–3.

Pineda M. H. & Ginther O. J. (1972) Inhibition of oestrous and ovulation in mares treated with an antiserum against an equine pituitary fraction. *Am. J. Vet. Res.* **33,** 1775–80.

Pineda M. H., Ginther O. J. & McShan W. H. (1972) Regression of corpus luteum in the mare treated with an antiserum against an equine pituitary fraction. *Am. J. Vet. Res.* **33,** 1767–73.

Purvis A. D. (1972) Elective induction of labour and parturition in the mare. *Proc. 18th Ann. Conv. Am. Assoc. Equine Pract.* 113–17.

Reddy S. M. & Khan C. K. A. (1976) Oestrogen injection test for early pregnancy diagnosis in mares. *Curr. Sci.* **45,** 519–20.

Robinson J. R. (1977) Use of chlomiphene citrate to induce oestrous in anoestrous mares. *VM/SAC,* **72,** 605–7.

Roser J. F., Evans J. W., Keifer B. L. *et al* (1980) Reproductive efficiency in mares with anti-HCG antibodies. *9th Int. Congr. Anim. Reprod. A.I. (Madrid)* **3,** 194.

Roser J. F., Keifer B. L., Evans J. W. *et al* (1979) The development of antibodies to human chorionic gonadotrophin following its repeated injection in the cyclic mare. *J. Reprod. Fert.* (Suppl.) **27,** 173–9.

Rossdale P. D. & Jeffcott L. B. (1975) Problems encountered during induced foaling in pony mares. *Vet. Rec.* **97,** 371–2.

Rossdale P. D., Jeffcott L. B. & Allen W. R. (1976) Foaling induced by a synthetic prostaglandin analogue (fluprostenol). *Vet. Rec.* **99,** 26–8.

Rossdale P. D., Pashen R. L. & Jeffcott L. B. (1979) The use of Synthetic prostaglandin analogue (fluprostenol) to induce foaling. *J. Reprod. Fert.* (Suppl.) **27,** 521–9.

Saltiel A. & Camberos L. O. (1979) Efecto de la gonadotrophina coriónica humana sobre diferetes parámetros reproductivos en la yegua: un análisis de 416 registros. *Veterinaria (Mexico)* **10 (3),** 210.

Scheffrahn N. S., Wiseman B. S., Vincent D. L. *et al* (1980) Ovulation control in pony mares during early spring using progestins, $PGF_{2\alpha}$ HCG & GnRH. *J. Anim. Sci.* **51,** (Suppl) 325.

Shepherd G. E., Findlay J. K., Cooper M. J. *et al* (1976) The use of synthetic prostaglandin analogue to induce oestrous in mares. *Aust. Vet. J.* **52**, 345–48.

Shilova A. V., Platov E. M. & Lebendev S. G. (1976) The use of human chorionic gonadotrophin for ovulation date regulation in mares. *8th Int. Congr. Anim. Reprod. A.I. (Crackow)* **III**, 204–7.

Short R. V. (1965) Recent advances in equine reproductive physiology. *BEVA 4th Annual Congress* p. 51.

Spincemaille J., Coryn M., Vandekerckhove D. *et al* (1975) Use of $PGF_{2\alpha}$ in controlling oestrous cycle of the mare and steroid changes in peripheral blood. *J. Reprod. Fert.* (Suppl.) **23**, 263–7.

Squires E. L., Stevens W. B., McGlothlin D. E. *et al* (1979a) Effect of an oral progestin on the oestrous cycle and fertility of mares. *J. Anim. Sci.* **49**, 729–35.

Squires E. L., Stevens W. B., McGlothlin D. E. *et al* (1979b) Control of oestrous and ovulation with a progestin. *Proc. 3rd Int. Symp. Equine Med. Control (Lexington)* 219–24.

Stolla R. & Leidl W. (1979) Substitution of progesterone in $PGF_{2\alpha}$-treated mares during early pregnancy. *Münch Tiérärztl. Wschr.* **92**, 309–12.

Sullivan J. J., Parker W. G. & Larson L. L. (1973) Duration of oestrous and ovulation time in non-lactating mares given human chorionic gonadotrophin during three successive oestrous periods. *JAVMA* **162**, 895–8.

Threlfall W. R. (1980) Intrauterine therapy in the brood mare. *Proc. 26th Ann. Conv. Am. Assoc. Equine Pract.* 155–9.

Thompson F. N. & Witherspoon D. M. (1974) Induction of luteolysis in the mare with a prostaglandin analogue. *Theriogenology* **2**, 115–9.

Tolksdorff E., Jölche W., Lamond D. R. *et al* (1976) Induction of ovulation during the postpartum period in the thoroughbred mare with a prostaglandin analogue, Synchrocept. *Theriogenology* **6**, 403–12.

Tsukada T., Ikemoto Y. & Kawagughi M. (1975) Effects of higher doses of PMS and HCG combined or not combined with intrauterine infusion on the hypovaria in light breed mares. *Jap. J. Anim. Reprod.* **21**, 12–17.

Turner D. D., Garcia M. C., Webel S. K. *et al* (1981) Influence of follicular size on the response of mares to allyl trenbolone given before the onset of the ovulatory season. *Theriogenology* **16 (1)**, 73–84.

Vanderplassche M., Spincemaille J. & Bouters R. (1971) Aetiology, Pathogenesis and treatment of retained placenta in the mare. *Equine Vet. J.* **3**, 144–7.

Van Niekerk C. H., Courrough R. I. & Doms H. W. H. (1973) Progesterone treatment of mares with abnormal oestrous cycles early in the breeding season. *J. S. Afr. Vet. Assoc.* **44**, 37–45.

Van Niekerk C. H. & Morganthal J. C. (1976) Plasma progesterone and oestrogen concentrations during induction of parturition in mares with flumethasone and prostaglandins. *8th Int. Congr. Anim. Reprod. A.I. (Crackow)* **III**, 386–9.

Vernon M. W. (1980) The role of prostaglandins in the utero-ovarian axis of the cycling and early pregnant mare. *Diss. Abstr. Int.* **B. 40 (8)**, 3607.

Vivrette S. L. & Irvine C. H. G. (1979) Interaction of oestradiol and gonadotrophin-releasing hormone on LH release in the mare. *J. Reprod. Fert.* (Suppl.) **27**, 151–5.

Voss J. L., Pickett B. W., Burwash L. D. *et al* (1974) Effect of human chorionic gonadotrophin on duration of oestrous cycle and fertility of normally cycling, non-lactating mares. *JAVMA* **165**, 704–6.

Voss J. L., Wallace R. A., Squires E. L. *et al* (1979) Effects of synchronisation and frequency of insemination on fertility. *J. Reprod. Fert.* (Suppl.) **27**, 257–61.

Wearly W. R., Murdick P. W. & Hensel J. D. (1972) A five year study of the use of post-breeding treatment in mares in a standardbred stud. *Proc. 17th Ann. Conv. Am. Assoc. Equine Pract.* 89–96.

Webel S. K. (1975) Estrus control in horses with a progestin. *J. Anim. Sci.* **41**, 385.

Webel S. K., Ellicott A. R. & Dziuk P. J. (1970) Control of ovulation and maturation of pony eggs. *J. Anim. Sci.* **31**, 1036.

Wesson J. A., Miller K. F. & Ginther O. J. (1980) Response of plasma LH and FSH to gonadotrophin-releasing hormone in pony foals and ovariectomised pony mares. *Theriogenology* **14 (2)**, 113–21.

Witherspoon D. M., Lamond D. R., Thompson F. N. *et al* (1975) Efficacy of a prostaglandin analogue in reproduction in the cycling mare. *Theriogenology* **3**, 21–9.

Woodley S. L., Burns P. J., Douglas R. H. *et al* (1979) Prolonged interovulatory interval after estradiol treatment in mares. *J. Reprod. Fert.* (Suppl.) **27**, 205–9.

Zerobin K. (1969) Ovulation, Ei-und spermientransport. *Schweiz. Arch. Tierhk.* **111**, 305–21.

13

Pharmaceutical control of reproduction in farm animals

C.D. MUNRO & SUSAN E. MARRINER

This chapter reviews the principal uses of hormones in the treatment of reproductive disorders in cattle, sheep, pigs and goats. Besides their use in the correction of clinical defects, much of the current interest in pharmaceutical preparations to regulate reproduction in farm animals centres around their application in modifying normal reproductive events for management reasons. To a major extent their use is dictated by the changing economic considerations of meat and milk production and by associated agricultural trends. In addition, as an extension of their role in management regulation, techniques continue to be developed to augment reproductive efficiency in an effort to overcome the limitations on productivity set by normal breeding methods and by natural reproduction.

Based on the regulatory role of the endocrine system on reproduction the majority of compounds used for pharmaceutical control of these processes are either synthetically prepared, homologous hormones, synthetic derivatives of these hormones, or heterologous endocrine preparations with biological actions in other species. Following from this there are two general principles governing their use. Firstly, reflecting the above, in many cases these hormone preparations have a variety of actions in addition to the usually specific effect required when they are administered. Besides the consequences of this multiplicity of actions for veterinary use, the possible extension of these other effects through residues to consumers can, due to legislative control, restrict the availability of a compound for regulation of animal reproduction, e.g. the stilbenes. Secondly when using these compounds it must always be borne in mind that their effectiveness is entirely dependent on both the presence and, more specifically, the responsiveness of the target organ or organs for the preparation. Besides genotype, the level and type of husbandry coupled with relevant veterinary examinations at appropriate times are major determinants in the preparation and identification of potentially responsive animals. In all cases where these compounds are used for management control or augmentation of normal reproduction a

244

high standard of husbandry is essential to permit their potential advantages to be realised.

Control of the timing of parturition

The process of parturition can be considered as the active superimposition of a series of events that are designed to disrupt the balance that has existed between dam and foetus throughout the period of gestation. At the end of pregnancy, the changes in the tubular genitalia that provide an expulsive force to the foetus and permit its passage to the environment reflect alterations in the endocrine status of both dam and foetus. Pharmaceutical techniques attempting to control the timing of parturition are based either on premature disturbance of the foeto–maternal balance or on postponement of the normal process of pre-partum disruption. It is therefore of relevance to consider, prior to a discussion of these techniques, both the endocrine factors maintaining the latter stages of pregnancy and the subsequent changes that occur in the endocrine system in association with spontaneous foetal expulsion.

Endocrine factors maintaining pregnancy

Progesterone appears essential to maintenance of pregnancy in all species. Its major role in this respect is to ensure relative uterine quiescence by its adverse effect on repolarisation of the myometrium. Amongst farm animals there are species differences in the major source of this steroid in late gestation. In the cow, pig and goat ovarian luteal tissue is of continuing importance, whereas in the sheep from about day 50 placental progesterone suppresses uterine contractions. These species differences are continued as regards the plasma oestrogen concentrations in the dam. In cattle and pigs, oestrogens are elevated for a considerable time prior to term but, in sheep, basal oestrogen concentrations are present until the final few days of pregnancy. In all species an alteration in the absolute concentrations of progesterone and/or oestrogen concentrations in maternal plasma occurs in the immediate pre-partum period.

Foetus-associated endocrine factors in parturition

Following the initial studies of Liggins *et al* (1973) in sheep there is now considerable support for the concept that in cattle, sheep, pigs and goats the foetus initiates the sequence of events that leads to its expulsion from the uterus. The ability of exogenous ACTH and glucocorticoids infused to the foetus to start parturition, coupled with clinical observation of prolonged gestation in association with pituitary/adrenal defects, illustrates the essential involvement of this system as the initial trigger to the process of birth. In spite of a variety of suggestions, such as placental insufficiency, the stimulus leading to activation of the foetal hypophyseal-adrenal system as a prelude to birth remains undefined.

In the bovine foetus there is a ten-fold increase in the plasma corticosteroid concentrations over the last ten days of pregnancy, with peak concentrations being reached on the day of birth. In association with this increase there is a shift from corticosterone to cortisol secretion. Maternal plasma progesterone concentrations, from the corpus luteum, decline gradually over the last two months of gestation. Superimposed on this gradual decline, which possibly reflects an increasing utilisation of precursors for oestrogen synthesis, a precipitous decline in the circulating concentration of progesterone occurs 24–48 hours before foetal expulsion. A decline in progesterone synthesis in the cow is a prerequisite to normal foetal expulsion. In the non-pregnant cyclical cow, uterine $PGF_{2\alpha}$ has been confirmed as the luteolytic factor (Nancarrow *et al* 1973). At term, maternal plasma concentrations of the main $PGF_{2\alpha}$ metabolite, 15-keto-13, 14-dihydro-$PGF_{2\alpha}$ (PGFM), have been reported to be elevated prior to or simultaneously with the marked progesterone decline, supporting a similar luteolytic mechanism as in the non-pregnant animal (Edqvist *et al* 1980). Following initial release, PGFM concentrations continue to increase markedly to the time of foetal expulsion. The already elevated maternal plasma oestrogen concentrations increase over the last few days of pregnancy reaching peak concentrations just before or at parturition. In the cow these oestrogens are of placental origin, with the foetus appearing not to be involved in the provision of precursors. Evidence supports the concept that following increased adrenocortical activity by the foetus, glucocorticoids act to further stimulate placental oestrogen synthesis which in turn brings about uterine $PGF_{2\alpha}$ release and subsequent luteolysis.

In sheep, parturition is preceded by a decline in maternal plasma progesterone commencing during the last five days before foetal expulsion and a dramatic increase in circulating oestrogens over the last three days of pregnancy. Foetal plasma cortisol concentrations initially increase from four days to one day pre-partum, with a marked increase during the final 24 hours of pregnancy (Comline *et al* 1970). It has been proposed that the enhanced foetal cortisol secretion activates enzymic formation of oestrogens from placental progesterone which, in turn, causes the decrease in progesterone in the maternal plasma. Although progesterone normally declines in the maternal circulation, the sheep differs from the cow in that this alteration does not appear to be a prerequisite to the process of birth. In the sheep, the concentration of PGFM has been observed to increase during first-stage labour with the concentrations being closely related to the magnitude of uterine contractions. It is probable that the primary role of the late pregnancy increase in oestrogen synthesis is to stimulate $PGF_{2\alpha}$ synthesis and that the cotyledonary/caruncle complex is the major source of this initial oestrogen-stimulated $PGF_{2\alpha}$ release. The essential role of $PGF_{2\alpha}$ release in parturition has been demonstrated by suppressing parturition with meclofenamic acid (a non-steroidal anti-inflammatory drug inhibiting prostaglandin synthesis).

In the pig, events initiating parturition appear similar to those in the cow with a gradual decrease in circulating progesterone over the last two weeks of gestation followed by a rapid decline within the final 24 hours, an increasing concentration of total oestrogens over the complete period, and a marked increase in maternal plasma prostaglandins over the final 24 hours of pregnancy (Silver *et al* 1979). Similarly in the goat, luteolysis is a prerequisite to parturition but, in this species, it appears that the continuing elevation of maternal circulating oestrogens is in response to oestrogen precursors controlled or produced by the foetus.

Other factors in parturition

Following alteration of the progesterone:oestrogen ratio, an integrated series of endocrine-mediated changes occurs (supplemented latterly by neuroendocrine and neural controlled events) to ensure expulsion of the foetus. As regards myometrial contractility, prostaglandins can induce uterine contractions and elevated oestrogen concentrations enhance spontaneous contractility. In addition there is evidence that prostaglandins in turn are capable of releasing oxytocin which, from studies in sheep, can, in a self-reinforcing feedback system, lead to further marked release of myometrial prostaglandins. Independent of the probable role of prostaglandins, release of oxytocin is ensured by the neuroendocrine system triggered by anterior vaginal distension.

In addition to the expulsive forces required for delivery, the lower genital tract must be capable of permitting passage of the foetus. Some of the details associated with the ultimate distension of the cervix have been established mainly in experimental studies in sheep and goats. It is apparent that the direct cause of cervical dilation at term is uterine contractility but it is clear that this can only take place subsequent to increased tissue compliance. Changes in compliance have been shown to reflect alterations in cervical collagen which in turn is related to changes in the glycosaminoglycans and water content of the ground substance. This pre-partum softening of the cervix has, in the sheep, been induced by systemic and intracervical infusion of $PGF_{2\alpha}$ to pregnant ewes while treatment with a PG synthetase inhibitor reduces the rate of softening and dilation of the cervix in sheep undergoing glucocorticoid-induced parturition. A capacity of the ovine cervix in the late pregnancy to synthesise both PGE and PGF has reinforced the concept of a functional involvement of these substances in increasing tissue compliance at term. Similar structural changes have been observed following intracervical oestrogen injections to late-pregnant ewes linking, with the previous observations, these alterations to the other components of the parturition process. In the pig, and possibly in other farm species, a role has been proposed for the ovarian polypeptide hormone relaxin in pre-partum softening of the birth canal. Plasma relaxin concentrations in the pig increase rapidly in the 14 days preceding parturition with $PGF_{2\alpha}$ stimulating relaxin release.

Not only must maternal changes in the tubular genitalia be coordinated to ensure that foetal expulsion occurs, but these in turn must obviously be integrated with the ability of the neonate to survive. Again such factors as foetal lung maturation and closure of the ductus arteriosus are linked to the endocrine events of term, the former being induced by cortisol and the latter by prostaglandins (PGE).

Induction of parturition

If the criterion for successful induced parturition is birth of a healthy offspring without damage to the dam or the neonate, then it must be appreciated that the time of birth can be best regulated by controlling the time of mating and therefore of conception. However, a limited ability to regulate the time of parturition by directly initiating the process of birth does have potential management benefits both for individuals and groups of animals. One example is where parturition can be programmed to occur coincident with labour availability both for reasons of convenience and to ensure improved supervision of birth. Extension of these techniques to groups of animals permits a degree of batch management of neonates and dams.

Greater flexibility in the time when foetal expulsion can be programmed to occur can be obtained if the criterion for successful induction is altered to diminish the necessity of neonatal survival. This may be considered where, for example, productivity of the dam, coordinated to the availability of foodstuffs and profitability of product, represents a sufficiently great finan-cial advantage to permit sacrifice of a proportion of offspring.

Besides management purposes, elective termination of gestation can be employed in a variety of clinical circumstances: to save the dam or foetus in life-threatening situations, to treat pathologically prolonged pregnancies, or in attempts to reduce the incidence of dystocia.

In considering any technique to control the timing of parturition the following factors must be assessed: effectiveness of the technique; cost-benefit of its application; dam and neonatal survival; subsequent productivity and fertility of the dam. No matter what technique is employed, the overall aim should be to make the process of parturition as normal as possible.

Duration of gestation

The duration of normal gestation in farm animals is influenced by many factors. These include breed, genotype of sire and foetus, number and sex of foetuses, and parity of dam. In addition environmental influences appear to play a role with season of calving affecting gestation length in cows, and temperature and altitude influencing gestation lengths in other species. Due to the need to relate the timing of induction regimens to the normal period of foetal expulsion, an appreciation of the average and range of gestational lengths in the various species of farm animals is relevant.

In *cattle* average gestational lengths for various breeds are from 275 to 290 days. Under typical UK conditions, gestation lengths range from Aberdeen Angus and Ayrshire 279 days, through the Friesian 281 days, to the large continental beef breeds, e.g. Blonde Aquitaine and the South Devon 287 days and 285 days respectively. For practical purposes these figures can be reduced by 2 days for heifer dams and by 3–6 days for twin calves.

In *sheep* pregnancy in various breeds lasts on average 144–153 days. Medium wool breeds (e.g. Dorset Horn) have shorter whereas long wool breeds (e.g. Romney) have longer gestation periods.

In *pigs* the average duration of gestation is 111–119 days. It is essential in any scheme to apply induction regimens in this species to compute the gestation period for the individual pig unit. This can be accomplished by a 6-month retrospective analysis of breeding records.

In *goats* pregnancy lasts on average, 150 days with a range from 147–155 days. Interbreed differences are slight.

Cattle

Application of induction regimens in cattle can be considered for management and therapeutic reasons. In the former category, calvings avoiding antisocial times and parturition relative to grassland availability or alternative cheap feed sources have been investigated. A variety of conditions directly and indirectly associated with pregnancy have also been treated by induction, e.g. prolonged gestation, hydrops allantois, mummified foetus, traumatic reticulitis, and excessive udder oedema. In addition it can be applied where a life-threatening situation exists in the late-pregnant dam and salvage of the foetus is applicable, e.g. fractures. Undoubtedly the major current interest in the UK lies in the potential of these regimens to reduce birth weight of the calf and so, together with increased calving supervision, reduce the incidence of dystocia. Increased dystocia risk is associated with the use of large continental beef breeds on smaller UK breeds. In addition a substantial dystocia risk also arises from the current practice of using Friesian/Holstein bulls on dairy heifers which in turn are expected to calve at approximately 24 months of age. There is no doubt that foetal weight increases dramatically in the final stages of gestation and that premature termination of the pregnancy can lead to a reduction in birth weight. This assumes a comparable reduction in foetal skeletal proportions, especially at the critical points of the foetus as regards its transpelvic passage — this, unfortunately, may not occur. Studies have shown that, following induction by the techniques described below, the overall rate of dystocia in a herd may not be reduced but there is some evidence to suggest that severe dystocias involving excessively forced extraction or Caesarean section are reduced. The studies of Hindson (1978) based on identification of foetal/maternal dysproportion should be referred to for a predictive technique for assessing the likely occurrence of dystocia in individual animals.

Corticosteroids

The administration of corticosteroids to cattle after an appropriate time of pregnancy will prematurely induce foetal expulsion. Under normal circumstances parturition in the cow is associated with an increase in maternal plasma corticosteroid concentrations. This increase is variable amongst cows and probably reflects a response of the dam to the process of birth rather than being an integral part of the process. The placenta appears to act as an efficient barrier to transplacental passage of steroids and prevents the substantial late pregnancy cortisol increase in the foetus concurrently elevating maternal blood concentrations of this steroid. Studies on the pattern of maternal plasma progesterone, oestrogens and PGFM have confirmed that the foeto-placental unit in the late-pregnant cow recognises a synthetic glucocorticoid given to the dam in the same way as it recognises the foetal signal. Using the short-acting glucocorticoid, dexamethasone, the maternal hormone changes normally spread over the last 20–30 days of pregnancy are condensed over a 5–7 day period preceding foetal expulsion (Edqvist *et al* 1980).

Two groups of corticosteroids have been investigated for their ability to induce parturition. These are the short-acting compounds such as dexamethasone or betamethasone, which are normally administered as free alcohols or soluble esters, and the long-acting preparations, such as dexamethasone trimethyl acetate, which are usually in the form of insoluble esters or suspensions. Given at an appropriate stage of pregnancy, the short-acting drugs lead to parturition in roughly 2–4 days whereas the long-acting preparations take 2–3 weeks.

Although glucocorticoids are capable of initiating foetal expulsion from the time maternal oestrogen levels become elevated during pregnancy (in the mid-trimester of gestation), their use as agents to induce parturition is restricted by the considerably later time that a consistently viable foetus can be expelled. Calf survival at day 260 or earlier is poor. In practice, the use of corticosteroids is normally limited to foetal expulsion from day 270, although even this figure would be too early when dealing with the large continental beef breeds. As a general rule, for maximum success parturition induction should be restricted to the last 10–14 days of predicted gestation. Provided this guideline is adhered to, the ability of the calf to absorb colostrum and its chances of neonatal survival and growth rate are similar to those of control animals.

Short-acting compounds. The average 2–3 days between the use of a short-acting glucocorticoid and foetal expulsion varies in individual animals, different breeds, and different types and dose of preparations. In general the interval decreases as treatment nears the time of natural birth. Retention of the foetal membranes is a consistent side-effect of the use of short-acting glucocorticoids and, although its incidence is inversely related to the day of gestation when induction is carried out, even with foetal expulsion around day 270 it has been reported as occurring at a frequency of 60% or more. There is possibly also a breed difference in its occurrence: in one study Holsteins were shown to have a greater incidence than Angus cows. Various efforts have been made to resolve this problem: synthetic and natural oestrogens have been given before or concurrent with the short-acting glucocorticoids. However, these have had, in general, no effect on the rate of retained foetal membrane and have resulted in an increase in the incidence of difficult births. Although the significance and treatment of retained foetal membranes remains controversial, it is of relevance to record that Wagner *et al* (1974) found no differences in the fertility of induced cows suffering from retained foetal membranes compared to those that expelled their membranes normally.

Following glucocorticoid-induced parturition at day 260 onwards, colostrum immunoglobulin content is normal. Although milk yield may be initially reduced, 305 day yields are not depressed. Double injections of short-acting glucocorticoids have been used to induce parturition in cows at an earlier stage of pregnancy than that recommended above with the treatments separated by a week for cows failing to respond to the first treatment.

Long-acting formulations of glucocorticoids can be administered prior to day 260 with a view to inducing parturition. Although these are capable of resulting in a lower incidence of retained foetal membranes than the short-acting compounds, they suffer the disadvantage of a very variable time from treatment to birth. Combinations of a long-acting glucocorticoid followed either by a short-acting glucocorticoid or prostaglandin, for those cows not calving within 7–12 days of the first treatment, have provided an alternative system for early induction. However, these regimens are impractical where calf survival is important in view of the unacceptably high calf mortality with some combination and times of treatment (Day 1977, Murray *et al* 1981).

Other regimens. Both prostaglandin $F_{2\alpha}$ and analogues of this compound can induce parturition in cattle. Whereas corticosteroids require functional placentomes to induce calving and cannot therefore be used when the calf is dead (e.g. a mummified foetus), prostaglandins act to trigger the process of birth independent of these tissues. Following injection of prostaglandins luteolysis appears to occur and is associated with a decline in plasma progesterone followed by foetal expulsion within 2–3 days. Like glucocorticoids, their effectiveness is related to the stage of pregnancy when they are administered — with similar guidelines to the use of short-acting glucocorticoids being applicable to their use in the production of viable offspring. Endogenous oestrogens appear to play a permissive role in determining the effectivenes of prostaglandins used for parturition induction (Hendricks *et al* 1977). It may be that the effectiveness of combined glucocorticoid–prostaglandin regimens for earlier induction is due to the glucocorticoids initially increasing endogenous oestrogens. The interval between injection and foetal expulsion is related to the stage of prematurity at treatment with longer, more variable, intervals being associated with earlier treatment. Although some studies have shown diminished pelvic ligament relaxation and vulva oedema compared to glucocorticoid inductions, parturition appeared normal in animals treated late in pregnancy. As with short-acting glucocorticoids, placental retention is the major problem associated with prostaglandin induction.

Goat

Relatively little work has been done on the induction of parturition in goats. Glucocorticoids, oestrogen and $PGF_{2\alpha}$ each appear capable of inducing birth but treatments seen to result in live birth only if foetal expulsion occurs after day 139 (Currie & Thorburn 1977). Parturition occurs on average 30.8 hours after injection of 20 mg prostaglandin $F_{2\alpha}$ intramuscularly in the latter stages of pregnancy (Umo & Fitzpatrick 1976).

Pig

Reflecting the dependence of the late-pregnant pig on luteal progesterone production both short-acting glucocorticoids, $PGF_{2\alpha}$ and its analogues are capable of inducing parturition. The marked variability in the interval from treatment to foetal expulsion has rendered the use of glucocorticoids impractical. Using $PGF_{2\alpha}$ or the analogue, cloprostenol, much more accurate timing of paturition can be achieved so that, unlike the cow, it becomes possible to programme parturition to occur at a period of the day convenient for supervision of birth. The stage of gestation, the compound, the dose, and possibly the litter size influence the response, but not the age of the sow. If treated within the last two days of gestation, the majority of sows farrow in 19–29 hours. Earlier treatment extends the interval to foetal expulsion whereas later treatment, due to some sows farrowing spontaneously, increases the variability of response within animals treated in late pregnancy. There appears to be no significant difference between the interval from injection to farrowing with cloprostenol and $PGF_{2\alpha}$. In spite of this apparent precision of response, variable results have been obtained in programming farrowing to occur within working hours in commercial piggeries. For example, Einarsson (1981), in one 500 pig unit, found that although 79% of $PGF_{2\alpha}$ and 100% of cloprostenol-treated sows farrowed within 36 hours of treatment, the proportions giving birth within working hours, i.e. 22–32 hours after a morning treatment the previous day, were only 34% and 61%, respectively.

When pigs are treated within the last two days of gestation farrowing is normal, and piglet birth weight, the percentage of stillborn piglets and piglet losses to weaning are at least similar to controls. Some studies have reported an increased percentage of piglets reared to weaning and a decrease in stillbirths and crushed piglets — presumably due to associated improved supervision. Treatment with prostaglandins earlier than two days before term results in an increase in perinatal and postnatal mortality and a decrease in birth weight compared to controls. Increasing the dose of prostaglandin advances the time of onset of parturition as does larger compared to smaller litters. Although side-effects, in the form of cage biting and increased respiratory rate, appear more common with $PGF_{2\alpha}$ than cloprostenol, these responses are not severe.

Sheep

Prostaglandin $F_{2\alpha}$ is relatively ineffective as a drug to induce parturition in sheep. For example 15 mg of $PGF_{2\alpha}$ given on day 141 resulted in only 33% of ewes lambing within three days of treatment (Harman & Slyter 1974). Short-acting glucocorticoids in contrast are effective when used within the last five days of pregnancy. A single injection of 6–12 mg dexamethasone given on day 142 of gestation to 20 ewes from a flock with a 145-day average led to parturition occurring 46.42 hours after treatment (sem 2.29 hours) (Haresign & Webster 1981). Due to the limited period when these drugs are effective in ensuring good neonatal survival, their major application lies in parturition synchronisation of groups of animals with similar, known mating dates rather than as agents to significantly reduce the length of gestation. Retained placenta is not a problem in the sheep treated with glucocorticoids. Unlike the cow, parturition can be induced in the sheep with exogenous oestrogens close to expected term. In one study of sheep, at least 136–141 days pregnant, injecting 20 mg stilboestrol led to 75% of ewes lambing in response to increased myometrial activity 24 hours after treatment. Cervical dystocia unfortunately occurred in the remaining 4 ewes (Hindson *et al* 1967).

Induction of abortion and prevention of pregnancy

Under circumstances where it is desired purely to terminate pregnancy in an animal, e.g. mismating, some of the techniques mentioned in the foregoing section on parturition induction may be applicable. The appropriate technique is a function both of the species under consideration and the stage of gestation.

In all species in very early pregnancy prostaglandin $F_{2\alpha}$ can be used to terminate the luteal lifespan and therefore prevent the establishment of a pregnancy. If used in this manner it must be remembered that all farm animals have a period after ovulation when the corpus luteum is not responsive to $PGF_{2\alpha}$. An interval of about a week should therefore be allowed to elapse between the last opportunity the animal had to become pregnant and the injection of $PGF_{2\alpha}$. Exceptions to this include the pig, where the luteal tissue appears insensitive to $PGF_{2\alpha}$ for a longer time than the other farm animals, and sheep and goats, where experimental data are limited and for which the manufacturers do not recommend $PGF_{2\alpha}$ for abortion induction. Effectiveness of treatment should, if possible, be assessed by observing the return of the animal to oestrus. In the absence of adequate data on the effectiveness of the drug after this early stage of possible pregnancy in pigs, its use after this time cannot be recommended. Similarly the onset of placental progesterone production after the first third of pregnancy in sheep prevents the application of this drug as an agent to induce abortion.

In cattle, luteolysis and termination of pregnancy using cloprostenol gives acceptable results when the drug is injected up to day 150 of pregnancy (Day 1977). Using 500 μg cloprostenol in 18 heifers 119–129 days pregnant, Schultz & Copeland (1981) reported an abortion rate of 83.3%. In some cases evidence of foetal expulsion may be missed if the animals are at pasture or if the foetus is expelled and lodges in the vagina. Abortion normally occurs within seven days. After day 150, variable results in the effectiveness of $PGF_{2\alpha}$ and its analogues to abort cows have been reported, with extension of the interval from injection to abortion being observed compared to earlier abortions. Resumption of cyclical ovarian activity occurred sooner in earlier compared to later abortions.

In later pregnant goats preliminary evidence suggests that prostaglandin analogues will be effective but further data are required (Holst & Nancarrow 1975).

Stimulation of uterine contractions

As previously mentioned, oxytocin from the posterior pituitary is released during second stage labour and plays a role in the integrated series of endocrine events associated with myometrial contractility. Synthetic oxytocin preparations can be used to stimulate uterine contractions in cases of uterine inertia. Oxytocin acts on an oestrogen-primed uterus in the absence of progesterone. The dangers of administering this drug in the presence of an incompletely dilated cervix should always be recognised.

Postponement of parturition

In most species of farm animals, in recognition of the suppressant effects of progesterone on birth, attempts have been made to control the timing of foetal expulsion by administering progesterone, and thus prolonging pregnancy, until a convenient time. Almost invariably these techniques have met with little success with animals going into labour in spite of the administered drugs and with a substantial increase in stillbirths.

Temporary postponement of parturition has been reported in cattle and in sheep using clenbuterol. This acts on the β_2 adrenergic receptors of the myometrium to inhibit uterine contractions. If given to a cow during first-stage labour, a delay of 6–8 hours in foetal expulsion can result. It appears that softening of the lower birth canal continues to occur during this period. With progression to the time of parturition, the duration of suppressant action of clenbuterol is reduced. In some studies use of this drug has been associated with a high percentage of cows that required assistance at calving. Further data on its application on farm are required.

Treatment of hydrops allantois and mummified foetus in cows

Cases of hydrops allantois have been treated successfully with both dexamethasone and prostaglandin $F_{2\alpha}$. Using the short-acting glucocorticoid Christianson & Hansen (1974) induced parturition within four days of treatment in five out of seven cows with hydrops with one of the cows dying after calving. Two cows treated with prostaglandins expelled the fluids and foetus around 82 hours after treatment (Memon *et al* 1981). Retained foetal membranes occurred in almost all animals with both treatments. In contrast to hydrops allantois, cases of mummified foetus will not respond to glucocorticoid treatment in view of the requirement for a functional placenta with the latter drugs before these preparations can be effective. Case reports of mummified foetus treated with prostaglandin $F_{2\alpha}$ indicate that the foetus is usually not fully expelled but requires to be manually removed from the posterior uterus, cervix or vagina around three days after treatment (Talbot & Hafs 1974, Daykin 1976). Comparison of results with the established treatment of mummified foetus involving administration of large amounts of oestrogens will require more extensive studies.

Control of the timing of oestrus and insemination in cycling animals

In the normal cyclical animal, the intervals between periods of oestrus and ovulation are controlled in the main by the period of persistence of functional luteal tissue in the ovaries. Progesterone, secreted by the corpus luteum, exerts an inhibitory influence on the release of pre-ovulatory amounts of gonadotrophins and prevents the occurrence of oestrus. Removal of the progesterone effect, following luteolysis, allows final follicular development to occur; also oestrogens from the developing follicles elicit a positive feedback by way of the hypothalamus on the pituitary leading to an LH/FSH surge and oestrogens initiate oestrus behaviour and ovulation. This natural regulation of the times of occurrence of oestrus and ovulation can be exploited in two ways to artificially control the time of occurrence of these events. Firstly, luteolysis can be induced by injection of a luteolytic agent such as prostaglandin $F_{2\alpha}$ or an analogue of this compound. Secondly, the suppressant effects of progesterone can be employed to hold in check the occurrence of oestrus and ovulation, following spontaneous luteolysis, until the required time for these to take place. These techniques are applicable both to individual animals and to synchronising the occurrence of oestrus and ovulation in groups. Numerous potential benefits result from the ability to regulate the time of insemination in farm animals, e.g. batch management of dams and neonates. In addition, should the interval between

Table 13.1 Luteolytic action of $PGF_{2\alpha}$ or $PGF_{2\alpha}$ analogues.

Species	Corpus luteum responsive to $PGF_{2\alpha}$ from	Oestrus
Bovine	day 5*	48–72 hours, but very variable
Ovine	day 5	29–48 hours, varies with breed
Porcine	day 11–12	5–7 days
Caprine	day 5	53 ± 2 hours

*Oestrus = day 0.

treatment and the following ovulation be consistent and predictable, insemination can be carried out without recourse to the detection of oestrus — fixed time AI.

Induction of luteolysis — prostaglandin $F_{2\alpha}$ and analogues ($PGF_{2\alpha}$)

Table 13.1 summarises the periods within the oestrous cycle of farm animals when the corpus luteum has been found to be responsive to injected $PGF_{2\alpha}$ and the interval between treatment and oestrus. When used in a group of randomly cycling animals, not all individuals will have a responsive corpus luteum at the time of first injection either because they are in the period when a corpus luteum is forming in the ovaries or because their corpus luteum has been acted on by endogenous prostaglandin and is undergoing or has undergone regression. Attempts to synchronise oestrus and ovulation in a group must therefore employ a second injection carried out after a sufficient interval to ensure that all animals have formed a responsive corpus luteum in their ovaries. That this is possible in farm animals, with the exception of the pig, reflects the relative constancy and predictability of the period of follicular growth leading to oestrus and ovulation after luteolysis.

Extension of the luteal phase — progesterone and progestogens

If the aim is to suppress oestrus and ovulation solely due to the action of the administered hormone, this can be most conveniently accomplished by ensuring that the hormone continues to exert its effect beyond the period when natural luteolysis takes place. A range of compounds with some of the physiological effects of progesterone, but modified in various ways to decrease undesirable properties of the parent compound, have been developed — the progestogens. Such compounds can be administered either by the intravaginal route (as can progesterone) or unlike progesterone, orally.

Although at least partly applicable to regulation of oestrus and ovulation in pigs and sheep, this technique in the cow is associated with depressed fertility at the following oestrus. Accordingly in cattle efforts have been directed towards reducing the period of endogenous progesterone with an attendant improvement in fertility. Unfortunately, when administered for a period of time less than the duration of the luteal phase, some animals may not have undergone luteolysis when the treatment is stopped and therefore their oestrus will not be sufficiently synchronised either to others in the group or within the individual to allow for fixed time AI. Specifically, although progesterone administration for 12 days will be effective in suppressing oestrus and ovulation in animals treated after spontaneous luteolysis and in cows treated around mid cycle, it will not be effective in animals treated in the early luteal phase. Efforts have therefore been directed towards the development of techniques to induce premature luteolysis in this latter group of animals. The administration of oestrogens along with progesterone in the early luteal phase was found to be capable of shortening the cycle. Such observations led to the development of the progesterone-releasing intravaginal device (PRID) for use in cows. This consists of a stainless steel coil coated with silicone rubber containing dissolved progesterone. Oestrogen is provided by a gelatin capsule containing oestradiol benzoate attached to the coil. When inserted to the vagina, progesterone levels increase in the blood within one hour and the gelatin capsule also dissolves within this short time. Such a regimen allows the coil to be effective in suppressing oestrus and ovulation in the majority of cows in a group when inserted for 12 days.

Cattle

The potential management benefits resulting from synchronised mating regimens in groups of cows have been summarised by Cooper (1980). In contrast Roche (1979) comments on how far these theoretical benefits have been achieved in practice.

A variety of treatment regimens have been proposed for the use of prostaglandins in groups of cattle (Cooper 1981). These involve a range of treatments from two injections 11 days apart to all animals followed by a fixed time AI, to techniques such as oestrus detection or palpation of corpora lutea to identify potentially responsive animals in the group (Table 13.2). After treatment of cows with a responsive corpus luteum, oestrus normally occurs after 2–3 days. Endocrinologically the sequence of ovarian events after prostaglandin-induced luteolysis has been shown to be similar to that found at the end of the normal cycle. Following a single prostaglandin injection to a group of cows with responsive corpora lutea there is, however, much greater variability in the interval from luteolysis to ovulation than after two prostaglandin injections 10–12 days apart. When used as a single

Table 13.2 Some treatment regimens using prostaglandins allowing restricted mating of groups of cows. (Adapted from Cooper 1981).

Selection of animals	2 injections 11 days apart, fixed time AI or 1 injection, 2nd injection to cows not AI d after 11 days
Potentially responsive cows Rectal palpation to detect CL	1 injection, AI at oestrus. If no response repeat examination/treatment after 7 days
Over 5 days AI cows in oestrus	1 injection, AI cows over following 5–7 day heat detection period
Oestrus detection for 10 days, cows in oestrus during 10 days	Leave for 5 days then 1 injection.

injection regimen in the former case it is therefore essential to inseminate cows twice for maximum fertility or to serve at observed oestrus.

Most studies agree that the fertility of induced oestrus in beef cows and in heifers is normal, with the obvious proviso that animals are cyclical when treated. However a degree of controversy still remains as regards the subsequent fertility of dairy cows injected then inseminated at a fixed time. Although in general the weight of evidence favours these cows as having normal fertility, other studies have cast doubts on the ability of all dairy cows to meet the provision of synchrony required for fixed time AI. In low-fertility groups of dairy cows, a proportion of animals were failing to become synchronised with a considerably greater spread of returns to oestrus than in high-fertility groups (Saunders 1980). It has been reported that 10–18% of cows will exhibit oestrus four or more days after the second prostaglandin injection. A possible explanation for this occurrence in dairy cows has been provided by the work of Jackson *et al* (1979). These authors found that 18% of dairy cows treated with two injections of prostaglandin failed to synchronise to the second injection and that this was associated mainly with prolonged periods of low levels of progesterone in plasma after the initial treatment. Should such animals therefore have a corpus luteum of less than five days old at the second injection, they will obviously fail to respond. A similar incidence of prolonged low progesterone concentrations in plasma was found in normal cyclical cows but, in this latter case, there was no effect on fertility as oestrus was similarly delayed in these animals. In situations where fertility is depressed after the use of prostaglandins and fixed time AI, it is considered likely that factors other than the prostaglandins *per se* contribute, e.g. non-cyclical cows, poor nutrition.

Similar controversy exists about the need to use two inseminations compared to one for fixed time AI after double prostaglandin regimens. The alternatives include either double AI at 72 and 96 hours after prostaglandin injection or a single AI after 78 hours. In general it appears that a slight improvement in conception rate occurs with two fixed time AIs compared to a single insemination, although a recent study (Young & Henderson 1981) failed to show any significant effect of single, compared to double, AI or to AI of untreated controls. In all situations where prostaglandins are used to batch mate cows, it is relevant to remember that first service conception rates using AI at natural oestrus are frequently around 50%.

Synchronisation of groups of cows with a PRID inserted for twelve days is followed by either fixed time at 56 hours or double AI at 48 and 72 hours. Aversion of farmers to the vulvar discharge that is often associated with PRID removal can be countered by evidence of fertility of treated cows. Coil retention is good and appears to be related to the dimensions of the PRID. Earlier studies reported a coil loss rate of 4%. A major problem when the PRID is used to synchronise heats in groups of cows is that 10% of cows can show oestrus 1–4 days after fixed time AI (Roche 1979). Failure to re-inseminate these animals in heat more than 24 hours after the previous service results in poor fertility. Those that fail to synchronise to coil removal have elevated plasma progesterone concentrations after withdrawal of the PRID. Animals with the PRID inserted early in the cycle are most likely to have a delayed oestrus. Fertility after the use of the PRID in dairy cows appears normal, although results have again been below expectations in some studies.

A recent development in synchronising mating in groups of cows combines the use of the PRID and prostaglandins, with the PRID inserted for a much shorter time (e.g. 7 days) and the prostaglandins being used on day 6 to ensure all cows are free from a functional corpus luteum at removal.

Sheep

Information on the use of prostaglandins to synchronise oestrus in sheep has recently been summarised by Thimonier (1981). The luteolytic effectiveness was demonstrated by injection of the prostaglandin analogue cloprostenol to luteal phase ewes. This led to 84% of animals being detected in oestrus 29–48 hours later (Trounson *et al* 1976), using absence of oestrus over the previous 5 days to select potentially responsive animals. Other workers have been less successful in achieving a controlled oestrus following a single prostaglandin injection. It has been suggested that the time of onset of oestrus is shorter when the injection is given early in the cycle. The similarity between natural and prostaglandin-induced pre-ovulatory LH peaks and luteal phase plasma progesterone concentrations was recorded by Haresign & Acritopoulou (1977) confirming, as for the cow, the lack of effect of this compound on events other than luteolysis. To synchronise oestrus in a group of randomly cycling ewes requires two injections of prostaglandins at an approrpriate interval; various studies have used intervals ranging from 7 to 15 days. It is unlikely that an interval as short as 7 days would be relatively effective in view of the interval between treatment and re-formation of a responsive corpus luteum in animals that responded to the initial treatment. Conversely it is likely that, when a 14–15 day interval is used, some animals will undergo spontaneous oestrus prior to, or at least independent of, the second injection. At present, the studies using prostaglandins to control service in sheep are characterised by marked variation of fertility. In general, oestrus must be detected for best fertility. Higher fertility has been reported with two injections 14 days apart than with an 8 day interval (Fairnie *et al* 1977). However, using a 9 day interval and hand mating treated animals, Haresign & Acritopoulou (1977) found no differences in conception; studies are obviously required to define the criteria for optimum synchronisation and fertility in ewes more closely.

Progestogen-impregnated intravaginal sponges containing, for example, medroxyprogesterone acetate, are effective in synchronising oestrus in ewes if inserted for a period of time at least equal to the length of the luteal phase. After about 13–14 days with the sponge in place, oestrus usually follows two days after sponge removal, although fertility may be reduced at this first oestrus. A variety of factors have been proposed as possibly explaining this effect. These include impaired gamete transport and disorders in the timing of oestrus and ovulation. Unlike cattle, if mating is postponed to the second oestrus after sponge removal, due to the relative constancy in length of the oestrous cycle in sheep, synchrony is maintained. By combining pregnant mare serum gonadotrophin (PMSG) injections with sponge removal, conception rates have been improved and synchrony is sufficiently precise to give acceptable results with fixed time AI. Insemination with fresh diluted semen at 48 and 58 hours, or at 48 and 62 hours after sponge removal, gave similar pregnancy percentages of around 68%. Comparable results with a single AI at 55–57 hours were around 11% lower, although there are some data to suggest that this figure could be improved by increasing the sperm numbers at AI (Gordon 1976).

Goats

Little work has been done on synchronisation of oestrus in goats. A double prostaglandin injection regimen comprising two treatments 11 days aparts with 8 mg $PGF_{2\alpha}$ injected twice at four hourly intervals at each treatment has been described. 85% of goats exhibited oestrus 53 ± 2 hours after the first injection (Ott *et al* 1980).

Pigs

Following the withdrawal of the non-steroidal pituitary suppressant agent methallibure, there is currently no commercially available product to synchronise oestrus in groups of gilts. A variety of, generally impractical, proposals have been outlined to overcome the fact that the corpus luteum exhibits a delayed responsiveness to prostaglandins and to enable all animals in a group to have potentially responsive corpora lutea at treatment. These include serving at spontaneous oestrus then using prostaglandins to abort all animals after day 12 of pregnancy and synchronise the following oestrus; inducing accessory corpora lutea to form with PMSG and the LH-like hormone, human chorionic gonadotrophin (hCG), given after day 8 of the cycle — which will prolong the cycle by 5–15 days; and prolonging the luteal phase by administering oestrogens between days 10 and 14.

Recently encouraging results have been obtained during trials with an orally active progestogen, allyl trenbolone, following 'long term' use of this compound.

In post-partum sows, synchronised weaning can lead to synchronised oestrus. For example, after a 5–8 week lactation, oestrus occurs 4–7 days after weaning. With early weaning the interval from weaning to oestrus is longer and more variable. PMSG followed either at the onset of oestrus or after an interval of 96 hours by hCG, gives a more precise control of the time of ovulation. Variable results have been reported and further studies are required to permit routine application of this technique.

Therapeutic aspects of luteolysis using prostaglandins

There are a variety of circumstances, especially in dairy cattle practice, where the ability to induce luteolysis is an appropriate treatment. It should be remembered that, in all cases, prostaglandins can act only on luteal tissue; their efficiency, in clinical practice, is determined primarily by the ability of the clinician to select appropriate cases for treatment by detection of potentially responsive luteal tissue. In addition, when used in clinical practice the effectiveness of prostaglandins in inducing luteolysis should not be taken as the end point of treatment. Rather, in all cases, the effect of the drug in returning the animal to normal and allowing service and conception should be considered.

Anoestrus in the cow

Besides their use in batch mating to ensure groups of animals meet their reproductive targets, treatment of individual cows failing to achieve first service or pregnancy in a given target period is often carried out. Defining anoestrus as absence of oestrus for longer than the normal cycle, such cases can be divided into four categories:

1 Those with anoestrus due to quiescent ovaries.

2 Those where the lack of observed oestrus is due to the cow either showing weak or silent oestrus.

3 Those where ovarian cycles have ceased due to persistence of luteal structures on the ovaries.

4 Those with ovarian pathology not covered by the above, e.g. some types of non-luteal cystic ovarian disease.

Recognition of the underlying type of anoestrus is imperative if prostaglandins are to be used logically and effectively. Specifically, differentiation of cows in categories two and three must be made for these are liable to respond to prostaglandins, while treatment of those in groups one and four will not be effective. Identification of suitable animals for treatment is normally based on the detection of luteal tissue *per rectum,* although milk progesterone assays have been employed in some cases.

The efficiency of rectal examination as a means of identifying potentially responsive corpora lutea has been investigated. Both slaughterhouse surveys and comparison with blood and milk progesterone assays have shown that inaccuracies in the detection of mature (i.e. potentially responsive) corpora lutea are around 25% for experienced clinicians. When used as a treatment for anoestrus cows found to have a palpable corpus luteum, 66.8% of cows ($n = 253$) were detected in oestrus within 1–8 days of injection (Eddy 1977). Almost certainly inaccuracies in detection of responsive corpora lutea contributed towards this result. To be regarded as effective this treatment must result in the cow being served. The relative inefficiency of heat detection (50%) on many dairy farms obviously also poses limitations. Application of aids to heat detection (e.g. tail paste and KaMar heat mount detectors) should be considered as part of the treatment package for such animals. Also, as these animals have generally failed to meet their reproductive targets, at the time of treatment every effort should be made to ensure the maximum chance of conception, i.e. they should be served at observed oestrus or, failing that, have fixed time AI at 72 and 96 hours.

Persistence of the corpus luteum beyond the normal lifespan has been found in non-pregnant cows to be a relatively rare reason for anoestrus (1.9% cows, Bulman & Wood 1980). In all cases prior to prostaglandins being used to terminate anoestrus, examination of the tubular tract should be carried out to eliminate pregnancy. It is generally recognised that persistence of the corpus luteum does not occur in cows with a normal tubular tract — persistence resulting either from acquired lesions of the uterus interfering with prostaglandin synthesis or release. Such persistent corpora lutea retain their responsiveness to prostaglandins.

Within the cystic ovarian disease syndrome, luteal cysts have been found to be appropriate cases for treatment using prostaglandin $F_{2\alpha}$. In a small scale trial with a group of veterinary practices, Booth (1981) found, determining the functional status of ovarian cysts by milk progesterone assay, that 44% of clinically identified luteal cysts were misdiagnosed. Other workers have, however, reported a higher accuracy in identification, on clinical grounds, of luteal cysts (Hoffmann *et al* 1976, Eungler & Schallenberger 1981), highlighting the lack of agreed characteristics to allow a consistently accurate diagnosis of this condition. Unfortunately, response to prostaglandin treatment does not necessarily confirm the diagnosis of luteal cysts. In a slaughterhouse survey AI-Dahash & David (1977) found that 30.7% of cysts were accompanied by corpora lutea. Existence of a concurrent responsive corpus lutem in a cow with a cyst in its ovaries would be associated with an apparent response of the cyst to prostaglandin. As an extension of this, the occurrence of cysts in the ovaries of cyclical animals has been described (Boyd & Munro 1979). In the presence of relatively inefficient oestrus detection it would be quite possible to ascribe anoestrus in such a cow as reflecting the abnormal function of a cyst on the ovaries. In this context (Dawson 1975) reported that the presence of a cyst on the ovaries increased the chances of a corpus luteum on the same ovary not being palpable. Within the limited data available on the effectiveness of $PGF_{2\alpha}$ treatment, results have ranged from 85% pregnant at an interval from treatment to conception of 42 days (Booth — endocrinological confirmation of diagnosis) to a similar pregnancy rate but with an average interval to conception of 19.4 days (Eddy — clinical diagnosis). Gunzler & Schallenberger (1981) divided luteal cysts further on the basis of milk progesterone concentrations into moderate and high progesterone level groups. The latter was associated with milk progesterone levels equivalent to those found with a mature corpus luteum in the ovaries. Best results to treatment with the $PGF_{2\alpha}$ analogue, cloprostenol, in terms of expression of oestrus and conception rate were obtained in high-level cows. Defects in re-formation of corpora lutea appeared to occur in the moderate-level group and were associated with a conception rate to first service of 24% though, again, only small numbers of cows were involved in this latter figure.

Chronic endometritis in the cow

Both chronic non-specific endometritis in cycling cows and pyometra associated with persistence of the corpus luteum can be treated with $PGF_{2\alpha}$ or an analogue.

In the case of pyometra, a high success rate (85–91%) has been reported for returning the cow to oestrus and/or a profuse discharge of mucopurulent material from the vulva — the latter usually occurring within 3–4 days of injection (Gustafsson *et al* 1976, Jackson *et al* 1977). Repeated treatment, after an interval of at least 7–10 days, has been shown to clinically resolve the condition in the majority of cows failing to respond to the initial injection. That, in the main, the uterine damage associated with pyometra in the cow is not permanent is apparent from data on the subsequent fertility of treated animals. For example 13 of 20 treated cows which responded became pregnant with an average number of 2.3 inseminations/conception. In addition in most cases, having re-initiated cycling, oestrous cycles continue to show in the majority of animals after treatment. The relative advantages of this technique over the traditional approach of oestrogen therapy have been demonstrated by De Kuif *et al* (1977) and Duncanson (1980).

The rationale for the use of prostaglandins in cycling animals with non-specific endometritis lies in the beneficial influences of endogenous oestrogens on the uterus. Such a hypothesis follows from the early experiments of Rowson *et al* (1953) who demonstrated the resistance of the uterus during the oestrogenic phase of the cycle to the introduction of infection compared to the relative ease with which infection could establish itself during the luteal phase. The effectiveness of this treatment for non-specific endometritis has recently been demonstrated by inseminating cows at the first oestrus after prostaglandin treatment. In general, however, insemination is delayed until the second oestrus with the nature of the vulvar discharge at oestrus being used to confirm the clinical response of the cow.

In herd fertility control work, controversy remains about the optimal time of treatment of non-specific endometritis during the service period. The question of the need to treat cases observed in the pre-service period remains open to investigation. Furthermore it should be noted that, in spite of empirical claims to the contrary, there is no current published evidence to support the use of prostaglandins to treat endometritis in non-cycling cows.

Therapeutic uses of ovulation–luteinisation induction

The ability to induce ovulation and luteinisation has therapeutic applications in cases of abnormal or suppressed follicular development.

Cystic ovarian disease in cows

This is by far the most common pathological condition of the ovaries found in dairy cattle. Within the cystic ovarian disease complex two types of cysts are found: those secreting significant amounts of progesterone where the behavioural history is of anoestrus, and a second group not associated with significant levels of progesterone in the peripheral plasma where the presenting signs are either excessive, abnormal oestrus behaviour or anoestrus. For conveniency these two types of cysts are often referred to as luteal and follicular, respectively. The treatment of luteal cysts with prostaglandin $F_{2\alpha}$ has already been mentioned.

Although the condition of cystic ovarian disease is considered as an ovarian defect, it would be more appropriate to regard it as a hypothalamic pituitary disorder. Recent studies have examined the peripheral plasma gonadal steroid concentrations of follicular cyst cows showing nymphomania. Although in some (65.5%) nymphomaniac cows oestradiol-17β concentrations are higher than the concentrations recorded during the preovulatory increase in normal cows (Saumande *et al* 1979), other studies have found no difference compared to normal cows and no difference between follicular cyst cows showing anoestrus or excessive oestrus (Nessan & King 1981). During the normal oestrous cycle, elevated concentrations of plasma oestrogens, in the absence of a progesterone block, would elicit an LH surge from the pituitary by positive feedback on the hypothalamus. The LH surge would in turn suppress oestrogen synthesis by the follicle and initiate the process of final follicular maturation and ovulation. The ability of exogenous LHRH to induce an LH discharge from the pituitaries of cows with cystic ovarian disease confirms that lack of pituitary LH is not a basic part of the pathogenesis of this condition.

Therapy for follicular cysts comprises either giving a direct luteotrophic stimulus, usually in the form of hCG in some cases combined with progesterone, or stimulating the endogenous luteotrophin, LH, by injecting LHRH. In addition, progesterone treatment over a period of time approaching the duration of the normal luteal period has been employed both in the past by daily injections and currently using a more practical approach with the PRID (with the oestradiol capsule removed). Following successful treatment with either LHRH or hCG, oestradiol concentrations in the peripheral plasma decline and progesterone levels increase within 5–9 days to levels similar to those during the oestrous cycle. Progesterone then remains elevated for approximately a normal luteal phase before declining and allowing the animal to return to oestrus. Throughout the period of elevated progesterone concentrations, oestrus behaviour will obviously be suppressed, although in view of the irregular pattern of oestrus shown by some of these cases, absence of oestrus does not necessarily indicate effective treatment.

If the criterion for successful treatment is taken as a re-establishment of ovarian cycles, then several studies have shown that hCG and LHRH are equally effective, with around 80% cases responding (Elmore *et al* 1975, Sequin *et al* 1976). However Nakao *et al* (1979) found a lower recovery rate after hCG and observed that nearly half of the cows that failed to respond to this treatment subsequently responded to LHRH 10 days later. Whether the latter result demonstrates refractoriness to hCG or whether it reflects the effect of two luteotrophic stimuli is not clear. In a small study of combined hCG–progesterone treatment (Nymfalon) and LHRH, Booth (1981) reported no significant difference between the two treatments using increased milk progesterone concentrations as the criterion for success.

Although fertility of treated cystic ovarian disease cows may be depressed compared to normal animals, recent data give cause for a certain amount of optimism. Using the LHRH analogue, buserelin, acceptable first service conception rates were observed in a clinical trial involving 724 cows. Similarly acceptable fertility was reported in the small-scale trial of Booth (1981) using hCG–progesterone or LHRH. This is not to underestimate the significance of the condition both to the veterinary surgeon, who will undoubtedly encounter individual cows that fail to respond to treatment and animals that fail to conceive, or to herd economics, where unsuccessfully treated cows have to be culled and where the delay in getting successfully treated cows served and pregnant constitutes a serious economic loss. Until we know what governs whether an individual cow responds to treatment in practice, unresponsive cases are normally re-treated, increasing the dosage of hCG or using an alternative (with PRIDs now being added to the list). Further basic research on the defect is required to allow a more logical selection of appropriate treatment. Following the latter point above about the effects on herd economics, results from the combined use of LHRH followed after nine days by prostaglandin $F_{2\alpha}$ are of interest. Using this approach, the interval from treatment to conception was reduced by 11 days compared to LHRH alone (Garverick *et al* 1976).

With the combined approach, luteal cysts, whether or not they respond to LHRH, would be optimally treated at the time of the prostaglandin injection. Follicular cysts responding to the LHRH would have luteal tissue responsive to prostaglandins at the second treatment. In addition the detection of oestrus would be facilitated by the prostaglandins allowing attention to be concentrated on the animals over a limited period of time.

Initiating ovarian cycles in non-cyclical animals

Non-cyclical ovaries associated with anoestrus occur physiologically in animals prepubertally, post partum and during the non-breeding period of seasonal breeders.

From an endocrinological point of view there are many similarities between recurrent anoestrus after parturition and the anoestrus of prepubertal life. In the cow, for example, the post-partum period is characterised by a relatively early resumption of follicular development after calving which is often followed, prior to the first post-partum ovulation, by transient luteal structures developing in the ovaries. Ultimately growth of follicles culminates in ovulation which, in dairy cows at least, is often associated with absence of normal expression of oestrus. In contrast, the second ovulation, occurring after a cycle that can be shorter and associated with a smaller corpus luteum than usual, is usually accompanied by normal signs of oestrus. A comparable series of events whereby ovarian cycles are gradually established occurs over the transitional period from pre- to post-pubertal life in the calf. Similarly the re-initiation of normal reproductive function in seasonal breeders is a gradual process.

Initiating ovarian cycles in post-partum cows

First ovulation in dairy cows, following a normal parturition, normally occurs 15–36 days post-partum. In contrast the time of first ovulation in suckled cows is more variable, although recent data (Peters 1982) have contradicted the findings of previous studies that the interval from calving to first oestrus is consistently delayed compared with milked cows. In either group, however, variable percentages of cows have been reported as being acyclic around the time they require to be bred in aiming for a 365 day calving interval. Within dairy cows, marked variation in the incidence of non-cycling in the period around 50 days post partum has been reported ranging from 4 to 26.2% in UK and Irish herds (e.g. Munro *et al* 1982). Similarly in beef herds it has been found that onset of cyclical activity, is often delayed until around 60 days after calving. Currently two endocrine treatments are available that have had a degree of success in initiating cycling in non-cycling cows — the progesterone releasing intravaginal device (PRID) and LHRH.

PRID

As previously mentioned, many post-partum cows experience a transient plasma progesterone increase prior to the first post-partum ovulation. Current evidence suggests that this progesterone increase, arising from luteinised follicles, serves to modulate the pituitary LH release pattern such that a subsequent growth of follicles is capable of triggering (by the oestrogens exerting a positive-feedback) an LH surge and hence ovulation. However, as a transient progesterone increase is not a consistent feature of the return to cycling after calving, it cannot be regarded as an essential prerequisite. Nevertheless it is probable that the PRID acts to initiate cycling in non-cycling animals by stimulating this transient endogenous progesterone increase.

When used in dairy cows around 50–60 days post partum, the PRID (inserted for 12 days and followed by fixed time AI at 56 hours after removal) appeared beneficial in that only one in 19 of non-cyclical untreated cows became pregnant to service over a 24-day observation period whereas seven of 19 non-cyclical animals conceived to the induced ovulation (Drew *et al* 1978). In contrast Bulman & Wood (1980) found no difference in the average interval between calving and conception in non-cyclical untreated compared to treated cows where the PRID was inserted at a similar time after calving to the above. Similarly Peters (1982) provided indirect evidence on its lack of applicability to the beef herd by observing no consistent effect on calving interval by routinely treating suckler cows with the PRID 40 days after calving compared to controls. The apparent beneficial effects of ensuring cyclical ovarian activity early after calving when PRIDs are inserted around 20 days post-partum are valid when attempts are being made to tighten up the calving pattern in a herd by ensuring early service of late calvers (Drew 1980).

LHRH

LHRH injected to a cow with a responsive pituitary leads to a rapid release of LH to the peripheral blood with peak concentrations being reached about 2–4 hours after injection. Current evidence suggests that, at least in the cow and sheep, LHRH releases both FSH and LH from the pituitary. In the post-partum dairy cow, the peripheral plasma LH profile is characterised by a relatively brief period of basal LH concentrations, followed by a series of short-lived spikes of the hormone which occur at increasing frequency and increase in magnitude with extension of the post-partum interval. Similarly spikes of LH occur prior to the time of first post-partum ovulation in the beef suckled cow. In contrast, FSH appears to remain at a relatively constant elevated concentration during most of the post-partum acyclic period (Peters 1982).

Exogenous LHRH injected to dairy cows has been shown to be capable of eliciting a maximal LH discharge from the pituitary as early as 12–15 days post partum. In contrast, in the suckled cow, maximal pituitary responsiveness is delayed till 20–30 days post calving. In the anoestrous dairy cow, a single injection of LHRH has been shown (when given around day 50 after calving) to be capable of initiating ovulation and resumption of ovarian cycles (Lamming & Bulman 1976). In contrast in the suckled beef cow, a single injection of LHRH, although in many cases resulting in ovulation, was not followed in the majority of instances by a normal luteal phase. A second injection after 10 days or when the transient increase in progesterone returned to basal concentrations, appeared necessary in suckled cows to re-initiate cycling after calving (Webb *et al* 1977).

Attempts have been made to adapt these original observations to the routine treatment of non-cyclical cows. As for PRID treatment Bulman & Wood (1980) found no benefit in treating acyclic dairy cows 50 days or more after calving with LHRH compared to untreated controls. Similarly in beef cows, Peters (1982) found treatment to have been of no benefit. In contrast in dairy cows, combining LHRH treatment with milk progesterone monitoring to assess its effectiveness and to dictate subsequent action (no increase — repeat LHRH; prostaglandin treatment of responding cows not observed in oestrus) was found to be more effective in reducing the treatment–conception interval than a single treatment and AI at observed oestrus. In addition, in the monitored cows the calving–conception interval was reduced compared to untreated controls (Humblot & Thibier 1980). Whether such monitoring could be carried out by rectal examination at appropriate intervals after treatment remains to be established, although in the absence of on-farm progesterone assays this would seem the most logical adjunct to injection of the drug.

Effectiveness of treatment

In the absence of recognised standard treatment for non-cyclical cows there is a continuing need to critically determine the effectiveness of both the drugs mentioned previously and new additions to the range, e.g. LHRH analogues. Assesssing the effectiveness of treatment in turn demands that cows are identified as non-cyclical prior to injection. The need to carry out at least two examinations at an appropriate interval to differentiate cyclical cows around oestrus fron non-cyclical animals and the limitations of this technique have been commented on by Munro *et al* (1982).

In considering any treatment for non-cycling animals it must always be remembered that, on a herd basis, the incidence of non-cycling decreases with increasing time after calving. This may well account for the lack of apparent beneficial effects found when non-cyclical cows were treated by the PRID or LHRH in some previous studies. It is unlikely that, in the absence of an aetiological agent being identified to explain the acyclical state in a large percentage of non-cyclical cows, any single endocrinological treatment will ever be consistently effective. As an example, current studies have demonstrated that cows suffering from sub-nutrition, recognised in turn as being associated with acyclicity, have adequate pituitary LH in their plasma to recommence cycling but apparently suffer diminished ovarian responsiveness. As such it would be most unlikely that either LHRH or PRID would be effective in treating such cases. Whether, however, techniques such as body condition scores or weighing can identify all such potentially unresponsive cows or whether these can be identified from the ovarian characteristics remains to be determined.

An alternative application of techniques to initiate cycling lies in the blanket treatment of all post-partum cows at a relatively early stage post partum. This has potential advantages in reducing the incidence of post-partum diseases associated with non-cycling. In a preliminary study, Holstein cows were injected with LHRH 8–23 days after calving. The number of cases of cystic ovarian disease was reduced in treated compared to controls and there were fewer culls for infertility. The incidence of post-partum uterine infection was, however, unaffected (Britt *et al* 1977). Conversely a recent study has shown the apparent beneficial effects of treating non-cyclical cows affected by non-specific endometritis with LHRH.

Out-of-season breeding of sheep

PMSG is capable of inducing ovulation in the anoestrous ewe. This hormone is normally used in conjunction with intravaginal progestogen sponges; the progestogen appears to play a role in ensuring that the induced ovulations are accompanied by oestrus and also in modifying hypothalmic responsiveness to follicular oestrogens. There is some evidence that teasing of progestogen-primed anoestrous ewes can induce ovulation independent of the use of PMSG. The effectiveness of these PMSG–progestogen regimens is affected by several factors both in terms of the oestrus-inducing ability of the technique and subsequent fertility of the induced oestrus. In general, the ability of these methods to induce heat is related to the stage of treatment within the anoestrous period; best results being obtained as the onset of the normal breeding period is approached. Although the progestogen is normally administered for 14–15 days, to achieve optimum results the dosage of PMSG must be varied to take account of the season of the year, the breed of the ewe, and whether the ewe is lactating. In the spring and in lactating ewes conception rates are lower than in the summer/autumn period and in dry ewes. Further details of the technique and results can be obtained in the work of Gordon (1975). The combined use of modification of the photoperiod and progestogen priming in suitable breeds can give two lamb crops per year (Robinson *et al* 1975).

Augmentation of normal fertility

The availability of techniques to improve the prolificacy of farm animals is an attractive concept. Methods have been, and continue to be, investigated to improve fertility in association with AI and to increase the number of young born over a certain period of time — with the attendant long term benefit in some cases of a decrease in generation interval. In the main these techniques have centred around either an increase in the number of ovulations in individual cyclical animals or ensuring that ovulations, and therefore the chances of conception, occur when the animal's reproductive system is normally quiescent. As for other aspects of the artificial control of reproduction, the interplay between genotype, environment, and the endocrine treatment employed is a major determinant of the success of these techniques. In some cases management alterations (e.g. modifying lighting or improving nutrition) are alone sufficient to augment fertility but will not be considered in detail here, although often a satisfactory response to administered hormones necessitates the application of similar management systems.

Augmenting conception rate in cattle

The ability of LHRH and its synthetic analogues to bring about an LH surge in the cow has been investigated as a technique for improving conception rates in dairy cattle routinely presented for AI. Improvements in conception rate of around 15% have been reported following the use of the LHRH analogue buserelin in this way, with the compound being administered on the day of AI. The effectiveness of a compound of this nature implies that it will act to correct defects in endogenous LH release in cows (delayed ovulation being the most obvious of the disorders that might be appropriate to this form of treatment). Estimates of the incidence of delayed ovulation in cattle are widely variable, probably reflecting to a large extent differences in the criteria used to identify the condition. It is possible, under certain circumstances where delayed ovulation is a problem in a herd, that blanket treatment of cows will improve conception rate; however, considerably more information is required to identify appropriate herds for treatment and the optimum time for administration of the drug. For example it may be more appropriate, in view of the delay between LH release and ovulation, to consider injecting the compound early in oestrus to ensure LH release at the normal time rather than delaying treatment until the day of AI when some cows, due to the conduct of the commercial AI services, will be the latter stages of oestrus or beyond the end of heat. However, against this, the potential disadvantages of creating a premature LH surge by injecting cows prior to the time of their endogenous pre-ovulatory LH discharge must be considered.

Superovulation

An increase in the number of ovulations at oestrus is the basis of many techniques to augment fertility. The number of ovulations occurring at any oestrus reflects the extent of follicular development which in turn is controlled by ovarian responsiveness, predetermined by genotype and the availability of gonadotrophins. In general, an increase in gonadotrophic stimulation allows the ovaries to exceed their normal limit for production of mature follicles.

As follicular development during the oestrous cycle is controlled by anterior pituitary gonadotrophins, it would seem logical to consider administration of these substances as the initial approach to superovulation. This view is further substantiated when it is appreciated that there are differences in the relative amounts of the polypeptide gonadotrophins LH and FSH in the pituitaries of farm animal species. However several factors have prevented this approach being routinely employed. Firstly, these hormones can only be obtained from anterior pituitary tissue by sophisticated extraction and isolation techniques, rendering them prohibitively expensive in purified form. Secondly, as polypeptides of a relatively low molecular weight (approximately 30 000), they have a short half-life and must be given by frequent injections. Nevertheless, crude extracts of horse and sheep pituitary tissue have occasionally been employed in studies of superovulation in farm animals. In addition, pituitary FSH derived from the increased amounts of this substance in post-menopausal human females' urine — human menopausal gonadotrophin (hMG) — has occasionally been used in studies in cattle.

In the main, however, commercially orientated work in this field has concentrated on the more readily available placental gonadotrophins derived from pregnant mare serum and human pregnancy urine. Pregnant mare serum gonadotrophin (PMSG) consists mainly of FSH-like activity with a minor LH activity, whereas the hormone from human pregnancy urine — human chorionic gonadotrophin (hCG) — consists of LH activity.

Although of equine and human origin, these gonadotrophins exhibit biological activity in all farm animals. Besides availability, a further consideration to the use of PMSG as an FSH substitute is its longer half-life of 40–125 hours (Menzer & Schams 1979), necessitating less frequent administration to supplement circulating gonadotrophins.

PMSG

In all cyclical female farm animals, the use of PMSG to induce superovulation follows certain common principles and is subject to certain limitations. Although experimentally normal follicular development during the luteal phase can be augmented using PMSG, these follicles neither ovulate nor trigger behavioural oestrus due to the suppressant effects of endogenous progesterone. The practical use of PMSG is therefore restricted to enhancing the normal follicular development, ovulation and the associated oestrus that occurs during the follicular phase. In general a single subcutaneous injection of the hormone is given just prior to the end of the luteal phase to coincide with the commencement of a wave of follicular growth at this time. It appears that the response to PMSG is greater when injected early rather than later in the follicular phase as suppression of the quantitative aspects of follicular development is a feature of the terminal stages of this period. Table 13.3 summarises the stage of the cycle when the hormone is normally administered on the assumption that the treated individuals have an average cycle length for the species.

As an alternative, the duration of the luteal phase can be artificially controlled to ensure the correct temporal relationship to the administration of PMSG. Both progesterone–progestogen administration and the use of prostaglandin $F_{2\alpha}$ have been employed. In cattle, PMSG administered at day 9–12 of the cycle is normally followed by a luteolytic prostaglandin injection 40–45 hours later. There is evidence to suggest that inducing luteolysis at mid-cycle is associated with a higher yield of embryos in the following luteal phase than in cows treated with PMSG in the natural late luteal period

Table 13.3 Timing and dosage of PMSG for super ovulation.

Species	PMSG injected (day of cycle)	Dosage for embryo transfer (IU)
Bovine	16–17	1500–2500
Ovine	12–13	1200–1700
Caprine	17–18	1500
Porcine	15–16	750–1500

(Seidel *et al* 1978). Alternatively the PRID can be used to control the length of the luteal phase. In sheep, intravaginal polyurethane sponges impregnated with a progestogen are normally employed. By inserting these for 14–16 days, the random distribution of ovulations in a group of cycling ewes can be synchronised. The effectiveness of the prostaglandin analogue cloprostenol in terminating the luteal phase of sheep injected with PMSG 1–3 days earlier allows scope for an alternative approach.

A contraindication to the widespread use of PMSG for superovulation is the unpredictability of the response. Besides dosage of the drug, various factors have been identified as modifying the number of follicles that develop in response to a fixed amount of PMSG. These include breed, age, the time of injection during the oestrous cycle and nutrition. This lack of precision of response extends not only to animals of the same breed but also, as has been demonstrated in cattle, between treatments in the same animal (Newcomb *et al* 1979). The disadvantages of an imprecise response are two-fold: firstly inadequate superovulation can render the exercise pointless, secondly excessive superovulation can result in reduced fertility of the embryos. It has been suggested that, with excessive follicular development, the ovaries are of such a size that the fimbrae of the oviduct are incapable of encompassing them and so picking up ovulated eggs. In addition the percentage of immature or atretic eggs increases with excess superovulation, e.g. in the sow this has been reported with superovulatory responses in excess of 25 (Hunter 1966). A third disadvantage is that there is some circumstantial evidence, based on endocrine profiles of superovulated cattle, that abnormal gonadal steroid secretion could interfere, by acting on the oviduct, with gamete transport. Due to this variation in response, techniques allowing an estimate to be made of the extent of follicular development or superovulation would form a useful part of these systems. In cattle, palpation of the ovaries *per rectum* and an estimate of the number of corpora lutea can be carried out, although this can underestimate results and is obviously not applicable to other farm animals. As an alternative, in cattle the peripheral plasma concentrations of progesterone and oestrogens over the period before and after superovulation have been examined. Unfortunately the correlation between corpora lutea numbers and embryos recovered from the uterus is poor. As regards oestrogen secretion during the follicular phase, although some studies have reported a positive relationship, this has not been substantiated in other investigations (Sreenan *et al* 1978; Kelly *et al* 1981). Table 13.3 gives an indication of the dosages of PMSG normally employed for superovulation, where the technique is used prior to embryo transfer and the aim is to produce up to 10–15 ovulations.

In general it appears that there is no need to administer excess LH, in the form of hCG, to ensure that ovulation follows PMSG induction of excess follicular growth. Should hCG be injected it would logically be used to supplement the existing endogenous pre-ovulatory LH surge. Difficulty can be experienced in this respect in cattle in timing the hCG administration to coincide with the LH surge which occurs just before or at the onset of oestrus. There are potential disadvantages in the premature administration of exogenous hCG including luteinisation of follicles without ovulation and release of immature eggs. In addition it has been shown that hCG given to the cow during pro-oestrus can inhibit the endogenous LH surge and terminate oestradiol secretion by the follicles (Dobson & Fitzpatrick 1975). It is possible that this termination of oestradiol secretion would be sufficient to prevent this hormone triggering the behavioural state of oestrus.

Prepubertal ovulation

Prepubertal ovulation of female farm animals would allow the generation interval to be shortened and benefit progeny testing. Calves, ewes and lambs can all be induced to ovulate prior to the initiation of spontaneous oestrous cycles using PMSG, although very early life is characterised by a lack of ovarian responsiveness to exogenous gonadotrophins. These regimens normally involve administration of PMSG followed, after an appropriate interval of 2–5 days depending on the species, by hCG to ensure ovulation. Pretreatment with progestogens before PMSG has been employed in 10–16-week-old lambs to give a 77% fertilisation rate of recovered ova (Trounson *et al* 1977). In addition, the capacity for these embryos to produce viable lambs has been demonstrated. In calves induced to ovulate, pregnancy rates from transferred ova are low (Seidel *et al* 1971). In the prepubertal gilt, the success rate of PMSG and hCG in inducing precocious puberty is low. Although animals can be stimulated to ovulate, they do not consistently continue cycling (Paterson & Martin 1981) or, if inseminated, the corpora lutea did not always produce enough progesterone to maintain a pregnancy (Sega & Baker 1973). An alternative approach in gilts around 140 days of age involves the administration of oestrogens which, in preliminary experiments, resulted in an early synchronised first oestrus in 60% gilts when combined with the boar stimulation effect.

Increasing numbers of offspring per pregnancy

Lack of consistency in response to PMSG coupled with a uterine factor which restricts the number of embryos that can be carried to term has prevented the use of PMSG to increase the number of calves born per pregnancy in cows. In addition the problem of freemartinism in the females of dissimilar sexes *in utero* precludes this technique from being applied for offspring destined for breeding or milk production. Insertion of a single additional embryo into the uterine horn opposite to that containing a potential self-ovulated embryo has given encouraging results for induced twinning in cattle (Gordon 1976). In cycling sheep, the administration of PMSG in association with progestogen sponges for oestrus synchronisation may improve the lambing percentage. Besides stimulating excess follicular development, there is some evidence that PMSG may overcome a possible depression in fertility at the first oestrus after sponge removal. Doubling the dose of PMSG (750 IU), however, failed to improve the pregnancy rate or lambing percentage over a dose of 375 IU after progestogen sponges (Gordon 1976).

Embryo transfer

Should embryos be destined for transfer to recipient animals, it is essential for maximum success in establishment of pregnancies that the luteal phase of donor and recipients is synchronised. Although this can be achieved by selecting from a large group of suitable recipients those randomly in oestrus on the same day as the donor, it is often more convenient to synchronise the oestrous cycles of preselected recipient animals. Normally in cattle, prostaglandin $F_{2\alpha}$ or analogues are employed by one of the methods detailed previously. Advance planning is obviously essential to ensure that recipients have a potentially responsive corpus luteum at the time the donor animal commences the superovulatory treatment. In sheep and goats, where progestogen sponges are more likely to be used in the recipients, the sponges should be removed from these animals one day before the donor as PMSG advances the time of oestrus in the donor.

Reproduction in males

There is considerably less information about the normal physiological control of reproduction and the underlying causes of non-infectious infertility in male farm animals than about animals like the cow and ewe. Reflecting this lack of background knowledge there are, in general, no situations where hormone preparations are routinely used, with a physiological basis, to treat reproductive disorders in males.

For example, although androgens in sufficient amounts and after an appropriate latency period can induce male behaviour in castrates, their use to treat diminished libido in bulls on the basis of an unconfirmed testosterone deficiency being responsible for the condition is questionable for two reasons: firstly, because bulls with a complaint of this type commonly have normal plasma androgen profiles and, secondly, because of the potentially suppressant effect of androgens on pituitary gonadotrophins and the essential role of these latter hormones in normal spermatogenesis. Other sporadic therapeutic applications of hormones in males, such as the use of the luteinising hormone (LH)-like preparation hCG to induce descent of a cryptorchid testis, should be regarded with similar caution in the absence of documented physiological and clinical evidence to support their use.

There is a certain amount of experimental interest in managemental control of reproduction in males. Enhancement of sperm production in bulls and rams is under investigation. Although prostaglandins administered to these species gave encouraging results in that they increased sperm per ejaculate, current evidence would suggest that they achieve this transient efect by their action on the tubular genital tract rather than by stimulation of spermatogenesis. Conversely suppression of the behavioural components of male reproduction is being examined in bulls as a chemical alternative to castration. Efforts in this field are directed towards modification of the normal control mechanism for testicular androgen synthesis by immunisation with either hCG or synthetic androgens and hypothalamic LHRH — with this latter hormone rendered antigenic by coupling to a larger carrier protein. Although experimentally effective in regulating the prepubertal development of testes and production of androgens, such techniques are subject to the vagaries of biological variations as regards antibody production and until such problems are overcome they are unlikely to find economic application.

References

Bierschwal C. J., Elmore R. G., Brown E. M. *et al* (1980) Pathology of the ovary and ovarian disorders and the influence of ovarian abnormalities on the endometrium, including therapeutic aspects (cow). *Proc. 9th Int. Congr. Anim. Reprod. AI. (Madrid)* **1**, 193.

Booth J. M. (1981) Cystic ovaries — milk progesterone levels. In *Proc. Br. Cattle Vet. Assoc. 1980–81,* p. 71.

Boyd H. & Munro C. D. (1979) Progesterone assays and rectal palpation in pre-service management of a dairy herd. *Vet. Rec.* **104**, 341.

Bradford G. E., Taylor St. C. S., Quirke J. F. *et al* (1974) An egg-transfer study of litter size, birth weight and lamb survival. *Anim. Prod.* **18**, 249.

Britt J. H., Harrison D. S. & Morrow D. A. (1977) Frequency of ovarian follicular cysts, reasons for culling, and fertility in Holstein-Friesian cows given gonadotrophin-releasing hormone at two weeks after parturition. *Am. J. Vet. Res.* **38**, 749.

Bulman D. C. & Wood P. D. P. (1980) Abnormal patterns of ovarian activity in dairy cows and their relationship with reproductive performance. *Anim. Prod.* **30**, 177.

Christiansen I. J. & Hansen L. H. (1974) Dexamethasome-induced parturition in cattle. *Br. Vet. J.* **130**, 221.

Comline R. S., Nathanielsz B. P. W., Paisley R. B. *et al* (1970) Cortisol turnover in the sheep foetus immediately prior to parturition. *J. Physiol.* **210**, 141.

Cooper M. J. (1981) Cloprostenol as a tool in the management of dairy cattle. *Acta. Vet. Scand.* (Suppl.) **77,** 171.

Currie W. B. & Thorburn G. D. (1977) The foetal role in timing the initiation of parturition. In *The Fetus and Birth.* Ciba Symposium.

Al Dahash S. Y. A. & David J. S. E. (1977) Anatomical features of cystic ovaries in cattle found during an abbatoir survey. *Vet. Rec.* **101,** 320.

Dawson F. M. L. (1975) Accuracy of rectal palpation in the diagnosis of ovarian function in the cow. *Vet. Rec.* **96,** 218.

Day A. M. (1977) Cloprostenol for termination of pregnancy in cattle. *N.Z. Vet. J.* **25,** 136.

Daykin J. M. (1976) Prostaglandin and the bovine mummified foetus. *Vet. Rec.* **98,** 37.

Dobson J. & Fitzpatrick R. J. (1975) The effect of hCG on endogenous gonadotrophin in normal bovine follicular activity. *J. Reprod. Fert.* **43,** 337.

Drew B. (1980) The effect of progesterone treatment on fertility of dairy cows. In *31st Ann. Meeting Eur. Assoc. Anim. Prod.* Paper GC2:33.

Drew S. B., Gould C. M. & Bulman D. C. (1978) The effect of treatment with a progesterone releasing intravaginal device on the fertility of spring calving Friesian dairy cows. *Vet. Rec.* **103,** 259.

Duncanson G. R. (1981) Retained placenta and endometritis — treatment and control. In *Proc. Br. Cattle Vet. Assoc. 1980–81* p. 58.

Einarsson S. (1981) Comparative trial with natural prostaglandin and an analogue (Cloprostenol) in inducing parturition in sows. *Acta Vet. Scand.* (Suppl.) **77,** 321.

Eddy R. G. (1977) Cloprostenol as a treatment for no visible oestrus and cystic ovarian disease in dairy cows. *Vet. Rec.* **100,** 62.

Edqvist L. E., Lindell J. O. & Kindahl H. (1980) Premature and normal term delivery in the cow: Role of the $PGF_{2\alpha}$. *Proc. 9th Int. Cong. Reprod. & AI (Madrid)* RT.-A-5, 41.

Edqvist L. E., Lindell J. O. & Kindahl H. (1981) Prostaglandin $F_{2\alpha}$ release at premature and normal term deliveries in the cow. *Acta Vet. Scand.* (Suppl.) **77,** 267.

Elmore R. G., Bierschwal C. J., Youngquist R. S. *et al* (1975) Clinical responses of dairy cows with ovarian cysts following treatment with 10 000 IU hCG or 100 mcg GnRH. *Vet. Med/Sm. Anim. Clin.* **70,** 1346.

Fairnie I. J., Wales R. G. & Gherardi P. B. (1977) Time of ovulation, fertilisation rate, and blastocyst formation in ewes following treatment with a prostaglandin analogue (ICI 80996). *Theriogenol.* **8,** *183* (abstr.).

Gaverick H. A., Kesler D. J., Cantley T. C. *et al* (1976) Clinical and endocrine responses of dairy cows with ovarian cysts to GnRH and $PGF_{2\alpha}$. *J. Anim. Sci.* **46,** 719.

Gordon I. (1975) Hormonal control of reproduction in sheep. *Proc. Br. Soc. Anim. Prod.* **4,** 79.

Gordon I. (1976) Progress towards fixed-time sheep AI and twinning in beef cattle. *Wld. Rev. Anim. Prod.* **12,** 33.

Gunzler O. & Schallenberger E. (1981) The treatment of ovarian cysts in cattle with prostaglandins — possibilities and limitations. *Acta. Vet. Scand.* (Suppl.) **77,** 327.

Gustafsson B., Backstrom G. & Edqvist L. E. (1976) Treatment of Bovine pyometra with prostaglandin $F_{2\alpha}$: an evaluation of a field study. *Theriogenol.* **6,** 45.

Haresign W. & Acritopoulou S. (1977) Paper presented to 28th Meeting European Association for Animal Production, Brussels.

Haresign W. & Webster G. M. (1981) The induction of parturition in ewes with dexamethasone. In *Prog. & Papers Sums. Br. Soc. Anim. Prod.* (Harrogate). paper no. 56.

Harman E. L. & Slyter A. L. (1974) Induction of parturition in the ewe. *J. Anim. Sci.* **39,** 989.

Hendricks D. M., Rawlings N. C. & Ellicott A. R. (1977) Hormone levels in beef heifers during prostaglandin-induced parturition. *Theriogenol.* **7,** 17.

Hindson J. C. (1978) Quantification of obstetric traction *Vet. Rec.* **102,** 327.

Hindson J. C., Schofield B. M. & Turner C. B. (1967) The effect of a single dose of stilboestrol on cervical dilation in pregnant sheep. *Res. Vet. Sci.* **8,** 353.

Hoffman B., Gunzler O., Hamburger R. *et al* (1976) Milk progesterone as a parameter for fertility control in cattle; methodological approaches and present status of application in Germany. *Br. Vet. J.* **132**, 469.

Holst P. J. & Nancarrow C. D. (1975) Intramuscular administration of a prostaglandin analogue during pregnancy in the goat. *J. Reprod. Fertil.* **43**, 403.

Humblot P. & Thibier M. (1980) Progesterone monitoring of anestrus dairy cows and subsequent treatment with a prostaglandin $F_{2\alpha}$ analog or gonadotropin-releasing hormone. *Am. J. Vet. Res.* **41**, 1762.

Hunter R. H. F. (1966) The effect of superovulation on fertilisation and embryonic survival in the pig. *Anim. Prod.* **8**, 457.

Jackson P. S. (1977) Treatment of chronic post partum endometritis in cattle with cloprostenol. *Vet. Rec.* **101**, 441.

Jackson P. S., Johnson C. T., Bulman D. C. *et al* (1979) A study of cloprostenol-induced oestrus and spontaneous oestrus by means of the milk progesterone assay. *Br. Vet. J.* **135**, 578.

Kelly E. F., Renton J. P. & Munro C. D. (1981) Assessment of oviduct patency in the cow. *Vet. Rec.* **108**, 357.

Kesler D. J., Garverick H. A., Elmore R. G. *et al* (1979) Reproductive hornones associated with the ovarian cyst response to GnRH. *Theriogenol.* **12**, 109.

Kruif A. De., Wiel N. J. G. J. van der, Brand A. *et al* (1977) Oestrogens and prostaglandins in the treatment of cattle with pyometra. *Tijdschr voor Diergeneesk.* **102**, 851.

Lamming G. E. & Bulman D. C. (1976) The use of milk progesterone radioimmunoassay in the diagnosis and treatment of subfertility in dairy cows. *Br. Vet. J.* **132**, 507.

Liggins G. C., Fairclough R. J., Grieves S. A. *et al* (1973) The mechanism of initiation of parturition in the ewe. *Rec. Prog. Horm. Res.* **29**, 111.

Memon M. A., Lock T. F. & Nelson D. R. (1981) Induction of parturition with prostaglandin $F_{2\alpha}$ in cows with hydroallantois. A case report. *Theriogenol.* **16**, 681.

Menzer C. & Schams D. (1979) Radioimmunoassay for PMSG and its application to in-vivo studies. *J. Reprod. Fertil.* **55**, 339.

Munro C. D., Boyd H., Martin B. *et al* (1982) Monitoring pre-service reproductive status in dairy cows. *Vet. Rec.* **110**, 77.

Murray R. D., Smith J. H. & Harker D. B. (1981) Use of cloprostenol with dexamethasone in the termination of advanced pregnancy in heifers. *Vet. Rec.* **108**, 378.

Nakao T., Tsurubayashi M., Horiuchi S. *et al* (1979) Effects of a systemic application of human chorionic gonadotrophin, gonadotrophin-releasing hormone analog and bovine anterior pituitary gonadotrophin in cows with cystic ovarian disease. *Theriogenol.* **11**, 385.

Nancarrow C. D., Buckmaster J., Chamley W. *et al* (1973) Hormonal changes around oestrus in the cow. *J. Reprod. Fertil.* **32**, 320.

Nessan G. K. & King G. J. (1981) Relationship of peripheral oestrogens and testosterone concentrations to sexual behaviour in normal and cystic cows. *Can. Vet. J.* **22**, 9.

Newcomb R., Christie W. B., Rowson L. E. A. *et al* (1979) Influence of dose, repeated treatment and batch of hormone on ovarian response in heifers treated with PMSG. *J. Reprod. Fertil.* **56**, 113.

Ott R. S., Nelson D. R. & Hixon J. E. (1980) Peripheral serum progesterone and luteinizing hormone concentrations of goats during synchronization of oestrus and ovulation with prostaglandin $F_{2\alpha}$. *Am. J. Vet. Res.* **41**, 1432.

Paterson A. M. & Martin G. B. (1981) Induction of puberty in gilts (3). *Anim. Prod.* **32**, 55.

Peters A. R. (1982) *Ovarian activity in the post-partum suckling cow.* FRCVS thesis.

Robinson J. J., Fraser C. & McHattie I. (1975) The use of prostaglandins and photoperiodism in improving the reproductive rate of the ewe. *Ann. Biol. Anim. Biochem. Biophys.* **15**, 345.

Roche J. F. (1979) Control of oestrus in cattle. *Wld. Rev. Anim. Prod.* **15**, 49.

Rowson L. E. A., Lamming G. E. & Fry R. M. (1953) The relationship between ovarian hormones and uterine infection. *Vet. Rec.* **22**, 335.

Saumande J., Le Coustumier J. & Marais C. (1979) Oestradiol-17β and progesterone in nymphomaniac cows. *Theriogenol.* **12**, 27.

Saunders R. W. (1980) The impact of prostaglandins on the AI service. In *Proc. Upjohn Symposium on Prostaglandins.* Stoneleigh, p. 29.

Schultz R. H. & Copeland D. D. (1981) Induction of abortion using prostaglandins. *Acta Vet. Scand.* (Suppl.) **77**, 353.

Segal D. H. & Baker R. D. (1973) Maintenance of corpora lutea in pre pubertal gilts. *J. Anim. Sci.* **37**, 762.

Seidel G. E. Jr., Elsden P. P., Nelson L. D. *et al* (1978) In *Current topics in veterinary medicine. 1.* Control of reproduction in the cow, ed. J. M. Sreenan. Martinus Nijhoff, Hague.

Seidel G. E. Jr., Larson L. L., Spilman C. H. *et al* (1971) Culture and transfer of calf ova. *J. Dairy Sci.* **54**, 923.

Sequin B. E., Convey E. M. & Oxender W. D. (1976) Effect of gonadotrophin-releasing hormone and human chorionic gonadotrophin on cows with ovarian follicular cysts. *Am. J. Vet. Res.* **37**, 153.

Silver M., Barnes R. J., Comline R. S. *et al* (1979) Prostaglandins in the foetal pig and prepartum endocrine changes in mother and foetus. *Anim. Reprod. Sci.* **2**, 305.

Sreenan J. M., Beehan D. & Gosling J. P. (1978) In *Control of Reproduction in the Cow,* ed. J. M. Sreenan, Commission of the European Communities, Luxembourg, p. 144.

Talbot A. C. & Hafs H. D. (1974) Termination of a bovine pregnancy complicated by mummified foetus. *Vet. Rec.* **95**, 512.

Thimonier J. (1981) Practical uses of prostaglandins in sheep and goats. *Acta. Vet. Scand.* (Suppl.) **77**, 193.

Trounson A. O., Willadsen S. M. & Moor R. M. (1976) Effect of prostaglandin analogue Cloprostenol on oestrus ovulation and embryonic viability in sheep. *J. Agri. Sci.* **86**, 609.

Trounson A. O., Willadsen S. M. & Moor R. M. (1977) Reproductive function in prepubertal lambs: ovulation, embryo development and ovarian steroidogenesis. *J. Reprod. Fert.* **49**, 69.

Umo I. & Fitzpatrick R. J. (1976) Induction of parturition in goats with prostaglandin $F_{2\alpha}$. In *Proc. VIIIth Intern. Congr. Anim. Reprod. AI* (Cracow) **3**, 411.

Wagner W. C., Willham R. L. & Evans L. E. (1974) Controlled parturition in cattle. *J. Anim. Sci.* **38**, 485.

Webb R., Lamming G. E., Haynes N. B. *et al* (1977) Response of cyclic and post partum suckled cows to injections of synthetic LHRH. *J. Reprod. Fertil.* **50**, 203.

Young I. M. & Henderson D. C. (1981) Evaluation of single and double artificial insemination regimens as methods of shortening calving intervals in dairy cows treated with dinoprost. *Vet. Rec.* **109**, 446.

PART 5
NUTRITION, METABOLISM AND FLUID BALANCE

14

Nutrition of the horse

D.L. FRAPE

Maintenance of the appetite of a horse during extended periods of maximum work is an art, but a knowledge of the established facts of nutritional physiology may enable the horse more nearly to achieve its genetic potential during these periods.

Eating behaviour

The horse has evolved as a browsing herbivore consuming small and frequent feeds of lush leafy vegetation. The principal carbohydrates of these feeds are cellulose, hemicellulose forming the structural elements of plant cells, and some soluble sugars. It has been said that the structural carbohydrates, termed vegetable fibre, are essential to the life of all herbivores, but this is only true in the sense that herbivores are better adapted than other animals to their efficient use and not that herbivores are unable to survive in their absence. The leaves of herbage and arborial species contain hundreds of organic substances and, although some of these are hazardous, this food source meets all the daily nutritional needs of the horse. Frequent grazing and browsing ensures that the microbial flora of the gastrointestinal tract are maintained in a state of happy equilibrium without overloading or deprivation of the population in any section; the fibre also provides bulk which promotes peristalsis without causing blockage.

Functioning of the gastrointestinal tract

Stomach

A characteristic of all herbivores is enlargement of some part of the gastro-intestinal tract to accommodate fermentation of the digesta by micro-organisms. In the horse it is the caecum and colon which are especially enlarged. The adult horse has a stomach of relatively small capacity and food empties from it more rapidly than from that of the foal. In contrast to the ruminant animal therefore, saliva in the horse plays a different role and is

Table 14.1 Mean concentrations of electrolytes in gastrointestinal tract liquor (mEq/l). Data from *Progress in Nutrition and Allied Sciences*, courtesy of Oliver & Boyd.

	Sodium	Potassium	Chloride	Phosphate	Bicarbonate
Stomach	58	28	85	12	7
Jejunum	112	24	65	18	15
Cranial ileum	118	18	76	15	27
Caudal ileum	126	15	48	16	80
Caecum	122	17	30	16	65
Ventral colon	105	29	15	28	50
Dorsal colon	80	44	3	58	27
Small colon	47	53	4	55	18

secreted in response to the mastication of food. It is a source of hypotonic fluid and of sodium, potassium, bicarbonate, and chloride ions (Table 14.1). The buffering power of saliva favours some fermentation in the stomach since it retards the rate at which the pH of the digesta decreases. There is, nevertheless, a considerable stratification of the digesta in the stomach marked by differences in pH and this, together with the small capacity, must ensure that in quantitative terms there is only partial digestion and fermentation (Kern *et al* 1974). Gastric fermentation primarily yields lactic acid on account of the generally low pH (Elsden *et al* 1946, Alexander & Hickson 1970). Little proteolytic activity occurs in the fundic region but more has been observed in the pyloric region (Kern *et al* 1974).

Small intestine

Proteolytic activity per ml of digesta increases by a factor of ten in the ileum in comparison to the pyloric region and this is attributable mainly to secretions of the succus entericus (Kern *et al* 1974, Table 14.2). Large quantities of pancreatic juice are also secreted as a result of the presence of food in the stomach in response to stimuli mediated by vagal fibres and by endocrine activity, but the enzyme activity of this secretion is of a low order (Comline *et al* 1963). It does, nevertheless, provide large amounts of fluid and sodium — potassium and chloride ions affording a suitable medium for the functioning of the enzymes secreted by the villi of the small intestine (Table 14.1). Secretions from the bile duct and pancreas are stimulated by gastric hydrochloric acid and gastric juice — secretions which cease after a fast of 48 hours (Comline *et al* 1963). Brush border glucoamylase from the intestinal mucosa complements the activity of pancreatic alpha-amylase (Roberts 1974). Ileal juice has been demonstrated to be relatively high in amylase, lactase, and maltase activity, but to contain less protease and peptidase activity (Baker *et*

Table 14.2   Proteolytic activity of ingesta of ponies given Timothy hay. (Data from Kern *et al* (1974) *J.Anim. Sci.* **38**, 559–64.)

	Activity*	NH₃-N (mg/100 ml)
Stomach (fundic pH 5.4)	3	2.9
Stomach (pyloric pH 2.6)	54	3.9
Ileum	530	5.2
Caecum	12	2.9
Terminal colon	15	5.4

*1 unit = $0.045\mu g$ protein hydrol./mg ingesta/minute.

al 1972). Pancreatic juice contains bicarbonate which raises the pH of the gastric ingesta for the optimum functioning of these enzymes; however its concentration is lower than that of chloride (Comline *et al* 1969).

β-galactosidase declines in activity from birth to 3–4 years of age. Diarrhoea in foals sometimes results from a deficiency in the enzymic digestion of lactose and it has been proposed by Roberts (1974) that an oral tolerance test, in which foals are given 1 g lactose/kg body weight (as a 20% solution) could be of clinical value in determining small intestinal mucosal damage. A glucose tolerance test at the rate of 1 g glucose/kg body weight given by stomach tube has also been suggested as a means of diagnosing diabetes mellitus. In normal animals a peak in blood glucose occurs at two hours and normal levels are regained within four hours of dosing.

A large flux of phosphate is apparent throughout the intestines and net movements indicate a voluminous endogenous secretion into the jejunum and caecum with a large net absorption in the dorsal and small colons (Schryver *et al* 1972) (Table 14.1). A considerable ileal influx and secretion of NaHCO₃ probably functions as an effective buffer during microbial fermentation in the caecum facilitating organic absorption, and large amounts of sodium, chloride, and bicarbonate ions are removed from the colon, whereas potassium and phosphate ions tend to increase — the latter acting as a buffer in the dorsal colon (Alexander 1963, Schryver *et al* 1972, Argenzio 1975). Intestinal movements are greatly affected by intestinal blood flow and by endocrine secretions — adrenaline inhibits the movement of the stomach, ileum, and large intestine.

Large intestine

In the adult horse, feed first appears in the caecum 45 minutes after eating and digesta remain in the gastrointestinal tract for approximately one-third the time they are resident in the tract of the ruminant. Partly for this reason dietary fibre appears to be digested to only 60–80% of that in the ruminant

(Van der Noot & Trout 1971). Both the residence time and the microbial concentration in the caecum and colon of the horse are, in general, less than they are in the rumen (Meyer 1980). Chromic oxide recovery shows almost complete passage of digesta within 72 hours in the horse although our own evidence indicates detectable amounts occurring up to 14 days following feeding (Frape *et al* 1982). Rate of passage of digesta is not significantly affected by the chemical composition of the diet but, as in the ruminant, it is affected by its physical form (Wolter *et al* 1974). Rate of passage is faster with pelleted feed and ground and wafered hay than with loose hay, suggesting that expulsion decreases the time for which micro-organisms may act on the digesta and so decreases the extent of roughage digestion (Wolter *et al* 1975). However, the effect is small and the overall influence of pelleting on diet utilisation is beneficial. Rolling or cracking of grain also assists its digestion, especially when horses' teeth are unsound, by allowing enzymes access to the endosperm.

The diet of the working horse

Domestication

Man has modified the diet of domesticated horses in order to make possible increased work rates and to decrease the time devoted to feeding. This has entailed a partial or total replacement of herbage by cereals, their byproducts, and conserved dry hay. This alteration to the natural diet has achieved its objectives, but it has been accompanied by physiological problems. Much of this chapter will be devoted to the problems which have been encountered following man's intervention. Nevertheless, one physiological advantage of the development has been that feeds containing less than approximately 15% crude fibre are digested with an efficiency approximating to that of cattle and sheep, whereas diets containing more than this amount possess an organic matter and crude fibre digestibility approximately 85% of that in sheep and 75% of that in cattle.

Nutrient requirements

Water economy

The caecum is the primary site of net water absorption and the horse's large intestine has as a critical function the storage and absorption of large volumes of fluid — particularly of water and sodium ions, reflecting organic acid production and reaction with bicarbonate (Argenzio 1975). Horse faeces usually contain 66–76% water, though that voided by ponies and donkeys may be drier. A high grain diet decreases faecal water content and pelleted foods tend to increase faecal moisture although, after acclimitisation, differences may be small. Wet bran mashes are sometimes given in an endeavour to increase the moisture content of faeces but, in fact, they do not alter those produced by horses given dry bran with access to water (Hintz *et al* 1975).

Fluid loss in the horse can result from either water deprivation or excessive, unreplenished loss. There is little published information on the extent to which horses may become dehydrated whilst remaining fit. It has, on the other hand, been demonstrated that appetite fails in the Somalian donkey when 22% of bodyweight is lost through dehydration but it can lose up to 30% of its body weight and successfully recuperate and recover normal weight by drinking 24–30 litres in a period of 2–5 minutes. These animals can also survive and withstand the effects of drinking saline solutions containing up to 1% salt and many Arab horses have had no alternative but to drink brackish water in the desert (Maloiy 1970).

Scientific evidence in the horse has been limited to observing alterations in the composition of the blood during extended work. The interpretation of evidence from endurance exercise is complicated by changes in general metabolism during work, movements of fluid and electrolytes in particular into and out of the blood pool, losses of fluid, electrolytes and plasma proteins from the body and, in the thoroughbred in particular, splenic contraction. Horses subjected to endurance rides show rises in packed cell volume and total plasma protein (TPP). The former may rise by 20–30% and the latter by 7–10%. The change in TPP probably represents the extent of dehydration. Despite the haemoconcentration, sodium and chloride levels in the plasma fall during protracted work largely as a result of sweating. Plasma chloride may fall by 10 mEq/l (10–11%) and sodium by 4 mEq/l (approximately 3%). Metabolic alkalosis also normally occurs with blood pH rising to 7.44 or greater. In horses which become exhausted these changes are more variable (packed cell volume in exhausted horses may rise fractionally by 45% and plasma protein by as much as 20% (a rise of 1.4 g/100 ml)). As a consequence of the loss of electrolytes from the blood, only a part of the water loss is replaced voluntarily since that proportion of the thirst drive which is mediated by hypertonicity is markedly reduced. Thus, full repletion will require the administration of electrolytes as well as water in order to restore homeostasis (Rose *et al* 1977, Frape *et al* 1979).

It is frequently stated that horses should be watered *before* being fed so that the water does not dilute the digesta and reduce the efficiency of digestion. However, it has been established that, when the stomach is full of digesta, water passes over the lesser curvature directly into the intestine without mixing. Nevertheless, some mixing does occur if only a little food is present in the stomach.

Estimates of how much water the working horse needs obviously depend upon the degree of work and the prevailing atmospheric temperature and insolation. Requirements can rise to as much as 75–80 kg/day, whereas for fattening under good conditions the requirement may be in the region of 25–30 kg/day, and in mares during late pregnancy it may be 40 kg/day. Lactating mares may need up to 55–60 kg/day (Caljuk 1961).

Protein metabolism

Protein digestion

In the ruminant herbivore, especially when it is not receiving large amounts of dry matter, most dietary protein is deaminated by the microbial flora. On the other hand, approximately 70% of crude protein digestion occurs in the horse before digesta reaches the region of active microbial deamination (Frape 1975) (Table 14.2). Despite these anatomical and mechanistic differences between the horse and the ruminant, the overall efficiency of crude protein digestion is similar (Van der Noot & Gilbreath 1970). The proteolytic activity in several regions of the gastrointestinal tract in the horse has been measured and, although proteolysis occurs in the pyloric region of the stomach, the major activity apparently takes place in the ileum as a consequence of the action of enzymes of the succus entericus — pancreatic trypsin probably playing a lesser role (Kern *et al* 1974).

Dietary requirement for protein and amino acids

The adequacy of dietary protein is a function of the amount present, relative to the energy content of the diet, of its digestibility and amino acid balance (Reitnour & Salisbury 1976), and of the horse's need for protein. Mature horses are relatively indifferent to the protein quality of the diet. However, insufficient dietary protein will have a severe effect on growth of the foal. For this growth most proteins are limiting in their lysine content and the hind gut is insufficiently developed for the foal to make any practical use of dietary inorganic nitrogen. Growing colts and fillies respond to the addition of lysine to their diet when the dietary crude protein content is 12–14% based upon linseed meal (Hintz *et al* 1971). Such supplementation increases both daily liveweight gain and nitrogen retention. These responses may also be increased by substituting better quality proteins for the linseed meal.

In the adult, it is likely that the daily requirement for protein increases as work demand increases owing to an increase in amino acid metabolism which accompanies an increase in the processes liberating energy. Nevertheless, as the daily requirement for energy rises with work load, it is very unlikely that there is any need for an increase in the concentration of protein in the diet at this time. Work carried out forty years ago (Axelsson 1943) led to the conclusion that the horse's requirement for protein during work was a constant proportion of the energy requirement and so increased as the rate of work increased in accord with the above conclusions.

Utilisation of non-protein nitrogen

It has been suggested that supplementation of diets with non-protein nitrogen sources (NPN), such as urea, may allow the exclusion of expensive protein concentrates. Urease is not synthesised by the tissues of higher animals so that utilisation of urea depends upon the intervention of the gut microflora (Fig. 14.1) and either the subsequent digestion of those organisms and the absorption of the amino acids derived, or the direct use by the host of ammonia released during the microbial hydrolysis of urea. A feeding value for NPN also requires that the daily needs are not already met by pre-formed dietary protein. Under normal conditions the only animals likely to fulfil these requirements are rapidly growing young stock, who have a fully developed hind gut, and lactating mares. An increase in nitrogen retention has been demonstrated in such animals given low protein basal diets (Slade *et al* 1970, Godbee & Slade 1981), but under practical conditions in the UK it is unlikely that NPN sources could play any important part in horse feeding. That the quality of the dietary protein exerts a major influence is demonstrated by an

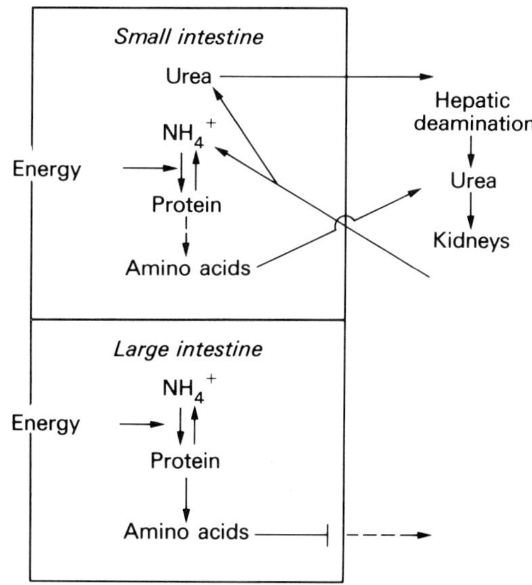

Fig. 14.1 Microbial protein metabolism in the gastro-intestinal tract of the horse.

association between the amino acid distribution of dietary protein and that of the free amino acids in blood, indicating that dietary proteins are to a significant extent hydrolysed in the small intestine with the absorption of their constituent amino acids (Reitnour *et al* 1970).

Probably important to protein metabolism and to the utilisation of NPN is the functioning of the urea cycle (Fig. 14.1). Whereas in the ruminant dietary and salivary urea are exposed to attack by rumen bacteria before reaching the absorptive surfaces of the intestine, most urea from these sources is likely to be absorbed from the small intestine of the horse and not utilised for protein synthesis until secreted into the small intestine and carried into the large intestine, hydrolysed to ammonia, and synthesised into microbial protein. The hydrolysis of proteins of either dietary or microbial origin in the small intestine will yield amino acids which can be absorbed through the wall. The greater part of the microbial activity of the equine GI tract occurs in the caecum and colon where microbial protein is formed from inorganic nitrogen sources, from nitrogen of endogenous origin, and from food protein residues. As the supply of dietary proteins and NPN is increased, the nitrogen content of the substrate for this activity generally rises. The rate of microbial protein synthesis in the hind gut, however, probably depends to a greater extent on the energy supply than on the circulating level of blood urea and its rate of secretion into the lumen of the gut.

Growth of the intestinal microflora and the utilisation of their protein

It has been clearly shown that both protein and NPN are utilised in the hind gut for synthesis of microbial protein (Prior *et al* 1974, Wootten & Argenzio 1975). Three questions of considerable economic and biological significance arise from this: 1 Does this activity increase the supply of amino acids in the blood circulation of the horse? 2 Can amino acids resulting from the hydrolysis of proteins be absorbed through the wall of the hind gut (Fig. 14.1)? 3 Can dietary NPN affect the nitrogen economy of the horse, either independently of the microflora or through its activity? There are several pathways by which NPN can lead to the synthesis of protein available to the host without postulating the necessity for amino acids absorption through the wall of the hind gut. Small quantities of ammonium compounds can be utilised in transamination reactions, principally in the liver of the adult, leading to the synthesis of dietary non-essential amino acids. However, as a consequence of normal deamination which occurs in the liver, it is unlikely that additional supplies of ammonium ions will increase the yield unless the horse is receiving a low protein diet. Under such conditions the administration of urea has been demonstrated to cause a rise in circulating glycine, thus implicating hepatic transaminations (Reitnour 1978).

It has been calculated that, in the pony, between 0.4 and 2.9 g of endogenous urea secreted into the gut daily is synthesised into microbial protein (Prior *et al* 1974) (Table 14.3). Twenty per cent of the caecal bacteria, in addition to the ciliate protozoa, exhibit proteolytic activity in the horse (Kern *et al* 1973), thus providing a mechanism for the hydrolysis of microbial protein in the large intestine. Nevertheless, the proteolytic activity in the hind gut is probably less than 4% of that in the small intestine. The economic importance of the mechanism is therefore, not likely to be large, although amino acids present in the lumen of the caecum can be absorbed and detected in the blood vessels draining the region (Slade *et al* 1971). Under conditions of deprivation, this source of amino acids probably represents a means of survival in many herbivores, but under normal domestic conditions it is likely to represent a less important source of sustenance. Deprivation under range conditions also normally entails the consumption of poor quality roughage. In order to digest this fully, the microflora require adequate nitrogen for their growth. Poor quality roughage contains little nitrogen so that both its fibre and the total organic matter are poorly digested by the domesticated horse.

Ammonia and urea toxicity

A theory that excessive dietary protein poisons horses may stem from the fear of the consequences attendant upon increased urea production. On the contrary, however, the horse would appear to be less subject to such toxicity than the ruminant, largely for anatomical reasons. Urea itself is a fairly innocuous compound and toxic episodes are precipitated only by the action of urease-releasing ammonia, unless very high blood levels of urea are reached. Urea is a highly soluble compound which, if present in the diet, is mainly absorbed through the wall of the small intestine (Fig. 14.1), avoiding significant deamination by the intestinal microflora. Much of this urea is subsequently excreted through the kidneys unless renal damage is present. However, in the absence of dietary urea it can be calculated that a 500 kg horse

Table 14.3 Rate of degradation of endogenous urea by intestinal microflora in ponies. (Data from Prior *et al* (1974) *J.Anim.Sci.* **38**, 565–71.)

Dietary protein (%)	Urea production rate (mg/kg/hr $BW^{10.75}$)	Degradation rate of urea in GI tract (production rate– excretion rate)
6	42.7	27.7
9	59.1	33.0
13	78.7	38.8
18	133.3	49.5

receiving a diet of normal protein content secretes 88 g of urea daily, or approximately half the urea synthesised systemically into the lumen of the intestinal tract (Prior *et al* 1974). This is a process which proceeds reasonably steadily throughout the 24 hours so that the intestinal bacteria are not presented with sudden increases in urea concentrations leading to greater rates of ammonia production than they can utilise in the slower, and energy-demanding, anabolic process of protein synthesis. The horse is, therefore, less subject to ammonia toxicity than is the ruminant animal. It has been shown that ammonia intoxication of the horse requires as much as 3 g urea/kg body weight in one dose. This greatly exceeds any amount likely to be found even in ruminant feed.

Carbohydrate metabolism

Depot fat in the horse is more unsaturated than fat situated at comparable sites in the ruminant. This is related to the fact that more dietary fat in the ruminant is metabolised by micro-organisms before it is digested and absorbed by the host. The digestion of starches and sugars follows a parallel fate. Consequently, more glucose is absorbed and enters the portal vessels in the horse than in the ruminant and the pattern of carbohydrate metabolism in the horse is intermediate between that of the ruminant and that of non-ruminants such as the pig (Argenzio & Hintz 1972) (Fig. 14.2). Although all three groups of animals utilise glucose and the volatile fatty acids — the end

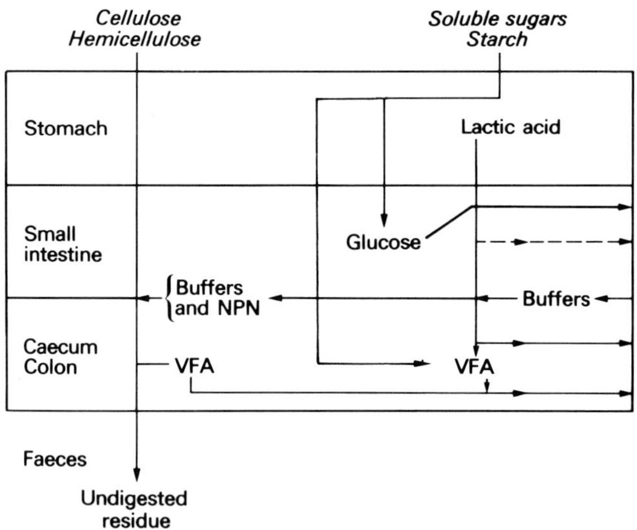

Fig. 14.2 Carbohydrate digestion in the horse.

products respectively of mammalian digestion of starch and of microbial metabolism of all carbohydrates — with a similar efficiency, the horse adapts readily to the metabolism of widely variable proportions of glucose and VFA within the majority of its tissue cells demanding energy. Metabolic ailments associated with carbohydrate metabolism result from subjecting the horse to rapid changes in the dietary sources from which these end products arise.

The dietary ratio of starch to fibre

The digestion of starchy diets mainly takes place in the small intestine, whereas that of fibre occurs in the hind gut. It has been shown that 70% of the available carbohydrate from maize is digested proximal to the caecum as compared to 40% of that from lucerne (Hintz *et al* 1971). Horses given the former feed derive most of their energy from glucose, while those given the latter derive it predominantly from the metabolism of volatile fatty acids (VFA). The efficiency of digestion of cellulose and other fibrous components in hay and similar materials is influenced by the familiarity of the microflora with the substrate. A sudden switch from a starchy to a fibrous diet can lead to poor utilisation of the fibre in the second diet because of a sparsity of cellulolytic organisms. Hence, the proportions of starch to fibre should remain relatively constant over long periods in order to retain a relatively high level of fibre digestibility. Starch-fermenting organisms have a higher rate of metabolism than those which ferment fibre and, when the former are encouraged by a rich starchy substrate, they overwhelm the slower growing cellulolytic organisms. In general, however, following acclimatisation to the diet, there appears to be no effect of forage-to-grain ratio on the digestibility of fibre of each type if the nutrient requirements of the flora are met. The adjustment which is necessary in the species distribution and population size of the hind gut microflora following a dietary change is undoubtedly less in the horse than in the ruminant because, within reasonable limits, the composition of the digesta entering the caecum changes to only a small extent in these circumstances when compared with that entering the rumen.

As the quantity of feed given to the horse increases, the rate of passage of digesta through the gastrointestinal tract also increases and, as the proportion of starch in the diet is raised, it appears that more starch reaches the caecum undigested (Hintz *et al* 1971, Kern *et al* 1973). Large numbers of Gram-positive and -negative bacilli grow in the caecum of the pony and bacterial numbers increase following the replacement of one quarter of the hay by crimped oats (Kern *et al* 1973, 1974). This suggests that a proportion of the starch is subjected to microbial metabolism with the production of VFA (Table 14.4) and lactic acid. Ciliate protozoa have also been observed in the caecum and this supports the same inference (Kern *et al* 1973).

Table 14.4 Molar percentages of VFA in rumen fluid and pony caecal fluids after feeding diets with differing proportions of hay to grain. (Data from Hintz & Schryver (1978) *J.Equine Med. Surg.* **2,** 147–50.)

Hay:Grain		Acetate	Propionate	Butyrate
			Molar percentage	
1:0	Pony	73	17	8
	Cattle	74	18	8
1:4	Pony	59	25	11
	Cattle	62	22	16

The extent of fibre digestion is not only dependent on its chemical nature but is also influenced by how long the digesta are in the gastrointestinal tract and by the efficiency, or rate, of degradation. Evidence is conflicting on the relative efficiencies of forage degradation by ruminal and equine microbes, but residence time is appreciably less in the horse than in the ruminant. Differences between the ruminant and the horse in the extent of fibre digestibility therefore favour the ruminant but are not as extreme as might be supposed from differences in residence time. Most evidence indicates that the horse digests fibre with an efficiency approximating to 70% of that in the ruminant (Frape & Boxall 1974, Frape 1975). Early evidence (Axelsson 1943) demonstrated that, as dietary fibre level increased, digestibility of organic matter declined both in horses and cattle, but that the reduction was greater in the horse. The relationship derived between crude fibre content (X) and coefficient of digestibility of organic matter (Y) is given below:

for horses $Y = 97.0 - 1.26\ X$

for cattle $Y = 86.0 - 0.66\ X$.

Microbial fermentation of starch and fibre

Mammals secret no enzymes capable of degrading the cellulose and hemicellulose abundant in forages, and depend on microbes for their degradation. These organisms obtain energy for their growth from this fermentation process and the VFAs and lesser quantities of other short chain fatty acids, produced as byproducts, are absorbed and utilised by the host. The small intestine of all mammals secretes amylases capable of hydrolysing starch, but in addition some starch is acted on in the horse by Lactobacilli and Streptococci in the saccus caecus of the stomach and in the caecum, with the formation of lactic acid. Following a starch meal there is a fall in the pH and an increase in the molar proportion of valerate and propionate relative to acetate in the VFA of the caecal fluid (Hintz & Schryver 1978) (Table 14.4). The implication is that starch is present in the caecal fluid, although an alternative explanation for the presence of these acids is that they may be derived from bacterial reduction of lactate. Significant effects of dietary starch concentration on the population of faecal ciliate protozoa have been demonstrated (Frape *et al* 1982) from which one may infer that the amount of starch entering the large intestine can be influenced by diet.

Certain differences exist between the ruminant and the horse in the metabolism of VFA. Whereas butyrate is metabolised to ketones in the wall of the rumen, it is absorbed more or less unchanged from the hind gut of the horse. Furthermore, the digestion of cellulose in the horse caecum, in contrast to that in the ruminant, is predominantly carried out by Gram-negative bacilli (Kern *et al* 1973). Microbial fermentation is most active in this organ but the total production of VFA is approximately four times greater in the colon because of its greater size and approximately half the horse's maintenance energy requirements are furnished by nutrients absorbed from the large intestine (Frape 1975, Meyer 1980).

The rapid production of acids during fermentation can be harmful and therefore, under normal circumstances, the secretion of buffers is important. The principal buffer in the caecum and ventral colon is bicarbonate, whereas in the dorsal colon it is phosphate; however, both are present throughout the hind gut (Alexander 1963) (Table 14.1). Substantial quantities of bicarbonate are secreted in the caudal ileum accompanied by an absorption of chloride. This bicarbonate reacts with organic acid facilitating the absorption of both as CO_2 and organic acid anion.

Intermediary metabolism of the end products of carbohydrate metabolism

Under full feeding the horse is similar to other non-ruminants in insulin secretion and sensitivity but fasting leads to a lower glucose tolerance (Argenzio & Hintz 1972) (Table 14.5) and the administration of relatively large doses of insulin fails to cause convulsions. Nevertheless, glucose appears to be a preferred energy source in most tissue cells because, during extended work, plasma glucose concentration decreases whilst that of free fatty acids increases (Argenzio & Hintz 1970, Mehring & Tyznik 1970, Madigan & Evans 1973, Ralston *et al* 1979). This does not mean that depot fats are inefficiently metabolised by horses trained to extended work and endurance rides (Goodman *et al* 1973, Frape *et al* 1979).

Tissues utilise several substrates as sources of energy. These include glucose, fatty acids and amino acids. The efficiency of the catabolism of these substrates with the formation of ATP differs; for instance, glucose is utilised more efficiently per unit of gross energy than acetic acid. Acetate which

Table 14.5 Effect of glucose and VFA infusions on blood glucose levels (mg/100 ml) in fasted and fed ponies. (Data from Argenzio & Hintz (1970) *J.Anim.Sci.* **30**, 514–18.)

	Time after infusion (min.)						
	0	5	10	20	30	60	120
Fasted							
Acetate	63	57	56	59	58	66	54
Propionate	70	66	66	67	64	81	84
Butyrate	64	59	65	62	65	54	51
Glucose	69	576	446	276	251	200	168
Fed							
Acetate	85	75	74	77	66	69	76
Propionate	83	86	75	75	76	70	79
Butyrate	89	68	72	75	76	71	71
Glucose	89	551	419	294	232	168	114

predominates as an end product of roughage degradation is therefore likely to be less desirable in the racehorse trained for maximum performance linked to muscular effort. Of the circulating fatty acids and VFAs derived from microbial metabolism, only propionate is glucogenic and therefore raises blood glucose levels (Table 14.5). In addition to yielding glucose, starchy foods produce less water-absorbing residue in the hind gut and therefore less total body weight would be represented by non-muscular material, causing a lower weight handicap. When overheating and hyperexcitability result from the consumption of large quantities of starchy foods, this is less likely to be a consequence of differential efficiencies in ATP formation than of differences in the rate of digestion and fermentation of the two types of feed— the rapid degradation of starch yielding both glucose and VFA.

Carbohydrate-derived ailments

The conditions of laminitis and lymphangitis undoubtedly arise as a result of excessive carbohydrate, and particularly starch, consumption (Garner *et al* 1975, 1977). By the provision of bran mashes, one endeavours to decrease the intake of total dry matter and starch and to increase the rate of passage of digesta, thus providing some partial benefit. Breeds of ponies and horses subsisting on poor grazing possess a gut microflora which, without a protracted period of adjustment, is inappropriate to the utilisation of large quantities of starch.

Starchy foods are subjected to gastric fermentation in the horse. The relatively low pH of the succus caecus supports a population of the order of 10^8 Lactobacilli per ml and somewhat fewer Streptococci, and produces lactic

Table 14.6 Mean caecal pH values following feeding. (Data from Willard *et al* (1977)
J.Anim.Sci. **45**, 87–93.)

Hours after feed	Nature of feed	
	Hay	Concentrate
0	7.14	7.22
1	7.16	7.24
3	7.01	6.77
5	6.89	6.27
7	6.75	6.19
9	6.96	6.44
11	7.12	6.82

acid as a major product of starch and sugar fermentation (Alexander &
Davies 1963). Lactic acid is not well absorbed from the intestine and any lactic
acid which, together with starch, reaches the large bowel, acts as a substrate
for further bacterial metabolism, yielding VFA (Fig. 14.2). Facultative
anaerobic Streptococci occurring in this region ferment the starch together
with a range of sugars, so producing lactic acid. This acid is partly metabolised
before absorption and one organism which has been shown to possess this
capacity is *Veillonella gazogenes* (Alexander 1963). When large quantities of
the substrate are available, the production of lactic acid is greater than the rate
of further metabolism and the pH falls (Willard *et al* 1977) (Table 14.6).
Relatively large quantities of the acid then accumulate and are absorbed into
the circulatory system. Furthermore, and probably of equal importance, the
more rapid rate of VFA production from starch fermentation than from fibre
fermentation contributes to the metabolic effects of lactate. Blood lactate
may rise considerably with an associated fall in blood pH, and acids which
cannot be metabolised are excreted by the kidneys in conjunction with cations
such as sodium ions. In addition, there is an increased loss of carbon dioxide
through the lungs.

Microbially derived lactic acid is the racemic mixture of the D- and
L-forms; it therefore differs from the L-lactic acid produced normally during
muscular work. The D-form is only slowly metabolised by mammalian cells
and therefore contributes to the sustained metabolic effects. There is thus a
considerable loss of alkali reserve. Dehydration occurs 1 as a result of
increased urine production, 2 from the osmotic attraction of fluid to the VFA
in the lumen of the large intestine and, 3 through loss of fluid to tissues from
blood. In consequence, increased concentrations of total serum protein and
blood haemoglobin occur. Indigestion is accompanied by anorexia, reduced
water intake, apathy, muscular tremors, and general discomfort (Table 14.7).
As the pH of the ingesta falls, there is an increasing shift in the population of

Table 14.7 Progressive effects of acidosis.

Metabolic effects	Clinical effects
Gas production	Wood chewing
Intestinal acidity	Coprophagy
Gut erosion	Lymphangitis
Fall in blood pH	Laminitis
Loss of sodium	Cardiac failure
Fluid loss	
increased urine flow	
tissues (decarboxylations)	
gut lumen (osmosis) — leading to fall in	
blood pressure and anaemia of GI tract	

Table 14.8 Plasma lactate (mmol/l) in 31 horses following a carbohydrate overload of the gastrointestinal tract. (Data from Garner *et al* (1977) *J.Anim.Sci.* **45**, 1037–41.)

	Condition of horses		
Hours after starch gruel*	No laminitis (5 animals)	Laminitis (21 animals)	Death (5 animals)
0	1.0	0.7	0.7
8	1.2	0.9	1.0
16	1.4	1.2	1.7
24	1.6	1.6	2.7
32	1.3	1.7	2.7
40	1.6	2.5	3.9
48	1.1	2.4	Death
56	1.4	2.0	

*Corn starch–wood-flour gruel given via stomach tube at rate of 17.6 g/kg body weight.

micro-organisms to Gram-positive Streptococci and more particularly to Lactobacilli. Lactic acid formation in the digesta is often accompanied by amino acid decarboxylation (such as that of histidine to histamine), although it is more likely that increased capillary permeability of peripheral tissues is initiated by locally produced histamine. Some evidence suggests that an endotoxaemia-based pathogenesis may be a primary cause of laminitis in horses (Moore *et al* 1981). A fall in blood pressure, circulatory collapse, and death appear to be closely associated with blood lactate levels (Garner *et al* 1977) (Table 14.8). Wood chewing and coprophagy in acidotic animals have been reduced by infusions of sodium carbonate into the caecum in order to arrest the fall in pH (Willard *et al* 1977). Some cases of gastric tympany may be caused by excessive gastric fermentation, since the associated gas production may not escape through the cardia.

Other diet-related ailments

The aetiology of *azoturia* is still undefined. Although the condition may be precipitated by certain drugs, a dietary cause is uncertain. The symptoms of lameness and myoglobinuria are thought to occur particularly in hard-working horses who are rested whilst maintained on a full diet. Opinion has it that a breakdown of muscle glycogen to lactic acid in this situation is a cause of the symptoms. The replacement of concentrated feeds by bran is thought to provide a sufficient reduction in starch intake and gut lactic acid production to suppress the condition.

In addition to acidosis, which may cause coprophagy and wood chewing, *coprophagy* has been induced by providing mature horses with diets containing inadequate quantities of protein. Another possibility is that failure to provide long hay causes boredom which in turn precipitates wood chewing. Stabled horses given similar quantities of total fibre in ground or long forms will consume the former more rapidly (Meyer *et al* 1975) leaving more time for the development of vices.

Colic precipitated by sudden changes in diet is readily understandable in terms of the above discussion. It has already been stated that highly indigestible lignified long fibrous roughages may cause blockage at certain critical points along the gastrointestinal tract and horses which are prone to eat too quickly or which have defective teeth may insufficiently masticate feed and hence be subject to this type of colic.

Some instances of 'tying up' have responded, it is claimed, to selenium supplementation of the drinking water although, in cases investigated by the author (unpublished data), no beneficial change has followed supplementation of horses showing the condition. However, it is undoubtedly true that, in a number of localities in the world where the herbage is deficient in selenium, cases of white muscle disease and failure of proper muscular development in foals have resulted from the dam providing an inadequate supply of selenium. It is thought that the minimum requirement for selenium is of the order of 0.6 mg/100 kg body weight daily, however there is no direct experimental evidence in the horse.

Vitamin B requirements

Whether or not the diet satisfies the vitamin B requirements of the horse depends upon a number of inter-related factors which include: the dietary content and availability of each vitamin; their rates of synthesis, utilisation, and destruction by the gut microflora; the extent to which the net amount synthesised is absorbed by the host; and the gross requirement of the host as influenced by its rate of cellular metabolism. This latter is generally increased over and above the maintenance demand during growth and in late pregnancy, lactation and work. Thiamine, riboflavine, pantothenic acid, nicotinic acid, pyridoxine, folic acid, biotin, and cyanocobalamin are synthesised in the intestinal tract, but the population size and species distribution of the microflora are influenced by dietary constitution, so that diet indirectly affects the net synthesis of vitamins. When large doses of antibiotics are given, dramatic changes in the species distribution of the microflora can be seen and severe diarrhoea thus occurs (Cook 1973), affecting both the synthesis and absorption of B vitamins. Acute diarrhoea, as in so-called colitis 'X', must be treated promptly to restore fluid and electrolyte balance; however, if anorexia persists, death will ensue apparently as a result of failure to repair damaged tissues. Before this occurs complete intravenous feeding should be instituted.

Young and rapidly growing horses seem to have an insufficiently well developed hind gut for synthesis to meet their cyanocobalamin requirement without dietary supplementation. On the other hand, no dietary requirement in the adult has been demonstrated, with the possible exception that a supplement for horses which are out of condition is thought to improve appetite. All horses require a dietary source of thiamine (Carroll 1950), although approximately one-quarter of the thiamine synthesised in the caecum is absorbed (Linerode 1966). Opthalmia is claimed to have been caused by riboflavine deficiency (Cunha 1969), distinct from that caused by Leptospirosis or Microfilaria infection. No dietary requirement for pantothenic or nicotinic acid has been demonstrated, but horses which are confined to the stable, deprived of grazing, and which consume large quantities of oats may benefit from folic acid supplementation.

Vitamins A and E requirements

The horse's ability to convert β-carotene to retinol (vitamin A) is apparently somewhat poorer than that of several other domesticated species (Fonnesbeck & Symons 1967). However a deficiency is unlikely to occur except in animals grazing in parched, desiccated regions or those receiving a cereal-based diet with hard hay. Some evidence exists of inadequacies amongst horses in training. The requirement for the adult is assumed to be approximately 600 μg retinol/kg diet, but some recent evidence suggests that concentrations up to ten times as great may be needed for maximal haematological development (Donoghue *et al* 1981). This evidence requires confirmation. Mild toxity occurred when 1.2 mg retinol per kg body weight was given daily in the diet.

Reports of an α-tocopherol (vitamin E) selenium deficiency syndrome have been made in foals out of mares receiving feed which is deficient in selenium (Caple *et al* 1978). Whether muscle function of horses subjected to extreme work loads, as in training, demands elevated intakes of α-tocopherol has yet to be demonstrated (Brady *et al* 1978). However, cereal grains which have been harvested in good condition and milled shortly before feeding should satisfy normal demands as long as they have not been grown on selenium-deficient soils. Moulded grain is a different story. Unsaturated oils are also safe as long as they are not rancid and contain appropriate amounts of α-tocopherol. Compounded feeds should contain adequate amounts of stable esters of α-tocopherol.

Dietary fat digestion and fatty acid metabolism during work

Very little work has been conducted on the value of dietary fat to the horse. Normal dietary regimens provide the horse with small quantities of relatively unsaturated fat which, as already mentioned, is to a large extent deposited unchanged. The horse does not have a gall bladder — bile is secreted continuously and a high rate of enterohepatic cycling of bile acid has been reported. This does not appear to hinder the digestion and absorption of fat. Supplementary fat is utilised well and it has been suggested that high fat diets may reduce the incidence of founder (Hintz *et al* 1978), although conclusive evidence is lacking.

Dietary fat has little effect on plasma free fatty acids, but these are increased during exercise when the horse draws on its reserves as a readily available source of energy. The proposal has been put forward that the monitoring of plasma lipids may be a useful tool in gauging the metabolic response to disease. In fasted horses, the concentration of plasma free fatty acids is much higher than in fully-fed horses, but ketone levels appear to be unaffected. Hyperlipidaemia has been observed in fasting healthy ponies and up to 7 g total lipids per 100 ml of plasma have been noted by comparison with approximately 0.5 g per 100 ml in the normally fed horses (Naylor *et al* 1980). This metabolic response is similar to that seen in parasite-infested individuals.

The metabolism of free fatty acids is an aerobic process yielding more ATP per unit of mass than can be derived from carbohydrate. It is therefore ideal for meeting the energy expenditure of continuous moderate exertion. Training for continuous hard work, such as that to which endurance horses are subjected, leads to a metabolic adaptation in which relatively more body fat, in addition to glucose, is catabolised, yielding ATP to meet the increased demand. In the UK, horses are subjected to greater and more variable amounts of exercise or work than is the ruminant. Exercise itself has little effect upon the efficiency of digestion. In fact, light exercise may slightly improve it, apparently through a decrease in the rate of passage of digesta.

 Chapter 14

Mineral nutrition

Calcium and phosphorus deficiency

Probably more has been written on mineral nutrition, and in particular the calcium and phosphorus requirements of the horse, than on any other nutritional theme. Despite this, large numbers of horses in temperate latitudes given cereal-based diets are deprived of an adequate intake of calcium. The horse has evolved as a browsing animal, consuming leaves which contain a proper balance and adequate amounts of calcium and phosphorus. Furthermore, the phosphorus is in a form which is readily utilised. With the advent of domestication, cereals and cereal by-products have formed a major component of the diet. These materials are lacking in significant quantities of calcium while the phosphorus is in the form of phytic acid-salts, which are not only poorly utilised but also depress the utilisation of dietary calcium by increasing its faecal excretion. Hay given to horses, and in particular hard hay given to thoroughbreds in training, is a stemmy material containing few legumes and consequently inadequate concentrations of calcium and phosphorus when it is used as a supplement to cereals. In agricultural terms, these hays are of relatively low nutrititional quality, compounding the problem imposed by the cereal component of the diet.

It has been suggested that a rapid growth rate in the foal is undesirable; this is particularly true when the dietary amounts of calcium and phosphorus and their ratio are unsatisfactory since this will increase the incidence of skeletal problems, such as epiphysitis. It should be noted that direct experimental evidence for this is lacking in the horse. However, it has been clearly demonstrated (Schryver *et al* 1971, Jordan *et al* 1975) that an inadequate consumption of calcium or phosphorus and wide dietary ratios of these substances cause inadequate net retention of calcium, phosphorus, or both, depending on the precise circumstances. A significant anatomical change in nutritional secondary hyperparathyroidism following an extended dietary calcium deficiency, is the resorption of the outer circumferential lamellae of long bones (Krook 1968). When the calcium intake of ponies is excessive for considerable periods of time, but dietary phosphorus adequate, the medullary region of bones is relatively large and the cortical region relatively small (Jordan *et al* 1975).

Epiphysitis is sometimes apparent in the spring and early summer, particularly where animals have been kept indoors during the winter and given roughages of poor quality, little vitamin D or calcium, and large amounts of cereals, bran, and linseed. On the other hand, horses receiving diets consisting solely of poor roughage may suffer from phosphorus-deficiency rickets. Thus, unsupplemented feed offered to horses may have either a very high or a very low calcium:phosphorus ratio. This should be

Table 14.9 Net fractional absorption (%) of calcium and phosphorus from the gastro-intestinal tract of the horse. (Data from Schryver *et al* (1974) *Corn. Vet.* **64**, 493.)

	Ca	P
Small intestine I	40	−15
Small intestine II	23	17
Caecum	− 5	−18
Ventral colon	−17	− 2
Dorsal colon	9	40
Rectum	− 7	23

rectified but the provision of slightly elevated amounts of calciferol will assist in correcting the effects of diets having a low calcium:phosphorus ratio, especially in seasons and latitudes of low solar elevation.

Calcium and phosphorus absorption and metabolism

Phosphorus, and to a lesser extent calcium, are not only absorbed from but also secreted into the gastrointestinal tract. Measurements have been made of the net absorption in various regions of the gut and, although phosphorus is secreted into and absorbed from all regions of the GI tract, it is apparent that a major site of net phosphorus absorption is the dorsal and small colon (Schryver *et al* 1974). By contrast, a major site of net calcium absorption (and also of magnesium, zinc and copper) is the upper part of the small intestine, little detectable calcium being absorbed from the large intestine (Schryver *et al* 1970, 1974a) (Table 14.9). These facts possibly explain why excessive calcium intake has little effect on phosphorus absorption whereas excessive phosphorus (especially that of cereal origin) depresses calcium absorption in the horse.

The absorption and metabolism of calcium is under the control of parathormone, calcitonin, and thyroxine secreted by the parathyroid and thyroid glands. The efficiency of calcium absorption from the gut depends upon the mucosal content of calcium binding protein—the synthesis of which is dependent upon a dietary supply of vitamin D. An excessive dietary content of vitamin D can have a similar ultimate effect to that of a deficiency by stimulating the synthesis of excessive amounts of calcium binding protein in the bone, which leads to their rarefication. Under normal conditions, hormonal regulatory mechanisms maintain homeostasis of blood calcium levels even during times of calcium deprivation, as with high grain-supplemented diets. Under these conditions, the parathyroid undergoes hyperplasia and hypertrophy. There does appear, nevertheless, to be a small fall in blood calcium concentration at this time but this is probably not sufficient for plasma

Table 14.10 Mineral composition of growing horses (mat. wt. 500 kg). (Data from Schryver *et al* (1974) *J.Nutr.* **104**, 126.)

Calcium and phosphorus percentages of air dry diets	Carcass Ca (mg/g fat-free tissue)	$\left(\dfrac{\text{Fresh wt}}{\text{body wt}}\right) \times 100$	Spec. grav.	Ca mg/ Ash g
		Limb-bones composition		
Ca 0.7%, P 0.6%	64.1	19.6	1.440	385
Ca 2.8%, P 0.6%	71.7	21.7	1.466	381
Ca 2.7%, P 1.1%	67.7	19.0	1.462	385
Ca 0.7%, P 1.4%	65.0	21.4	1.437	382

calcium to be used as a measure of calcium adequacy in individual horses receiving adequate amounts of vitamin D. There are laboratory methods for using blood calcium levels as a measure of calcium status, but these are unsuited to clinical application (Argenzio *et al* 1974). Present evidence indicates that the urinary ratio of inorganic phosphate to creatinine may be a useful measure of the horse's status for the adequacy of calcium (Coffman 1980).

Experiments have shown that both calcium content and density of long bones continue to rise as dietary calcium levels are increased to levels much higher than those used in practice (Schryver *et al* 1974b) (Table 14.10). High concentrations of dietary calcium are inadvisable because they tend to decrease the availability of other dietary minerals such as iron, zinc, and copper, and may also lead to the development of brittle bones (osteopetrosis). An adequate dietary level of calcium may be defined as that level beyond which no improvement is obtained in the conformation of bones and in the incidence of fractures and similar ailments of the legs.

Magnesium, sodium and chloride

As for calcium, the minimum daily amount of magnesium required to prevent acute clinical symptoms (ataxia, hyperpnoea, etc.) and depressed serum magnesium levels is fairly well established. Magnesium retention may be increased, at least over short periods, by raising dietary magnesium to quite high levels. However, no particular benefit appears to accrue from such increases and symptoms of magnesium tetany (hypomagnesaemia) which are observed in lactating dairy cows do not appear to have been encountered in the mare.

Sodium and VFA are major ions absorbed from the hind gut which in turn may control water movements in that region (Argenzio 1975). It has been shown that 96% of the sodium and chloride and 75% of the soluble potassium and phosphate entering the large bowel are absorbed in horses receiving a conventional diet (Hintz *et al* 1978). Persistent enteric infections and other causes of diarrhoea in horses interfere with this absorptive process and indicate the need for therapy with sodium, potassium, and chloride ions. Another cause of hypokalaemia and electrolyte loss generally is high work output in hot weather. The reason for this is twofold: firstly, large quantities of sodium, potassium, chloride, and water are lost in sweat, so that rehydration should be accompanied by electrolyte replacement therapy; secondly, an increased work load is inevitably accompanied by increased energy demands which are met by greater proportions of cereal grain and less hay in the diet. This change indirectly decreases the potassium, sodium, and chloride content of the unsupplemented diet. A forage diet, on the other hand, contains vastly more potassium than is needed. A farinaceous diet therefore requires supplementation with sodium chloride and, in periods of high potassium loss, additional potassium may also be required.

Only limited studies have been conducted into trace element deficiencies and toxicities in horses. The available evidence indicates that deficiency symptoms are unlikely to occur in horses receiving considerable amounts and varieties of concentrated feeds. On the other hand, equids restricted to grazing may be subject to pathological changes similar to those seen in other grazing herbivores, although the dietary thresholds precipitating deficiencies differ in several respects. Investigations currently being undertaken in this laboratory indicate that seasonal fluctuations in the circulating blood levels of several trace elements occur.

Drug–diet interactions

For the purposes of this discussion a drug may be defined as a chemical which is not required for normal growth and reproduction or a chemical which is so

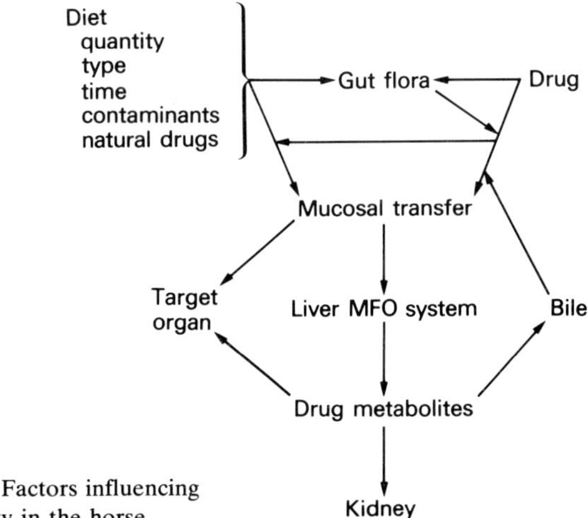

Fig. 14.3 Factors influencing drug toxicity in the horse.

required, but is given in quantities vastly exceeding those needed for these purposes. It is of interest to consider here the effect of diet on the response to drugs used pharmacologically (Fig. 14.3).

Much has been written both about the effects of diet and nutritional status on the responses of man and animals to drugs, and conversely, on the effects some drugs may have on dietary utilisation and nutritional status. Nearly all this work has been carried out on animals other than equine species, so that tentative conclusions only may be drawn concerning the horse. Several detailed reviews provide useful reference sources (Oltersdorf *et al* 1977; Theuer & Vitale 1977, Newberne *et al* 1978).

There are a large number of drugs present in natural foods including the lathyrogens, solanum alkaloids, goitrogens, and cyanogenetic glycosides. Both natural and synthetic drugs are metabolised by enzyme systems, those of the endoplasmic reticulum of the cells of several tissues being especially important, and the principal site of this metabolism being the liver. The enzyme complex known as the mixed function oxidase system (MFO) may be stimulated or induced both by drugs and by certain dietary nutrients. Metal poisons such as lead and mercury act as potent inhibitors of MFO induction. The principal dietary components stimulating the system are protein (Basu 1977) and, to a lesser extent, fats (Wade & Norred 1976, McLean 1977). Animals receiving diet poor in protein are less capable of metabolising many drugs. Energy deprivation, by inducing breakdown of tissue protein, also decreases synthesis of the enzymes of the MFO system. Whether drug activity is thereby increased or decreased depends upon whether the product is more or less active than the administered drug. However, the increased oral toxicity of β-adrenoceptor stimulants in fasted animals is considered to be a consequence of accelerated gastric emptying and increased intestinal absorption (Kast & Nishikawa 1981).

Both drugs and diet may influence the species' distribution of the microflora and fauna of the gastrointestinal tract which may in turn influence the host's reaction to the drug and its vitamin B and vitamin K status. Deficiencies of several B vitamins, especially of riboflavine, cause a decrease in the activity of enzymes of the hepatic microsomal MFO system and prolong the sleeping time induced in rats by pentobarbitone (Miltenberger & Oltersdorf 1978), α-tocopherol has also been demonstrated to be a specific MFO stimulator (Zannoric & Sato 1976) and several mineral elements, at higher than normally required levels, including selenium and calcium, provide protection against heavy metal toxicities (Levander 1977). Persistent use of certain drugs may induce vitamin deficiencies (Clark 1976). Specific dietary fibre sources (Kritchevshy 1977, Frape *et al* 1981, 1982) also influence the absorption and toxicity of orally administered drugs. This effect may be independent of the capacity of the intestinal wall to metabolise drugs which can, however, be influenced by several other non-nutrient components of natural feedstuffs (Pantuck *et al* 1977).

When drugs are given orally, the extent to which they are absorbed may be affected by the time of dosing relative to feeding (Kast & Nishikawa 1981) and by the digestibility and fatty acid composition of the fat component of the diet (McLean 1977). Some drugs may induce malabsorption of nutrients (Truswell 1974) while others can increase or decrease appetite and impair glucose tolerance (Marks 1974). Purgatives and certain diuretics, if used persistently, may cause hypokalaemia through an increased rate of faecal or urinary potassium loss.

Dietary allergies

Certain horses are particularly prone to allergic reactions associated with diet, and amongst sensitive animals some are more strongly reactive than others. Effects may occur in the skin (where small oedematous lumps can be seen) and lungs. Evidence from this laboratory shows that circulating antibodies in sensitive horses react with specific uncooked foods, the removal of which from the diet generally leads to a regression of the lesions. The most critical allergy is chronic obstructive pulmonary disease (COPD), which results from a sensitisation to inhaled mould spores — particularly those of *Micropolyspora faeni* and *Aspergillus fumigatus* (McPherson *et al* 1979), which are present in large quantities in badly harvested, damp and overheated hay. These spores react with the lung tissue to induce precipitating antibodies. The reaction becomes worse with repeated exposure and the most rapid recovery is brought about by removing all hay and straw bedding and providing the horse solely with pelleted feed together with haylage or soaked hay. This may require taking the horse to another stable if the premises are heavily contaminated with the spores in question or turning the animal out to grass. All hay and straw contains mould spores — some samples are simply worse than others. The danger of producing a hay with high moisture content and therefore prone to excessive moulding, is increased when it contains large quantities of leafy leguminous material. This is possibly why horse owners are reluctant to use legume hays.

In the past, COPD was likened, erroneously, to alveolar emphysema in man, but recent studies have shown that bronchiolitis is the major pathological feature with emphysema being absent or confined to small areas of the lung (Nicholls 1978). Treatment with bronchodilator drugs brings about a temporary improvement in the clinical condition (Murphy *et al* 1980) and control may be achieved by repeated inhalation of sodium cromoglycate (Thomson & McPherson 1981). (For further discussion see Chapter 25).

References

Alexander F. (1963) In *Progress in Nutrition and Allied Sciences,* D. P. Cuthbertson (ed.). Oliver and Boyd, Edinburgh.

Alexander F. (1972) *Equine Vet. J.* **4,** 166–9.

Alexander F. & Davies E. M. (1963) *J. Comp. Path.* **73,** 1–8.

Alexander F. & Hickson J. C. D. (1970) *Proc. IIIrd Internat. Symp. Camb. 1969.* Oriel Press, Cambridge.

Argenzio R. A. (1975) *Cornell Vet.* **65,** 303–29.

Argenzio R. A. & Hintz H. F. (1970) *J. Anim. Sci.* **30,** 514–18.

Argenzio R. A. & Hintz H. F. (1972) *J. Nutr.* **102,** 879–92.

Argenzio R. A., Lowe J. E., Hintz H. F. *et al* (1974) *J. Nutr.* **104,** 18–27.

Axelsson J. (1943) *Nodisk Rotograsyr.* Stockholm, Hästarnas ut fodring och skötsel.

Baker J. P., Lieb S., Crawford B. H. Jr. *et al* (1972) *Proc. 27th Distillers Feed Conf.* 28–33.

Basu T. K. (1977) *J. Human Nutr.* **31,** 449–58.

Brady P. S., Ku P. R. & Ullrey D. E. (1978) *J. Anim. Sci.* **47,** 492.

Caljuk E. A. (1961) *Tr. Vses. Instit. Koneoodstoo.* **23,** 295.

Caple I. W., Edwards S. J. A., Forsyth W. M. *et al* (1978) *Aust. Vet. J.* **54,** 57–60.

Carroll F. D. (1950) *J. Anim. Sci.* **9,** 139.

Clark F. (1976) *J. Human Nutr.* **30,** 333–7.

Coffman J. (1980) *Vet. Med. (Small Animal) Clin.* April 671–6.

Comline R. S., Hall L. W., Hickson J. C. D. *et al* (1969) *Proc. Physiol. Soc. J. Physiol.* **204,** 10–11.

Comline R. S., Hickson J. C. S. & Message M. A. (1963) *Proc. Physiol. Soc. J. Physiol.* **170,** 47–8.

Cook W. R. (1973) *Vet. Rec.* **93,** 15–17.

Cunha T. J. (1969) *Feedstuffs* **41,** 19.

Donoghue S., Kronfield D. S., Berkowitz S. J. *et al* (1981) *J. Nutr.* **111,** 365–74.

Elsden S. R., Hitchcock M. W. S., Marshall R. A. *et al* (1948) *J. Exp. Biol.* **22,** 191–202.

Fonnesbeck P. V. & Symons L. D. (1967) *J. Anim. Sci.* **26,** 1030–8.

Frape D. L. (1975) *Equine Vet. J.* **7,** 120–30.

Frape D. L. & Boxall R. C. (1974) *Equine Vet. J.* **6,** 59–68.

Frape D. L., Peace C. K. & Ellis P. M. (1979) EAAP Harrogate H6–5.

Frape D. L., Tuck M. G., Suttcliffe N. H. *et al* (1982) *Comp. Physiol. Biochem.* **72A,** 77–83.

Frape D. L., Wayman B. J. & Tuck M. G. (1981) *Br. J. Nutr.* **46,** 315–26.

Frape D. L., Wayman B. J., Tuck M. G. *et al* (1982) *Br. J. Nutr.* **48,** 97–110.

Garner H. E., Coffman J. R., Hahn A. W. *et al* (1975) *Am. J. Vet. Res.* **36,** 441–4.

Garner H. E., Hutcheson D. P., Coffman J. R. *et al* (1977) *J. Anim. Sci.* **45,** 1037.

Godbee R. G. & Slade L. M. (1981) *J. Anim. Sci.* **53,** 670–6.

Goodman H. M., Noot G. W., Van der., Trout J. R. *et al* (1973) *J. Anim. Sci.* **37,** 56–62.

Hintz H. F., Hogue D. E., Walker E. F. Jr. *et al* (1971) *J. Anim. Sci.* **32,** 245–8.

Hintz H. F., Ross M. W., Lesser F. R. *et al* (1978) *Feedstuffs* March **20,** 27–8.

Hintz H. F. & Schryver H. F. (1978) *J. Equine Med. Surg.* **2,** 147–50.

Hintz H. F., Schryver H. F. & Lowe J. E. (1971) *J. Anim. Sci.* **33,** 1274.

Hintz H. F., Schryver H. F. & Lowe J. E. (1973) *Feedstuffs* July **2,** 25–31.

Hintz H. F., Schryver H. F. & Stevens C. E. (1978) *J. Anim. Sci.* **46,** 1803–7.

Jordan R. M., Myers V. S., Yoho B. *et al* (1975) *J. Anim. Sci.* **40,** 78.

Kast A. & Nishikawa J. (1981) *Lab. Anim.* **15,** 359–64.

Kern D. L., Slyter L. L., Effele E. C. *et al* (1974) *J. Anim. Sci.* **38,** 559–64.

Kern D. L., Slyter L. L., Weaver J. M. *et al* (1973) *J. Anim. Sci.* **37,** 463–9.

Kritchevsky D. (1977) *Fed. Proc.* **36,** 1692–5.

Krook L. (1967) *Cornell Vet.* LVIII, 59–73.

Levander O. A. (1977) *Fed. Proc.* **36,** 1683–7.

Linerode P. A. (1966) PhD dissertation, Ohio State University.

Madigan J. E. & Evans J. W. (1973) *J. Anim. Sci.* **36,** 730–3.

Maloiy G. M. (1970) *Am. J. Physiol.* **219,** 1522–7.

Marks V. (1974) *Proc. Nutr. Soc.* **33,** 209–14.

McLean A. E. M. (1977) *Fed. Proc.* **36,** 1688–91.

McPherson E. A., Lawson G. H. R., Murphy J. R. *et al* (1979) *Equine Vet. J.* II, 159–66.

Mehring J. S. & Tyznik W. J. (1970) *J. Anim. Sci.* **30,** 764.

Meyer H. (1980) *Tierernährg* **8,** 123–50.

Meyer H., Ahlswede L., Reinhardt H. J. (1975) *Deut. Tierärztl. Wochenschr.* **82,** 54–8.

Miltenberger R. & Oltersforf U. (1978) *Br. J. Nutr.* **39,** 127.

Moore J. N., Garner H. E. & Coffman J. R. (1981) *Equine Vet. J.* **13,** 240–2.

Murphy J. R., McPherson E. A. & Dixon P. M. (1980) *Equine Vet. J.* **12,** 10–14.

Naylor J. M., Kronfield D. S. & Acland H. (1980) *Am. J. Vet. Res.* 899.

Newberne P. M., Gross R. L. & Roe D. A. (1978) *Wld. Rev. Nutr. Diet.* **29,** 130–69.

Nicholls J. M. (1978) PhD thesis, University of Glasgow.

Noot G. W. Van der & Gilbreath E. B. (1970) *J. Anim. Sci.* **31,** 351–5.

Noot G. W. Van der & Trout J. R. (1971) *J. Anim. Sci.* **33,** 38–41.

Oltersdorf U., Miltenberger R. & Garner H. D. (1977) *Wld. Rev. Nutr. Diet.* **26,** 41–134.

Pantuck E. J., Hsiao K. C., Loub W. D. *et al* (1976) *J. Pharm. & Exp. Therapeut.* **198,** 278–83.

Prior R. L., Hintz H. F., Lowe J. E. *et al* (1974) J. Anim. Sci. **38,** 565.

Ralston S. L., Van Denbrock G. & Baile C. A. (1979) *J. Anim. Sci.* **49,** 838–45.

Reitnour C. M. (1978) *Equine Vet. J.* **10,** 65–8.

Reitnour C. M., Baker J. P., Mitchell G. E. Jr. *et al* (1970) *J. Nutr.* **100,** 349–53.

Reitnour C. M. & Salisbury R. L. (1972) *J. Anim. Sci.* **35,** 1190–3.

Reitnour C. M. & Salisbury R. L. (1976) *Am. J. Vet. Res.* **37,** 1065.

Roberts M. C. (1974) *Res. Vet. Sci.* **17,** 400–1.

Rose R. J., Purdue R. A. & Hensley W. (1977) *Equine Vet. J.* **9,** 122–6.

Schryver H. F., Craig P. H., Hintz H. F. *et al* (1970) *J. Nutr.* **100,** 1127–32.

Schryver H. F., Hintz H. F., Craig P. H. *et al* (1972) *J. Nutr.* **102,** 143–8.

Schryver H. F., Hintz H. F. & Lowe J. E. (1971) *Equine Vet. J.* **3,** 102–9.

Schryver H. F. & Lowe J. E. (1974a) *Cornell Vet.* **64,** 493.

Schryver H. F., Hintz H. F., Lowe J. E. *et al* (1974b) *J. Nutr.* **104,** 126–32.

Slade L. M., Bishop R., Morris J. G. *et al* (1971) *Br. Vet. J.* **127,** XI–XIII.

Slade L. M., Robinson D. W. & Casey K. E. (1970) *J. Anim. Sci.* **30,** 753–60.

Theuer R. C. & Vitale J. J. (1977) In *Nutritional Support of Medical Practice.* Sneider *et al* (eds.) 297–305. Harper & Row, New York.

Thomson J. R. & McPherson E. A. (1981) *Equine Vet. J.* **13,** 243–6.

Truswell A. S. (1974) *Proc. Nutr. Soc.* **33,** 215–24.

Wade A. E. & Norred W. P. (1976) *Fed. Proc.* **35,** 2475–9.

Willard J. G., Willard J. C., Wolfrann S. A. *et al* (1977) *J. Anim. Sci.* **45,** 87–93.

Wolter R., Durix A. & Letourneau J. C. (1974) *Ann. Zootech.* **23,** 293–300.

Wolter R., Durix A. & Letourneau J. C. (1975) *Ann. Zootech.* **24,** 237–42.

Wootton J. F. & Argenzio R. A. (1975) *Am. J. Physiol.* **229,** 1062–7.

Zannoni V. G. & Sato P. H. (1976) *Fed. Proc.* **35,** 2464–9.

15

Metabolic disorders of cattle: current trends in treatment and prophylaxis

P.A. MULLEN

Metabolic disorders of farm animals now number at least 14, an expansion from earlier days when only four were considered. Among cattle, disorders associated with imbalances of water, calcium and phosphorous, magnesium, sodium, protein and energy are recorded. These disorders may be associated either with an excess or a deficiency of a prime component, or with an imbalance that may arise during digestion and/or subsequent metabolism when adequate quantities have been consumed.

A metabolic disease has been described as a '. . . disturbance of the internal homeostasis of the body brought about by an abnormal change in the rate of one or more critical metabolic processes' (Payne 1977). This definition unites two important concepts. Firstly, metabolic disease involves an abnormal change in the internal environment of the body and, secondly, this change is brought about by an alteration in the dynamic equilibrium of metabolic processes.

Metabolites in the blood, body fluids and various organs are in a state of continuous interchange. Their concentrations in the blood are controlled by careful and selective adjustments to the rates of input and output, in a system which has a rapid throughput. The final effect of such changes is that, if uncompensated, they lead to a change in concentration of the metabolite, and disorder of the internal environment ensues. Cattle, like other animals, have evolved complicated endocrinological mechanisms to regulate metabolic processes. Sometimes, however, owing to unusually severe demands or stress, the capacity for adjustment becomes overwhelmed and a change in the internal environment occurs. This change, if uncorrected, results in metabolic disease (Payne 1977).

In most instances metabolic disorders of cattle are not primarily due to inherent defects in the animal's biochemical pathways and this is in contrast to many metabolic disorders in man. Rather, they result from a breakdown in the animal's ability to cope with the metabolic demands of high production, coupled with the strain of modern intensive husbandry and feeding systems. In summary, metabolic disease derives from a failure to compensate for

"

imposed and man-made demands on livestock.

The current trends in both treatment and prophylaxis of imbalances in calcium and phosphorous, magnesium, protein and energy will now be considered.

Hypomagnesaemia

The term hypomagnesaemia refers solely to a biochemical state in which blood magnesium concentrations are subnormal. It is not synonymous with tetany. An acceptable serum magnesium concentration range for cattle in the UK national herd is 2.0–3.5 mg/100 ml (0.822–1.4385 mmol/l) (Payne *et al* 1970).

In a herd of hypomagnesaemic cows, clinical or subclinical signs may be present. Subclinical effects may include slight nervousness, depressed appetite, and a lowered milk yield, which may fall by 13–20%. These effects may occur in the absence of tetany and, indeed, hypomagnesaemic herds may show no signs of ill-health whatsoever.

The aetiology of magnesium deficiency is an inadequate absorption of magnesium from the digestive tract. Magnesium absorption occurs mainly from the fore-stomachs and not the small intestine. No active mechanism controlling magnesium homeostasis has yet been identified and the concentration in plasma varies within wide limits depending upon magnesium intake and availability. In contrast, serum calcium concentrations remain within a much narrower range, regardless of the dietary intake.

Some 70% of the magnesium in the body resides in the skeleton, yet these reserves are not readily mobilised, for normal magnesium concentrations are present in the bones of cattle after several months of chronic hypomagnesaemia (Allcroft 1960). In emergencies only about 0.5 mg/kg/day can be mobilised from bone. Magnesium is lost with the faeces, urine and milk. Thus, a high-yielding cow secretes approximately 3 g/day of magnesium into her milk. Since the magnesium concentration in milk remains reasonably constant (9–16 mg/100 ml), a sudden increase in secretion of magnesium by the udder is unlikely to be an important aetiological factor in clinical hypomagnesaemia. On the other hand, the faecal output does vary and altered losses in faeces together with a steady milk loss may reduce the extracellular fluid reserves, and this at a time when dietary input may be in critically short supply. The system of magnesium homeostasis is therefore fundamentally unstable, a factor which emphasises the importance of steady and continuous intake from the alimentary tract. Urinary output of magnesium appears to be significant only as a means of eliminating excess magnesium. The renal threshold is met when plasma concentrations exceed 1.8–2.0 mg/100 ml

(Storry & Rook 1962). Urinary losses of magnesium are not important in the development of hypomagnesaemia. The absence of magnesium from the urine is, rather, an indication of insufficiency.

The optimal content of magnesium in the diet is 0.25% of dry matter, the range in most diets being 0.10–0.30% of dry matter. For cows not receiving supplementary magnesium, their daily intake can vary between 10 and 40 g. On spring and late autumn pasture, daily magnesium intake is 13–23 g, whereas summer pasture provides 20–30 g/day. The absorption of magnesium from the diet varies widely (5–35% of intake) but more commonly it is in the range 15–25%, the lower availabilities occurring on spring grass and with winter diets.

Cows not receiving a magnesium supplement on late spring grass absorb only 3–4 g magnesium each day as compared with 5–7 g/day on summer pasture. Factors which reduce the availability of magnesium from the diet fed are: high concentrations of potassium, nitrogen and fat, and low levels of energy. With a magnesium requirement of 3.6 g for 10 litres of milk each day which increases to 5.8 g for 30 litres, the need for supplementary feeding of magnesium becomes apparent.

Diagnosis

Hypomagnesaemia is commonly seen in lactating cows soon after turnout to spring grass. The problem also arises in autumn calving herds and in suckler cows on autumn aftermath. Throughout the year it may be seen in suckler cows kept outdoors and receiving inadequate amounts of hay and silage. The clinical signs, grazing history, fertilizer history and time of year are the main criteria used to diagnose hypomagnesaemia. Determination of the serum magnesium concentration in affected animals, and from fellow cattle showing no clinical signs, will usually support the diagnosis and confirm its presence on a herd basis, i.e. < 1.8 mg/100 ml (0.822 mmol/l) and in tetany cases < 1.0 mg/100 ml (0.41 mmol/l). Occasionally cattle show extreme clinical signs yet when sampled just prior to treatment may show normal serum concentrations. This highlights the need to sample within the herd and not solely from single clinical cases. If calcium concentrations are determined, these may also be below the normal range and this change may have an important bearing upon the development of clinical signs (Blood & Henderson 1974).

A good correlation has been found between urine magnesium concentration and the amount of magnesium absorbed from the diet. Urine magnesium output is a more sensitive indicator of magnesium absorption than blood concentrations. Magnesium surplus to requirements is excreted in the urine; its absence from urine may therefore be considered an indication of insufficient magnesium content in the diet and/or its absorption.

Treatment

Treatment depends on the acuteness of the clinical signs presented. The acute case, as well as requiring the administration of magnesium salts, may require sedation or even anaesthesia. In the less acute case sedation is probably unnecessary. The replacement of magnesium salts may be by the use of magnesium sulphate or magnesium chloride. Some clinicians prefer a combination of calcium salts to which magnesium hypophosphite is added, e.g. 20% PM (Astra Chemicals). The final choice remains with the clinician, but when the clinical manifestations are clear-cut the intravenous administration of magnesium sulphate alone should be considered. The intravenous administration of this salt is not without an element of risk, but up to 400 ml of a 25% solution (or less) administered slowly into a vein and accompanied by careful monitoring of the heart can be performed with confidence. Sufficient should be given to reduce the heart rate to within its normal range (60–80 beats/minute) and then administration is stopped. This will raise the circulating magnesium level quickly. The remainder of the 400 ml solution should then be administered subcutaneously for later absorption. An alternative treatment is the slow i.v. administration of 400 ml 20% PM solution, followed by 400 ml 25% magnesium sulphate solution subcutaneously. Irrespective of which treatment is chosen, dietary supplementation of magnesium (calcined magnesite) must begin at once and be continued for a variable time depending on the season. Sedatives available include xylazine and chloral hydrate. A solution of chloral hydrate and magnesium sulphate can be given intravenously both to sedate and to raise the magnesium levels. However the hazards from nerve and/or muscle trauma to a recumbent cow should be recalled.

The use of solutions containing glucose may be contraindicated for, in some cases of hypomagnesaemia, a concomitant hyperglycaemia has been found (Barker 1939).

Prevention

Magnesium supplementation prevents hypomagnesaemia by increasing the amount of magnesium available for absorption, so that there is an excess of magnesium above normal requirements. In spring a daily supplement of 30 g magnesium is usually adequate to maintain normal blood levels. In recovered tetany cases, and in cattle during the winter, higher levels of supplementation are required. It is more difficult to prevent hypomagnesaemia than it is to prevent tetany. As little as 5 g magnesium supplementation/day will usually prevent tetany, whereas 30 g magnesium/day may be required to prevent hypomagnesaemia.

Magnesium supplementation may take any one of five forms:

1 Direct feeding in concentrates—.a cake containing 57 g calcined magnesite (or its equivalent in magnesium) daily is recommended.

2 Pasture dusting with calcined magnesite (15 kg/hectare)—the fields are dusted when a dew is on the grass or during light rain, just prior to the cows going into them. Alternatively, a week's supply of pasture can be dusted ahead of the cattle. This method will not be effective if the pasture is bare, if the grass is less than 4 inches (10 cm) long, or if granular magnesite is used.

3 Water medication—.a suitable magnesium salt (acetate, chloride, or sulphate) is added to the water. A single source of water must be available and this should contain a constant concentration of magnesium. Alternatively, a dispenser adding a predetermined amount of magnesium each day (20 g/cow) should be available. This is the maximum quantity of magnesium which should be provided, since larger amounts may cause scouring.

4 Freely available molasses-based magnesium salts—.the disadvantage of this method is that intake can vary widely between cows, with some animals receiving none. Also the contents of the containers must be mixed daily to keep the supplement uniformly suspended.

5 Magnesium bullets placed into the rumen—.this novel method of supplying daily magnesium requirements over prolonged periods will represent a considerable advance once field experience clearly establishes that persistence of the bullets in the rumen can be relied on.

Summary

Cows with high milk yields have high requirements for magnesium. The absorption of magnesium may be decreased by many factors, including low intake and low availability of ingested magnesium. Lush pasture and shortage of dietary energy reduces magnesium availability. Several forms of supplementation are available.

Parturient paresis (milk fever)

Parturient paresis (milk fever) as presented to the veterinary clinician is usually a very rewarding condition to treat, yet the cause(s) of the disease remain obscure. While much information of practical value has been accumulated from research in many centres during the past fifteen years, we are probably now only a little further forward in our understanding of parturient paresis than in the period immediately after Little & Wright (1925) in America and Dryerre & Greig (1925) in the UK, independently recorded the central role of calcium in the syndrome. Since then many clinical observa-

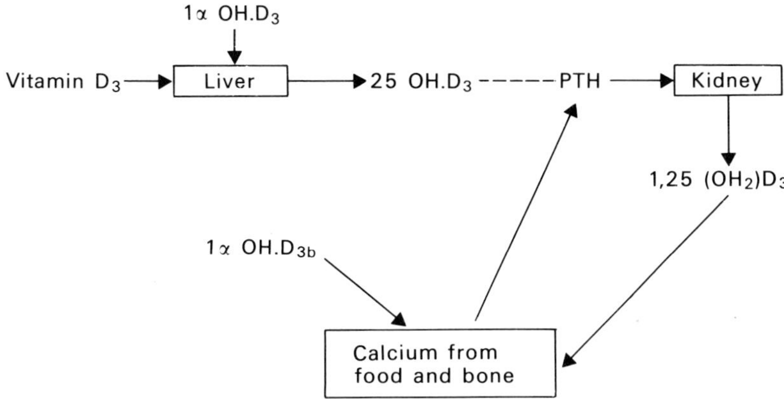

Fig. 15.1 Relationships of calcium, vitamin D₃ and analogues.

tions have been made, especially by Barker (1939), and there have been several studies of the biochemistry of milk fever (Robertson 1948, Marr *et al* 1955, Moodie *et al* 1955).

From the 1950s onwards, fewer clinical biochemical studies were undertaken, while observations and experiments on feeding behaviour before and after parturition took place. Most recently, further biochemical studies to re-examine the original observations of parathyroid involvement in calcium release have been made. In addition, the role of thyrocalcitonin has been explored. These investigations have utilised radioisotope techniques which have allowed measurements to be made of calcium movements, its mobilisation, and its distribution. Readers should refer to Kronfeld (1971) and Payne (1977) for a complete description of these investigations.

The plasma calcium concentration is regulated by parathormone, which is released in response to decreases in plasma calcium concentration, and by thryrocalcitonin which is secreted in response to increases in plasma calcium. In addition, a further regulatory component is vitamin D (and its metabolites), analogues of which are now becoming available commercially (Fig. 15.1). The physiological role of thyrocalcitonin is not exactly clear, for while its main action is to inhibit resorption of calcium from bone and lower the concentrations in plasma of calcium and phosphorous, it may also respond to high levels of calcium in the circulation to counter parathyroid activity.

The cost of milk fever in the UK in 1977 was estimated by Mullen (1977a) to be £6 000 000 for that year. Figures of its UK incidence vary from 3.4% (Leech *et al* 1960) to 8.79% (Mullen 1975). This latter figure is considered by some to be high, and the work was confined to dairy herds from areas where cases of the disease were being sought. Nevertheless, a figure of 8.79% is still low if incidence is gauged by known sales of treatments for parturient paresis. A wastage rate from culling of 1.5% from the national dairy herd was recorded by Beynon & Howe (1974).

Cows from their third lactation onwards are those most likely to be affected, with occasional cases reported at an earlier age. However, these are often among cows who, though calving for their second time, should by their age be calving for the third time. Cases occur mainly within 48 hours of calving, although cases before and after this period are not uncommon. For example, the frequency of hypocalcaemia some 12–16 weeks after calving which responds to calcium therapy, is increasing in some high-yielding dairy herds. The distribution of milk fever cases among the different breeds appears to mirror the position held in the national herd by a particular breed. Channel Isle breeds do not appear to be incriminated today as frequently as they once were; however the Guernsey breed certainly seems to show a predisposition to relapse (Mullen 1975). A relapse case is one which, after apparent clinical recovery, requires further treatment for hypocalcaemia, as recognised by clinical signs. A feature of these cases is a period of twelve hours which elapses before this second treatment is required, provided at least 8 g calcium has been administered by the intravenous route on the first treatment occasion (Mullen 1975).

At parturition in cattle there is physiological hypocalcaemia, hypophosphataemia, and hypomagnesaemia. These changes are relative and plasma levels of these ions may remain within normal ranges for cattle. Normal serum concentrations are: calcium 8.4 mg/100 ml (2.10 mmol/l), inorganic phosphate 6.0 mg/100 ml (1.938 mmol/l), and magnesium 2.3 mg/100 ml (0.945 mmol/l). Glucose concentrations tend to increase at parturition (Littledike *et al* 1969) and low glucose concentrations are of no clinical significance in parturient paresis (Fenwick 1978).

Calcium residing in bone tissues can be made available through the agency of parathyroid hormone. It is also available from the diet after absorption from the alimentary tract. Calcium is required for many purposes including foetal development, transfer to bone, and the normal functioning of all tissues. It is excreted in faeces and to a much lesser extent in urine (Fig. 15.2). The daily calcium requirement during pregnancy is approximately 10 g, but with parturition a major additional demand is imposed by milk production. Some 20–40 g calcium/day is required additionally for an average yielding cow (Fig. 15.2). The rate at which calcium can be mobilised after parturition is important in determining whether or not parturient paresis will occur. Present evidence shows a marked difference between the mobilisation rate in the pregnant and periparturient animal, to the disadvantage of the latter (Payne 1977).

At parturition a sudden demand for calcium occurs for lactation requirements (Fig. 15.2). However, the absorption of calcium from the digestive tract is impaired at this time and it may cease for a short period. The cow therefore moves from a state of dietary dependency to seeking calcium from bone stores through the agency of parathormone. Although parathormone is released in response to a falling calcium concentration in plasma, it appears to meet a non-responsive target bone. An appreciation of this situation underlies prophylactic measures which stimulate the parathyroid gland in the immediate pre-calving period (Pickard 1975).

A diet fed *pre partum* with an excess of calcium leaves the cow vulnerable to milk fever at parturition for the parathyroid/bone supply system will not

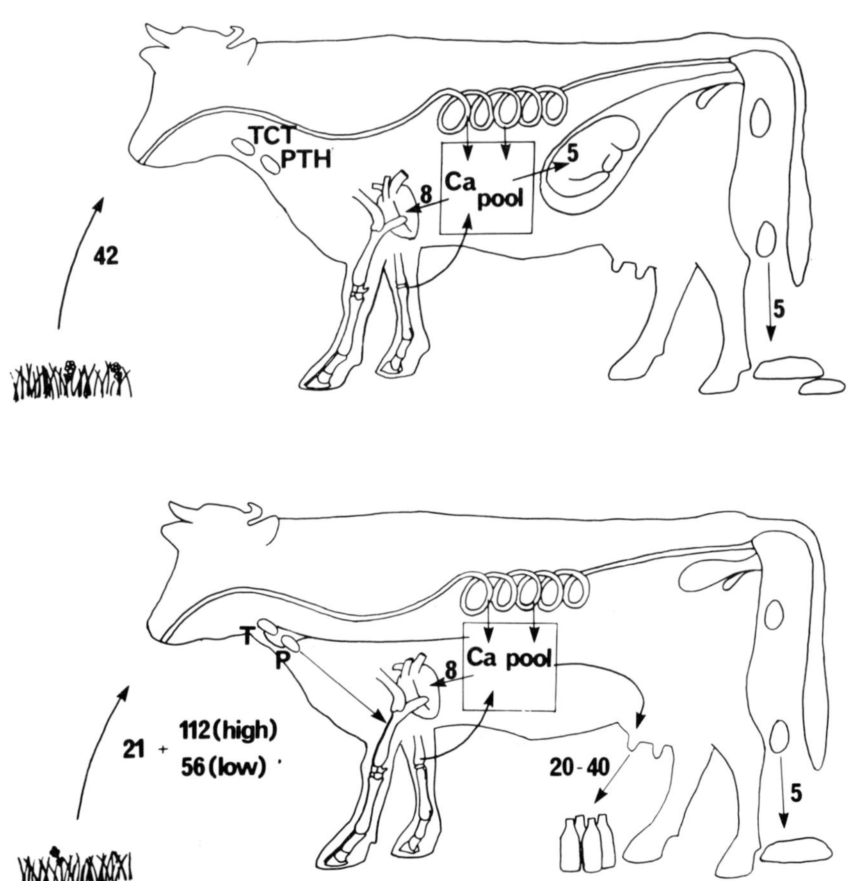

Fig. 15.2 Calcium requirements for the pregnant (*top*) and the lactating (*bottom*) cow. Measurements are in g/day.

Table 15.1 Approximate mineral content (g/kg) of common foods for dairy cattle.

Food	Calcium	Phosphorous
Young pasture grass Young pasture hay	4–6	2–3
Clover	15–20	2–3
Lucerne	25	2–3
Grass silage	6	3
Maize	0.2	3
Barley	0.5	4

have been primed for calcium release. Similarly, a high calcium diet will lower — whereas a low calcium diet will raise — 1,25 dihydroxycholecalciferol $(1,25(OH)_2D_3)$ in the circulation, with its recognised advantages. The early observations of Boda & Cole (1954) which suggested the value of a low calcium diet for some four weeks before parturition are now being tested on a world-wide basis, and such diets are worthy of local trials on individual farms where parturient paresis is a recognised problem. Where grass or its products are present in abundance there is fundamental difficulty, for with such feeds it is extremely difficult to obtain a low calcium concentration for the pre-partum diet (Table 15.1). It is important to consider absolute amounts of calcium, no more than 50 g/day being allowed (Pickard 1975), and not to rely on adjustments to the Ca:P ratio. Ideally, the diet should contain only 20 g calcium/day (Wiggers *et al* 1975).

Treatment

Since Little & Wright (1925) and Dryerre & Greig (1928) demonstrated the specific role of calcium deficiency in milk fever, all treatments have included calcium salts in various quantities, occasionally supplemented with magnesium and phosphate salts. In excess, calcium salts can be toxic (Bergman & Sellars 1953), whereas underdosing with calcium may be followed by a poor response or a relapse (Blood & Henderson, 1974). The dose used, therefore, is important. Calcium alone was the available element in the original treatment (Stinson 1929). It is still the principal element, but magnesium (Barker 1939) and phosphorous (Marr *et al* 1955) are also involved in the milk fever complex and they may now be incorporated in the treatment regimen. In particular, therapy with solutions combining magnesium and phosphorous with calcium should be more effective in preventing relapses than those containing calcium alone. However, comparative trials have failed to demonstrate a significant advantage for the addition of magnesium or phosphorous.

The quantitity of calcium first recommended to treat milk fever was 2.67 g calcium administered intravenously as a 10% calcium gluconate solution with an equal amount given subcutaneously (Stinson 1929). However, the quantity of calcium now administered to cases of parturient paresis in cattle varies with clinicians' preferences. While many clinicians use the intravenous route others prefer subcutaneous administration. In addition, it is not uncommon for a solution containing calcium salts to be given intravenously and a further solution, again containing calcium but frequently with magnesium and phosphorous salts as well, to be given subcutaneously on the same occasion. Practical considerations often govern the approach selected.

There are differing views of the advantage to be gained therapeutically for the cow rather than psychologically by the veterinarian from a treatment combining intravenous and subcutaneous calcium administration. Neither Van Meurs (1972) nor Mullen (1977a) found any advantage from the combination treatment: indeed, a greater relapse rate and a longer period before recumbency ended were observed in comparison with the response following a single intravenous administration (Mullen 1975). A recent report from Canada does not support these observations. Curtis *et al* (1978) reported a markedly better response with combined treatments (total of 16.87 g calcium). No explanation was offered for this difference but an examination of their data shows a difference from Van Meurs' and Mullen's work, namely that the serum inorganic phosphate concentrations before treatment were low (1.50 mg/100 ml) in the Canadian study.

The findings reported below were obtained from 'virgin' cases of milk fever, i.e. they exclude cases where the owner had given treatment before the veterinary surgeon arrived. Also, all cases received a single treatment with varying amounts of calcium salts (6.2 g,* 8 g,** 12.36 g,***) intravenously. If, after an initially favourable response to treatment, further treatment for hypocalcaemia was needed, the case was classed as a 'relapse'.

At the time of treatment 25% of the cattle were standing and of those recumbent 19% were comatose. Serum calcium concentrations varied widely before treatment, but the comatose cases had the lowest concentrations. Another common feature was their speedier response to treatment. A number of cases presented clinical signs of hypocalcaemia but biochemical confirmation was lacking, their calcium concentrations exceeding 8.4 mg/100 ml — the upper limit for hypocalcaemia. Their response to treatment was the anticipated one of a successfully treated parturient paresis case. Serum

---

* Astra Calc. No. 1 (20% Ca B) Astra Chemicals.
** Nova Calc. No. 1 (20% Ca B) Astra Chemicals.
*** Astra Calc. No. 2 (40% Ca B) Astra Chemicals.

calcium levels had increased in most cases 24 hours after treatment, the rise being significant with all three treatments. There was no significant difference between treatments. The pre-treatment hypocalcaemia, though improved, was still present in a very high proportion of cases 24 hours after treatment — even though clinical evaluation did not indicate a need for further treatment. This last observation suggests that both a clinician's and a diagnostic laboratory's time may be wasted determining blood calcium levels 24 hours after treatment for hypocalcaemia. Many cattle will still remain hypocalcaemic, regardless of whether the cow appears clinically normal or a relapse occurs. Hence, it is clinical judgement which determines whether further treatment is required.

With the 75% of cases recumbent when treated, the time before they regained the standing position varied. Five hours after treatment 90% were standing. Two peaks occurred: those standing within five minutes of completing treatment, and those at two hours after treatment. The response achieved within five minutes of treatment was best in cattle receiving 8.0 g calcium. The main therapeutic effect of 12.36 g calcium occurred two hours after treatment. The reason for this difference is not known.

There seems to be no sign, recognisable at the initial clinical examination, which can be used to predict potential relapses. Age appears to have no connection with predisposition to relapse. Moreover, response to treatment and a tendency to relapse are not influenced by the time of onset of disease. The majority (92%) of the relapses occurred within 48 hours of the initial treatment. At least twelve hours elapsed before a repeat treatment was needed for the relapse of persistent recumbency cases — a field observation reflecting the known rate of decline of serum calcium after treatment (Ramberg 1972).

The administration of calcium borogluconate to cases of milk fever brings about a significant increase in the serum concentration of inorganic phosphate. A similar response does not follow a similar calcium administration to dry cows (Hurwitz & Sachs 1973) which suggests that the value of polypharmacy preparations which include phosphorous with calcium may be limited. It may be preferable to leave to the clinician the decision to administer solutions of phosphorous such as sodium acid phosphate.

Serum magnesium concentrations increase at parturition. Frequently, following calcium borogluconate administration, a small but significant fall occurs. A study which appeared to show a benefit to cases of hypocalcaemia occurring in the spring from the inclusion of magnesium (Mullen 1975), was not confirmed on a subsequent occasion (Mullen 1977b).

The most important question for the clinician is, how much calcium should be administered as a routine treatment to produce a maximum clinical response (and a relapse rate not exceeding 20%) with the treatment being administered on a single occasion by the intravenous route. The following treatment is recommended: at least 8 g and not more than 12.36 g calcium. The 40% relapse rate with 6.2 g Ca (20% calcium borogluconate in 400 ml) is far too high; the relapse rate with 8 g and 12.36 g Ca (40% calcium borogluconate in 400 ml) is only 19%. On the other hand there are potential hazards with administering more than 12.36 g calcium, these include: 1 its natural toxicity, for example to excitable tissues like the heart; 2 the reduced response to further treatment (i.e. relapse) which occurs when large amounts of calcium are used at an early stage; and 3 the possibility that a hypercalcaemic cow may reman recumbent and unresponsive to treatment due to excess calcium. The longer the period of recumbency, the more at risk the cow remains to further muscle and nerve damage.

About 8 g calcium is close to the total amount of calcium present in the blood circulation of the normal cow. Administering this quantity by the intravenous route immediately raises the circulating level, and the response does not correlate well with the amount given; cures have followed treatment with as little as 1.9 g while some cases have required as much as 15.9 g. However, a minimum of 8 g does at least provide a consistent response. If calcium treatment is a stimulus rather than a replacement, the therapeutic response to a relatively small amount may be explained on the assumption of calcium exchange between compartments of the body's pool, as described by Ramberg (1972). The elevation caused by the therapeutic dose declines over six hours, but maintains levels high enough to prevent clinical signs. If the stimulus is sufficient to restore normal alimentary function, the intake of calcium from the gut will be enough to produce uncomplicated recovery in most cases.

Prevention

There is no well established preventive method for milk fever nor, of the methods available, one which gives superior results. The following may be considered: 1 oral dosing with calcium; 2 nutritional managements — low calcium diet *pre partum*, acid diets, or cereal feeding; 3 administration of vitamin D_3 or its analogues; and 4 breeding programmes. However, all these methods have deficiencies and none meets all the following criteria: prevention of hypocalcaemia, absence of prolonged hypocalcaemia, a rapid onset of action, a long duration of action (calving dates), simple and practical, and non-toxic.

1 Four 150 g doses of calcium chloride ($CaCl_2$) gel, given over two days by Jönsson & Pehrson (1970) commencing the day before calving, reduced the incidence of milk fever.

2 A diet fed *pre partum* which contains sufficient (or excess) calcium leaves

the cow vulnerable at parturition, because the PTH/bone supply system will not have been 'primed'. A high calcium diet will lower $1,25 (OH)_2D_3$ in circulation. On the other hand, a low calcium diet will raise circulating $1,25(OH)_2D_3$, with its recognised advantages. The original observations of Boda & Cole (1954) which suggested the value of a low calcium content in the diet for some four weeks before parturition are worthy of further trial. At the same time it is important to recognise the difficulty, with available feeds, of obtaining a low calcium content in the pre-partum diet (Table 15.1). A daily calcium intake of 18 g or less, given for two weeks *pre partum*, resulted in no milk fever cases in the study of Wiggers *et al* (1975). However, with a normal daily calcium intake of 40–46 g the incidence was 26%, and a high daily calcium intake gave an incidence of 41% (Table 15.2).

Determinations of plasma levels of parathyroid hormone and dietary calcium levels showed little or no influence on parathyroid activity nor when daily dietary intake of calcium ranged from 37 g to 150 g (Jönsson 1978). calving, have shown a beneficial effect in reducing milk fever incidence calcium commencing four weeks before the expected parturition date, then an increase of 50 g in the daily intake for the last two or three days before calving, have shown a beneficial effect in reducing milk fever incidence. (Table 15.3). However, this work has not been confirmed under controlled conditions (Ford 1978). In response to a low calcium concentration in the diet, a more efficient absorption of calcium from the intestines occurs, so circulating levels should immediately become higher. In addition, for three weeks the PTH/bone supply has been primed and thus remains responsive

Table 15.2 Experimental result of Wiggers *et al* relating dietary calcium intake and the incidence of milk fever.

Calcium intake (g/day)	No. of cows	Milk fever (%)
20	152	4.6
30–50	82	22.0
100–175	140	47.0

Table 15.3 Calcium and phosphorous requirements (g/day) for a 600 kg dairy cow.

Status	Calcium	Phosphorous
Maintenance	21	28
Pregnant (+M)	42	39
Lactating 20 l/day	56	34
Lactating 40 l/day	112	68

at parturition. The low calcium diet should only contain 20 g calcium; the UK forage diets make it difficult to provide a diet with less than 50 g.

Further dietary preventive measures include feeding acid diets designed to improve the amounts of calcium available to and within the body. For example, feeding ammonium chloride (25–100 g/day) for three weeks is helpful (Payne 1967). The alkalinity of the diet is determined by the amounts of Na^+ and K^+ as cations and SO_4^- and Cl^+ as anions it contains. By reducing these, so the diet becomes more acid. Most pre-partum diets are of high alkalinity, especially where beets are included. Originally grass silage preserved with mineral acid was the preventive, but this method is used less frequently today and instead salt mixtures are used. The most promising results have been obtained by dispersing on hay a solution of calcium chloride (33 g $CACl_2.2H_2O/l$ water) followed by a solution containing 130 g $Al_2(SO_4)_3.16H_2O$ and 80 g $MgSO_4/1.5$ l water (Dishington 1975). This 'acid' diet was given during the last four weeks before parturition. As an alternative, 100 g $CaCO_3$ was added daily to the diet, and this produced a better effect when compared to the former treatment.

Another recommendation is to add barley to the diet. This may act because of its low calcium content and also by causing acidosis in the rumen and so increasing calcium absorption.

3   The beneficial effect of large doses of vitamin D, given for 3–5 days before and two days after calving, was discovered by Hibbs & Pounden (1955). The major disadvantage of this method lies in predicting accurately the date of

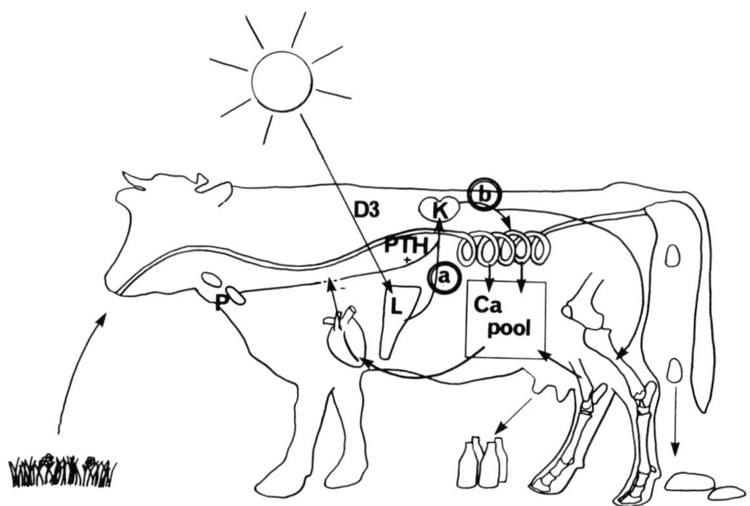

Fig. 15.3 Vitamin D metabolism showing the paths taken by 25,OH,D₃ (ⓐ) and by 1,25(OH)₂D₃ (ⓑ).

calving. A further disadvantage is the time elapsing from administration until the cholecalciferol is metabolised to its active form in the kidney (Fig. 15.3). This activation depends upon normal liver and kidney function and circulating levels of parathormone and calcium.

Analogues of vitamin D_3 have now been synthesised and from these eventually may arise prophylactic treatments. 1 K OH.D_3 is presently under close examination (Davies *et al* 1978). It has four main advantages which all useful analogues must have: it is highly active, it is quick acting, it is not dependent upon parathormone for its action or control (in contrast to vitamin D_3), and it raises quickly both calcium and phosphorous concentrations in serum. Its disadvantages are two-fold: timing its administration is not easy for the date of parturition may be uncertain, and it depresses serum magnesium concentrations (Sansom *et al* 1976, Mullen *et al* 1979). At present therefore its widespread application is not recommended.

4 Close examination of the influence of particular blood lines and a precise association with the incidence of milk fever with their progeny, although suggestive, has not yet given a conclusive link.

Acetonaemia (bovine ketosis)

All cattle suffering from primary spontaneous ketosis show strongly positive Rothera's test in the milk; blood glucose concentration is raised and ketone bodies in the blood, milk and urine show a fall. Excellent reviews of bovine ketosis with recommendations for control and treatment have been published (Baird *et al* 1974).

The majority of primary spontaneous ketosis cases occur between three and six weeks after calving. The prevalence of this condition nationally is not easy to ascertain, but the overt clinical syndrome is seen less frequently now than formerly. However, the extent of subclinical disease is considered to be widespread, and probably associated with heavy milk losses. Any condition (e.g. pyrexia) producing a temporary reduction in appetite in the newly calved cow can lead to a secondary ketosis. It is necessary, therefore, for an accurate diagnosis to distinguish between primary and secondary cases.

As primary ketosis progresses, ketotic cows refuse concentrated foods and, less frequently, hay. Additionally a pronounced loss of weight occurs, glazed faeces are seen and nervous symptoms are displayed by a large number of the more severely affected animals. Acetonaemia (ketosis) is not confined to those in poor bodily condition, although many cases do occur in high-yielding cows which are unable to conserve sufficient energy for their production and maintenance requirements. These animals are thin and may be regarded as being in a nutritional deficiency. The maximum milk yield in high-yielding cows may be reached in the third week of lactation, while maximum intake of digestible nutrient is not achieved until the seventh week (Reid *et al* 1966). On the other hand, ketosis may also be observed in the well fed and fat animal. This is especially true in the USA where the fat cow syndrome is more prevalent in corn-fed animals on rations which appear, on the basis of present knowledge, to be adequate (Curtis 1973).

The milk-producing potential of a cow is a characteristic of the individual and, even when food intake is inadequate, a high milk yield can be maintained for a limited period. Therefore, although the animal is losing weight, milk can be produced with body reserves providing the energy required for the synthesis of milk components. Many animals are able to continue in this state of negative energy balance with low carbohydrate reserve by mobilising depot fats without becoming clinically ketotic. This unstable situation, however, can rapidly develop into a severe clinical ketosis as a result of anything which causes a reduction of the animal's food intake. For example, the period of oestrus is accompanied by reduced intake for a short period.

Aetiology

At parturition a very high turnover of glucose occurs. A cow producing 20 litres of milk daily requires 17 000 kcal/day for production and maintenance, a need which increases until the peak of lactation is reached. Even though milk production in cows can be reduced by lowering the energy intake, this does not necessarily follow automatically or proportionally in early lactation, because hormonal stimulus for mammary gland activity overrides the effects of reduced food intake. This factor marks the difference between the ketosis of simple starvation and the more severe spontaneous ketosis of a high-producing cow in early lactation.

Studies by Baird *et al* (1968) and Baird & Heitzman (1970, 1971) of cows suffering from spontaneous ketosis, reveal an increase in the concentration of the ketone bodies in the liver which is accompanied by decreases in the steady state concentrations of several metabolites that are intermediate in the glucogenic pathway from the level of glucogenic amino acids through to glucose (Fig. 15.4). This includes decreases in the concentrations of a number of intermediates in the tricarboxylic acid cycle, which lie on the glucogenic route taken by carbon skeletons from such precursors as propionate and the glucogenic amino acids. One of the intermediates of the cycle which decreases in concentration is oxaloacetate. This compound is required to permit acetyl-CoA to enter the tricarboxylic acid cycle and be oxidised to carbon dioxide and water. If there is insufficient oxaloacetate, acetyl-CoA will be converted to the ketone bodies instead. The fact that oxaloacetate concentration falls suggests that oxaloacetate availability is decreased, and this would in

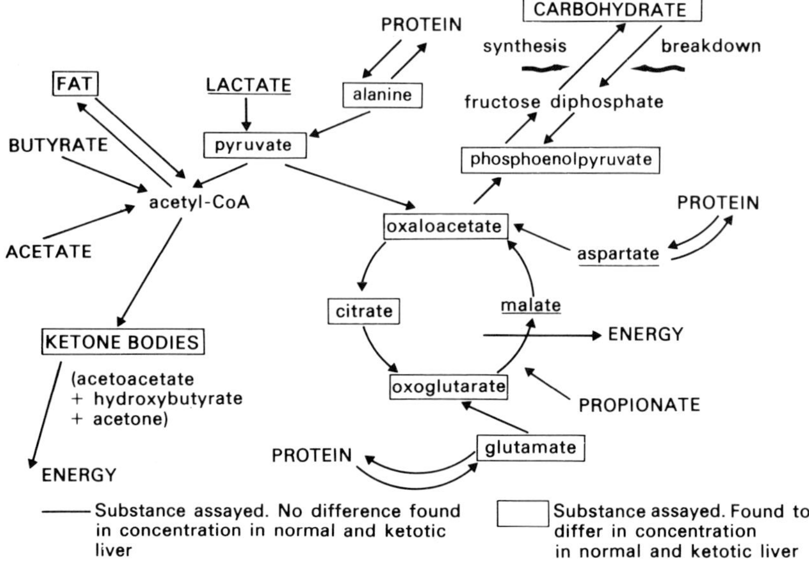

Fig. 15.4 The TCA cycle showing the influence of oxaloacetate.

itself lead to increased hepatic ketogenesis. However, fat oxidation and consequently acetyl-CoA production, is almost certainly much increased during spontaneous ketosis. An increase in acetyl-CoA production appears, therefore, to be occurring at the same time as a probable decrease in oxaloacetate availability. This coincidence of events leads to a profound increase in ketogenesis. Propionic acid, a glucose precursor formed in the rumen before entering the vascular system, is introduced into the tricarboxylic acid cycle eventually to become oxaloacetate. Thus the aetiology of bovine ketosis is becoming better understood.

Diagnosis and treatment

A diagnosis of ketosis is made on the basis of clinical signs together with the presence of ketone bodies in blood and milk. The concentration of ketone bodies in primary ketosis may exceed 100 mg/100 ml, whereas in secondary ketosis it does not usually exceed 50 mg/100 ml. The commercially available test (Rothera's) records the presence of acetone and acetoacetic acid, but not β-hydroxybutyric acid which may also be present. Milk is a suitable material for field examination and Shefki & Makinson (1974) found a good correlation between blood and milk ketone concentrations. In milk the colour requires some 30 seconds to develop. Measurement of the milk ketone concentration at intervals of 1–2 weeks, during the first twelve weeks of lactation, may be the ideal way to identify subclinical ketosis. Measuring these concentrations from a base of less than 5 mg/100 ml to higher concentrations as lactation progresses will detect developing subclinical ketosis and allow suitable dietary alterations to be made. Shefiki & Makinson (1974) found this approach to be more reliable than monitoring blood glucose concentrations, probably because glucose metabolism with higher levels of ketones present is disturbed, blood glucose being diverted from lactose synthesis to counter ketone production and so lower milk production.

Treatments available are many, but the principal aims are to increase the glucose concentration in the circulation and the production of propionic acid in the rumen.

1 Intravenous administration of glucose (400 ml of a 50% solution) will raise the oxaloacetate levels quickly, but the injection has to be repeated after 12–24 hours.

2 Glucocorticoid administration has been found to be one of the most beneficial treatments for primary bovine ketosis. The quantity of glucocorticoid to be administered depends on the weight of the animal, and reference should be made to individual manufacturer's instructions. Most treated cows show a marked improvement in condition, including a return of appetite, within 48 hours of this treatment. Following administration, a rise in blood glucose level and a fall in the level of ketone bodies occur, but there is no change in the concentration of free fatty acids, the main precursors of the ketone bodies (Baird & Heitzman 1971). This suggests a direct antiketogenic effect upon the liver itself. After 48 hours a significant increase of oxaloacetate, citrate, oxyglutarate and other intermediates of the tricarboxylic acid cycle are present. These workers concluded that the supply of oxaloacetate is of importance in regulating hepatic ketogenesis in the cow. Thus, when the concentrations of oxaloacetate and its precursors are high, ketogenesis will be reduced, and when they are low, ketogenesis will be increased if free fatty acids are available.

3 A major source of glucose in ruminants is propionic acid, and propionate precursors may be administered orally. Potassium chlorate has been recommended (Blackburn *et al* 1959). Three consecutive daily doses, each of 56 g, markedly reduce ketosis and increase the ratio of propionic acid relative to acetic and butyric acids produced from rumen fermentation. If administered for a longer period, this salt is toxic to the rumen microbial population (Barry *et al* 1978).

Prevention

A ten point programme has been recommended by Baird *et al* (1974). A summary of their proposals follows.

1 In the second half of lactation, the diet of a dairy cow should contain a greater proportion of home grown foods with a lower digestibility than that in the diet fed during peak lactation. Feeding in excess of requirements must be avoided during the second half of lactation.

2 At the beginning of the dry period, the cows should not be in fat condition.

3 'Steaming up' should not commence until 4–5 weeks before the expected date of parturition.

4 During the 'steaming up' period the production concentrate ration should be introduced to the cow, commencing with 2–4 lbs (1–1.8 kg) concentrate a day in the first week and rising to, but not exceeding, 8–10 lbs (3.6–4.5 kg) per day in the week before calving. Throughout this period the hay and silage to be fed during production should be included in the ration.

5 After calving, the quantity of production ration fed should be steadily increased as the milk production increases.

6 The overall protein concentration in the production concentrate ration should not exceed 16–18%. The carbohydrate in the ration should be readily digestible. Production concentrates should contain a balanced vitamin and mineral supplement.

7 Care must be taken that, when the milk yields are highest and the cows are being fed up to a maximum dry matter intake, they are managed in such a way that they can consume, if not all, as much of their ration as possible.

8 During the first three months of lactation, high-yielding animals should not be subjected to sudden changes in ration. A change in the source of a concentrate ration, i.e. from one manufacturer to another, can present dietary problems.

9 After the first 10–12 weeks of lactation, the feeding routine of the high yielders can be modified. The more expensive highly digestible carbohydrates in the ration can be replaced gradually by cheaper cereals such as barley.

10 In all stages of lactation attention must be paid to the quality of the foods fed to a dairy herd. Silage and hay quality is frequently overrated by the farmer, leading to inadequate intake for the animal's requirements. Silage may contain a high proportion of butyric acid and this may lead to accretion of ketone bodies and a lack of glucose precursors.

Attention to these ARC recommendations will help to reduce the incidence of bovine ketosis and bring about a more efficient use of the foods provided and an increased yield of milk both in quantity and quality.

References

Allcroft R. (1960) Prevention of Disease. *Br. Vet. Assoc. Conference on Hypomagnesaemia*, pp. 102–19. BVA, London.

Baird G. D. & Heitzman R. J. (1970) Gluconeogenesis in the cow. The effect of a glucocorticoid on hepatic intermediary metabolism. *Biochem. J.* **116**, 865.

Baird G. D. & Heitzman R. J. (1971) Mode of action of the glucocorticoid on bovine intermediary metabolism: possible role in controlling hepatic batogenesis. *Biochem. Biophys. Acta* **252**, 184.

Baird G. D., Heitzman R. J., Hibbitt K. G. *et al* (1974) Bovine Ketosis: a Review with Recommendations for Control and Treatment. *Br. Vet. J.* **130**, 214–20.

Baird G. D., Hibbit K. G., Hunter G. D. *et al* (1968) Biochemical Aspects of Bovine Ketosis. *Biochem. J.* **107**, 683.

Barker J. R. (1939) Blood plasma changes and variations in the female bovine toxaemias. *Vet. Rec.* **51**, 575–80.

Barry T. N., Harte F. J., Perry B. N. *et al* (1978) Some effects of Potassium Chlorate administration on in vitro and in vivo rumen fermentation. *J. Ag. Sci.* **90**, 345–53.

Bergman E. N. & Sellars A. F. (1953) Studies on intravenous administration of calcium, potassium and magnesium to dairy calves. Some biochemical and general toxic effects. *Am. J. Vet. Res.* **14**, 520–9.

Beynon V. H. & Howe K. S. (1974) The Disposal of Dairy Cows in England and Wales 1972–73. *Univ. Exeter Ag. Econ. Unit*, p. 32.

Blackburn P. S., Castle M. E. & Drysdale A. D. (1959) Treatment of ketosis in dairy cows by potassium chlorate. *Vet. Rec.* **71**, 665.

Blood D. C. & Henderson J. A. (1974) In *Veterinary Medicine*, 4th ed., p. 683. Bailliere Tindall, London.

Boda J. M. & Cole H. H. (1954) The influence of dietary calcium and phosphorous on the incidence of milk fever in dairy cattle. *J. Dairy Sci.* **37**, 360–72.

Curtis R. A. (1973) Prevention of retained foetal membranes in cattle. *Vet. Rec.* **92**, 291–2.

Curtis R. A., Cote J. F., McLennan M. C. *et al* (1978) Relationship of methods of treatment to relapse rate and serum levels of calcium and phosphorous in parturient hypocalcaemia. *Canadian Vet. J.* **19**, 155–8.

Davies D. C., Allen W. M., Hoare M. N. *et al* (1978) A field trial of 1 α-hydroxycholecalciferol (1 α-OH D$_3$) in the prevention of milk fever. *Vet. Rec.* **102**, 440.

Dishington I. W. (1975) Prevention of milk fever (hypocalcaemic paresis puerperalis) by dietary salt supplements. *Acta Vet. Scand.* **16**, 503–12.

Dryerre H. & Greig J. R. (1925) Milk fever: its possible association with derangements in the internal secretions. *Vet. Rec.* **5**, 225–31.

Dryerre H. & Grieg J. R. (1928) Further studies in the etiology of milk fever. *Vet. Rec.* **8**, 721–8.

Fenwick D. C. (1978) Parturient paresis of cows: blood glucose levels. *Austral. Vet. J.* **54**, 4.

Ford E. J. H. (1978) 1 α-hydroxycholecalciferol in the prevention of milk fever. *Vet. Rec.* **102**, 442.

Hibbs J. W. & Pounden W. D. (1955) Studies on milk fever in dairy cows. IV Prevention by short term, pre-partum feeding of massive doses of vitamin D. *J. Dairy Sci.* **38**, 65–72.

Hurwitz S. & Sachs M. (1973) The effect of the administration of calcium by different routes on the plasma calcium levels of normal cows. *Refuah Veterinarith* **30**, 44–50.

Jönsson G. (1978) Milk fever prevention. *Vet. Rec.* **102**, 165.

Jönsson G. & Pehrson B. (1970) Trials with prophylactic treatment of parturient paresis. *Vet. Rec.* **87**, 575.

Kronfeld D. S. (1971) Parturient hypocalcaemia in dairy cows. *Adv. Vet. Sci.* **15**, 133–57.

Leech F. B., Davis M. E., Macrae W. D. *et al* (1960) *Disease wastage and husbandry in the British dairy herd. Survey 1957–58.* HMSO, London.

Little W. L. & Wright N. C. (1925) The aetiology of milk fever in cattle. *Br. J. Exp. Path.* **6**, 129–34.

Littledike E. T., Whipp S. C. & Schroeder L. (1969) Studies on parturient paresis. *J. Am. Vet. Med. Assoc.* **155**, 1955–62.

Marr A., Moodie E. W. & Robertson A. (1955) Some biochemical and clinical aspects of milk fever. *J. Comp. Path. & Therap.* **65**, 347–65.

Moodie E. W., Marr A. & Robertson A. (1955) Serum calcium and magnesium and plasma phosphate levels in normal parturient cows. *J. Comp. Path. & Therap.* **65**, 20–36.

Mullen P. A. (1975) Clinical and biochemical responses to the treatment of milk fever. *Vet. Rec.* **97**, 87–92.

Mullen P. A. (1977a) Milk fever: influence of treatment before the clinician's visit. *Vet. Rec.* **101**, 366–7.

Mullen P. A. (1977b) Milk fever: a case against polypharmacy solutions. *Vet. Rec.* **101**, 405–7.

Mullen P. A., Bedford P. G. & Ingram P. L. (1979) An investigation of the toxicity of 1 α-hydroxycholecalciferol to calves. *Res. Vet. Sci.* **27**, 275–9.

Payne J. M. (1967) The cause and prevention of milk fever. *Vet. Rec.* **82**, Supplement 1.

Payne J. M. (1977) *Metabolic Diseases in Farm Animals.* William Heinemann, London.

Payne J. M., Dew S. R., Manston R. *et al* (1970) The use of a metabolic profile test in dairy herds. *Vet. Rec.* **87**, 150–8.

Pickard D. W. (1975) An apparent reduction in the incidence of milk fever achieved by regulation of the dietary intake of calcium and phosphorous. *Br. Vet. J.* **131**, 744.

Ramberg C. F. (1972) Kinetics of hypocalcaemia in cows fed high and low calcium diets. *VII World Association Buiatrics Conference,* p. 317. BCVA, London.

Reid J. T., Moe P. W. & Tyrrell H. F. (1966) Energy and protein requirements of milk production. *J. Dairy Sci.* **49**, 215.

Robertson A. (1948) Some observations on milk fever. *Vet. Rec.* **61**, 333–7.

Sansom B. F., Allen W. M., Davies D. C. *et al* (1976) Use of 1 α-OH cholecalciferol in preventing post parturient hypocalcaemia and its potential value for the prevention of milk fever in dairy cows. *Vet. Rec.* **99**, 310.

Shefki D. & Makinson M. (1974) Subclinical acetonaemia. *Vet. Rec.* **95**, 498.

Stinson O. (1929) A further communication on calcium therapy in milk fever. *Vet. Rec.* **9**, 741–2.

Storry J. E. & Rook J. A. F. (1962) Effects of large intraruminal additions of volatile fatty acids on the secretion of milk constituent. *Dairy Science Abstracts,* pp. 64–70.

Van Meurs G. K. (1972) The dosage in the treatment of parturient paresis in the cow. *Tijdschr. voor Djergeneesk.* **96**, 1649–53.

Wiggers K. D., Nelson D. K. & Jacobson N. L. (1975) Prevention of parturient paresis by a low-calcium diet pre partum: a field study. *J. Dairy Sci.* **58**, 430.

16

Anabolic agents in farm animals

R.J. HEITZMAN

The use of anabolic agents to increase animal production is not new and it was the development in the early 1950s of inexpensive synthetic oestrogens, especially the stilbenes, which led to their initial use. Most anabolic agents have some properties in common with the sex steroids and there is now a wide selection of agents available for use in farm animals (Fig. 16.1). These compounds act by changing the intermediary metabolism of the animal, while other anabolic substances like monensin alter the metabolic processes which occur in the digestive tract. These latter drugs are not discussed here. The synthetic oestrogens based on the stilbene molecule are still the least expensive but the potential health hazard associated with diethylstilboestrol (DES) (Roe 1976) has resulted in the development of alternative agents which, although more costly, are thought to be safer for the consumer.

Anabolic agents are used throughout the world, and the largest single use involves the production of beef steers in the USA. In some European countries the use of anabolic agents is banned whereas in others, particularly the UK, there is a widescale use.

This chapter discusses the efficacy of the anabolic agents in different species and also considers the safety of the agents, both for man, the consumer, and the recipient animals. Finally, the obscure area of their mode of action as growth promoters in farm animals is discussed and compared with their action in laboratory animals.

Anabolic agents in farm practice

Administration

Anabolic agents may be administered either orally or parenterally. They are given orally as feed additives to pigs and this will be the route of choice if they are developed for use in intensive methods of fish husbandry. They are usually administered either as subcutaneous implants to cattle, sheep, and poultry or injected as oily solutions to horses and some veal calves. Table 16.1 shows preparations commonly used in the western world.

333

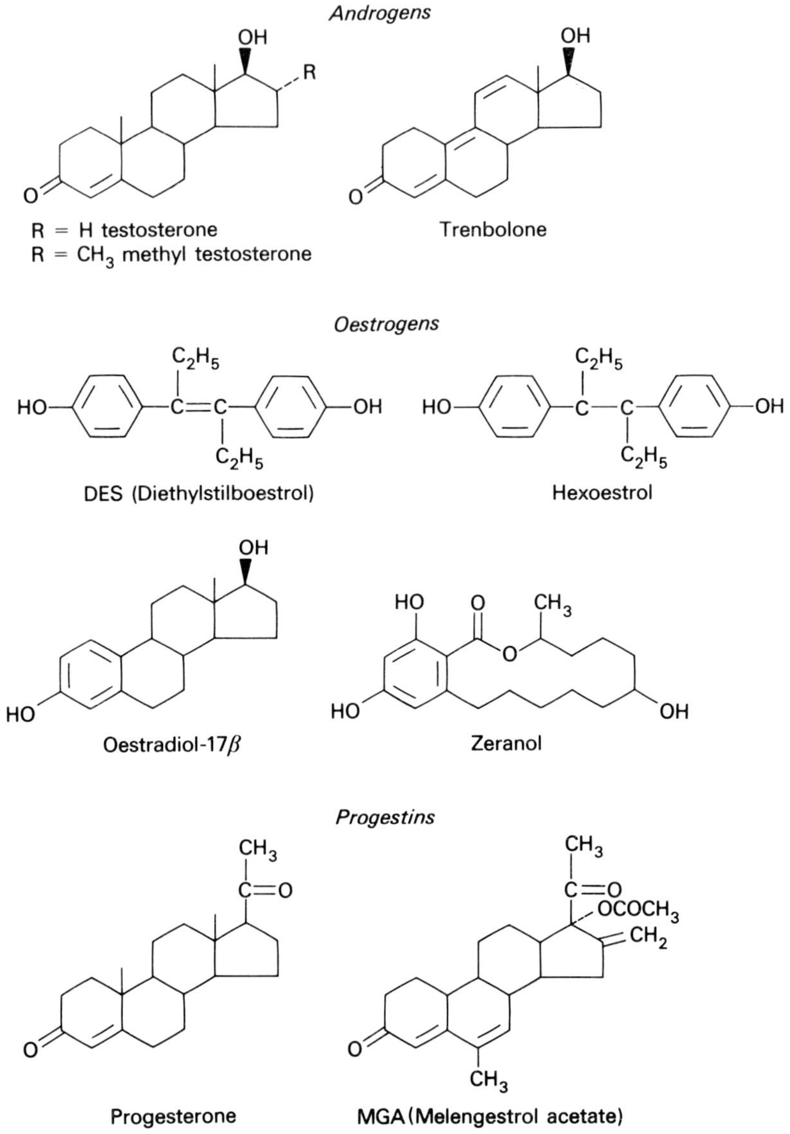

Androgens

R = H testosterone
R = CH$_3$ methyl testosterone

Trenbolone

Oestrogens

DES (Diethylstilboestrol)

Hexoestrol

Oestradiol-17β

Zeranol

Progestins

Progesterone

MGA (Melengestrol acetate)

Fig. 16.1 Ababolic agents used in farm animal production.

Formulation

Because the testing of efficacy at different doses and in various formulations is very expensive in large farm animals, there have been few critical studies of optimum formulation. The formulation should allow the absorption of an effective dose over a long period of time. This is best achieved either with

Table 16.1 Anabolic agents used in farm animals.

Agent	Dose	Form	Main use	Trade name
Androgen				
Trenbolone acetate	300 mg	Implant	Heifers, cull cows	Finaplix*
Oestrogen				
Diethylstilboestrol†	30–60 mg	Implant	Steers	
Diethylstilboestrol† and esters		Oily solution	Veal calves	
Diethylstilboestrol†	10–20 mg/day	Feed additive	Steers	
Hexoestrol†	12–60 mg	Implant	Steers, calves, sheep, poultry	
Zeranol	12–36 mg	Implant	Steers, sheep	Ralgro*
Oestradiol	30–50 μg/day	Silicone implant	Steers	Compudose*
Progestins				
Melengestrol acetate		Feed additive	Heifers	
Combined implants				
Trenbolone acetate	140 mg	Implant	Bulls, steers,	Revalor
+ oestradiol	20 mg		calves, sheep	
Trenbolone acetate	300 mg	Implant	Steers	
+ hexoestrol†	30–45 mg			
Trenbolone acetate	300 mg	Implant	Steers	
+zeranol	36 mg			
Testosterone (propionate)	200 mg	Implant	Heifers, calves	Implix-BF*
+ oestradiol (benzoate)	20 mg			Synovex-H
Progesterone	200 mg	Implant	Steers	Implix-BM*
+ oestradiol (benzoate)	20 mg			Synovex-S
Methyltestosterone		Feed additive	Pigs	Maxymin
+ diethylstilboestrol†				
Testosterone	120 mg	Implant	Calves	Rapigain
+diethylstilboestrol†	25 mg			

*products licensed in Great Britain, †agents banned in EEC countries and USA

Table 16.2 Absorption of trenbolone acetate by farm animals.

Animal	Formulation	Dose (mg)	Persistence of detectable residues* in plasma (days)
Steer	implant	200	~ 140
Cow	implant	300	140–200†
Calf	implant	300	100
Calf	implant	140	80
Sheep	implant	140	80–120
Cow	i.m.	3 × 120 mg	10–20
Horse	i.m.	90	7
Steer	oral	4 mg/day	7–14**

*Trenbolone was measured by a radioimmunoassay method in jugular vein plasma except in the cows implanted with 300 mg.
†In this case H^3-trenbolone acetate was implanted in cows and residual radioactivity in the plasma was measured.
**The period after withdrawal of oral trenbolone acetate.

preparations administered as subcutaneous implants which are effective for several months, or as orally administered feed additives given daily. Intramuscular injections are active only for a few weeks. These effects are illustrated in Table 16.2 which gives the persistence of detectable residues (*see* p. 346) of trenbolone acetate in the plasma of animals treated with the same drug by three different routes. It is clear that the duration of absorption is longer in animals receiving implants than in those given intramuscular injections.

The rate of absorption of an agent from an implant can be altered by a number of factors, including implant size, shape, and hardness, and the nature of the base materials used. An interesting phenomenon is that the rate of absorption of one agent can be changed by the presence of a second agent. Single implants of oestradiol-17β administered to sheep and cattle are absorbed in about 40 days. However, when a second steroid, either testosterone, trenbolone acetate, or progesterone, is combined with the oestradiol and administered at the same site, the rate of absorption of the oestradiol is delayed and complete absorption takes about 100 days (Fig. 16.2). This is a physical effect at the site of implantation, since the rate of absorption of oestradiol from a single implant is unaffected by implantation of another steroid at a different site.

This effect on absorption of oestradiol in a combined implant contributes to the improved efficacy of combined implants (Heitzman *et al* 1981).

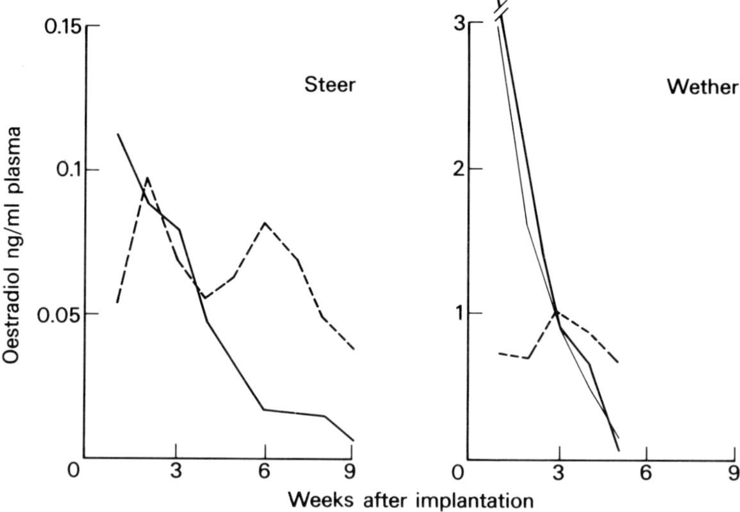

Fig. 16.2 Absorption of oestradiol from implants in cattle and sheep. Concentrations of oestradiol-17β are the mean values for three steers or wethers per treatment group. The implants were placed subcutaneously at the base of the ear(s) and plasma samples were taken from the vein ipsilateral to the oestradiol implant. The treatments were — 20 mg oestradiol-17β, ---- 20 mg oestradiol-17β combined with 140 mg trenbolone acetate, — 20 mg oestradiol-17β implanted in one ear and 140 mg trenbolone acetate implanted in the opposite ear. The concentration of oestradiol-17β was measured by a radioimmunoassay method.

Use and efficacy

Anabolic agents are used primarily for improving meat production in ruminants; they were used to a lesser extent in pigs and on a very small scale in poultry. They are also effective growth promoters in horses and fish. Anabolic agents used in ruminants increase live weight gain (LWG) and feed conversion efficiency (FCE). However, in poultry the oestrogenic anabolic agents were used for chemical caponisation, while in pigs the main action of anabolic agents is to improve the lean muscle tissue content of the carcase and reduce the unwanted fat content.

Definition of terms

LWG is the live weight gained by an animal in a set time, e.g. 10 kg in a week. ADLG is the live weight gained by an animal divided by the number of days during which the weight gain has been measured. FCE is a measure of the efficiency with which feed is converted to a component of animal growth, and may be measured in many ways. Feed may be total amount of wet feed, amount of dry matter, or the amount of protein, carbohydrate, or fat in feed. Growth may be measured as LWG, fat, protein or skeleton growth. In summary it is the amount of material ingested to give a unit increase in a component of growth. The units of measurement are always the same because the FCE is a ratio.

Cattle

Anabolic agents have been most successfully used in cattle, particularly in intensive rearing systems. One hypothesis for the role of anabolic agents as growth promoters in cattle suggested that both androgens and oestrogens were necessary to realise maximum growth rate (Heitzman 1976). The concentrations of steroids in blood which result in the fastest growth rates correspond approximately to a combination of the androgen level in a growing bull and the oestrogen level in a young cow. Thus theoretically, the ideal steroids for treatment should maintain this natural hormone status for as long as possible, preferably for several months. If this hypothesis is valid the greatest benefits would be seen in heifers and cows administered androgen, in steers treated with androgen combined with an oestrogen, and in bulls treated with oestrogen. The results which follow illustrate that, in practice, the hypothesis is valid.

Steers

Steers implanted with both androgen and oestrogen had higher LWG than steers treated with either androgen or oestrogen alone. Table 16.3 shows LWG and FCE in trials using trenbolone acetate as the androgen and hexoestrol, oestradiol-17β, or zeranol as the oestrogen. Stollard *et al* (1977) recorded similar results in a very large scale trial ($>$ 1500 animals) when they treated steers with single or combined implants of trenbolone acetate and hexoestrol.

Heifers and cows

Beranger & Malterre (1968) reported that trenbolone acetate improved LWG of cull cows, and there are several reports that androgens improve the LWG and FCE of heifers (Burris *et al* 1952, Best 1972, Heitzman & Chan 1974, Galbraith 1980). Fig. 16.3 shows the increased LWG of heifers treated with trenbolone acetate compared with controls. The measurements were made over an unusually long period but illustrate that the benefit obtained during the initial months after implantation has not diminished after one year;

Table 16.3 Average daily weight gains and feed conversion ratios in steers following administration of anabolic agents. (Data from Heitzman *et al* 1981.)

Trial	Treatment	Dose (mg)	No. of animals	Period of trial (days)	Average daily live weight gain kg/day	FCR[†]
1	Control	–	15	64	0.84	–
1	Trenbolone acetate	300	15	64	0.91	–
1	Hexoestrol	36	15	64	0.94	–
1	TBA/hexoestrol	300/36	15	64	1.17*	–
2	Zeranol	36	8	71	0.76	–
2	Trenbolone acetate/zeranol	300/36	8	71	1.00	–
3	Control	–	6	100	0.79	9.3
3	Trenbolone acetate	140	6	100	0.89	8.5
3	Oestradiol	20	6	100	0.88	8.8
3	Trenbolone acetate/oestradiol	140/20	6	100	1.15*	6.9*

*$p < 0.05$ compared with control value.

[†]FCR is feed conversion ratio, i.e. the amount of unit feed consumed to produce one unit of live weight gain.

The steers in trials 1 and 2 were fed 3 kg concentrates per day and maize silage *ad libitum*. The steers in trial 3 were fed hay and concentrate according to body weight.

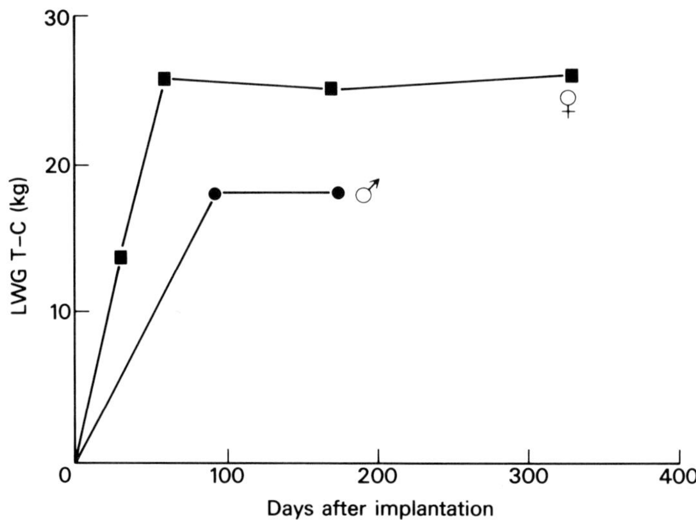

Fig. 16.3 Increased LWG of treated animals compared with controls (T–C) are the mean values of 15 steers and 6 heifers per treatment group, respectively. The treated steers received 300 mg trenbolone acetate plus 36 mg hexoestrol and the heifers were given 300 mg trenbolone acetate.

similar observation (Fig. 16.3) was made in steers treated with trenbolone acetate plus hexoestrol (Heitzman *et al* 1977b).

Bulls

In mainland Europe most beef is produced from bulls and there is an increasing use of this method in the USA and to some extent also in the UK. Anabolic agents are only occasionally used in bulls but the results of some initial trials suggest that LWG and FCE are improved in bulls treated with combined implants (Szumowski & Grandadam 1976, Galbraith 1979). Oestrogens suppress the gonadal secretion of testosterone and thus exogenous androgen is necessary to achieve the optimum circulating concentrations of both androgens and oestrogens.

Veal calves

Veal production, especially in Europe, is concentrated into intensive units and anabolic agents have been used successfully to increase productivity under these systems of management. The efficacy of anabolic agents in veal calves has been discussed by Van der Wal (1976) and a summary of his investigation is shown in Table 16.4. The maximum improvements in LWG

Table 16.4 Effects of anabolic agents on the performance of veal calves. (Data from Van der Wal *et al* 1975.)

Treatment	Dose (mg)	Difference in LWG compared to control (range in kg)	No. of experiments	Time after treatment (wks)
DES	25	4.9–9.1	3	4–5
Oestradiol	20	4.1	2	3–4
Zeranol	36	0.5–3.4	2	6
Testosterone	200	7.6–9.7	4	3–4
+ oestradiol	20			
Trenbolone acetate	140	9.0–15.8	5	4–5
+ oestradiol	20			
Progesterone	200	4.6–7.6	3	3–5
+ oestradiol	20			

Friesian bull calves were implanted with anabolic agents at 11 weeks of age. The number of animals used in the study was 563. LWG is live weight gain.

and FCE were obtained when bull calves were treated with combined preparations of androgen plus oestrogen.

Sheep

Zeranol and hexoestrol have been used to improve the production of wether lambs, but the responses and economic returns are not sufficient to encourage widescale use. However, Szumowski & Grandadam (1976) and Coelho *et al* (1978) have demonstrated that LWG and FCE are improved with combined preparations of androgen and oestrogen.

Pigs

The improvement of lean:fat tissue ratio is the main benefit derived from treating pigs with anabolic agents. Fowler *et al* (1978) showed that oral administration of ethyl-oestradiol combined with trenbolone acetate or methyl testosterone reduced fat tissue in castrate males but not females. Van Weerden & Grandadam (1976) observed improvements in LWG, FCE, nitrogen retention, and lean:fat tissue ratio in castrate male pigs receiving either implants of trenbolone acetate and oestradiol or oral administration of trenbolone acetate plus ethyl-oestradiol. Implants are not yet used commercially in pigs and oral administration of anabolic agents is no longer practised because the use of orally active DES is prohibited throughout the western world.

Poultry

Nesheim (1976) reviewed the effectiveness of anabolic agents as growth promoters in poultry and concluded that sex steroids, growth hormone, and thyroid-active compounds were without effect. More recent studies (Ranaweera 1978, Ranaweera & Wise 1981) did, however, suggest that the androgen, trenbolone acetate, improved LWG and FCE in turkeys. The stilbene-oestrogens were used for the chemical caponising of chickens. The main response to oestrogen administration is not to increase LWG and FCE but to produce a fat cover on the birds which improves their presentation and acceptability. Clearly, the mode of action of oestrogens in poultry is not the same as in ruminants.

Other species

Horses and rabbits provide only a small percentage of human dietary protein and, although anabolic agents are used to promote growth and condition in race horses, they are not used in farm practice for these species.

Fish farming is an expanding industry. Anabolic agents can be administered easily to fish as a feed additive. Some initial trials in young trout receiving synthetic androgens in the feed resulted in large increases in the growth rate of treated fish. This is an area of farming which may develop in the future and anabolic agents, if allowed as feed additives for fish, could improve the efficiency of protein production.

Conclusions

Anabolic agents are being used on an increasing scale to improve growth rate and FCE in farm animals. The greatest benefits have been obtained in cattle, especially veal calves, beef steers, and heifers. Some benefits are possible from their use in bulls, pigs, sheep, turkeys, and trout but investigations in these species are still at the developmental stage.

Safety of anabolic agents

Many anabolic agents are potent sex steroids and some are potential carcinogens. Therefore it is important that the potential hazards of these drugs are fully investigated. Both the parent compounds and their metabolites must be tested to ensure that there are neither undesirable side-effects in the recipient animals nor a public health hazard to consumers. Decisions have to be made between the clear benefits of using anabolic agents to improve animal production and the potential hazards to human health. Some countries ban the use of anabolic agents and in others there is legislation restricting their use.

Hazards to farm animals

The hazards most likely to occur in farm animals following administration of anabolic agents are those associated with the hormonal activity of the drug or its metabolites. There is no evidence that at, the recommended dose rates, the drugs are toxic or in any way adversely affect the health of the animal. The main hazards observed in meat-producing animals are changes in behaviour and interference with reproductive function in breeding animals.

Behavioural changes

In a survey of 1.9 million cattle to determine the cause of illness and deaths among feedlot steers in the USA, bulling and riding was found to be one of the major problems (Pierson *et al* 1976). During 1968–70, bulling was responsible for 1.5% of illness and death in feedlot steers and, over the next four years, the incidence of illness and death from bulling rose to 3.7%. The authors suggested that the increases were associated either with the increasing use of oestrogens (in particular the increase from feeding 10 mg DES daily to 20 mg DES) or with the introduction of implants containing other oestrogens.

In the UK bulling has also been a problem in some steers treated with hexoestrol, either as a single implant or combined with trenbolone acetate. Normally, these problems are only seen for 1–2 weeks immediately after treatment and with careful management the problem is not difficult to overcome.

The use of androgens in steers and heifers tends to produce a more aggressive and active animal while, on the other hand, oestrogens are believed to be useful in making bulls easier to handle.

Changes in reproductive function

The use of hormones to regulate reproductive function has been investigated extensively. Oestrogens and progesterone are used to synchronise oestrus in cattle and sheep without adversely affecting future reproductive performance. However, the use of hormones to obtain early puberty has met with little success. There appears to be no advantage in using oestrogens and progestins to induce early oestrus in beef heifers (Neville *et al* 1974) or young lambs (Cooper, Pers. Commun.) and there are real disadvantages in using androgens to obtain rapid growth and early puberty in dairy heifers (Heitzman *et al* 1979).

Friesian heifer calves were implanted at four months and again at seven months of age with trenbolone acetate or a combined preparation of trenbolone acetate and oestradiol. In comparison with untreated controls there was: an increase in growth rate; a delay of 3–6 months in the onset of puberty; an increased incidence of dystocia; a severe reduction in milk production; and virilisation of genitalia (Fig. 16.4).

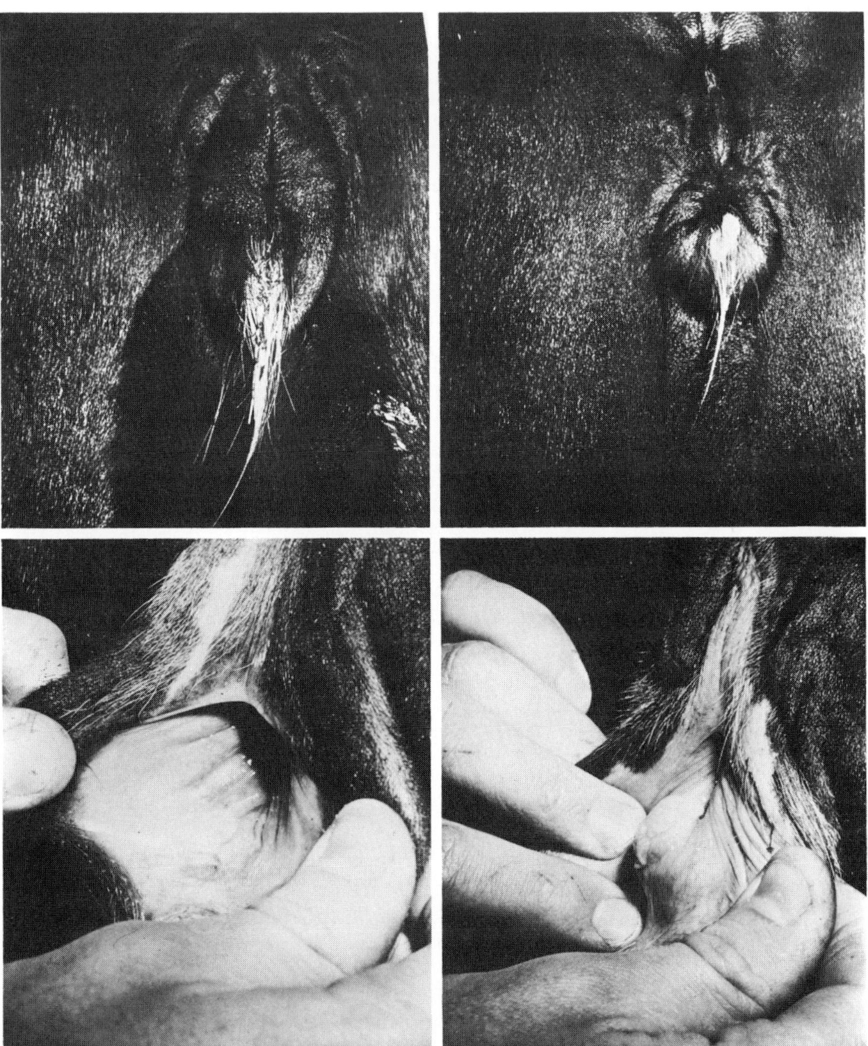

Fig. 16.4 Changes observed in the external genitalia of one-year-old heifers implanted with 300 mg trenbolone acetate at 4 months and again at 7 months of age. Above are the vulva of control (left) and treated (right) animals, below are the clitoris in control (left) and implanted (right) animals, respectively.

Trenbolone acetate has also been shown to interfere with oestrous cycling in mature cows (Heitzman *et al* 1977a) and to reduce the number of oestrogen receptors in the uterus of young calves (Kryein & Hoffman 1976). Thus, anabolic agents which are potent androgens should not be used in female animals intended for breeding purposes.

Public health considerations

The greatest potential hazard from the use of anabolic agents is that meat products from treated animals may contain amounts of the agent or its derived metabolites (residues) which are harmful to the consumer. (Residues are defined as the amount of the anabolic agent (parent compound) and its metabolites remaining in the tissues at any given time.) The metabolism of an agent in farm animals can be quite different from its metabolism in laboratory animals and man and thus it is essential that the residues of the anabolic agent are fully defined.

The metabolism of oestradiol (Hendricks & Torrence 1977, Dunn *et al* 1977, Bottoms *et al* 1977) and progesterone (Estergreen *et al* 1977) in farm animals has been thoroughly investigated and the residues identified. However, not all of the metabolites of the stilbene derivatives and zeranol have been identified.

An example of the between-species differences in the metabolism of an anabolic agent is summarised in Table 16.5. Trenbolone acetate (17β) is excreted in the bile of rats as metabolites with either a 17β-hydroxy or 17-ketone functional group; however, in cows, the major metabolites are derivatives of 17 α-hydroxy trenbolone.

Table 16.5 Metabolites of trenbolone acetate in bile of rats and cows. (Data from Pottier *et al* 1981.)

Functional group at 17 position	% Initial dose in bile	
	Rat	Cow
β-acetate	0	0
β-hydroxy	35	<1
α-hydroxy	<1	40
Ketone	23	3

Animals were administered H^3-trenbolone acetate as a pulse injection into a jugular vein. Bile was collected for 24 hours by a chronic catheterisation technique. The total recovery of radioactivity in bile over a 24-hour period was 80% and 84% from a heifer and rats, respectively.

Determination of residues

Although radiotracer studies provide the methods of choice for investigations of absorption, excretion, total residues, and metabolites (Aschbacher *et al* 1975, Pottier *et al* 1975, 1978), radioimmunoassay (RIA) and chromatographic methods are also used (Hoffman & Oettel 1976, Hoffman & Karg 1976, Heitzman & Harwood 1977, Harwood *et al* 1981, Hoffmann & Laschutza 1980).

Implants of anabolic agents are absorbed over several months and it is therefore likely that there will be residues in edible tissues, urine, faeces, and blood at slaughter. The concentration of residues in edible tissues is similar to that of the naturally-occurring sex steroids in farm animals and is <1 ppb. RIA is the only method sufficiently sensitive to measure these low levels and it is now possible, using RIA methods, to measure residues of DES, hexoestrol, dienoestrol, trenbolone, oestradiol, progesterone and testosterone in edible tissues, biological fluids, and faeces. A RIA method for zeranol is currently being developed (Dixon 1981).

Monitoring of residues in animals and tissues

Regulation of the use of anabolic steroids is difficult and requires a monitoring system covering both imported meat and animals sent for slaughter. Clearly, in those countries where millions of animals are slaughtered annually, only a small percentage can be monitored in detail. It is possible in some countries to operate a monitoring system but this can only be done where there is an efficient veterinary inspection of animals and carcases at the slaughterhouse and where there is a rapid analytical system available in the central laboratories.

Carcinogenicity of anabolic agents

The carcinogenicity of anabolic agents has been reviewed extensively in the IARC monograph (1974) and Roe (1976), in a short review, defines a carcinogen as '... an agent which under defined conditions increases the age-standardised risk of development of, or death from, one or other form of malignant disease as compared with matched control subjects or animals not exposed to the agent.' Roe concludes that, at very high dose levels, the anabolic agents DES, oestradiol, and testosterone are carcinogens and that there is not sufficient proof to confirm that trenbolone acetate, zeranol and melengestrol acetate are not carcinogens. The question must be asked whether the residues in animal products are at concentrations which would be carcinogenic to the consumer. In the case of the naturally-occurring steroids, testosterone, oestradiol and progesterone, this seems most unlikely but there is a potential hazard from residues of synthetic anabolic agents. The synthetic anabolic agents and their metabolites should perhaps be fully evaluated in long term, multi-generation laboratory animal studies. In France, anabolic agents are tested by so-called 'relay toxicity trials' (see Ferrando & Truhaut 1976) in which lyophilised meat from treated farm animals is fed to several generations of rats and any adverse effects recorded. The author believes this method represents a valuable assessment of risk because it is almost the only one which exposes the test animal to all the residues present in meat from treated animals.

Conclusions

Some countries restrict the use of anabolic agents because they believe there is a high risk to public health, while other nations allow their use believing the benefit outweighs the risk. Meat products will be deemed safe when it can be shown that:
1   there are negligible residues in the meat;
2   the concentration of residues of anabolic agents which are natural steroids are at levels similar to those found in farm animals; or
3   the residues of synthetic anabolic agents are known and demonstrated to be safe in terms of toxicity and carcinogenicity.

There are negligible hazards to animals associated with the use of anabolic agents for meat production but there are serious hazards when they are used in animals intended for breeding purposes.

Mode of action of anabolic agents

The exact modes of action of anabolic agents still remain unclear and it is difficult to identify a simple single mode of action. The common action of all anabolic agents is to increase nitrogen retention. Nitrogen balance studies have confirmed that anabolic agents with sex steroid-like activity, when administered parenterally, do increase nitrogen retention but they do not alter absorption or metabolism in the alimentary tract (Chan *et al* 1975).

Hormonal regulation of protein metabolism

In presenting current concepts of the way in which hormones regulate protein metabolism, it should be emphasised that most of the investigations have been carried out in laboratory animals. We do not know how far this work is applicable in farm animals.

Two modes of action of anabolic hormones can explain the increase in protein accretion in muscle tissue. Anabolic hormones can act directly on the muscle cell to regulate protein synthesis and degradation but they can also act indirectly by modification of a second growth-promoting hormone. Both are likely actions of the anabolic hormones.

An anabolic hormone in the vicinity of the muscle cell has two possible actions. Either it recognises a specific receptor on the cell surface and attaches itself to the outer surface membrane or it enters the cells where it combines with a specific cytoplasmic receptor to form a complex. In both cases it is the attachment to a specific receptor which initiates the events leading to increased protein accretion (for review see Mainwaring 1977).

It is thought that, in cells lacking specific receptors, there is little direct activity of the hormone. Thus, muscle cells must have specific receptors for either the primary hormone in the case of a direct action or for the secondary hormone in an indirect mode of action. An androgen receptor has been reported for rat muscle cells (Michel & Beaulieu 1976) and for porcine muscle cells (Snochowski *et al* 1981).

The distribution of receptors may be determined by the sex of the animal and this might explain the relative responses of the sexes to different sex steroids.

Protein accretion

Proteins are continually being synthesised and degraded in muscle cells and the rates of these processes determine the protein turnover rate. When synthesis exceeds degradation there is an increase in the net amount of protein and this is called protein accretion. However, protein accretion is a very inefficient process because of high turnover rates. Anabolic hormones are known to increase protein accretion and they may also reduce protein turnover rates (Vernon & Buttery 1976). This means that more protein is laid down at a lower energy cost. This action may explain why feed conversion efficiency is so dramatically improved by anabolic agents.

Mode of action of oestrogens

Considerable evidence supports the view that oestrogens (and progesterone) exert their primary effect at the level of chromatin transcription and gene expression in cell nuclei of particular target tissues. These include the uterus, liver, and chick oviduct. In contrast, little is known of the action of oestrogens in skeletal muscle. Studies to date indicate that oestrogens probably act through the secondary hormones, growth hormone, and insulin.

The combination of increased growth hormone (GH) and insulin concentration at the muscle cell is thought to increase protein accretion (Trenkle

1976). Injections of GH increase LWG in pigs and probably in young cattle as well (Machlin 1976).

The implantation of oestradiol-17β in wether sheep caused significant increases in the plasma concentration of GH and insulin (Donaldson 1977). A similar effect was observed with DES in cattle (Trenkle 1976). The primary action of the oestrogen is thought to be on a factor controlling the secretion of GH from the pituitary. The effects on growth of exogenous oestrogen and GH are similar and it is concluded that one of the main actions of oestrogens, especially in castrate males, is the increased production of GH and insulin.

Mode of action of androgens

The evidence is not conclusive but it is possible that androgens act directly on the muscle cell (Young & Pluskal 1977, Mainwaring 1977). Androgens regulate protein synthesis and degradation, promoting protein accretion and decreasing protein turnover rate (Vernon & Buttery 1976). Ranaweera (1978) suggested that they are more anticatabolic than anti-anabolic. Mainwaring (1977) has reviewed the possible mechanisms of action of androgens when they enter their target cells and form complexes with specific androgen receptors. These complexes can enter the nucleus of the cell and alter DNA replication and stimulate RNA synthesis, which in turn modifies protein synthesis.

A second possible mode of action is on the rate of protein degradation. Androgens, but not oestrogens, are known to displace corticosteroids from their receptor sites (Mayer & Rosen 1975). Corticosteroids are potent catabolic agents and may serve a regulatory and suppressive role in normal growth. It is not inconceivable that androgens may limit this role in animals by substitution at the receptor site. However, other workers have found that there is very little competition between androgens and corticosteroids for the same binding sites in pig muscle cells (Snochowski *et al* 1981).

A third possible mode of action of androgens is that they act indirectly by regulating the circulating levels of thyroxine. It is known that total circulating levels of thyroxine are dramatically decreased both in cattle (Heitzman *et al* 1977) and sheep (Donaldson 1977) in the presence of androgens. More recently it was shown by Heitzman *et al* (1980) that the levels of thyroxine binding globulin were not reduced in androgen-treated steers and heifers, but the free thyroxine index was significantly decreased (Fig. 16.5). Thus the free active thyroid hormones are lowered and this may be a factor in regulating protein turnover in muscle cells.

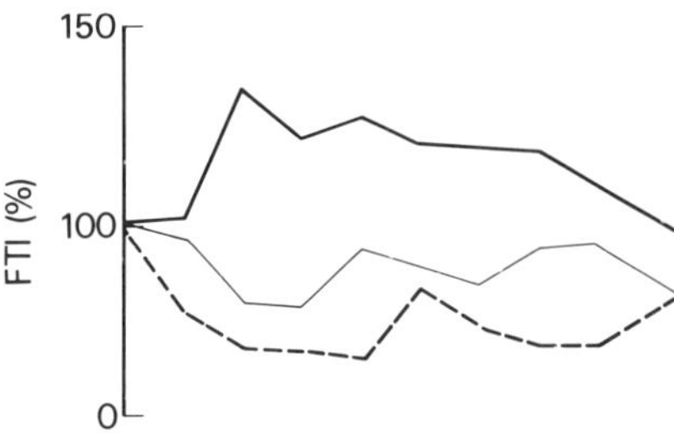

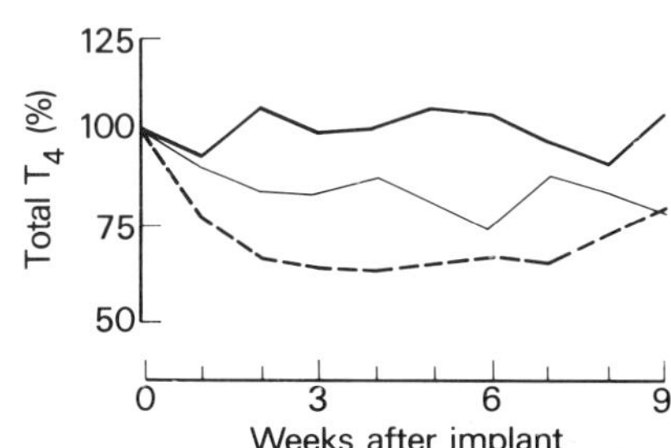

Fig. 16.5 The free thyroid index (FTI) and total plasma concentration of thyroxine (T₄) as a percentage of the value observed before implantation. There were three steers in each group and the treatments were — control; — 20 mg oestradiol-17β plus 140 mg trenbolone acetate; and ---- 300 mg trenbolone acetate.

Conclusions

The proposed differing modes of action of androgens and oestrogens in the regulation of protein metabolism offer biochemical support for the hypothesis that, to obtain maximum growth, the optimum steroid treatment would maintain maximum physiological concentrations of both androgens and oestrogens in circulating body fluids.

References

Aschbacher P. W., Thacker E. J. & Rumsey T. S. (1975) Metabolic fate of diethylstilboestrol implanted in the ear of steers. *J. Anim. Sci.* **40,** 530.

Beranger C. & Malterre C. (1968) Influence d'un stéroide trienique à activité anabolisante sur l'egraissement des vachesteries. *C. R. Soc. Biol. de Clemont Ferrand* **162,** 1157.

Best J. M. J. (1972) The use of trenbolone acetate implants in heifer beef production at pasture. *Vet. Rec.* **91,** 264.

Bottoms G. D., Coppoc G. L., Monk E. *et al* (1977) Metabolic fate of orally administered estradiol in swine. *J. Anim. Sci.* **45,** 674.

Burris M. J., Bogart R. A., Oliver A. W. *et al* (1952) The effects of testosterone propionate on rate of gain, feed efficiency and carcass quality of beef heifers and steers. *J. Anim. Sci.* **39,** 170.

Chan K. H., Heitzman R. J. & Kitchenham B. A. (1975) Digestibility and N-balance studies on growing heifers implanted with trienbolone acetate. *Br. Vet. J.* **131,** 170.

Coelho J. F. S., Galbraith H. & Topps J. H. (1978) The effect of a combination of trienbolone acetate and 17β-oestradiol on the performance, carcass composition and blood characteristics of castrated male lambs. *Anim. Prod.* **26,** 360.

Dixon S. N. (1981) Radioimmunoassay of the anabolic agent zeranol. I. Preparation and proprties of a specific antibody to zeranol. *J. Vet. Pharmacol. & Therap.* **3**, 177.

Donaldson I. A. (1977) The action of anabolic steroids on nitrogen metabolism and the endocrine system in ruminants. PhD thesis, University of Reading.

Dunn T. G., Kaltenbach C. C., Kortinik D. R. *et al* (1977) Metabolites of estradiol-17β and estradiol-17β-benzoate in bovine tissues. *J. Anim. Sci.* **45**, 65.

Estergreen C. V. L., Lin M. T., Martin E. L. *et al* (1977) Distribution of progesterone and its metabolites in cattle tissues following administration of progesterone-4-^{14}C. *J. Anim. Sci.* **45**, 642.

Ferrando R. & Truhaut R. (1976) Considerations toxicologiques specialies sur les anabolisants toxicite de relais. In *Anabolic Agents in Animal Production.* F. C. Lu & J. Rendel (eds.), Environmental Quality and Safety.

Fowler V. R., Stockdale C. L., Smart R. I. *et al* (1978) Effects of two androgens combined with oestrogen on the growth and efficiency of feeds. *Anim. Prod.* **26**, 358.

Galbraith H. (1979) Growth, metabolic and hormonal response in blood of British Friesian entire male cattle treated with trenbolone acetate and hexoestrol. *Anim. Prod.* **28**, 417 (Abs. 14).

Galbraith H. (1980) The effect of trenbolone acetate on growth, blood hormones and metabolites, and nitrogen balance of beef heifers. *Anim. Prod.* **30**, 389.

Harwood D. J., Heitzman R. J. & Jouquey A. (1981) A radioimmunoassay method for the measurement of residues of the anabolic agent hexoestrol in tissues of cattle and sheep. *J. Vet. Pharmacol. & Therap.* **3**, 245.

Heitzman R. J. (1976) The effectiveness of anabolic agents in increasing the growth rate of farm animals; report on experiments in cattle. In *Anabolic Agents in Animal Production.* F. C. Lu & J. Rendel (eds.), Environmental Quality and Safety, Suppl. V, p. 89.

Heitzman R. J. & Chan K. H. (1974) Alterations in weight gain and levels of plasma metabolites, proteins, insulin and free fatty acids following implantation of an anabolic steroid in heifers. *Br. Vet. J.* **130**, 532.

Heitzman R. J., Chan K. H. & Hart I. C. (1977) Liveweight gains, blood levels of metabolites, proteins and hormones following implantation of anabolic agents in steers. *Br. Vet. J.* **133**, 62.

Heitzman R. J., Donaldson I. A. & Hart I. C. (1980) Effect of anabolic steroids on plasma thyroid hormones in steers and heifers. *Br. Vet. J.* **136**, 168.

Heitzman R. J., Gibbons D. N., Little W. *et al* (1981) A note on the comparative performance of beef steers implanted with the anabolic steroids trenbolone acetate and oestradiol-17β, alone or in combination. *Anim. Prod.* **32**, 219.

Heitzman R. J. & Harwood D. J. (1977) Residue levels of trenbolone and oestradiol-17β in plasma and tissues of steers implanted with anabolic steroid preparations. *Br. Vet. J.* **133**, 564.

Heitzman R. J., Harwood D. J., Kay R. M. *et al* (1979) The effects of implanting prepuberal dairy heifers with anabolic steroids on hormonal status, puberty and parturition. *J. Anim. Sci.* **48**, 859.

Heitzman R. J., Harwood D. J. & Mallinson C. B. (1977a) The effect of an anabolic steroid, trenbolone acetate, on oestrus cycling in dairy cows. *Abs. XIth Acta Endocrinol. Congress.* p. 42.

Heitzman R. J., Harwood D. J. & Mallinson C. B. (1977b) Liveweight gain in steers treated with single or repeated implants of trenbolone acetate and hexoestrol. *Abs. 69th Ann. Mtg. Am. Soc. Anim. Sci.* p. 44.

Hendricks D. M. & Torrance A. K. (1977) Endogenous estrogens in bovine tissues. *J. Anim. Sci.* **45**, 652.

Hoffman B. & Karg H. (1976) Metabolic fate of an anabolic agent in treated animals and residue levels in their meat. In *Anabolic Agents in Animal Production.* F. C. Lu & J. Rendel, (eds.) Environmental Quality and Safety, Suppl. V, p. 181.

Hoffman B. & Laschutza W. (1980) Entwicklung eines Radio-immunotests zur Bestimmung von Diäthylstilböstrol im Blutplasma und essbaren Geweben vom Rind. *Archiv. für Lebensm. Hygiene.* **31,** 77.

Hoffman V. & Oettel G. (1976) Radioimmunoassays for free and conjugated trienbolone and for trienbolone acetate in bovine tissues and plasma samples. *Steroids* **27,** 509.

I.A.R.C. (1974) International Agency for Research on Cancer Monographs on the Evaluation of Carcinogenic Risk of Chemicals to Man: *Sex Hormones.* **6,** 1.

Kyrein H. F. & Hoffman B. (1976) In vitro und in vivo Beeinflussung uteriner cytoplasmatischer Östrogenrezeptoren bei weiblichen Kälbern durch hormonale Anabolika. *Adv. Anim. Phys. Nutr.* **6,** 91.

Machlin L. J. (1976) Role of growth hormone in improving animal production. In *Anabolic Agents in Animal Production.* F. C. Lu & J. Rendel, (eds.). Environmental Quality and Safety, Suppl. V, p. 43.

Mainwaring P. (1977) In *The Mechanism of Action of Androgens.* Springer Verlag, New York.

Mayer M. & Rosen F. (1975) Interaction of anabolic steroids with glucocorticoid receptor sites in rat muscle cytosol. *Am. J. Phys.* **229,** 1381.

Michel G. & Beaulieu E. E. (1976) An approach to the anabolic action of androgens by an experimental system. In *Anabolic Agents in Animal Production.* F. C. Lu & J. Rendel, (eds.). Environmental Quality and Safety, Suppl. V, p. 54.

Nesheim M. C. (1976) Some observations on the effectiveness of anabolic agents in increasing the growth rate of poultry. In *Anabolic Agents in Animal Production.* F. C. Lu & J. Rendel, (eds.). Environmental Quality and Safety, Suppl. V, p. 110.

Neville W. E., Williams D. J. & Witherspoon D. M. (1974) Effect of hormones on certain factors affecting reproduction in prepuberal Hereford heifers. *Am. J. Vet. Res.* **35,** 1057.

Pierson R. E., Jensen R., Braddy P. M. *et al* (1976) Bulling among feedlot steers. *J. Am. Vet. Med. Assoc.* **169,** 521.

Pottier J., Busigny M. & Grandadam J. A. (1975) Plasma kinetics, excretion in milk and tissue levels in the cow following implantation of trenbolone acetate. *J. Anim. Sci.* **41,** 962.

Pottier J., Heitzman R. J., Cousty C. *et al* (1981) Metabolites of trenbolone acetate in the bile of the cow and the rat. *Xenobiotics* **11,** 489.

Ranaweera P. (1978) The effects of trienbolone acetate in growing turkeys. DPhil thesis, University of Cambridge.

Ranaweera K. N. P. & Wise D. R. (1981) The effects of trienbolone acetate on carcass composition, conformation and skeletal growth of turkeys. *Br. Poult. Sci.* **22,** 105.

Roe F. J. (1976) Carcinogenicity studies in animals relevant to the use of anabolic agents in animal production. In *Anabolic Agents in Animal Production,* F. C. Lu & J. Rendel, (eds.). Environmental Quality and Safety, Suppl. V, p. 227.

Snochowski M., Lundstrom K., Dahlberg E *et al* (1981) Androgen and glucocorticoid receptors in porcine skeletal muscle. *J. Anim. Sci.* **53,** 80.

Stollard R. J., Kilkenny J. B., Kathieson A. A. *et al* (1977) The response to anabolic steroids in finishing steers. *Anim. Prod.* **24,** 132.

Szumowski P. & Grandadam J. A. (1976) Comparison des effets du diéthylstilboestrol (DES) et de l'acetate de trenbolone (TBA) seul ou associé à l'oestradiol-17β (TBA-E) sur le croissance et l'engraissement des ruminants. *Rec. Vet. Med.* **152,** 311.

Trenkle A. (1976) The anabolic effect of oestrogens on nitrogen metabolism of growing and finishing cattle and sheep. In *Anabolic Agents in Animal Production.* F. C. Lu & J. Rendel, (eds.). Environmental Quality and Safety, Suppl. V, p. 79.

Van der Wal P. (1976) General aspects of the effectiveness of anabolic agents in increasing protein production in farm animals, in particular in bull calves. In *Anabolic Agents in Animal Production,* F. C. Lu & J. Rendel, (eds.). Environmental Quality and Safety, Suppl. V, p. 60.

Van der Wal P., Berende P. M. & Sprietsma J. E. (1975) Effect of anabolic agents on performance of calves. *J. Anim. Sci.* **41,** 978.

Van Weerden E. J. & Grandadam J. A. (1976) The effect of an anabolic agent on N-deposition, growth and slaughter quality in growing castrated male pigs. In *Anabolic Agents in Animal Production*, F. C. Lu & J. Rendel, (eds.). Environmental Quality and Safety, Suppl. V, p. 115.

Vernon B. G. & Buttery P. J. (1976) Protein turnover in rats treated with trienbolone acetate. *Br. J. Nutr.* **36,** 575.

Young V. R. & Pluskal M. G. (1977) Mode of action of anabolic agents, with special reference to steroids and skeletal muscle: a summary review. Abs. 2nd Int. Symp. on Protein Metabolism and Nutrition. *Eur. Ass. Anim. Prod.* (Biddinghuizen).

17

Fluid therapy in calves

W. VANDAELE

Although diarrhoea is important in all young animals, the problem has been studied most extensively in calves, probably because dehydration as a consequence of diarrhoea in calves is still an important cause of death (Edwards & Williams 1972). Indeed, in many European countries, 10% of newborn calves are lost each year.

Treatment of the diarrhoeic animal is always a complex problem and a multitude of different drugs are still used. They include antibiotics, sulphonamides, intestinal protectants, steroids, antihistamines, drugs to decrease intestinal motility and others to increase motility. Their efficacy appears to be inconsistent. For example, it is frequently recommended that antibiotics be administered parenterally, although their chief benefit when given in this way must be to prevent secondary infections, such as pneumonia, which are likely to occur because the resistance of the affected animal is greatly reduced. Anticholinergic agents and other drugs intended to decrease intestinal motility are contraindicated. Current evidence from both clinical and laboratory sources demonstrates that the gut becomes hypomotile in cases of diarrhoea: necropsy of an animal affected by acute scours reveals an intestine generally filled with fluid, very flaccid, and with no muscular tone. In France, Dardillet & Ruckebusch (1973) confirmed this clinical observation by means of electromyographic recordings from the intestine. All types of normal intestinal activity (peristaltic, propulsive, mixing) decline substantially in the diarrhoeic calf.

The first essential in the treatment of the diarrhoeic calf is provision of a suitable environment. The calf must be removed from cold, wet conditions, dried off and made warm. The second essential is to replace depleted body fluids and electrolytes. Although parenteral administration of water and electrolytes has been the classic method of rehydration, more recently the technique of oral administration of electrolytes has been developed, and early doubts of the efficacy of the oral technique have now been dispelled (Lewis 1975, Vandaele 1976, 1977). In this chapter the pathophysiology of fluid and electrolyte losses and appropriate fluid therapy will be considered in detail. Other facets of the management and treatment of diarrhoea in the calf are dealt with in Chapter 18.

Pathophysiological aspects of diarrhoea

The clinician needs to know how much fluid he should administer, the route by which he should administer it, and what the composition of the replacement fluid should be. The correct decisions can only be taken in the light of knowledge of the effects of diarrhoea upon fluid and electrolyte balance. These effects can be classified into three categories: water depletion, metabolic disturbances, and electrolyte imbalances.

Secretion and absorption both occur continuously through the entire ten metre length of the small intestine of the calf, absorption taking place primarily at the villus tips and secretion primarily in the crypts. Normally, 98% of ingested fluid is absorbed. Diarrhoea reduces absorption and increases secretion (Figs. 17.1–17.5) (Moon 1978).

Water depletion

Whereas water comprises approximately 70% of the weight of an adult animal, it represents between 73 and 85% of the weight of a calf (Fayet 1968,

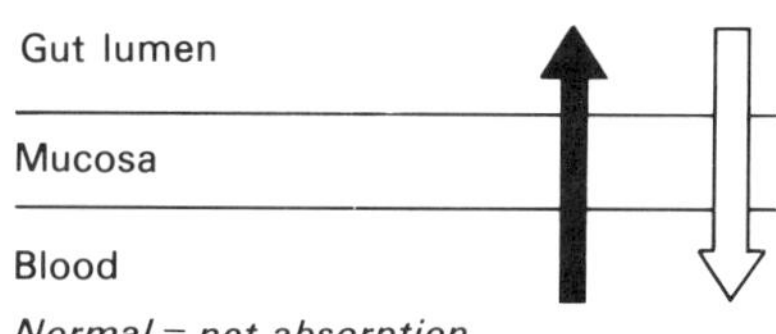

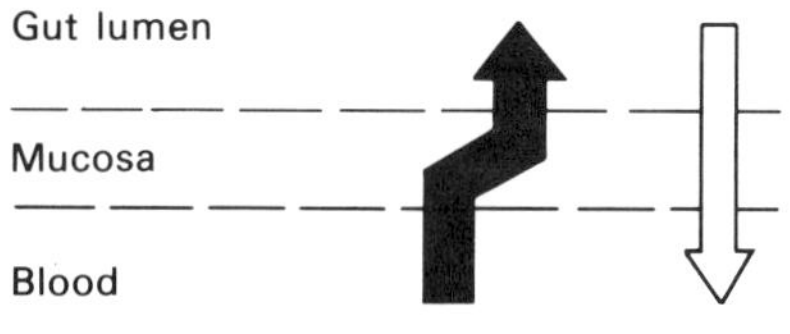

Fig. 17.1 Bidirectional water and electrolyte fluxes across intestinal mucosa. Normally, flux from lumen > flux to lumen = net absorption.

Fig. 17.2 Increased pore size of inflamed intestinal mucosa results in flux to lumen > flux from lumen. If pores are large enough to accommodate plasma proteins, exudation occurs.

Fig. 17.3 Crypt–villus unit in small intestines. Villous epithelial cells are the mature or oldest part of the population. They are differentiated to digest and absorb. The young undifferentiated crypt epithelial cells proliferate and are currently thought to be the major secretory cells of the intestines. Normally, flux from intestinal lumen to blood across villous epithelium > flux from blood to intestinal lumen across crypt epithelium = net absorption.

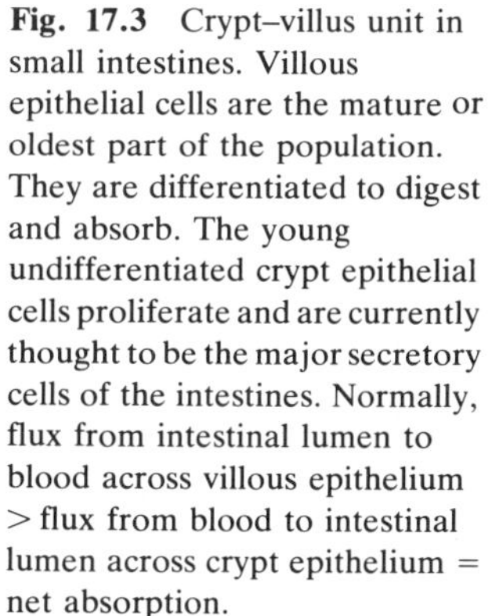

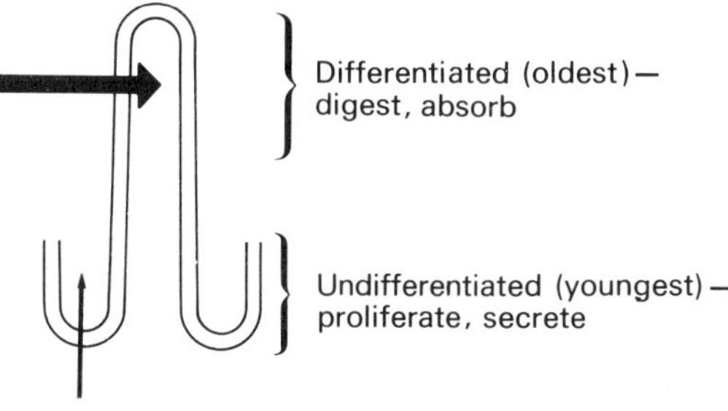

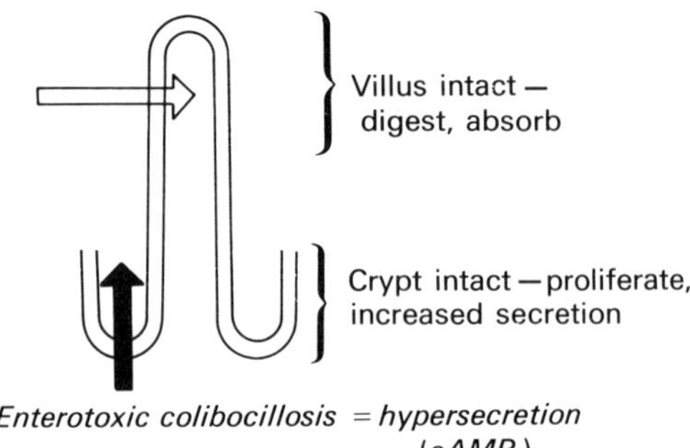

Fig. 17.4 Hypersecretory crypt–villus unit in enterotoxic colibacillosis. Villous epithelium and function are intact. However, increased secretory flux exceeds absorptive capacity. Hypersecretion probably occurs in crypts and is thought to be mediated by increased cellular cyclic adenosine monophosphate (cAMP).

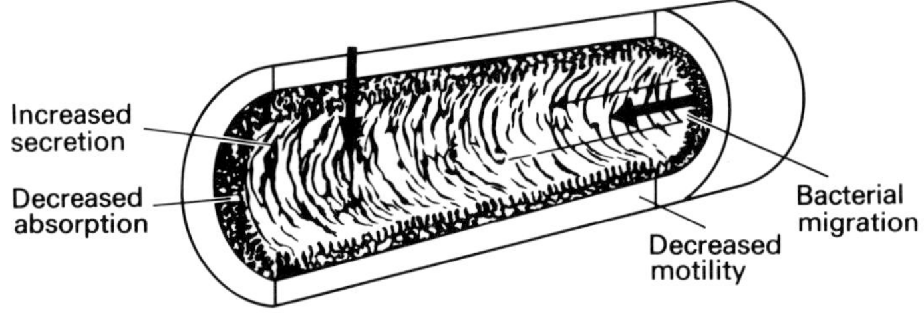

Fig. 17.5 Intestinal alterations as a result of diarrhoea. Either increased secretion or decreased absorption or both may occur. There is generally an increase in bacterial colonisation and a decrease in motility (Phillips & Lewis 1971).

Phillips & Lewis 1973). In an adult animal, 50% of body weight is intracellular fluid and 20% is extracellular fluid (15% interstitial water and 5% plasma; Fig. 17.6) but in a young calf the extracellular fraction is much greater, accounting for about 45% of body weight, whilst only about 30% is accounted for by intracellular fluid (Fayet 1978).

Diarrhoea may be regarded as a consequence of a lack of absorption of sodium and other electrolytes. This reduction in sodium absorption reduces the osmolarity of extracellular fluid. When this occurs, water from the interstitial and vascular compartments flows into the lumen of the gut, in response to the osmotic pressure gradient across the gut wall. 'Dehydration' therefore occurs from a loss of water, sodium, and chloride ions from the extracellular compartment and, in fact, preferentially from the blood vascular system (Fig. 17.7).

Calves require large volumes of water even when healthy. For example, calves of 100 kg need approximately 10 l/day. Such a calf would produce 8500 calories daily from metabolism when placed in a warm environment and thus it would need to eliminate 8.3 l water a day for temperature regulation, to which must be added a minimum of 1 l for urine production and 0.8 l for cell anabolism (Espinasse 1977).

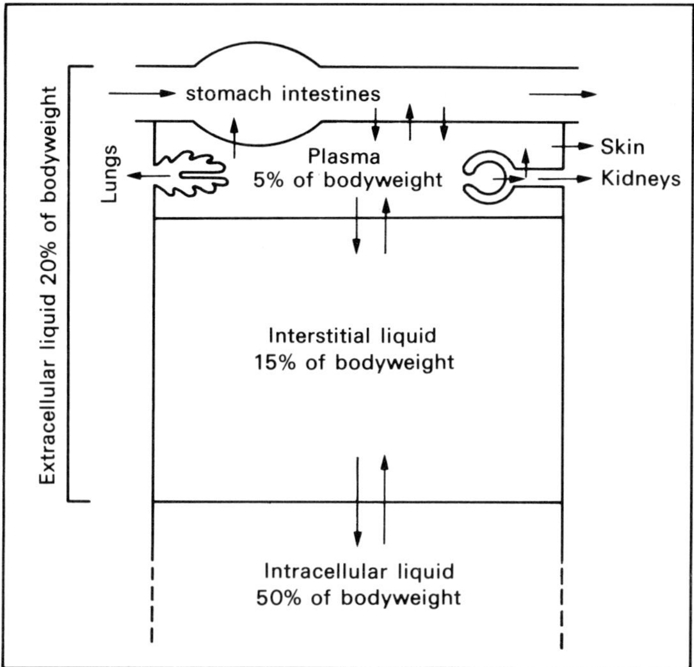

Fig. 17.6 Liquid compartments of the body. Arrows indicate water movements (Gamble 1954).

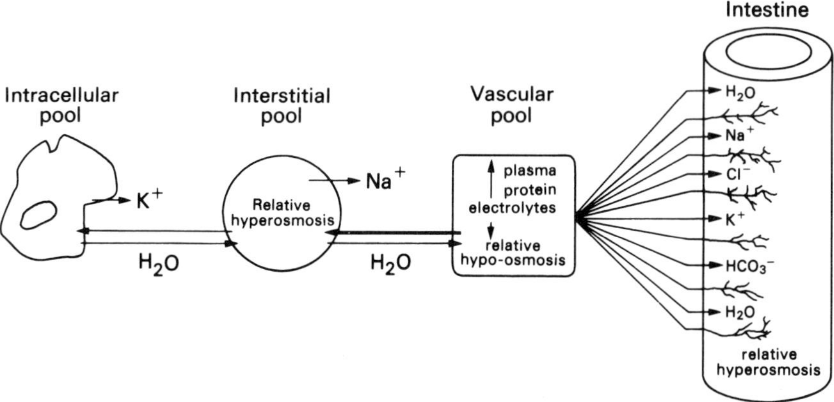

Fig. 17.7 A possible mechanism for preferential plasma fluid losses. Both water and electrolytes are lost from the body during diarrhoea, but the plasma electrolyte losses in excess of total body losses cause a relative hyposmosis in this compartment. This results in fluid being preferentially lost from the blood vascular system (Phillips & Lewis 1971).

The metabolic water requirement is greater in young animals than in adults because it is correlated with body surface area rather than body weight. For instance, an adult animal of 500 kg has an extracellular water volume of 100 l which is only 3–4 times the volume in a young calf although its body weight is ten times greater (Barragry 1974).

The extent of dehydration in water-depleted subjects can be estimated on the basis of body weight loss (Barragry 1974). There are several potential causes of water depletion. *1 Increased water content of the faeces.* The faeces of the normal calf contain 70–80% water but, in diarrhoea, the water content increases to 90–95% (Phillips *et al* 1973). In addition, the total volume of faeces is increased at least six-fold (Fayet 1968) and sometimes as much as thirty-fold (Fisher 1972) in diarrhoeic calves. Based on these figures, Phillips *et al* (1973) estimated that in calves with diarrhoea 96% of the body weight loss was water loss. *2 A reduction in milk intake.* Fisher & Martinez (1976) considered the reduction in milk uptake to be the most important reason for water loss. *3 Respiratory loss.* Respiration leading to loss of water by lung evaporation continues in the diarrhoeic animal and the process may be accelerated by the presence of fever or in a hot, dry environment.

The consequences of these losses (see Fig. 17.7) are, firstly increases in haematocrit, blood viscosity and plasma protein concentration (Phillips *et al* 1971, Phillips & Lewis 1973, Tennant *et al* 1972); secondly decrease in plasma osmolarity as a consequence of losses of electrolytes, especially sodium, which has an important role in the maintenance of osmotic pressure (Fayet 1971, Phillips *et al* 1971, Phillips & Lewis 1973); lastly at a later stage peripheral vasoconstriction induced by a decrease in blood volume and blood pressure (Phillips *et al* 1971). This is clinically detectable as coldness of the extremities and is accompanied by an increase in cellular catabolism (Michell 1967).

Metabolic disturbances

The most important change is acidosis, blood pH falling from 7.34–7.40 to 6.85–7.15 (Fayet 1968, Fisher 1965, Fisher & de la Cuente 1972, Tennant *et al* 1972) because of a number of factors.

1   A loss of bicarbonate ion (HCO_3^-) in the faeces (Lewis & Phillips 1972, Phillips & Knox 1969, Whitten & Phillips 1971). This loss leads to generation of H^+ from plasma bicarbonate, thus:

$$CO_2 + H_2O = H_2CO_3 = H^+ + HCO_3^- \text{ (intestinal loss).}$$

2   Production of lactic acid by anaerobic glycolysis (Oliva 1970) as a consequence of tissue hypoxia in both extracellular and intracellular compartments (Lewis & Phillips 1973). The hypoxia, in turn, is caused by reduced peripheral blood flow. The lactic acid ionises to produce lactate and hydrogen ions.

3 Not only is lactate production increased (Tennant *et al* 1972), but hepatic metabolism of lactate is reduced because of hepatocellular damage resulting from passive venous congestion. In consequence, blood lactate levels rise even further.
4 Organic acids are produced by the abnormal intestinal flora (Michell 1974).
5 When hypovolaemic shock occurs, respiratory function is also compromised and further retention of H^+ follows.

In addition to acidosis, in cases of dehydration, hypoglycaemia (Lewis *et al* 1975, Tennant & Reina Guerra 1968, Tennant *et al* 1972), and uraemia (Tennant *et al* 1972) also occur.

Electrolyte losses and imbalances

Fig. 17.8 and Table 17.1 show the diarrhoea-associated changes in electrolyte balance demonstrated by workers in the USA in calves and Table 17.2 illustrates further data obtained from a French study. Whilst the American study describes the changes which occur in the whole animal, the French study reports plasma concentrations of electrolytes.

The most widely documented electrolyte losses are of sodium and bicarbonate ions. Sodium concentrations in plasma fall from 135–140 mEq/l to 125–130 mEq/l and bicarbonate from 25–30 mEq/l to 8–15 mEq/l. The rapid transit of intestinal contents and loss of intestinal secretions lead also to a loss of potassium or, at least, to a marked reduction in net potassium gain in those animals which continue to feed.

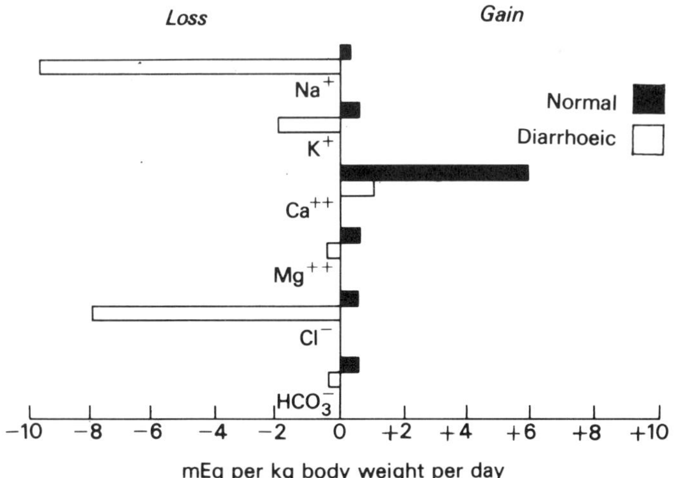

Fig. 17.8 Changes in body electrolyte balance as a result of acute infectious diarrhoea in six calves, as measured by radioactive tracer techniques (Lewis & Phillips 1972).

Table 17.1 Water * and electrolyte ** balance in normal and diarrhoeic calves (Lewis & Phillips 1972).

	Normal	Diarrhoeic	Number of calves (normal — diarrhoeic)
Total water	+ 22.3 ± 5.6	− 72.3 ± 8.8	8 — 8
Insensible water	− 16.8 ± 0.7	− 16.8 ± 0.7	7 — 7
Sodium	+ 8.4 ± 2.5	−235.2 ± 45.8	6 — 8
Potassium	+ 28.8 ± 9.6	− 65.5 ± 15.0	8 — 8
Chloride	+ 20.4 ± 11.8	−280.4 ± 65.8	8 — 6
Calcium	+121.6 ± 30.6	+ 22.1 ± 7.9	3 — 3
Magnesium	+ 7.4 ± 3.0	− 5.7 ± 0.4	3 — 3
% body weight change/day	+ 0.9 ± 0.4	− 7.9 ± 1.8	8 — 8

*In g per kg body weight per day (mean ± s.e.)
**In mg per kg body weight per day (mean ± s.e.)

Table 17.2 Plasma concentrations (mmol) of Na^+, K^+, Cl^- and HCO_3^- and plasma pH in 20 normal and 30 diarrhoeic calves (Fayet 1968).

	Normal calves	Diarrhoeic calves	Statistical significance
Na^+	140 ± 4.1	129 ± 4.8	$p<0.001$
K^+	5.2 ± 0.6	6.2 ± 1.8	$p<0.01$
Cl^-	100 ± 4	106 ± 10	$p<0.05$
HCO_3^-	26.3 ± 2.7	14.8 ± 3.9	$p<0.001$
pH blood	7.34 ± 0.03	7.15 ± 0.09	$p<0.001$

Fig. 17.9 illustrates how the changes in electrolyte balance interact at the cellular level. It will be seen that acidosis tends to increase the degree of potassium loss from the intracellular compartment. The decrease in intracellular potassium levels is particularly detrimental because a normal concentration of this ion is necessary to maintain the normal electrical potential across the cell membrane. The effect of decreasing membrane potential is manifested clinically by muscle weakness, lethargy and cardiac dysfunction, as indicated by bradycardia, arrhythmias and other electrocardiographic changes (Lewis 1977).

This review is primarily concerned with fluid therapy in the diarrhoeic animal but the general principles of fluid replacement are the same for horses that have become dehydrated as a result of exercise (Lewis 1977). The competition horse, for instance, experiences the same predominant loss of water from extracellular fluid as the diarrhoeic calf, and the major electrolyte

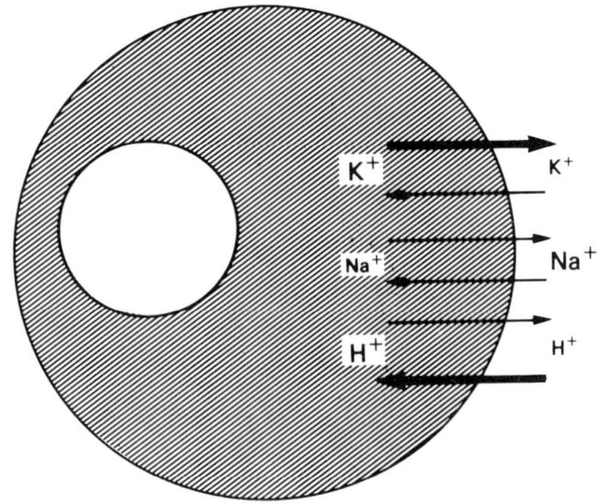

Fig. 17.9 Tissue buffering in acidosis. As a result of the increased hydrogen ion concentration in extracellular fluid, these ions move into the cells. This movement of positively charged ions causes potassium ions to move out of the cells to maintain electrical neutrality (Lewis & Phillips 1971).

losses are also very similar. Calcium losses may be more severe, resulting in hypocalcaemic tetany. Physiologically, exercise alters intestinal absorption because sympathetic nervous system activity reduces gastrointestinal blood flow during periods of exertion.

Therapeutic aspects of diarrhoea

Initially one must evaluate the degree of dehydration and then follow a rehydration 'plan'. Donawich & Christie (1971) proposed a simple system based on the weight of the animal and the extent of dehydration, expressed as a percentage of body weight loss. Initial weight of the animal × % dehydration would equal litres lost and/or quantity of fluid to be given. For example, a calf of 50 kg with a 5% loss in weight would receive 50 × 0.05 = 2.5 l. An approximate estimate of the degree of dehydration can be made on the basis of clinical signs as follows:

slight dehydration — loss of 2.5–5% of weight (Watt 1965)

moderate dehydration — loss of 5–10% of weight

severe dehydration — loss greater than 10% of weight.

On this basis, Lewis (1978) developed a table of clinical signs by which the degree of dehydration can be assessed (Table 17.3, Fig. 17.10).

In calculating the volume of fluid to be given, it is most important to remember to replace the continuing fluid losses since sick animals with diarrhoea are usually anorectic. It is therefore essential to meet continuing daily water and electrolyte requirements until such time as normal oral intake is resumed. As indicated above, a 100 kg calf may require as much as 10 l/day.

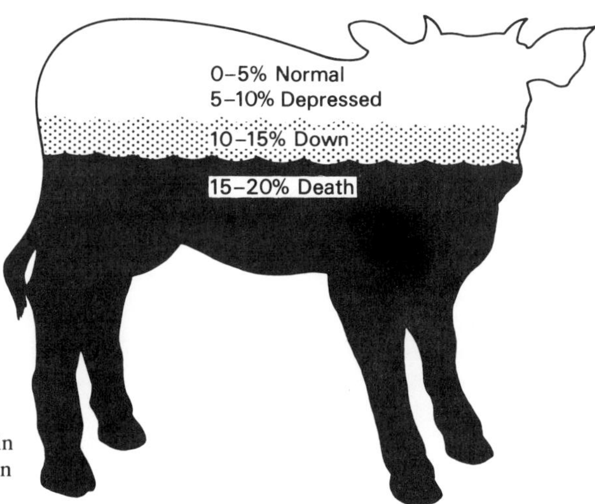

Fig. 17.10 Relationships
between percentage decreases in
body weight and clinical signs in
diarrhoeic calves.

Table 17.3 Clinical signs associated with various degrees of dehydration in the diarrhoeic calf
(Lewis 1978).

% loss in body weight	Clinical signs
0–5	None
6	Loss of skin elasticity, dry mouth, injected conjunctiva
8	Enophthalmous and increase in previous signs
10	Legs and oral cavity noticeably colder than rest of body, unable to stand and increase in previous signs
12	Shock, lying in lateral recumbency, unable to sit up unassisted and increase in previous signs
12 +	Fatal

The route of administration used in treatment depends on the calf's
condition, as indicated in Fig. 17.11.

Oral fluid therapy for the diarrhoeic calf

Early in dehydration or diarrhoea, oral therapy is often successful in replacing
lost body fluids and in meeting the calf's requirements until recovery. It is
always the route of choice unless there is persistent vomiting or upper
gastrointestinal tract obstruction, or under conditions so acute or so severe

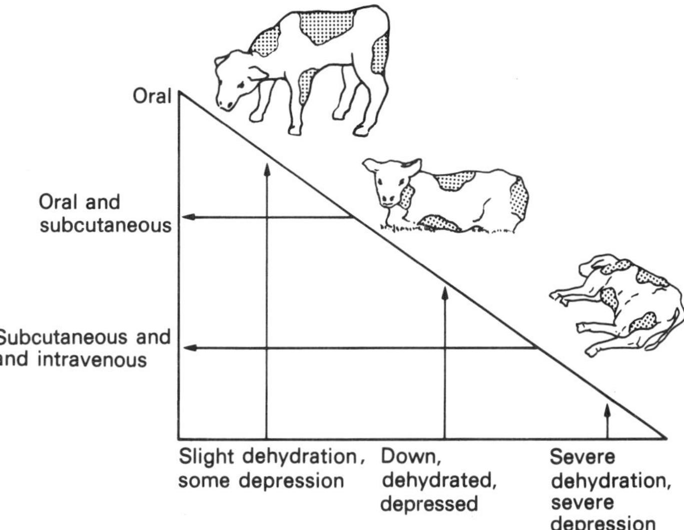

Fig. 17.11 Route of fluid therapy.

that the rate of intestinal absorption may not be sufficiently rapid to save the animal's life. In general, an animal with simple diarrhoea is likely to respond favourably to oral fluid administration, provided the degree of dehydration is 8% or less. Such treatment will suffice, for example, in cases of increased intestinal secretion, such as those due to *E. coli* enterotoxin, and in most but not all cases caused by a decrease in intestinal absorption, e.g. salmonellosis. It is the route of choice for several reasons: 1 The fluids are absorbed over a period of time, thus providing the animal with a sustained level of fluid input. 2 It is the safest route, in that the patient is able to absorb just those electrolytes which it requires, so there is little danger of overdosage. 3 Oral fluids do not need to be sterile and this greatly reduces costs. 4 The method is simple and the owner can initiate treatment himself as soon as he detects a case of diarrhoea, thus enabling an early start to treatment.

Factors affecting absorption

Next, it is necessary to consider how the fluid should be constituted to ensure maximum absorption. In order to derive the greatest benefit from oral fluids, formulations are required that utilise the interplay and synergistic effects that electrolytes and nutrients have on the absorption of each other and of water. Water absorption is a passive process, following entirely from the absorption of solutes. Thus, to obtain maximum water absorption, the fluid should be prepared to give maximum solute absorption. Solutes known to have a

Table 17.4 Concentrations of solutes (mmol/l) for optimal intestinal absorption (Lewis 1975).

Solute	Concentration
Glucose	1% or greater
Sodium	118
Glycine and imino amino acids	60–120
Other neutral amino acids	60–120
Bicarbonate	30 or greater
For diarrhoea therapy add:	
Additional bicarbonate	30–60
Potassium	25–30

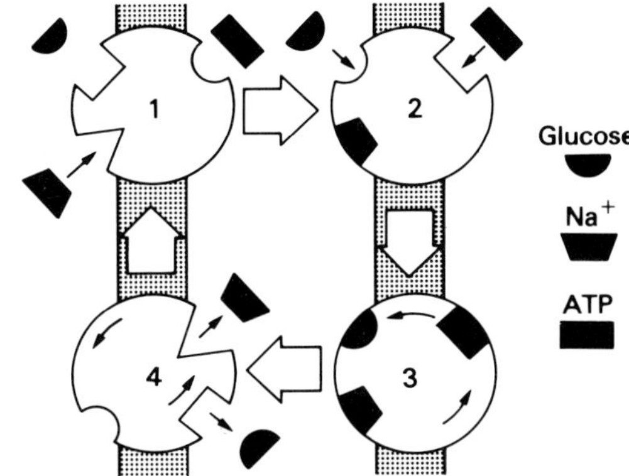

Fig. 17.12 Conformational change in a carrier protein induced by a solute (Na$^+$) which increases its affinity and therefore the rate of absorption of another solute (glucose) (Lewis 1978).

synergistic effect on the rate of absorption of each other and the concentrations presently thought to be optimal for maximum intestinal absorption are given in Table 17.4. For example, the presence of sodium in the intestinal lumen doubles the rate of glucose absorption, and the presence of glucose greatly increases the rate of sodium absorption. This synergistic effect that glucose and sodium have on the absorption of each other (and therefore of water also) occurs because the binding of one of these molecules to the carrier protein responsible for the solute's active transport across the gut wall causes a conformational change in that protein. This conformational change increases the affinity of that, or other carrier proteins, for other solutes (Fig. 17.12). The carrier protein is a part of the cell membrane.

Increasing the affinity of a carrier protein for its solute will increase that solute's rate of absorption. Thus, the binding of sodium to its carrier protein will greatly increase glucose absorption and vice versa. The presence of either glucose or sodium, or both, also increases the rate of glycine and amino acid absorption. In addition, the presence of glycine and amino acids will increase the rate of glucose and sodium absorption, and similarly with the other neutral amino acids and bicarbonate. Thus, *the simultaneous presence of all of these solutes will greatly increase the rate of absorption of each and that of water.*

Composition of replacement fluids

Solutions containing at least 1% glucose have been shown to be necessary for maximum sodium and water absorption and, conversely, solutions containing 118 mmol/l sodium have been used to result in maximum glucose and water absorption. The concentrations of amino acids required for maximum intestinal absorption have not been determined but total concentration is probably of the order of 60–120 mmol/l. It has, however, been shown that at least 30 mmol bicarbonate is needed for maximum sodium absorption. Additional substances needed by the patient may be added to the fluid composed on these lines. However, the total osmolarity should be kept as near isotonicity as possible. For the diarrhoeic animal 25–30 mmol potassium and an additional 50 mmol bicarbonate are needed to replace the extensive losses of these ions in the faeces (Table 17.4). Various commercial products have been produced on the basis of the above calculations and Lewis (1975) has reported on the value of one such product in clinical use in calves, horses and pigs in Europe (Table 17.5).

The present author (Vandaele 1976, 1977) has tested in extensive clinical trials a formulation containing:

Sodium chloride	11.64%	Potassium phosphate	8.68%
Calcium gluconate	2.2 %	Glycine	21.2 %
Magnesium sulphate	0.61%	Dextrose	55.67%

Table 17.5 Composition of an oral fluid replacement product (Lewis 1975).

	Optimum concentration	Composition of product (as reconstituted solution)
Glucose* (g/l)	56–170	56
Sodium* (mEq/l)	118	118
Glycine and imino amino acids** (g/l)	60–120	80
Other neutral amino acids** (g/l)	60–120	60
Bicarbonate (mEq/l)	80	80
Potassium (mEq/l)	25–30	29
Osmolality (mosm/l)	300–350	330

*Solutes with synergistic effect on one another, each increasing the intestinal absorption of the other.

**Solutes which are necessary for diarrhoeal therapy to correct acidosis and cellular losses.

Table 17.6   The composition (% w/w) of three commercially produced formulations for oral rehydration.

Constituent	Biodiet	Ion aid	Life guard
Dextrose	67.6	55.7	24.3
Glycine	10.3	21.2	46.5 (incl. prot.)
Sodium bicarbonate	–	–	16.3
Sodium chloride	14.3	11.6	3.6
Magnesium sulphate	–	0.6	1.0
Citric acid	0.8	–	–
Potassium citrate	0.2	–	–
Potassium chloride	–	–	4.6
Potassium phosphate	6.8	8.7	–
Calcium hydrogen phosphate	–	–	1.7
Calcium gluconate	–	2.2	–
Presentation	2 sachets	1 sachet (2 parts)	1 sachet

Clinical results with this solution were good. Relative to untreated controls, the treated animals showed lower mortality, higher weight gain, and shorter duration of antibiotic treatment. This formulation was also compared with a 'conventional' intravenous fluid in two groups of 100 calves, with very similar results (Vandaele 1976).

Table 17.6 lists the composition of three of the currently available formulations for oral rehydration. One of these contains citrate, which may enhance water absorption (Bywater 1977). Another contains bicarbonate for the reasons described above. Magnesium is included in some formulations as a prophylactic measure against the development of hypomagnesaemic tetany.

Administration of oral replacement fluids

As a rule of thumb Lewis (1975) advocates the administration of 2 l of oral fluids three times a day for the diarrhoeic calf (Table 17.7). It is preferable to

Table 17.7   Guidelines for oral fluid administration to diarrhoeic calves (Lewis 1975).

1   2 litres, 2–3 times a day
2   Preferably by bottle but by stomach tube if necessary
3   Leave calf on cow
4   If artificially feeding, stop milk administration during this period
5   Do not use these fluids alone for more than 2 days since fluids do not contain adequate energy. Dilute with milk after 2 days
6   Start early — before dehydration occurs
7   If treatment is not started early or calf's condition deteriorates, give fluids parenterally

allow the calf to suckle a nursing bottle in order to promote oesophageal groove closure and bypass of the rumen-reticulum. However, if the calf is not sucking, the fluid may be given as a drench; a human enema bag or oral feeding bag may be useful for this purpose. If the calf is sucking the cow it should be allowed to continue to do so. Radiostits (1973) has shown that there is no benefit in separating the diarrhoeic calf from the cow, since, if they are separated, the cow may not readily accept the calf when they are reunited. However, if the calf is being hand-fed, milk feeding should be discontinued during the treatment period.

A word of caution on the use of these oral fluids is required: the nutrients they contain are included to enhance the intestinal absorption of other solutes and water as previously discussed. They are *not* included as a source of energy and any energy the calf derives from them should be regarded as a bonus. Six litres of these fluids per day will provide less than 15% of the energy requirement of the growing calf. Hence, additional energy sources should be provided if the calf is still diarrhoeic after two days of treatment. In this case the fluid may be diluted with an equal volume of milk. If after a further 2–3 days of treatment the calf is still diarrhoeic, oral fluids should be discontinued and intravenous therapy initiated.

Treatment with oral fluids should commence when the calf first becomes diarrhoeic before there are any signs of dehydration, because it is better and easier to prevent the problems of dehydration than to treat them. The clinician should not wait until extensive fluid and electrolyte losses have already occurred and then try to recover lost ground. It is also worth pointing out that oral fluids are excellent media for microbial growth and are non-sterile, so that they should be refrigerated after making them up and, if not used after one day, discarded.

If the calf's condition deteriorates or if treatment is not started at an early stage, oral fluids by themselves may not be sufficient to balance the rate of water loss or they may not be absorbed rapidly enough to save the calf. Under such circumstances fluids should be given parenterally.

Parenteral fluid and electrolyte therapy

One advantage of using the intravenous route for fluid therapy is that the digestive tract can be 'rested' (Watt 1965). Intravenous solutions for rehydration have long been used by veterinarians and the most important factor to consider is the quantity which should be administered. This depends on the degree of dehydration, but a minimum of 2–3 litres daily is required (Vandaele 1968). Some authors go so far as to recommend, in severe cases, 85–150 ml/kg/24 hours (Massip 1977). Massip (1976, 1977) noted that 100 ml/kg administered over 4–6 hours was needed simply to correct an 8–10% deficit.

Thus, a calf which is severely dehydrated (10%) must receive 5 litres of intravenous electrolyte solution in the first 4–6 hours. To provide for daily requirements and to compensate for continuing losses, it is necessary to administer 140 ml/kg in the following 20 hours. However, if the diarrhoea ceases after the initial 4–6 hours, this quantity can be halved. Some 70% of dehydrated calves can be expected to respond in less than 24 hours to intravenous fluids. For the remaining 30%, another 24 hours' parenteral therapy is required and, if no improvement is seen by then, the prognosis is poor (Watt 1967).

The subcutaneous route can be used, if the volume is not too great, but hypertonic solutions must never be given by this route, since fluid is likely to accumulate at the injection site as a result of osmotic factors. Intraperitoneal injection has sometimes been recommended (Ketchell *et al* 1964) even with hypertonic solutions. However, since Lewis & Phillips (1971) and Tennant *et al* (1972) demonstrated that absorption from the peritoneum is reduced in diarrhoeic animals, this route has clear disadvantages.

Type of parenteral solution

Table 17.8 gives some examples of recommended parenteral solutions. To be of maximum benefit, parenteral therapy should aim at returning the blood volume to normal and correcting ion imbalances throughout the tissues. To accomplish this, the diarrhoeic calf requires a fluid similar in composition to extracellular fluid, such as Ringer's bicarbonate or lactate, sometimes with additional potassium and bicarbonate. As with oral replacement therapy, the problem of driving potassium back into the cells is a principal objective of fluid therapy (Lewis & Phillips 1972; 1973). Plasma potassium concentration may be nearly doubled in severe cases, in spite of large potassium losses from the body.

Because of its ability to enhance the movement of potassium into the cell, Lewis & Phillips include glucose in their fluid therapy regimens. However, since 97% of the total exchangeable potassium of the body is normally inside the cells (Edleman 1959), a movement of this ion back into the cells will rapidly deplete the very small extracellular potassium pool and still have relatively little effect on the intracellular potassium concentration. For this reason, it is also necessary to include potassium in the fluid given (Lewis & Phillips 1972) (see also Fig. 17.8). With this treatment, there is a potassium/hydrogen ion exchange at the cell membrane, with hydrogen leaving the cell as potassium enters; in other words, the reverse of what occurs in diarrhoea (Lewis 1977). Glucose should also be added to parenteral fluids to treat the hypoglycaemia which is frequently seen in the diarrhoeic calf (Lewis 1977). Bicarbonate administration is the treatment of choice for acidosis because its

Table 17.8 Examples of parenteral solutions.

Authors	Solution used	Na$^+$	K$^+$	Ca^{++}	Mg$^+$	Cl$^-$	Composition (mEq/l) Lactate	Acetate	HCO$_3^-$	Invert Sugar	Remarks
Tennant *et al* (1972)	Ringer's lactate	130	4	3	0	109	28	–	–	–	
Lewis (1978)	Ringer's lactate + 30 mEq NaHCO$_3$ and 10 mEq KCl	160	14	3	0	119	28	–	30	–	Subcutaneous injection
Lewis (1978)	Ringer's bicarbonate + 50 mEq NaHCO$_3$ and 20 mEq KCl	180	34	3	0	129	–	–	50	–	Intravenous injection only + glucose 50% 110 ml
Butler (1969)		139	10.2	1.4	1.5	97	55	–	–	50 g/l	
Radostits (1973)	Ionalyte	139	10	1.4	1.5	97	–	55	–	–	
Massip & d'Ieteren (1976)	Isotonax 37	139.8	10	5	3	102.8	55	–	–	–	
Vandaele (1968)	PO41 (+PO48)	56.5 (+83)	25	–	6	50	25	–	(+83)	100 g/l	

loss is the primary cause of the problem. The addition of 500 ml M/6 bicarbonate (83 mEq HCO_3) to the standard intravenous electrolyte solution is recommended (Vandaele 1968).

If lactate solutions are used, it is also advisable to include bicarbonate because lactate must first be metabolised to be of any benefit. In addition, some diarrhoeic calves have a lactic acidosis (Lewis 1977), indicating that they already have more lactate in their bodies than their livers are able to metabolise and, as noted above, hepatic metabolism of lactate may be compromised.

Dallenga (1975) tested several parenteral solutions and was able to establish limits for intravenous infusion. He proposed two types of parenteral solution, both to be given to the calf at the rate of 6 l/12 hours:

Type 1

Solution A			Solution B		
$NaHCO_3$		30g	$NaHCO_3$		14g
NaCl		9g	NaCl		12g
Water			Glucose		100g
to 15 drops/minute 3000 ml			Water		
			to 60 drops/minute 3000 ml		

Type 2

Solution A			Solution B		
$NaHCO_3$		30g	$NaHCO_3$		14g
NaCl		9g	NaCl		12g
Water			Glucose		100g
to 15 drops/minute 3000 ml			KCl		8g
			Water		
			to 60 drops/minute 3000 ml		

Thus, type 2 differs from type 1 in that solution B contains 8 g KCl. Solution type 1 was tested in 13 calves; 12 recovered and one died. Solution type 2 was tested in 48 calves; 44 recovered and 4 died. With both types of solution, the results were better than those obtained with bicarbonate solution alone (14 calves died, of 37 treated). Dallenga preferred solution type 2 because he obtained better clinical results, with the calves drinking more freely.

A recent development has been the introduction of a parenteral fluid which, in addition to replacing the fluid and electrolyte losses sustained by the patient, contains up to twelve times the extracellular fluid concentration of potassium, glucose and a buffering agent capable of interacting with the other ingredients to maintain a basic condition in which the pH does not exceed 10 (Phillips 1974, 1977). The dry ingredients are made up as a hypertonic solution for intravenous use and as an isotonic solution for subcutaneous administration. The composition is as follows:

K$^+$	23 mEq/l	Cl$^-$	64 mEq/l
HCO$_3$$^-$	80 mEq/l	Mg^{++}	6.4 mEq/l
Na$^+$	115 mEq/l	Glucose	6.8% w/v

In this fluid the glucose provides a source of energy and also facilitates potassium transport across the cell membrane. Without the presence of glucose, the high concentration of potassium would be lethal. Sodium is present in this solution as NaHCO$_3$ and as NaCl. Further bicarbonate is added as the potassium salt.

When the constituents are dissolved in 2.6 l of water, an almost isotonic solution results (osmolarity of approximately 285 mosm/l), which may be given subcutaneously (2.6 l/30 kg body weight). In the case of critically ill patients, the same weight of ingredients dissolved in only 1 litre of water can be administered intravenously for each 30 kg body weight. This solution is hypertonic, having an osmolarity of about 712 mosm/l. As such, it has the expected effect of drawing fluid from cells into the extravascular compartment.

In the cases of severe diarrhoea, when the patient is unable to rise for example, the preferred therapy is to administer the hypertonic (intravenous) and isotonic (subcutaneous) fluids in the recommended manner at the same time. Table 17.9 shows the effect of combined intravenous and subcutaneous therapy on 18 diarrhoeic calves.

General comments

Regardless of the route or type of fluid given, it is essential to warm it to body temperature. Cold fluids can produce local vasoconstriction and reduce the

Table 17.9 Intravenous and subcutaneous fluid therapy in 18 diarrhoeic calves.

Condition and treatment	Temperature (°C)	Plasma pH	Intracellular pH (muscle)	Plasma K$^+$ (mEq/l)	Intracellular K$^+$
Normal	37.6–36.4	7.441	7.011	4.62	167
Severe diarrhoea	33.6–30.7	7.042	6.784	8.06	147
i.v. treatment (4 hours after treatment)	+2.8 +1.9	7.111	6.878	−1.52	+7
s.c. treatment (4 hours after treatment)	+0.7 +1.9	7.142*	−	−0.5*	−

*Single measurement

rate of absorption. When given intravenously, cold fluids have an adverse effect on the sino-atrial node, and may produce arrhythmias and even cardiac arrest. This phenomenon has been well demonstrated in several studies (e.g. Le Roux 1965). Copping *et al* (1972) describe a study in which dogs were bled to produce a standard degree of haemorrhagic shock. When cold Ringer's lactate solution was taken from the refrigerator and administered intravenously, three of the five dogs died. However, when an equal amount of fluid was warmed to body temperature and administered at the same rate to five dogs, they all survived. Another important factor when fluids are administered intravenously is the rate of infusion. The rate may be expressed in *ml/minute* or as *drops/minute*. Buttler & Massip (1977) define a 'drop factor' which may be used to calculate how many drops of fluid per minute should be given. (The method is to calculate the number of drops contained in 1 ml, then divide 60 by that number, the result will give the 'drop factor'. The rate of dropping will then be in ml/hour: number of drops per minute × drop factor or, drops/minute = ml to be given in 1 hour/drop factor.

In practice, the recommended rate for calves is about 15 ml/minute. This can be raised to 25 ml/minute in critical cases (Vandaele 1968).

Conclusions

Current recommendations for the administration of fluids to calves can be summarised as follows (*see also* Fig. 17.11):

1   If the diarrhoeic calf is less than 5% dehydrated (i.e. showing no clinical signs of dehydration), 2 l of an oral nutrient-electrolyte fluid should be given by stomach tube or preferably by nursing bottle twice or three times a day.

2   If the calf is 6–10% dehydrated (i.e. able to stand and walk but showing clinical signs of dehydration, the limbs and oral cavity being at normal temperature), fluids should be given orally and, at the same time, 2 l of a specific electrolyte fluid should be given subcutaneously.

3   If the calf is more than 10% dehydrated (i.e. recumbent and unable to rise), fluids must be given intravenously. Intravenous therapy may be started at once, or 2 l may be administered subcutaneously initially and, after a two hour interval, a slow intravenous infusion may be started. The condition of the calf should be re-assessed 4–8 hours later and fluid therapy continued until the animal improves — when intravenous fluids may be discontinued and oral and/or subcutaneous therapy instituted. When the calf recovers further, oral fluids are continued alone until complete recovery or for 2–3 days, whichever is the shorter.

References

Barragry T. B. (1974) Some aspects of fluids and electrolyte imbalances in animals. *Ir. Vet. J.* **28**, 177.

Bywater R. J. (1977) Traitement de la diarrhée chez le veau avec des formulations orales réhydratantes. Symposium GTV, Octobre, Le Donjon.

Copping J. W., Mather G. G. & Winkler J. M. (1972) Physiologic responses to the administration of cold, room temperature and warm balanced salt solution in hemorrhagic shock in dogs. *Surgery* **71**, 206.

Dallenga H. W. (1975) Biochemische afwijkingen in het bloed van kalveren met diarrhee en hun correcties door middel van vloeistoftherapie. Thesis, Utrecht.

Dardillet C. O. & Ruckebusch Y. (1973) Functional characteristics of the gastroduodenal function of the newborn calf. *Ann. Rech. Vet.* **4**, 31–56.

Donawich J. & Christie B. A. (1971) Clinico-Pathologic Conference. *J. Am. Vet. Med. Assoc.* **158**, 501.

Edelman I. S. & Lederman J. (1959) The anatomy of body water and electrolytes. *Am. J. Med.* **27**, 156.

Edwards A. Y. & Williams L. L. (1972) Fluid therapy in treating dehydration from calf scours. *VM/SAC* **67**, 273–7.

Espinasse J. (1977) Physiopathologie générale du syndrome de deshydratation chez le veau. Symposium GTV, Octobre, Le Donjon.

Fayet J. C. (1968) Recherches sur le métabolisme hydrominéral chez le veau normal ou en état de diarrhée. *Rech. Vét.* **1**, 99, 109, 117.

Fayet J. C. (1971) Plasma and faecal osmolability, water kinetics and body compartments in neonatal calves with diarrhoea. *Br. Vet. J.* **127**, 37.

Fisher E. W. & Martinez A. A. (1976) Aspects of body fluid dynamics of neonatal calf diarrhoea. *Res. Vet. Sci.* **20**, 302.

Fisher E. W. & de la Fuente C. H. (1972) Water and electrolyte studies in newborn calves with particular reference to the effect of diarrhoea. *Res. Vet. Sci.* **13**, 315.

Ketchell R. J., Graham J. E. B. & Bodenistel J. K. (1964) Fluid and electrolyte therapy in small animals. *Canad. Vet. J.* **5**, 199.

Le Roux B. T. (1965) Emphysema Thoracis. *Br. J. Surg.* **52**, 89.

Lewis L. D. O. & Phillips R. W. (1972) Water and electrolyte cases in neonatal calves with acute diarrhoea. A complete balance study. *Cornell Vet.* **62**, 596–607.

Lewis L. D., Phillips R. W. & Elliot C. D. (1975) Changes in plasma glucose and lactate concentrations and enzyme activities in the neonatal calf with diarrhoea. *Am. J. Vet. Res.* **36**, 413.

Lewis L. D. (1975) *Treatment of the diarrhoeic calf.* Norden Laboratories.

Lewis L. D. (1977) Calf diarrhoea part II: effects of diarrhoea. Norden News, p. 20–2.

Lewis L. D. (1978) Calf diarrhoea part III: management, prevention and treatment of diarrhoea. Norden News, p. 22–5.

Massip A. (1976) La diarrhée du veau. Considerations physiopathologiques et notions de réhydration. *Ann. Med. Vet.* **120**, 9–26, 103–11.

Massip A. (1977) La diarrhée du veau. Aspects physiopathologiques et thérapeutiques. Symposium GTV, Octobre, Le Donjon.

Michell A. R. (1967) Body fluids and alimentary disease. *Vet. Rec.* **81**, 2.

Michell A. R. (1974) Body fluids and diarrhoea. Dynamics of dysfunction. *Vet. Rec.* **94**, 311.

Moon H.W. (1978) Mechanisms in the pathogenesis of diarrhea and review. *JAVMA* **172**, 443–8.

Oliva P. B. (1970) Lactic acidosis *Am. J. Vet. Med.* **48**, 209.

Phillips R. W. & Knox K. L. (1969) Diarrhoeic acidosis in calves. *J. Comp. Lab. Med.* **3**, 1.

Phillips R. W. & Lewis L. D. (1970) Diarrhoea in the calf. Part I: pathophysiologic changes and development, p. 104. *Proc. 4th Ann. Conv. Am. Assoc. Bovine Practit.*

Phillips R. W., Lewis L. D. & Know K. L. (1971) Alteration in body water turnover and distribution in neonatal calves with acute diarrhoea. *Ann. N.Y. Acad. Sci.* **176**, 231–43.

Phillips R. W. & Lewis L. D. (1973) Viral induced changes in intestinal transport and resultant body fluid alterations in neonatal calves. *Ann. Rech. Vet.* **4**, 87–98.

Phillips R. W., Lewis L. D. & Knox K. L. (1973) Alterations in body water turnover and distribution in neonatal calves. *Ann. Rech. Vet.* **4**, 87.

Phillips R. W. & Lewis L. D. (1976) Drugs affecting digestion and absorption. *Veterinary Pharmacology and Therapeutics,* 4th edn. eds. N. H. Booth and L. E. McDonald. Iowa State University Press, Ames, Iowa.

Radiostits O. M. (1973) Clinical management of diarrhoea in calves. *Bov. Pract.* **8**, 20.

Tennant B. & Reina-Guerra M. (1968) Hypoglycaemia in neonatal calves associated with acute diarrhoea. *Cornell Vet.* **38**, 136.

Tennant B., Harrold D. & Reina-Guerra M. (1972) Physiologic and metabolic factors in the pathogenesis of neonatal enteric infections in calves. *J. Am. Vet. Med. Assoc.* **161**, 993.

W. Vandaele (1968) *Solutions parentérales en médicine vétérinaire.* A. Chistiaens, Brussels.

Vandaele W. (1976) Nouvelle technique de réhydration par la voie orale: résultats des premiers essais réalisés en Europe dans le traitement des diarrhées des veaux. Internat. Congress of Diseases of Cattle, Paris. Proceedings pp. 305–11.

Vandaele W. (1977) Mise au point d'une formule pour la réhydration par voie orale et résultats des essais réalisés en Europe. Symposium GTV, Octobre, Le Donjon.

Watt J. C. (1967) Fluid therapy for dehydration in calves. *J. Am. Vet. Med. Assoc.* **150**, 742.

Whitten E. H. & Phillips R. W. (1971) In-vitro intestinal exchanges of Na^+, K^+, Cl^-, $3H_2O$ in experimental bovine neonatal enteritis. *Am. J. Dig. Dis.* **16**, 891.

18

Therapeutic agents in the treatment of diarrhoea in young farm animals

R.J. BYWATER

Diarrhoea in farm animals is no new problem. Tolnay (1799) described a diarrhoea in calves which probably differed little from the disease seen today, which is still only partly understood and still results in considerable morbidity and mortality. During recent years, however, some important progress has been made in the understanding of mechanisms involved in diarrhoea (Moon 1978) and this progress is being reflected in improved treatments.

Aetiology

In any disease, treatment should be related either to aetiology or symptomatology (preferably both), so it is worth briefly reviewing the present understanding of agents and mechanisms in diarrhoea. Firstly, diarrhoea clearly represents a net loss (secretion) of water and electrolytes. Any net absorption or secretion in the intestine is the result of two unidirectional fluxes, one from intestinal lumen to the blood, the other in the reverse direction. A net absorption results when the flux from the lumen is greater than the flux to the lumen, and vice versa. The fluxes are large and the difference between the net gain (healthy calf) and net loss (diarrhoeic calf) is small by comparison (Fig. 18.1). Thus the aim of therapy is to reverse the balance between the two fluxes, by reducing secretion, increasing absorption, or both.

Causative agents

It is now clear that many strains of *E. coli* possess factors which enable them to be pathogenic. These so-called 'virulence determinants' include the ability to cause intestinal secretion of fluid and electrolyte (governed by transmissible plasmids for enterotoxin production (Smith & Halls 1968)), and the ability to adhere to intestinal mucosa. This latter property is governed by the K88 and

375

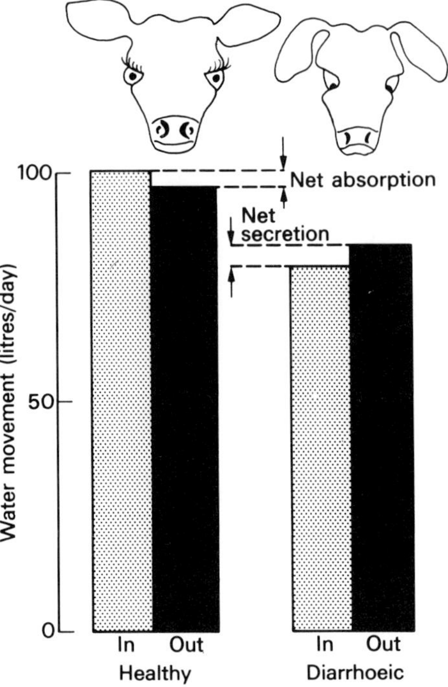

Fig. 18.1 Undirectional fluxes of water between intestinal lumen and blood in healthy and diarrhoeic calves. The columns marked 'In' show fluxes from lumen to blood. Those marked 'Out' show fluxes from blood to lumen. The net movement is the difference between the two unidirectional fluxes. (From Bywater & Logan 1974.)

987P antigens in pigs (Sojka 1971), and the K99 antigen in calves (Ørskov *et al* 1975).

The enterotoxins involved cause dilation when injected into ligated intestinal segments and have been divided into heat labile toxin/s of high molecular weight (Gyles & Barnum 1970) and heat stable toxin/s of low molecular weight (Smith & Halls 1967). However, subdivisions of these may occur (Burgess *et al* 1978). The activity of these two toxin types appears to differ, since the heat labile enterotoxin causes increased adenyl cyclase activity, with raised cyclic AMP (Dorner & Mayer 1975), while heat stable enterotoxin appears to act by increasing cyclic GMP (Hughes 1978, Newsome *et al* 1978) and/or calmodulin (calcium-dependent) regulator.

Salmonella infection has received rather less attention than *E. coli*. However, an enterotoxin has been described for *Salmonella enteritidis* (Koupal & Deibel 1975) as has adenyl cyclase stimulation by *Salmonella typhimurium* (Gianella *et al* 1975). Destruction of villus structure, which is not generally characteristic of *E. coli* infection, has been described in pigs affected by *Salmonella choleraesuis* (Arbuckle 1975) and seems likely to be a common feature of the disease. Such destruction has been associated with reduced β-galactosidase activity (Halpin & Caple 1976).

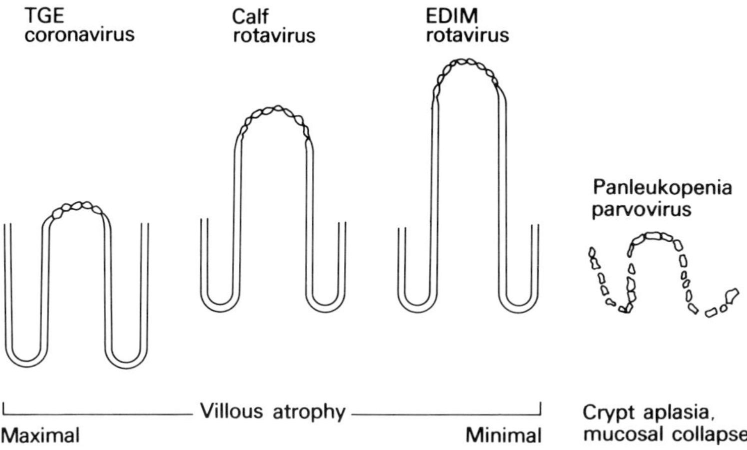

Fig. 18.2 Diagrammatic representation of damage to villi caused by different enteric viruses (Moon 1978). EDIM = Epidemic diarrhoea of infant mice.

Virus-induced diarrhoea has received considerable attention since it was shown (Mebus 1973) that rotavirus and coronavirus caused diarrhoea in calves and piglets. This diarrhoea resembled that caused by transmissible gastroenteritis (TGE) virus in pigs (Woode 1969).

Virus-induced diarrhoea typically involves disruption of villi, and Moon (1978) has noted that the damaged area of the villus varies between different agents. Thus rotavirus infection in calves damages the upper villus, while TGE damages the whole villus excluding the crypt. The most severe damage occurs with feline panleukopenia virus in cats (and parvovirus in dogs), where both villus and crypt are destroyed (Fig. 18.2).

The result in all cases represents a malabsorption, with decreased digestive enzymes such as β-galactosidase (lactase), as demonstrated (Fig. 18.3) by Bywater & Penhale (1968) and Halpin & Caple (1976). There is also a decrease in absorptive area due to flattening of villi. The pathogenesis of virus diarrhoea also involves a net secretion in the affected areas, possibly due to damage to the upper part of the villus which is the area most important in absorption, while the largely secretory crypt region remains intact.

The net secretion will combine with undigested food material reaching the caecum and colon. Here breakdown by micro-organisms to low-molecular-weight particles, osmotically and possibly pharmacologically active, will stimulate a fermentative diarrhoea (Weijers & Van de Kamer 1965).

The protozoa *Cryptosporidia* (Pohlenz *et al* 1978) have been found to cause diarrhoea in both calves and pigs, and indeed can be transmitted between the two species (Moon & Bemrick 1981). The mode of action appears, at least in part, to be villus damage with malabsorption.

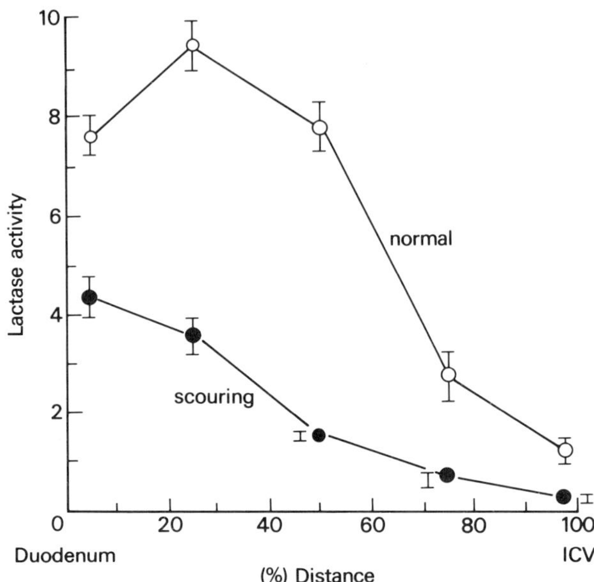

Fig. 18.3 Lactase (β-galactosidase, μM hydrolysed/mg/protein/hr) activity in the intestinal mucosa of healthy calves and calves dying after undifferentiated diarrhoea. Each point shows the mean of 10 observations. Vertical bars show s.e. ICV = Ileo-caecal valve. (Bywater & Penhale 1968.)

It has been found that where intensive examination of outbreaks has been carried out (Acres *et al* 1975, Moon *et al* 1978), the result has been a striking mixture of potential viral, bacterial, and protozoal pathogens. The implication for therapy is that specific treatments are likely to be of limited value (Tzipori 1981).

Therapy

While therapy should ideally be chosen following a specific diagnosis, this is often difficult for two reasons: firstly, because more than one pathogen may be present and contributing to the disease, and secondly, because the methods of diagnosis in the field (and even in the laboratory) are seldom such as to allow easy and accurate identification of pathogens. This being the case, therapeutic measures can usually only be chosen on the basis of experience, lack of specificity, and judged by their efficacy under both experimental and field conditions. There are six main types of treatment which will be discussed: antibiotics, motility-inhibiting drugs, intestinal adsorbents, fluid replacement (intravenous or oral), secretion-inhibiting drugs, and microbial implants.

Antibiotics

Antibiotics remain the most widely used treatment for diarrhoea in animals, and their use is logical in cases of bacterial disease caused by organisms such as enteropathogenic *E. coli*. It is the firm opinion of most practitioners that antibiotics are effective providing that the outbreak in question is caused by a sensitive strain of *E. coli*. However, there must be some doubts concerning efficacy of antibiotics in diarrhoea especially where viruses are implicated, although secondary bacterial involvement may still respond.

There have been few controlled trials of antibiotic efficacy in animals. Such trials are especially important in a disease where mortality and spontaneous recovery are very variable, so making it difficult to assess treatment efficacy in the absence of untreated controls.

Dalton *et al* (1960) carried out experiments which indicated that tetracyclines were effective as treatments for calf diarrhoea, but it was later suggested (Fisher & de la Fuente 1971) that the immune status of the calves was important in the outcome of these experiments. These authors also found that no beneficial effect was demonstrable following chloramphenicol or furazolidone treatment of diarrhoea in calves with low immunoglobulin levels. Similarly, Radostits *et al* (1975) could show no benefit from antibiotic treatment, with or without starvation.

However, successful antibiotic treatment in calves has been reported for apramycin (Pankhurst 1976), amoxycillin (Palmer *et al* 1977) and gentamicin (Jones *et al* 1977). Trimethoprim–sulphadiazine was also found effective (Daniels *et al* 1977) but only to a similar degree as milk reduction. This was rather similar to the finding (Bywater 1977) that, in experimental infection in calves, amoxycillin treatment, while significantly superior to a placebo, was by itself similar in efficacy to an oral glucose–glycine electrolyte formulation.

The use of antibiotics in piglet diarrhoea, although widespread, has received rather little experimental support. Ampicillin and sulphachlorpyridazine were compared as treatments for colibacillosis (Davis *et al* 1973) and it was concluded that there was no difference. However, no untreated control group was incorporated in this study.

An experimental infection model (challenge of colostrum-deprived piglets with enteropathogenic *E. coli*) was used by Keefe & Bywater (1976) to compare efficacy of amoxycillin and ampicillin with a placebo. Both antibiotics were found effective, with amoxycillin more so than ampicillin. Experimental infections were also used by Callear & Smith (1966), who demonstrated efficacy of furazolidone treatment of piglet colibacillosis, and by Ensley (1976) who reported gentamicin to be significantly more effective than chloramphenicol or oxytetracycline.

Such experimental infection studies, although not entirely typical of field infections, are nevertheless very useful as a means of carrying out controlled comparisons of different treatments.

Motility-inhibiting drugs

The use of drugs inhibiting motility (e.g. atropine, methscopolamine) is based on the assumption that diarrhoea is caused by excessive smooth muscle movement. Present understanding suggests that, at least in the colon, the opposite is true, and diarrhoea is associated with *decreased* motility (Waller & Misiewicz 1972). It is probable that most changes in small intestinal activity result from increased secretion causing dilation and reflex contraction. Anticholinergic agents such as atropine, methscopolamine, and benzetimide have been used in antidiarrhoeal remedies, and trial results with benzetimide (Symoens *et al* 1974) have shown that, in combination with antibiotics, it produced a more rapid return to normality. Used on its own, the drug controlled diarrhoea for 24 hours only.

Drugs having a specific constipating effect are available, e.g. loperamide (Niemegeers *et al* 1974) and diphenoxylate. These may have morphine-like actions — increasing smooth muscle tone and decreasing propulsion on the intestine. This type of symptomatic approach is not without risks since diarrhoea may be beneficial in removing toxins, and inhibition of movement may thus be counter productive (Dupont & Hornick 1973). It seems likely that reduced motility can have an effect similar to the adhesion factors (K88 antigen in pigs or K99 antigen in calves) in allowing enterotoxin-producing organisms to remain in the small intestine, where the fluid loss may then be increased. Moreover, in a trial in infants with diarrhoea, a diphenoxy-late–atropine combination was found no more effective than a placebo (Portnoy *et al* 1976). Loperamide, however, is interesting in that it has been shown (Sandhu *et al* 1979) to inhibit cholera toxin-induced secretion as well as having an effect on motility. It may therefore prove useful even in secretory diarrhoeas.

Intestinal adsorbents

Many antidiarrhoeal preparations contain kaolin, attapulgite, or other adsorbent agents. There are, however, few reports of experimental verification of their efficacy. The rationale for their use is adsorption of toxins within the lumen of the intestine and evidence has been presented to show that *E. coli* enterotoxins can be absorbed by attapulgite and charcoal (Drucker *et al* 1977, Gyles & Zigler 1978). However, the ability to adsorb toxins *in vitro* or in ligated loops may not be associated with therapeutic efficacy and kaolin or kaolin plus pectin were found ineffective in acute diarrhoea in infants

(Portnoy *et al* 1976). It has been suggested that the anionic adsorbing agent, cholestyramine, was useful in treatment of enteritis in infants (Berant *et al* 1976). Nevertheless, despite a demonstrable ability to adsorb enterotoxin and so to reduce secretory activity in animal models, cholestyramine was ineffective in preventing diarrhoea following oral challenge of piglets with enteropathogenic *E. coli* (Mullan *et al* 1979).

Fluid replacement

As dehydration and electrolyte loss are major factors in the pathogenesis of diarrhoea, so fluid replacement has been recognised as important in therapy. It was first considered that this must be intravenous, and an approach using either saline solutions or homologous plasma has been described (Watt 1967). However, the practical problems associated with prolonged intravenous therapy in calves or pigs mean that only a small proportion of animals can justify such measures. Despite this, it seems probable that intravenous rehydration remains a necessary part of therapy in severely affected collapsed animals.

Oral rehydration was first found effective in treatment of human cholera (Nalin *et al* 1970). The underlying principle was the continued active absorption of glucose, glycine, or both in the small intestine. This active absorption was accompanied by water and sodium, so that there was a net increase in absorption, with associated reversal of dehydration. A similar situation exists in diarrhoeic calves and pigs, where *E. coli* infection has been shown to have no effect on glucose or amino acid absorption (Whipp & Moon 1973, Bywater 1970). Thus oral rehydration should be an effective means of reversing dehydration, and this has been confirmed in diarrhoeic calves (Braun 1975, Hamm & Hicks 1975, Bywater 1977) and also in pigs (Bywater & Woode 1980).

This approach to the treatment of diarrhoea has the merit of being simple, soundly based, and generally effective, although Radostits *et al* (1975) were unable to show any benefit from temporary starvation (and oral electrolyte) in hospitalised calves. However, it is possible that 24 hours' withholding of milk (as used in these studies) was insufficient to allow restoration of normal digestion and absorption, and the electrolyte formulation may not have been ideal.

The principle that milk should be withheld during treatment is based on the lowered ability to digest lactose (Fig. 18.3), especially in the presence of virus damage to the intestinal mucosa (Pearson *et al* 1978). In this case, if copious milk feeding is continued, undigested milk reaching the large intestine results in a fermentative diarrhoea (Weijers & Van de Kamer 1965). However, milk withdrawal and substitution with water alone does not seem to be particularly effective compared with substitution of a glucose–glycine–electrolyte formulation. It was found that milk deprivation alone was of limited value in preventing mortality in experimentally challenged calves (Bywater 1980). Use of an effective oral glucose–glycine–electrolyte formulation as treatment for diarrhoea was found to be similar in efficacy to a broad spectrum antibiotic, while a combination of both forms of therapy was the most effective treatment (Bywater 1977).

Alkalinising substances, particularly sodium bicarbonate, have been included in some rehydration fluids (Radostits 1975) but excluded from others (Hamm & Hicks 1975).While the acidosis which is associated with diarrhoea suggests the need for such measures, bicarbonate may be inadvisable in that it reduces gastric pH, and so increases the possibility of re-infection with enteric pathogens (Nalin *et al* 1978). The palatability of alkaline solutions may also be low, and it is possible that their use is not required unless acidosis is severe. In the latter case, intravenous administration of alkalinising solutions is indicated.

Secretion-inhibiting drugs

Anticholinergic drugs such as atropine and methscopolamine have been used in combination with adsorbents or antibiotics in order to reduce secretion and suppress motility (despite increased motility being of questionable relevance). No evidence appears to have been presented to support the use of these compounds, although the anticholinergic drug benzetimide was found (Symoens *et al* 1974) to increase the rate of recovery when used with antibiotics to treat calf diarrhoea.

Anticholinergic drugs do not inhibit enterotoxin-induced secretion, but a number of drugs have been described which, at least experimentally, can be shown to reduce enterotoxin activity. For instance, cholera enterotoxin activity can be blocked by indomethacin (Gots *et al* 1974), ethacrynic acid (Carpenter *et al* 1969), methylprednisolone (Charney & Donowitz 1976), and aspirin (Farris *et al* 1976). In view of the similarities between cholera and coli toxins, it is possible that drugs may be used to inhibit the enterotoxin-induced secretion in *E. coli* and other diarrhoeas. Indeed, Jones *et al* (1977) have described inhibition of experimentally-induced colibacillosis in calves using flunixin meglumine which, like aspirin and indomethacin, is a non-steroidal anti-inflammatory agent inhibiting prostaglandin formation.

Chlorpromazine is known to affect calmodulin and there is evidence of reduced diarrhoea in piglets treated with the drug (Lonnroth *et al* 1979). However the accompanying sedation may be a practical problem.

Recent additions to the list of potentially effective anti-secretory drugs are those which mimic the α-2 effects of adrenaline (α-2-agonists), such as oxymetazoline, clonidine, and napthazoline. These have been shown experimentally to reduce enterotoxin-induced secretion in the intestine (Newsome *et al* 1981).

The recent demonstration of an antisecretory effect of loperamide (Sandhu *et al* 1979) implies that antimotility and antisecretory effects may coexist in the same drug.

Microbial implants

The use of lactic acid-producing bacteria to give increased growth rate and better health has been described (King 1968). It was assumed that the low pH and anti-*E. coli* activity were the likely explanations for the benefits described. Mitchell & Kenworthy (1976) have described a specific anti-enterotoxin activity in *Streptococcus faecium* and *Lactobacillus bulgaricus*. Both these agents have been used as supplements in animal feeds and it is possible that they may be producing a benefit both by lowering lumenal pH and antagonising enterotoxin. However, Turnbull *et al* (1978) could not confirm this finding using a strain of *E. coli* enterotoxigenic for man.

Conclusion

At present, the complexity of the causes of diarrhoea and the absence of a precise diagnosis — particularly under field conditions — lead to the use of non-specific and combined treatments. For the future, it is desirable to develop better diagnostic techniques and improve our understanding of the pathophysiology of the disease. More specific and efficacious treatments should then become available.

References

Acres S. D., Laing C. S., Saunders J. R. *et al* (1975) Acute undifferentiated neonatal diarrhoea in calves. I. Occurrence and distribution of infectious agents. *Can. J. Comp. Med.* **39**, 116–32.

Arbuckle J. B. R. (1975) Villus atrophy in pigs orally infected with *Salmonella choleraesuis. Res. Vet. Sci.* **18**, 322–4.

Bohl E. H., Kohler E. M., Saif L. J. *et al* (1976) Rotavirus as a cause of diarrhoea in pigs. *J. Am. Vet. Med. Ass.* **172**, 458–63.

Berant M., Wagner V. & Cohen N. (1976) Cholestyramine in the management of infantile diarrhoea. *J. Pediat.* **88**, 153.

Braun R. K. (1975) Peroral use of a special dietary food as a source of electrolytes in diarrhoeic calves. *Vet. Med./SAC* **70**, 601–6.

Burgess M. N., Bywater R. J., Cowley C. M. *et al* (1978) Biological evaluation of a methanol-soluble, heat-stable *E. coli* enterotoxin in infant mice, pigs and calves. *Infect. & Immunity* **21**, 526–31.

Bywater R. J. (1977) Evaluation of an oral glucose-glycine electrolyte formulation and amoxycillin for treatment of diarrhoea in calves. *Am. J. Vet. Res.* **38**, 1983–7.

Bywater R. J. (1980) Comparison between milk deprivation and oral rehydration with a glucose-glycine-electrolyte formulation in diarrhoeic and transported calves. *Vet. Rec.* **107**, 549–51.

Bywater R. J. & Keefe T. J. (1976) Amoxycillin as an antimicrobial agent in the control of colibacillosis in swine. *Proc. Int. Pig. Vet. Soc. Meeting.* Ames, Iowa.

Bywater R. J. & Logan E. F. (1974) The site and characteristics of intestinal water and electrolyte loss in *Escherichia coli*-induced diarrhoea in calves. *J. Comp. Path.* **80**, 599–610.

Bywater R. J. & Penhale W. J. (1968) Depressed lactase activity in the intestinal mucous membrane of calves dying after neonatal diarrhoea. *Res. Vet. Sci.* **10**, 591–3.

Bywater R. J. & Woode G. N. (1980) Oral fluid replacement by a glucose-glycine-electrolyte formulation in *E. coli* and rotavirus diarrhoea in pigs. *Vet. Rec.* **106**, 75–8.

Callear J. F. F. & Smith I. M. (1965) The effect of furazolidone on *Escherichia coli* infection of newborn piglets. *Br. Vet. J.* **122**, 168–76.

Carpenter C. C. J., Curlin G. T. & Greenough W. B. (1969) The response of canine Thiry Vella loops to cholera, and its modification by ethacrynic acid. *J. Inf. Dis.* **120**, 332–7.

Charney A. N. & Donowitz M. (1976) Prevention and reversal of cholera enterotoxin induced intestinal secretion by methyl prednisolone induction of $Na^+ - K^+$ ATPase. *J. Clin. Invest.* **57**, 1590–9.

Dalton R. G., Fisher E. W. & McIntyre W. I. M. (1960) Antibiotics and calf diarrhoea. *Vet. Rec.* **72**, 1186.

Daniels L. B., Fineberg D., Cockrill J. M. *et al* (1977) Use of trimethoprin suphadioxine in controlling calf scours. *Vet. Med/SAC* **72**, 93–5.

Davis W. I., Reynolds W. A. & Maplesden D. C. (1973) Comparison of ampicillin and sulphachlorpyridazine in treatment of colibacillosis in swine. *Vet. Med./SAC* **68**, 847–52.

Dorner F. & Mayer P. (1975) *Escherichia coli* enterotoxin: stimulation of adenylate cyclase in broken cell preparations. *Infect. & Immunity* **11**, 429–31.

Drucker M. M., Goldhar J., Ogra P. L. *et al* (1977) The effect of attapulgite and charcoal on enterotoxicity of *Vibrio cholerae* and *Escherichia coli* enterotoxins in the rabbit. *Infection* **5**, 211–13.

Dupont H. L. & Hornick R. B. (1973) Adverse effect of lomotil in shigellosis. *JAMA* **226**, 1525–8.

Ensley L. E. (1976) Gentamicin for the treatment and prevention of swine enteritis, colibacillosis and dysentery. *Proc. Int. Pig. Vet. Soc.* Ames, Iowa.

Farris R. K., Tapper E. J., Powell D. W. *et al* (1976) Effect of aspirin on normal and cholera toxin-stimulated intestinal electrolyte transport. *J. Clin. Invest.* **57**, 916–24.

Fisher E. W. & de la Fuente G. H. (1971) Antibiotics and calf diarrhoea — the effect of serum immune globulin concentrations. *Vet. Rec.* **89**, 579–82.

Gianella R. A., Gots R. E., Charney A. N. *et al* (1975) Pathogenesis of Salmonella-mediated internal fluid secretion. *Gastroenterology* **69**, 1238–45.

Gots R. E., Formal S. B. & Gianella R. A. (1974) Indomethacin inhibition of *Salmonella typhimurium, Shigella flexneri* and cholera-mediated rabbit ileal secretion. *J. Inf. Dis.* **130**, 280–3.

Gyles C. L. & Barnum D. A. (1969) A heat labile enterotoxin from strains of *E. coli* enteropathogenic for pigs. *J. Infect. Dis.* **120**, 419.

Gyles C. L. & Zigler M. (1978) The effect of adsorbent and anti-inflammatory drugs on secretion in ligated segements of pig intestine infected with *E. coli. Can J. Comp. Med.* **42**, 260–8.

Halpin I. & Caple I. W. (1976) Changes in intestinal structure and function of neonatal calves infected with rheovirus-like agent and *Escherichia coli. Aust. Vet. J.* **52**, 438–41.

Hamm D. & Hicks W. J. (1975) A new oral electrolyte in calf scours therapy. *Vet. Med./SAC* **70**, 279–82.

Hughes J. M. (1978) Role of cyclic GMP on the action of heat stable enterotoxins of *Escherichia coli. Nature.* **271**, 755.

Jones E. W., Hamm D., Corley L. *et al* (1977) Diarrhoeal diseases of the calf: observations on treatment and prevention. *N.Z. Vet. J.* **25**, 312–16.

Keefe T. J. & Bywater R. J. (1976) Amoxycillin as an antimicrobial agent in the control of colibacillosis in swine. *Proc. Int. Pig Vet. Soc.* Ames, Iowa.

King J. O. L. (1968) *Lactobacillus acidophilus* as a growth stimulant for pigs. *The Veterinarian* **5**, 273–80.

Koupal L. R. & Deibel R. H. (1975) Assay, characterisation, and localisation of an entero-toxin produced by Salmonella. *Infect. & Immunity* **11**, 14–22.

Lonroth I., Andren B., Lange S. *et al* (1979) Chlorpromazine reverses diarrhoea in piglets caused by enterotoxigenic *E. coli. Infect. Immun.* **24**, 900–5.

Mebus C. A. (1973) Viral agents in calf diarrhoea. *J. Am. Vet. Med. Ass.* **162**, 279.

Mitchell I. de G. & Kenworthy R. (1976) Investigations on a metabolite from *Lactobacillus bulgaricus* which neutralises the effect of enterotoxin from *Escherichia coli* pathogenic for pigs. *J. Appl. Bact.* **41**, 163–74.

Moon H. W. (1978) Mechanisms in the pathogenesis of diarrhoea: A review. *J. Am. Vet. Med. Ass.* **172**, 443–8.

Moon H. E. & Bemrick W. J. (1981) Fecal transmission of calf cryptosporidia between calves and pigs. *Vet. Pathol.* **18**, 248–55.

Moon H. W., McClurkin A. W., Isaacson R. E. *et al* (1978) Pathogenic relationships of rotavirus, *Escherichia coli* and other agents in mixed infections in calves. *JAVMA* **137**, 577–83.

Mullan N. A., Burgess M. N., Bywater R. J. *et al* (1979) The ability of cholestyramine resin and other adsorbents to bind *Escherichia coli* enterotoxins. *J. Med. Microbiol* **12**, 487–95.

Nalin D. R., Cash R. A., Rahman M. *et al* (1970) Effect of glycine and glucose on sodium and water absorption in patients with cholera. *Gut* **11**, 768–72.

Nalin D. R., Levine R. J., Levine M. M. *et al* (1978) Cholera, nonvibrio cholera and stomach acid. *Lancet* i, 856–9.

Newsome P. N., Burgess M. N. & Mullan N. A. (1973) Effect of *E. coli* heat stable enterotoxin on cyclic GMP levels in mouse intestine. *Infect. & Immunity* **22**, 290–1.

Newsome P. N., Burgess M., Holman G. D. *et al* (1981) α-2 adrenoceptors controlling intestinal secretion. *Biochem. Soc. Trans.* **9**, 413–4.

Niemegeers C. J. E., Lenaerts F. M. & Janssen P. A. J. (1974) Loperamide (R18553) a novel type of antidiarrhoeal agent. *Arzneimittel Forsch.* **24**, 1636–40.

Ørskov I., Ørskov F., Smith H. W. *et al* (1975) The establishment of K99, a thermolabile, transmissible *E. coli* K antigen previously called 'K Co' produced by calf and lamb enteropathogenic strains. *Acta Path. Microbiol. Scand. B.* **83**, 31.

Palmer G. H., Bywater R. J. & Francis M. E. (1977) Amoxycillin: distribution and clinical efficacy in calves. *Vet. Rec.* **100**, 487–91.

Pankhurst J. W. (1976) Trials with a new Gram negative antibiotic for enteric disease in calves. *Vet. Rec.* **99**, 107.

Pearson G. R., McNulty M. S. & Logan E. F. (1978) Pathological changes in the small intestine of neonatal calves naturally infected with rheo-like virus (rotavirus). *Vet. Rec.* **21**, 454–8.

Pohlenz J., Moon H. W., Cheville N. F. *et al* (1978) Cryptosparidiosis as a probable factor in neonatal diarrhoea of calves. *J. Am. Vet. Med. Ass.* **172**, 452–7.

Portnoy B. L., Dupont H. L., Pruitt D. *et al* (1976) Antidiarrhoeal agents in the treatment of acute diarrhoea in children. *JAMA* **236**, 844–6.

Radostits O. M. (1974) Treatment and control of neonatal diarrhoea in calves. *J. Dairy Sci.* **58**, 464–70.

Radostits O. M., Rhodes C. S., Mitchell M. E. *et al* (1975) Clinical evaluation of antimicrobial agents and temporary starvation in the treatment of acute undifferentiated diarrhoea in new born calves. *Can. Vet. J.* **16**, 219–27.

Sandhu B., Tripp J. H., Candy D. C. A. *et al* (1979) Loperamide inhibits cholera toxin induced small intestinal secretion. *Lancet* ii, 689.

Smith H. W. & Halls S. (1967) Studies on *E. coli* enterotoxin *J. Path. Bact.* **93**, 531–43.

Smith H. W. & Halls S. (1968) The transmissible nature of the genetic factor in *Escherichia coli* that controls enterotoxin production. *J. Gen. Microbiol.* **52**, 319–34.

Sojka W. J. (1971) Enteric diseases in newborn pigs, calves and lambs due to *Escherichia coli* infection. *Vet. Bull.* **41**, 509.

Stortz J., Kollier J. R., Eugster A. K. *et al* (1971) Intestinal bacterial changes in chlamydia-induced primary enteritis in newborn calves. *Ann. N.Y. Acad. Sci.* **176**, 162–75.

Symoens J., Geerts H. & Van Gestel J. (1974) Benzetimide in the treatment of diarrhoea in newborn calves and adult cattle *Vet. Rec.* **94**, 108–83.

Tolnay (1799) Arts veterinaria compendium pathologicum. Cited by Jensen (1893) *Mh Tierheilk* **4**, 97.

Turnbull P. C. B., Gerson P. J. & Stanley G. (1978) Inability of selected lactobacilli to inhibit the heat-labile or heat-stable enterotoxin effects of *Escherichia coli* B7A. *J. Appl. Bact.* **45**, 157–60.

Tzipori S. (1981) The aetiology and diagnosis of calf diarrhoea. *Vet. Rec.* **108**, 510–14.

Waller S. L. & Misiewicz J. J. (1972) Colonic motility in constipation or diarrhoea. *Scand. J. Gastroenterol* **7**, 93–6.

Watt J. G. (1967) Fluid therapy for dehydration in calves. *J. Am. Vet. Ass.* **150**, 742–50.
Weijers H. A. & Van de Kamer J. H. (1965) Alteration of intestinal bacterial flora as a cause of diarrhoea *Nut. Abs. & Reviews* **35**, 591–603.
Whipp S. C. & Moon H. W. (1973) Modification of enterosorption in experimental enteric colibacillosis of swine inoculated with *Escherichia coli. J. Infect. Dis.* **127**, 255–60.
Woode G. N. (1969) Transmissible gastroenteritis of swine. *Vet. Bull.* **39**, 239–48.

PART 6
OTHER PHARMACOLOGICAL AGENTS

19

Anti-inflammatory agents

D.H. SNOW

Drugs are frequently used to reduce the inflammatory response to injury whether it be traumatic or otherwise in origin. In large animal practice these therapeutic agents are an essential part of the armamentarium of equine practitioners, although they are used less frequently in the treatment of livestock. Because of the demands of racing and other equestrian disciplines it is not surprising that injuries promoting an inflammatory response are common. The frequency of drug usage to treat these conditions will vary from area to area since it is dependent on the drug doping legislation and drug detection capability of the state or country. As these agents interfere with the animal's natural defence mechanisms, the veterinarian often has to make decisions whether they should be employed at all, whether they should be used to provide relief in conjunction with a period of rest to allow healing, or used to return the animal to the performance arena as rapidly as possible. Arguments for and against the employment of anti-inflammatory agents to permit horses to compete have been considered by Snow (1981).

Although the major drugs selected for use in these species are similar to those developed in laboratory animals and used in man, data obtained cannot always be extrapolated from one species to another, as factors such as the mediators involved in the inflammatory process, and pharmacokinetic, pharmacodynamic and toxicological properties of the drugs will vary between species. For optimum efficacy therefore, these factors should be examined in the particular species in which they are to be used.

In this chapter the inflammatory process, the mediators involved, methods of assessment of efficacy of anti-inflammatory agents in the horse, and drugs commonly used will be described. In considering the use of therapeutic agents, those which are used in the treatment of a wide spectrum of inflammatory responses, and which are generally given systemically, will be mentioned first. A section will also be devoted to evaluating the usefulness of drugs that can be administered locally in the treatment of joint and tendon disorders — conditions of paramount importance to the equine practitioner.

Inflammation

Inflammation is the response of living tissue to an injury and consists of a series of events involving vascular and cellular changes to eliminate the noxious agent and repair any damage. The reaction gives rise to the cardinal signs of redness, heat, swelling, and pain; it may also lead to loss of function. The stimulus for inflammation can be either immunological or non-immunological in origin. The immunological mechanisms are outlined in Fig. 19.1 and the different types of hypersensitivity in animals are reviewed by Eyre (1980) and Hanna *et al* (1982). The initial response in the first few hours is similar, whatever the precipitating cause, but subsequent events will be largely dependent upon the severity, nature and duration of the injurious agent. If the cause is persistent, the later changes depend upon the nature of the noxious agent. For this brief review of the inflammatory response and mediators involved, information has been obtained from two comprehensive handbooks on the subject by Vane & Ferriera (1978) and by Houck (1979).

The initial pathological changes are related to alterations in the vascular bed, whist later ones are concerned with cellular events in the damaged tissue. The three processes involved are: 1 Increased blood flow to the injured area which results in the redness (erythema) and heat. 2 Increased vascular permeability, resulting in swelling (oedema). 3 Escape of leucocytes from blood into the extravascular tissue which, in some conditions, may contribute to the swelling.

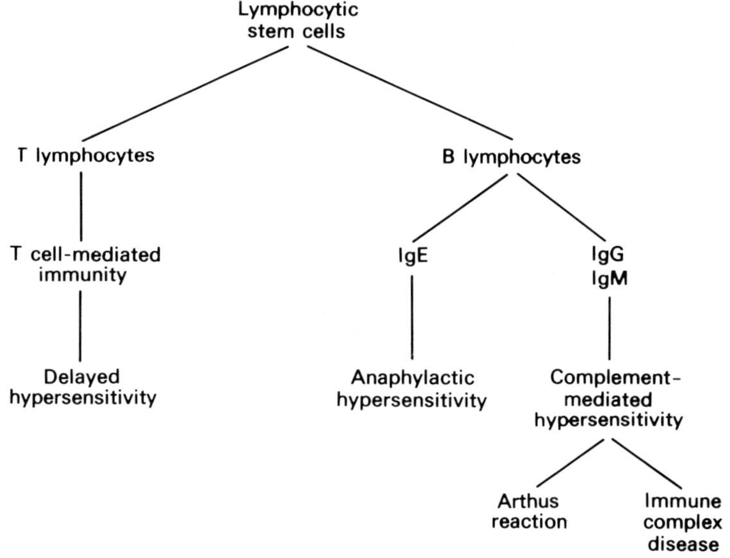

Fig. 19.1 Classification of hypersensitivity reactions. (From Turk & Willoughby 1978.)

The increased blood flow to the injurious area is brought about by dilatation of the arterioles. At first, blood flow is rapid through the injured area. However, after a varying period, there is a reduction in flow and eventual stasis may occur, possibly due to an increasing haematocrit as plasma escapes from venules.

In conjunction with, but separate from, the dilatation of the arterioles is the increase in vascular permeability leading to effusion and the production of oedema. This results from contraction of the endothelial cells of the venules to bring about a partial detachment of intercellular connections and the escape of protein and fluid.

Following these vascular changes, the process of leucocyte movement occurs and consists of the three stages of margination, emigration and chemotaxis. As the rate of blood flow decreases, leucocytes begin to appear in the marginal stream of the venules in the injured area and gradually adhere to the wall — a process referred to as margination or pavmentation. In the initial stages the adhering leucocytes are predominantly polymorpho-nuclears (PMNs) together with some eosinophils and monocytes, with lym-phocytes not being involved. This adhesion has been shown to depend on alterations in the vascular wall and not in the leucocytes. The leucocytes then emigrate from the venules by amoeboid movement, whilst any red cells escape due to entirely passive means. Once out of the vascular system, the movement of the leucocytes to the injured area occurs by chemotaxis.

The initial changes are generally of short duration and subsequent changes may follow one of four courses.
1 *Resolution,* in which complete restoration of the injured area to the normal state occurs. This is usually the sequel to mild chemical and physical injuries of brief duration.
2 *Healing* by scar tissue with or without regeneration of lost parenchymal cells.
3 *Suppuration,* where the nature of the injury, e.g. certain bacteria, results in the continued appearance of large numbers of PMNs.
4 *Chronic inflammation,* which occurs when there is a persistent irritation and results in the emigration of large numbers of leucocytes and can be characterised into those where granulomatous tissue forms and those where this does not occur. Granulation tissue results from the stimulation of fibroblast proliferation and secretion of mucopolysaccharides.

In the early stages of inflammation, the majority of emigrating cells are PMNs. These have a variety of activities; they are highly phagocytic and have the ability to discharge further mediators from their lysosomes. When emigration has finished they usually disappear from the injured area within 24–48 hours as they die and liberate their granules and cytoplasmic enzymes, which may play a role in mediating the later stages of inflammation. As the PMNs disappear, the mononuclear cells come to form an increasing proportion of those in the injured area. The main function of the mononuclear cells (monocytes, macrophages) is to eliminate material by phagocytosis or pinocytosis. Increasing numbers can move into the area as they are formed from bone marrow precursors.

In inflammation caused by cell-mediated immunity where, in contrast to other injuries, maximum intensity occurs only between 24 and 48 hours, the cellular infiltration initially consists mainly of PMNs and then later of monocytes, until by 48 hours there are equal proportions of small lymphocytes and monocytes.

Mediators

It is now well established that these inflammatory changes are brought about by the release of numerous substances that can mediate the various stages of inflammation. In addition, more than one mediator can usually bring about any one of these stages. The complexity of the multi-mediated early stages of inflammation is shown in Fig. 19.2. As well as this multitude of factors, the fact that the proportion of these different mediators involved in the response to injury varies with different noxious agents, between tissues, and between species adds to the complexity of the situation and helps explain why anti-inflammatory agents have varying efficacy in different tissues. However, a knowledge of the mediators involved does assist in the rational designs of drugs that may be useful as anti-inflammatory agents. For instance the recent identification of SRS-A, an important mediator of asthma in man, as a leukotriene (Samuelsson 1980) may aid in the discovery of more effective therapeutic/prophylactic agents for this condition. However as Ryan & Majno (1977) state ' . . . evolution has ensured that the acute inflammatory reaction takes place at all costs, if not by one mechanism then another. Although this is of great advantage in the evolutionary fight against infection, however, it complicates the problem of medicinal pharmacology.'

To further our understanding of the inflammatory response and means of modifying it, extensive work has been carried out in identifying the mediators involved. For a substance to be implicated as a mediator it has to satisfy the following four criteria: 1 It is released by an inflammatory stimulus. 2 Substances which inhibit its synthesis/release or antagonise its action *in vivo* should diminish the intensity of one or more components of the inflammatory reaction. 3 Administration of the substance should induce at least one of the components of the inflammatory reaction. 4 Administration of a substance which diminishes its destruction or uptake should enhance the inflammatory signs or symptoms.

Depending on their mode of action these mediators can be divided into three categories: those that act on pharmacological receptors, lytic enzymes of cell or plasma origin which cause direct damage to the integrity of tissue components and/or migratory cells, and chemotactic factors which stimulate cell migration to the site of inflammation. It appears that different factors are involved in the attraction of the various leucocytic cells.

A plethora of compounds, especially in the third category, have now been implicated as mediators and the more important are shown in Table 19.1. These various mediators act in a coordinated and sequential manner to bring about the pathological events seen in inflammation. At present most is known about the mediators that act on pharmacological receptors.

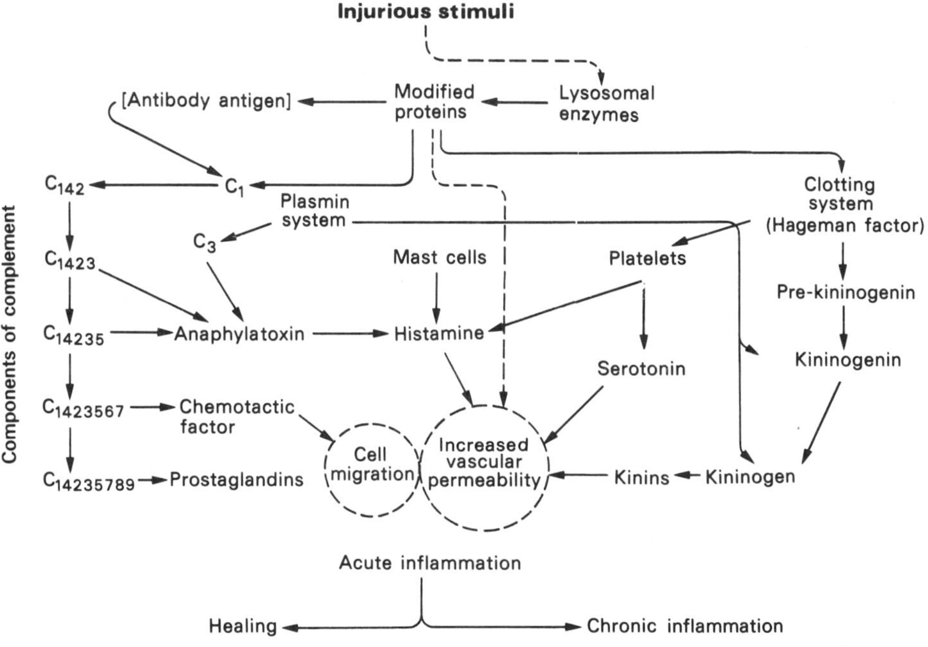

Fig. 19.2 Interaction of mediators of inflammation. (From Rocha e Silva 1978.)

Histamine

The release of histamine from mast cells and basophils causes inflammatory effects by its microcirculatory actions of vasodilation and increased permeability. It also stimulates sensory pain fibres. Histamine release in acute hypersensitivity reactions leads to more widespread responses, which can be life-threatening. The cellular effects of histamine have now been shown to be mediated via at least two receptor types, H_1 and H_2. The inflammatory responses are considered to be via H_1 receptors, and hence the effectiveness of the classical antihistamines (such as tripelennamine) against the early stages of acute inflammation and acute hypersensitivities. However, it has recently been shown that histamine can also behave in a fashion described as 'negative-feedback inhibition' by acting on H_2 receptors on mast cells, which results in inhibition of further release of histamine. This may explain why histamine release is only important in the initial stages of inflammation. Other modulating effects of histamine acting via H_2 receptors have been described (Busse 1979).

5-Hydroxytryptamine (5-HT; Serotonin)

This preformed vasoactive amine can be released in the early stages of the inflammatory response, although the extent varies considerably between species. Eyre (1972) has shown that it is released during immunologically-induced inflammation in ruminants. In most species its most important source is from damaged platelets. Its actions in the inflammatory response are similar to those of histamine.

Prostaglandins

Prostaglandins were first proposed as inflammatory mediators by Willis (1969) and, since that time, numerous studies have further elucidated their key role in the various stages of the inflammatory response. Because of their importance and the fact that the most commonly used anti-inflammatory agents exert their effect by preventing synthesis of these compounds, their actions will be considered in more detail.

Prostaglandins are not stored within cells but are synthesised in response to the appropriate stimulus. They are capable of being produced in all cells and the pathway of synthesis is shown in Fig. 19.3 The precursor of prostaglandins are three unsaturated C_{20} free fatty acids, of which by far the major one is arachidonic acid. This acid is only found free in cells in small amounts and is probably released as required from cell membrane phospholipids by

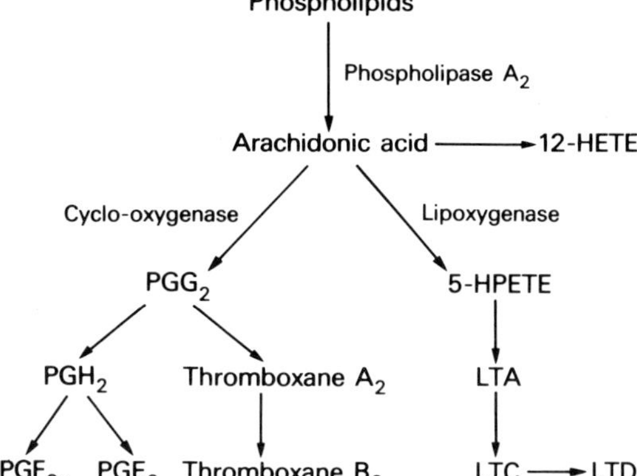

Fig. 19.3 Simplified scheme of transformation of arachidonic acid into prostaglandins, thromboxanes and leukotrienes (SRS-A).

the action of a membrane bound enzyme, phospholipase A_2. Cyclo-oxygenase, a multi-enzyme complex, then generate the intermediate endoperoxides (PGG_2 and PGH_2) which have very short half-lives and further enzymic action results in the production of thromboxanes and a series of prostaglandins. These have differing activity on various tissues and also between species. Different prostaglandins produced within one tissue can have opposing effects on that tissue. The complex of enzymes involved in the synthesis of these compounds from arachidonic acid are collectively referred to as prostaglandin synthetases, although this term has also often been used, in a more limited sense, synonymously with cyclo-oxygenases.

It is now apparent that these derivatives of arachidonic acid have an important place in the mediation and modulation of the inflammatory response, as well as numerous other physiological effects. Prostaglandins are named according to the substituents on the basic prostaglandin nucleus as belonging to series A–F with those of the E and F series being most abundant.

Vasodilation is caused by prostaglandins of the E series (PGE) whose action is of equal potency but, interestingly, of much longer duration than that of histamine or the kinins. PGE release is considered to be responsible for the maintenance of vasodilation after release of histamine, of 5HT, and of kinins has ceased.

Increased vascular permeability also occurs with PGE. However this is of a much shorter duration than the vasodilation it produces. As well as having a direct effect it appears that it also acts synergistically with the other mediators.

Hyperalgesia and *pain* can be produced by prostaglandins. However, during the inflammatory response it is thought that, in the quantities released, the major effect of PGE, PGI_2 and endoperoxide is the development of 'hyperalgesia'. This term refers to the production of a reduced threshold of the nocioceptors and therefore makes them sensitive to stimuli, both mechanical and chemical, which are normally non-painful. Therefore, pain can be perceived when bradykinin and histamine are released in concentrations which do not normally cause algesia.

Chemotaxis is only weakly produced with PGE having some chemoattractant activity for PMNs.

Granuloma formation has been shown to be enhanced by PGE which causes proliferation of fibroblasts.

Fever is now considered to be mediated by prostaglandin release raising the level of the thermoregulatory centre. The stimuli for the synthesis of the prostaglandin are endogenous pyrogens which are able to cross into the hypothalamus.

Slow reacting substance of anaphylaxis (SRS-A)

In addition to the major pathway of arachidonic acid metabolism described, it has now been shown that metabolism can occur via a complex of enzymes called lipoxygenases which result in the synthesis of the substance 12-hydroxy arachidonic acid (12-HETE) and of the recently isolated group of compounds, the leukotrienes (Fig. 19.3). Two of these leukotrienes have been identified as the substance previously known as SRS-A (Samuelsson 1980), and which plays an important role in immediate hypersensitivity in a number of species including cattle. This substance is synthesised in neutrophils and mast cells and, when released, has activities primarily on blood vessels and smooth muscle. 12-HETE has been found to exert pronounced chemotactic activity on neutrophils.

Kinins

These are linear polypeptides, which are released by the activation of proteases that are found in the plasma and in tissues. Most is known about the major kinin, bradykinin which is formed in plasma as a result of various stimuli. Its production results from activation of kininogens which act on bradykininogen. One of the activating factors is Factor XII or Hageman Factor, which is also important in the initiation of blood clotting and fibrin formation. The kinins formed have a short half-life due to their rapid inactivation by kinases; however, they are important mediators of the early events in acute inflammation. They are much more potent than histamine in causing vasodilation and increased vascular permeability. In addition they are a chemical irritant to pain receptors, although it is considered that normally a hyperalgesia due to prostaglandin release is necessary for the pain seen in inflammation. When released in the lungs during immediate hypersensitivity in a number of species they produce a marked broncho-constriction.

Complement

This is a system of factors that occur in normal serum. The activation of this system, resulting in the production of a number of biologically active substances during the complement cascade (Fig. 19.2), is brought about by interaction between antigen and antibody of IgG and IgM types. In addition, complement activation can occur via non-immune mechanisms such as bacterial endotoxins and related polysaccharides. The product of complement can cause lysis and cell destruction; the anaphylatoxins (C_{3a} and C_{5a}) may produce contraction of smooth muscle, chemotaxis of PMNs, and release of mediators from mast cell. Interactions can also occur between complement and the other blood systems of clotting, fibrin formation, and production of kinins.

Chemotactic factors

There are numerous substances which have been shown to exert an effect on the direction of movement of leucocytes once they have emigrated from the vascular system. Chemotaxis is considered the most important mechanism for the accumulation of leucocytes in the inflamed area and probably plays an important role in the maintenance of cells in the area during the chronic inflammatory state. A list of some of the substances incriminated as having chemotactic properties is shown in Table 19.1. Except for some activity by PGE, and 12-HETE, the immediate mediators of inflammation do not have chemotactic properties. However, substances with chemotactic properties have been identified as arising from a variety of sources, including products of complement, numerous lymphokines produced by lymphocytes, factors released by damaged or dying cells, factors generated during activation of enzyme cascades in plasma, and exogenous substances such as those released by some invading bacteria. These chemotactic factors may be either non-specific in that all leucocyte types are attracted or exert effects on a specific cell type.

Lysosomal enzymes

Within the granules of the PMNs and macrophages are hydrolytic enzymes

Table 19.1 Major mediators of the inflammatory response.

Mediating vascular changes
   Histamine
   5-Hydroxytryptamine
   Bradykinin
   Prostaglandins
   Leukotrienes

Mediating chemotaxis
   Anaphylatoxins
   12-HETE
   Lymphokines (numerous categories)

Lysosomal factors
   Cathepsins
   Neutral proteinases
   Cationic proteins

referred to as lysozymes. Although their mechanism of release and exact role in the inflammatory reaction are not fully understood, it is considered that they have both direct and indirect action in maintaining the inflammatory response. As well as enzymes being released from lysosomes, basic proteins devoid of enzymatic activity are also released which can enhance vascular permeability.

Testing for effective anti-inflammatory drugs

The detailed information on the sequence of the inflammatory response, variations resulting from type and site of injury, and mediators involved have been obtained from extensive investigations using models producing these responses in a number of laboratory animals. In addition, these models have also been used to assess the mode of action and relative potency of potentially clinically useful anti-inflammatory compounds. Although these tests are vital for the further development of these agents, because of well known variations in response between species, it is necessary that trials are carried out in the intended species. Tests should include those on efficacy since these also provide information on pharmacokinetics for formulation of correct dosage regimens, and toxicological studies. The latter aspects are extremely important for the classical non-steroidal anti-inflammatory drugs where it has been shown that marked differences exist between species.

The efficacy of a potential agent can be investigated either using appropriate inflammatory models in that species or by well controlled clinical trials.

In addition to having a model, it is important to have adequate criteria for assessment of the response. Although a number of clinical trials of new anti-inflammatory agents have been carried out in the horse, these have often been of only limited use due to lack of quantification of the inflammatory reactions, to the subjective rather than objective evaluation of response, lack of follow-up treatment, and lack of comparison to response with a placebo and/or drug of known efficacy. Various models have been developed in the horse to overcome this, with better methods of assessment of response. These have helped but, as very few comparative studies have been carried out, there is a large gap in our knowledge on the relative efficacy of these compounds except from personal experience and the often unsubstantiated claims of pharmaceutical companies. Today, this lack of information is not due to the inability to use adequate models or methods of assessment but the substantial costs required for carrying out such investigation.

Models for producing an inflammatory reaction in the horse include: 1 Myositis — injection of concentrated solution of lactic acid into the body of muscle. 2 Oesteoarthritis — removal of part of cartilage of joint, production of chip fractures, or injection of irritant substance or bacteria into a joint. 3 Tendinitis — injection of irritant substance around tendons.

Methods of evaluation of the response to an anti-inflammatory agent are dependent on the ability to assess alterations in the components of the inflammatory reaction, i.e. swelling, redness, heat, pain and loss of function. Recently a number of methods have been described in the horse that allow measurement of these components. These include *swelling* as quantified in the myositis model (Kilian *et al* 1974), *heat* which can be accurately determined by infra-red thermography (Purohit & McCoy 1980). This provides great promise for the future evaluation of anti-inflammatory drugs. Purohit & McCoy (1980) were able to demonstrate that heat still existed in lesions after observations indicated that the animals were clinically normal and suggested that thermography could be an extremely useful aid in helping decide when animals were fit to be returned to training/racing. *Loss of function* which is brought about by pain and other inflammatory events can also be readily assessed, if associated with lameness, by determination of alterations in stride length and pattern (Kilian *et al* 1974). Inflammatory processes in limbs also result in changes in the proportion of the body weight supported by each of the four limbs. The forces supported in each limb can be accurately determined by the use of force plate measurements (Pratt & O'Connor 1976).

Anti-inflammatory drugs

As the term 'anti-inflammatory drug' can be applied to any drug which inhibits any of the facets of inflammation, it is not surprising that an enormous number of compounds with diverse structures have been found to have some anti-inflammatory activity. The exotic potions and lotions used in the treatment of inflammatory conditions in the horse over the last few hundred years are legend. Still in use today are various counter-irritants, and blisters and firing which are employed to overcome or modify chronic inflammatory conditions. In addition to pure compounds from plant extracts, there are also available a large number of related synthetic compounds as well as preparations from animal tissues. The anti-inflammatory agents used can be broadly divided into two major groups: cyclo-oxygenase inhibitors (the classical non-steroidal anti-inflammatory drugs (NSAIDS); antipyretic analgesics) and corticosteroids. In addition there is a miscellaneous group which have varying actions and include hyaluronic acid and orgotein.

In the rational employment of these drugs it should be remembered that the veterinarian's role in treatment is two-fold in that symptomatic relief to reduce suffering is paramount but, in addition, steps to ensure correct diagnosis and removal of the underlying cause are generally necessary for the second purpose of healing. Unfortunately many of the compounds used to alleviate symptoms, by the very nature of their action may be contra-indicated for the second aim of healing and in the long term may result in exacerbation of the condition. Therefore, the aetiology of the condition, aim of treatment, and long term outlook should all be considered in deciding which therapeutic measures should be instituted.

Cyclo-oxygenase inhibitors (classical NSAIDs)

The oldest members of this large group of drugs are sodium salicylate and acetylsalicyclic acid, which were in therapeutic use in man before the turn of the century. Since then a large number of other groups of compounds exhibiting similar activity have been synthesised. Of the many drugs available for use in man, there are only a small number of veterinary importance and their structures are shown in Fig. 19.4. In the early 1950s the anti-inflammatory agent phenylbutazone was introduced into veterinary practice: its active metabolite oxyphenbutazone has also been used clinically, although specific veterinary preparations are unavailable. In the 1960s, synthesis of a large number of mainly acidic compounds with similar anti-inflammatory activity occurred. Of these, only three — meclofenamic acid, naproxen and flunixin meglumine — have been marketed for use in the equine, although some pharmacokinetic and metabolism studies have been

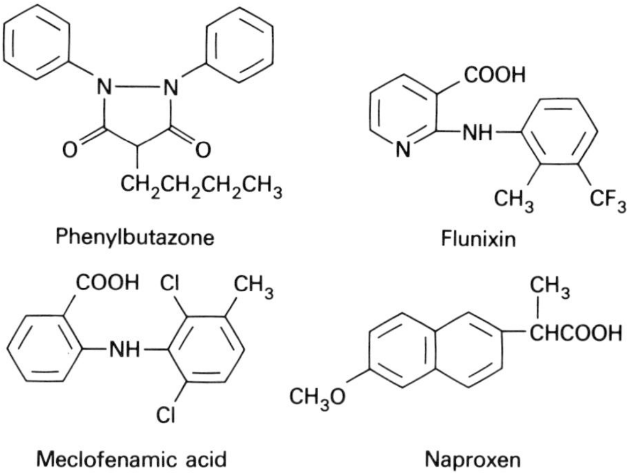

Fig. 19.4 Structure of the main non-steroidal anti-inflammatory drugs used in the horse.

carried out with acetylsalicylic acid (Davis & Westfall 1972, Jouany *et al* 1979), indomethacin (Phillips *et al* 1980, Lehmann *et al* 1981), fenamic acid (Lehmann *et al* 1981), and ibuprofen (Lambert *et al* 1979).

Chemical properties

All the compounds in this group are aromatic carboxylic acids with pKa values of 4.5 or less which result in a very low water solubility. To increase water solubility they are often administered as sodium salts, especially in formulations for parenteral use. Formulation as salts also increases the speed of absorption following oral administration. Their acidic nature has also been shown to aid their accumulation within inflamed tissue. With the exception of salicylate, which is approximately 50% bound to plasma proteins (Davis & Westfall 1972), the other compounds are extremely highly protein bound, being greater than 99% for meclofenamic acid (Snow *et al* 1981a) and naproxen. The extensive protein binding is of therapeutic importance as it is the non-protein bound or free drug that is associated with biological activity, either favourable or toxicological. Prior or concurrent administration of other drugs which are highly protein bound can, because of competition, lead to higher free levels of either drug, and in the case of very highly protein bound drugs, a decrease of 1% binding can result in markedly increased free drug concentration. Therapeutically this is of relevance in the possible administration of both warfarin and NSAIDs in the treatment of navicular disease since this could result in warfarin toxicity. In the dog the concomitant administration of these two drugs resulted in an elevation in the free fraction of warfarin in the plasma from 2.6 to 8.0% , as

well as a two-fold decrease in the plasma half-life of warfarin (Bachmann &
Burkmann 1975).

Mode of action

Although salicylates have been used throughout this century and phenylbutazone (PBZ) for the last 30 years, it has only been in the last decade that
the major mechanisms for their effective, anti-inflammatory, analgesic, and
antipyretic activities have been elucidated. Although previously numerous
actions such as stabilisation of lysosomal membranes and inhibition of
fibroblast activity have been attributed to this group, it has now been
extremely well documented that their primary activity is by their inhibition
of cyclo-oxygenase, and the prevention of the synthesis of various prostaglandins and their precursors. Thus this basic inhibitory mechanism can
account for the numerous beneficial activities attributed to this class of
compound (for details see Ferriera & Vane 1979).

Further support for the concept that this is the main mode of action
comes from the many studies which have generally shown that the in-vitro
cyclo-oxygenase inhibitory potency of the compounds is similar to the order
of potency of commonly used agents which is meclofenamic acid →
indomethacin → naproxen → phenylbutazone → acetylsalicylic acid. It is
thought that they competitively inhibit cyclo-oxygenase, by binding to the
active site, as the aromatic moieties in these compounds are sterically and
electronically similar to the polyene system in arachidonic acid (Shen 1979).
Some of these compounds have been shown to produce irreversible inhibition. Although this relative potency is generally true, differences have been
found between tissues and species, and may be attributed to the presence of
cyclo-oxygenase isoenzymes (Schror *et al* 1980).

In addition to their cyclo-oxygenase inhibitory activity, the fenamates,
including meclofenamic acid, have also been found to be prostaglandin
antagonists, as they also interact with prostaglandin receptors. Therefore
this class of compounds, but not the others, are able to prevent the action of
prostaglandins already present in the injured area, and hence may possibly
exert a more rapid diminution of inflammatory signs.

Metabolism and pharmacokinetics

With the exception of phenylbutazone, all the cyclo-oxygenase inhibitors
used in veterinary practice are degraded and/or conjugated to inactive
metabolites. However, phenylbutazone is partially metabolised to
oxyphenbutazone, a compound which also has anti-inflammatory activity.
Following a normal therapeutic dose in the horse, plasma oxyphenbutazone

concentration is approximately 10% of the phenylbutazone concentration, whilst repeated dosage at the highest recommended dose results in plasma concentrations as great as 25% of that of phenylbutazone (Gerring *et al* 1981).

The metabolites and small amounts of the parent anti-inflammatory drugs are excreted in the urine. Only small amounts of active drug are found in the urine and the rate of metabolism is the predominant factor responsible for the reduction in plasma concentrations after drug administration. Biliary excretion is also an important route of excretion in many species; however, this aspect has not been studied in the horse. Following biliary excretion of conjugated metabolites, they may be deconjugated within the intestine and re-enter the body via the enterohepatic circulation shunt. Because of their high protein binding only very small amounts are excreted in saliva and therefore saliva collection is of little use in detection of the illegal use of this group of drugs.

For the successful alleviation of inflammatory symptoms correct dosage is essential and this can only be brought about by a knowledge of factors that influence plasma concentrations following drug administration. Unfortunately due to scarcity of data, adequate plasma concentrations for any of these drugs associated with alleviation of symptoms are largely unknown; treatment is therefore often empirical. It is probable, because of the high protein binding characteristics, that therapeutic concentrations remain in tissues for a period after they are no longer detectable in plasma. This, together with the ability of some NSAIDs to irreversibly bind cyclo-oxygenase, may explain a residual effectiveness in certain conditions after cessation of therapy. Lehmann *et al* (1981) have shown that, following both phenylbutazone and naproxen administration, elimination was considerably slower from synovial fluid than serum (Fig. 19.5).

Intravenous administration

Although these drugs are not used intravenously in man, as the risks of side-effects far outweigh any need to obtain high plasma levels immediately, intravenous phenylbutazone preparations are available for use in the horse. These consist of phenylbutazone alone or its combination with another pyrazolone derivative, isopyrin, or a corticosteroid. Flunixin is also available for intravenous use.

Measurement of plasma concentrations following intravenous administration of these drugs allows their plasma half-lives to be determined accurately (Table 19.2). For phenylbutazone in the horse, a dose-dependent effect on plasma half-life occurs, possibly due to the inhibitory effect of the metabolite oxyphenbutazone. In support of this Tobin *et al* (1977) found

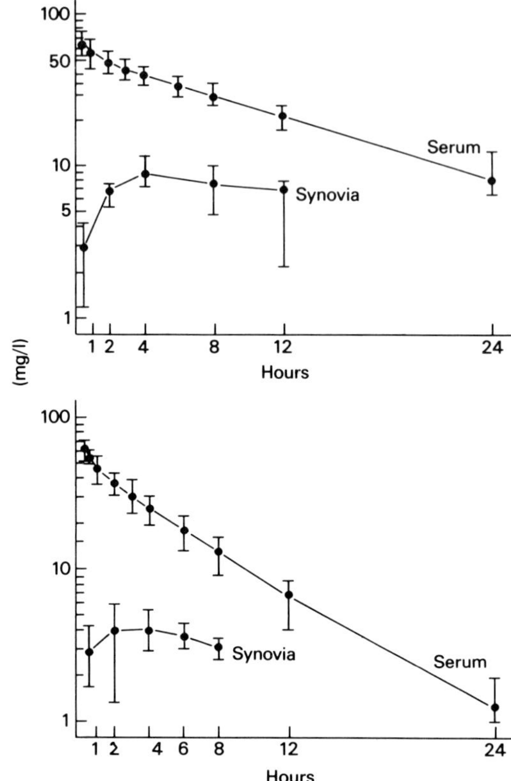

Fig. 19.5 Concentration of phenylbutazone (*above*) and naproxen (*below*) in serum and synovia following intravenous injection of 10 mg/kg.

that intravenous injection of oxyphenbutazone shortly before intravenous injection of PBZ resulted in prolongation of the latter's half-life. With a dose of 4.4. mg/kg i.v. the plasma half-life of phenylbutazone is of the order of 3–4 hours, whilst increasing the dose to 8.8 mg/kg doubles the half-life. The concurrent administration of phenylbutazone and isopyrin, another pyrazolone derivative, results in the prolongation of the half-life of both drugs due to competition for the metabolising enzymes responsible for their degradation (Jenny *et al* 1979). In cattle, the plasma half-life was found to range from 32 to 60 hours after an i.v. dose of 6 mg/kg (Eberhardson *et al* 1979). The considerably longer half-life was thought to be due to a slower rate of metabolism and may be connected with the finding that the metabolite, oxyphenbutazone, was absent from bovine serum.

Oral administration

Granules or powder preparations of meclofenamic acid, naproxen, phenyl-butazone and flunixin, are available for oral administration to horses. Both

Table 19.2 Plasma half-life and protein binding after intravenous administration of some non-steroidal anti-inflammatory compounds.

Drug	Dose (mg/kg)	Plasma $T\frac{1}{2}$ (hr)	% Protein binding	Reference
Acetylsalicylic acid	4.4	1.0	55	Davis & Westfall 1972
Phenylbutazone	4.4	3.5	0	Piperno *et al* 1968
	6.5	7.0	96	Gandal *et al* 1969
	6.0	6.2	–	Jenny *et al* 1979
	6.6	5.5	–	Snow *et al* 1981
	10	8.6	97–99	Lehmann *et al* 1981
Meclofenamic acid	2.2 & 4.4	1.0	>99	Snow *et al* 1981
Naproxen	10	4.7	99.6	Lehmann *et al* 1981
Flunixin meglumine	1.1	1.6	–	Houdeshell & Hennessey 1977

meclofenamic acid and naproxen are readily accepted in feed but palatability problems can be encountered with phenylbutazone. To overcome this, a paste preparation administered by a multidose applicator has been marketed recently; alternatively, the powder can be suspended in water and administered by syringe into the oral cavity.

Although the relationship of plasma drug concentration to pharmacological activity is not known for this group of drugs, F.E.I. regulations (1981) — allowing maximum plasma levels of 4 μg/ml for phenylbutazone — have made a knowledge of factors that can influence the rate and extent of absorption essential. Studies by Sullivan & Snow (1982) suggest that a number of factors will influence the absorption of both phenylbutazone and meclofenamic acid. Even under identical conditions of administration, large variations in rate of absorption, peak value concentrations and bioavailability occur for phenylbutazone. Irregular absorption is not surprising as it has been well documented in man that drug–food interactions can occur which can reduce, delay, increase, or have no effect on drug absorption (Toothaker & Welling 1980). Although NSAIDs are acidic and absorption can occur from the stomach, the majority is from duodenum (Moffat 1978). Therefore gastric emptying time, which is influenced by presence and nature of food, can affect absorption. For both phenylbutazone and meclofenamic acid delayed absorption with lower peak plasma concentrations have been reported following administration on a full compared to an empty stomach in the horse (Sullivan & Snow 1982). In addition, a lower bioavailability for PBZ and meclofenamic acid was seen in association with a full stomach. In some cases virtually no absorption has been found following the administration of either paste or powder preparations (5 mg/kg) to ponies allowed free access to hay (Snow, unpublished data). In comparing breeds it is possible that a lower bioavailability of both meclofenamic acid and PBZ occurs in ponies than larger breeds (Snow *et al* 1981a, Sullivan & Snow 1982), though the reasons for this are presently unknown. Studies on two commercially available powder preparations showed no difference in rate of absorption or bioavailability (Sullivan & Snow 1982), although a more rapid absorption and higher bioavailability on an empty stomach may be seen using the recently introduced paste preparation (Snow, unpublished data). Tobin has claimed that the bioavailability of naproxen is 50%; however, no details on the feeding regimen used are given (Tobin 1981).

Often a course of 5–10 days' treatment may be given with these drugs and, therefore, there is the possibility of increasing plasma concentrations. Gerring *et al* (1981) reported cumulation with sequential dosing twice daily at a dose rate of 4.4 mg/kg.

Intramuscular administration

With the exception of flunixin meglumine, the administration of these drugs by the intramuscular route is not recommended, probably because of the irritant nature of these acidic compounds. However, there are countries where the parenteral formulation of PBZ is injected intramuscularly, and recent studies indicate that slower absorption occurs using this route than by the oral route (Snow *et al* 1981a, Sullivan & Snow 1982).

Clearance from urine

In an attempt to control the use of medication in competing horses, many racing and equestrian authorities collect urine samples for analysis for the possible presence of prohibited drugs. Because of the concentrating properties of the kidneys, most drugs and their metabolites can be detected more readily and for a greater period of time in urine than in blood. Therefore, in using these drugs, the practising veterinarian needs to know how long they are likely to be detected, i.e. cleared in the urine. Unfortunately, due to the sensitivity of the analytical techniques used, animal variations, and other factors such as urinary pH, only approximate clearance times for therapeutic agents can be given. Moss & Hayward (1973) have shown that phenyl-butazone and its metabolites can be detected in urine for more than twice as long in horses producing acid than alkaline urine. Although horse urine is normally alkaline, in racing animals acidic urine is often produced (Moss 1976). In the UK there is the Royal College of Veterinary Surgeons' guidance that drugs should not be administered within eight days of racing. If this is followed, none of the NSAIDs in current use should be detected in urine with the present screening procedures.

Clinical use and efficacy

All the NSAIDs are claimed to be useful in numerous acute and chronic inflammatory conditions of both soft tissue and skeletal origin. From the limited clinical and experimental studies it appears that the different NSAIDs are more effective against some conditions than others. Mec-lofenamic acid has good efficacy against both acute and chronic laminitis, where noticeable improvement is seen 2–4 days after beginning treatment (Riley *et al* 1975). These investigators also found good efficacy against skeletal conditions including navicular disease (Riley *et al* 1971, Conner *et al* 1973). Naproxen has been reported to be more effective than phenyl-butazone against both experimentally-induced myositis and clinically occurring cases of 'tying-up' (Kilian *et al* 1974, Jones & Hamm 1978). Flunixin meglumine, a recently introduced compound, has extremely good analgesic activity and is effective in alleviating pain associated with colic, especially flatulant and spastic colic (Vernimb & Hennessey 1977). In these cases, the onset of response was very rapid, with horses showing an improvement in 15 minutes which lasted for 6–8 hours. Flunixin has also been shown to be more potent and more effective than PBZ in the treatment of an experimentally-induced lameness (Houdeshell & Hennessey 1977). Included in this report is an evaluation of 262 horses suffering from various soft tissue and inflammatory conditions: 74% of the treated animals had good or excellent response to flunixin, with remission of signs generally occurring after two or three days.

Although these newer agents are often claimed to be superior to phenylbutazone, just as aspirin is still the dominant NSAID in man, phenylbutazone is still the mose widely used and first choice NSAID despite the absence of either adequate clinical or experimental trials. The lack of good clinical trials probably results from the fact that this compound was marketed before data on efficacy were a prerequisite for drug registration. Its pre-eminence may be attributed to a number of factors, including clinical experience over 20 years which indicates its efficacy and dependability in a variety of conditions (Dunn 1972), the considerably lower costs for treatment, especially over any period of time (Table 19.3, p.414), and the establishment of 'Bute' as a household name.

The general selection of phenylbutazone as the best drug may have a sound pharmacological basis. Considerably lower dose rates of phenylbutazone are used in treating horses than other species, which is not true for other NSAIDs. In man it has been estimated that plasma concentration of about 50 μg/ml phenylbutazone is required for therapeutic effectiveness (Kampmann & Frey 1966). During equine therapy this concentration is never reached and it has been calculated that a minimal effective blood concentration of 7 μg/ml (approximately 11 μg/ml plasma) is necessary (Jenny *et al* 1979). The reason for this apparent increased potency is unknown. However, as discussed by Jenny *et al* (1979), it may be attributed partially to the fact that the plasma protein binding in the horse is lower than in man — 96.0% (Gandal *et al* 1969) and 98.8% (Kurz & Friemel 1967) respectively — leading to higher concentrations of the free drug responsible for pharmacological activity. For example, in the horse and man total plasma concentrations of 12 μg/ml and 50 μg/ml have a free concentration of approximately 0.5 μg/ml. It is also possible that equine cyclo-oxygenases are more readily inhibited by this drug.

Although these drugs are not marketed for use in cattle, there have been reports of their beneficial effects in treatment of certain bovine lameness (Weaver 1981). Because of the long half-life of PBZ in cattle, Eberhardson *et al* (1979) have recommended a dosage regimen of a priming oral dose of 9 mg/kg and maintenance doses of 4.5 mg/kg given orally every 48 hours.

Toxicity

Oral administration. PBZ has been used extensively in horses for over twenty years. Despite this widespread use and the fact that some animals have been maintained on the drug for several years, clinical reports on adverse side-effects following prolonged administration have been rare. This contrasts with the reports of a high incidence of minor side-effects in man, as well as with the low incidence of aplastic anaemia and agranulo-cytosis. Many of the side-effects reported in man can be related to the ulcerogenic property of PBZ. This activity is also shown by other cyclo-oxygenase inhibitors, the extent varying both within and between species (Wilhelmi 1974). These side-effects are considered to result from the inhibi-tion of the formation of prostaglandins, but the exact mechanism is unknown (Robert 1974).

Using high non-therapeutic doses, ulceration of the gastrointestinal tract has been reported in the horse following PBZ (Gabriel & Martin 1962) and meclofenamic acid (Riley *et al* 1971). With normal therapeutic regimens ulceration has not been considered a problem in the horse. However, recently it has been reported that, in ponies, oral dose rates of the order of 5 mg/kg twice daily will rapidly produce a protein-losing gastroenteropathy, with fatalities occurring after a period of administration as short as one week (Snow *et al* 1979, 1981b). Damage to the mucosa results in protein loss, ulceration being most pronounced in the large intestine where small ulcers converge to form a large area free of any epithelial lining. The impaired epithelial integrity is thought to result in absorption of toxins and the establishment of a terminal shock condition. Marked ulceration of the oral cavity and tongue can also be seen. Clinically the early signs of toxicity are anorexia, depression, ventral abdominal oedema, diarrhoea, and sometimes oral ulceration. The first indication on routine blood biochemistry is a progressive decline in total plasma proteins with both albumin and globulin fractions being equally reduced (Snow *et al* 1979, 1981b). With the appear-ance of clinical signs and weight loss (Fig. 19.6), an increase in plasma urea concentration occurs which probably results from tissue catabolism in an attempt to maintain normal plasma protein levels. As protein concentra-tions return to normal, urea concentrations decline. Recent studies (Snow, unpublished data) using a new paste formulation (5 mg/kg twice daily) have shown a plasma protein decrease with clinical signs of toxicity within two days of beginning treatment. Haematological studies in this investigation found that, in conjunction with the clinical signs, a degenerative shift to the left, with neutrophils containing toxic granules, as well as the occasional

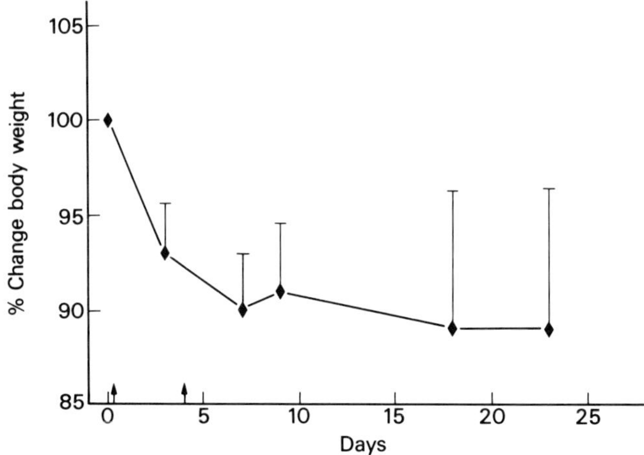

Fig. 19.6 Change in body weight of nine ponies (mean ± s.d.) after administration of phenyl-butazone (paste preparation). Dosage: day 1 5 mg/kg in morning; days 2 and 3 5 mg/kg morning and night; days 4 and 5 5 mg/kg in morning.

activated lymphocyte were produced. Alterations in red blood cell morphology occurred in association with the uraemia.

Although this toxic condition can be produced consistently in ponies, (Shetlands and larger breeds), a slightly lower dose rate of 8.2 mg/kg/day for up to two weeks in thoroughbreds did not produce similar clinical changes. However, in some animals, a decline in plasma proteins towards the end of the treatment period occurred (Snow *et al* 1981b). Similar effects of prolonged treatment on total plasma proteins have also been found by other workers (Gerber, Pers. Commun., Lees, Pers. Commun.). The reason(s) for the apparent greater susceptibility in pony breeds is presently unknown but studies suggest that it is due to local concentrations of the drug acting on the mucosa rather than high systemic blood concentrations. This is supported by the finding that there is no difference in the rate of metabolism of PBZ between breeds (Snow *et al* 1979, 1981b), that a similar dose rate intravenously does not produce these gastrointestinal changes (Snow, unpublished data), and by indications of a lower bioavailability in ponies than thoroughbreds (Sullivan & Snow 1982).

Although meclofenamic acid has been shown to cause ulceration at high doses (Riley *et al* 1971), both this compound and naproxen were shown to cause no obvious toxicity in ponies when administered for two weeks at a therapeutic dose rate followed by a further week's administration at twice this dose rate (Snow *et al* 1982).

Parenteral adminstration. Because of the acidic nature of PBZ, accidental extravascular injection following intravenous administration can lead to severe inflammation and sloughing at the injection site with phlebitis and, in some cases, permanent occlusion of the jugular vein (Gabel *et al* 1977). This can be avoided if cathetarisation is used for intravenous administration. If extravascular injection occurs steps should be taken to dilute and spread the drug at the site. Accidental injection of phenylbutazone into the carotid artery will cause immediate excitement, prostration, and sometimes death.

Although the intramuscular administration of phenylbutazone is not recommended, there are countries where this route is used. After intramuscular administration with either phenylbutazone or meclofenamic acid, pain and swelling occur at the site of injection, with elevated plasma CPK concentrations (Snow *et al* 1981b, Sullivan & Snow 1982). Flunixin meglumine (1.1 mg/kg) can be given safely by the intramuscular route.

Dosage regimens

Intravenous. Phenylbutazone can be administered by slow injection at a dose rate up to 5 mg/kg. Flunixin meglumine is given at a dose rate of 1.1 mg/kg.

Oral. It is recommended that an initial dose of up to 4.4 mg/kg twice daily be administered, following which the dose is halved for a further four days, then reduced again and given once daily or on alternate days, depending on effectiveness. Using low maintenance doses of the order of 2.2 mg/kg daily, horses have been treated for several years without ill effects. Because of the apparent increased susceptibility of ponies to phenylbutazone, a maximum dose of 2.2 mg/kg twice daily is now recommended. Meclofenamic acid is administered at a dose rate of 2.2 mg/kg once daily. A course of therapy is usually 5–7 days and, following this, the drug is administered at a frequency to provide effective prevention of recurrence of symtpoms. Clinical experience has shown that horses can be maintained on approximately twice weekly dosage for several years without side-effects. Naproxen is administered twice daily at a dose rate of 10 mg/kg for up to 14 days. However, as it is much more expensive than the preceeding two drugs, it is only used for prolonged administration in exceptional circumstances. The costs of a course of treatment with the three drugs presently available in the UK are shown in Table 19.3

Corticosteroids

This group of compounds is used frequently in the treatment of a variety of acute and chronic inflammatory conditions. The chemistry, administration,

Table 19.3 Cost (in 1982) of a 10 day course of oral treatment with non-steroidal anti-inflammatory drugs (450 kg horse).

Drug	Dosage regime	Cost (£)
Phenylbutazone	4.4 mg/kg twice daily for 4 days 2.2 mg/kg twice daily for 4 days 2.2 mg/kg daily for 2 days	1.56 powder 11.55 paste
Meclofenamic acid	2.2 mg/kg once daily	9.00
Naproxen	10 mg/kg twice daily	31.40

actions and uses will be considered in detail in Chapter 20. Although their pronounced anti-inflammatory effects have been attributed to a number of actions, recent studies indicate that one of the most important effects is their ability to decrease the synthesis of both prostaglandins and the leukotrienes. This results from the inhibition of phospholipase A_2 (Fig. 19.3) thus preventing the release of arachidonic acid. The corticosteroids do not cause this inhibition directly but, by acting at the genome, they initiate the synthesis of a substance that inhibits phospholipase A_2 (Flower 1981). Recent work (Flower & Blackwell 1979) has led to the isolation of such an inhibitor and to its identification as a polypeptide which was named 'Macrocortin' (Blackwell *et al* 1980). It has also been shown that, in addition to reducing prostaglandin synthesis, there is also an increase in the activities of enzymes which degrade prostaglandins (Moore & Hoult 1980).

Corticosteroids are employed in large animal practice in the treatment of numerous conditions (see Chapter 20), although their major use in equine practice is for their anti-inflammatory properties. For this purpose they are administered both systemically and locally. Because of their employment in equine practice and often prior to racing and other competitions, a knowledge of clearance times is required. Clearance times for corticosteroids in the urine of racing animals parallels their duration of activity. Chapman *et al* (1977) have presented details of the clearance of 14 proprietary preparations of corticosteroids as determined by a radioimmunoassay technique. Confirmation of identity using an on-line HPLC-mass spectrometer should lead to the identification of the illegal use of these compounds (Houghton *et al* 1981). Following therapeutic doses of dexamethasone, betamethasone and prednisolone, they could be detected in urine for 12.5, 14.5 and 27 hours respectively.

The side-effects that can be seen following corticosteroid therapy have been outlined in Chapter 20. It is generally considered that the single injection of even high doses of a corticosteroid is of little risk, the main exception being when infection is also present. In this situation, a bactericidal antibiotic should also be administered. However, in horses, the occurrence of laminitis has been reported after corticosteroid administration (Muylle & Oyaert 1973, Vernimb *et al* 1977). This may be due to the potentiating effect of corticosteroids on the vasoconstriction produced by adrenaline, noradrenaline and 5-hydroxytryptamine (Eyre *et al* 1979).

Local administration of anti-inflammatory agents

In addition to administration of these compounds for systemic distribution, discrete effects can be obtained by local application. This can be brought about by the incorporation of these substances, especially corticosteroids, in preparations that can be applied to inflamed skin or, much more commonly, local injections for the treatment of joint, tendon, and bursal inflammations.

Selection of therapeutic agents for local use

To help understand the possible rationale in the selection of various agents which can be used in the local treatment of joint diseases, a knowledge of the structures involved and their reaction to injury is important, and will be briefly described. Further details on this can be obtained from the excellent review by Nizolek & White (1981).

The synovial joint comprises the joint capsule and ligaments, the synovial membrane, synovial fluid and the articular cartilage. The joint capsule and ligaments form a sleeve around the articular cartilage and are endowed with both pain and proprioceptive end organs. The synovial membrane consists of an outer fibrous layer which is fused with the joint capsule and an inner (intimal) layer of synoviocytes of two main types in a loose connective tissue matrix. This layer is well vascularised. The functions of the synovial membrane are firstly production of synovial fluid and secondly removal of synovial fluid and detritus from the joint space. Synovial fluid in the joint space has two main functions: lubrication and nutrition of the joint tissues. The fluid is essentially a dialysate of plasma to which are added secretions of synoviocytes. The most important secretion is hyaluronic acid which is thought to be produced by the type A synoviocytes (Ghadially 1978). Hyaluronic acid is a high-molecular-weight polysaccharide, which consists of repeating units of a disaccharide of glucuronic acid and N.-acetyl glucosamine to form a long unbranched chain (Fig. 19.7). It is the hyaluronic acid which is responsible for the viscosity and thixotropism of synovial fluid. Contrary to earlier opinions, hyaluronic acid does not act as a lubricant for all structures of the joint, but is responsible only for lubrication of the soft tissues, whilst recent evidence indicates that lubrication of articular cartilage is dependent upon the presence of small amounts of a specific glycoprotein

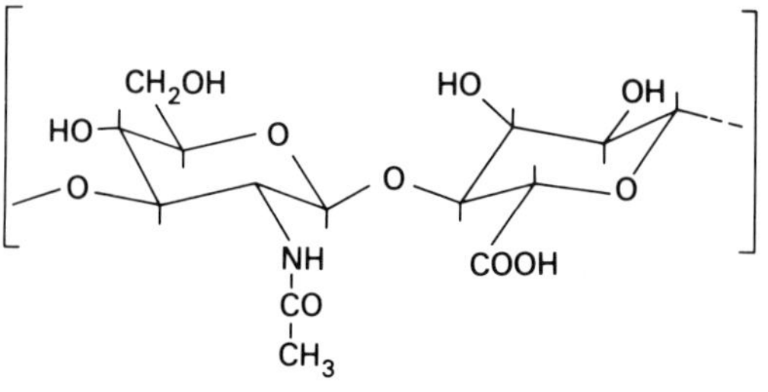

Fig. 19.7 — diagram (chemical structure)

Fig. 19.7 Disaccharide subunit of hyaluronic acid. $n = 2500$.

in synovial fluid (Swann 1978). Injury of the synovial membrane can arise from either external or internal (irritant substances or micro-organisms in the synovial fluid) insults and this leads to a typical inflammatory reaction. Synovitis leads to increased formation and decreased absorption of synovial fluid, resulting in increased synovial fluid. Associated with these changes in the amount of synovial fluid is an alteration in its composition (Nizolek & White 1981) and a decrease in its viscosity following a decrease in both quantity and quality of the hyaluronic acid due to its depolymerisation.

Articular cartilage is of the hyaline variety and serves a specialised biomechanical function in protecting the bones from abrasive damage, to dampen the force of impact, to distribute the load, and to facilitate movement between the articular surfaces. It consists of a relatively small number of cells (chondrocytes) within an extracellular matrix, composed of a meshwork of fine collagen fibres (type II) in which is entrapped the ground substance rich in water and aggregated proteoglycans. This matrix is synthesised and degraded by the chondrocytes. The proteoglycans are of high molecular weight, and form large aggregates by attachment to hyaluronic acid. Between 100 and 200 proteoglycan molecules are attached to a single hyaluronic acid molecule, which is synthesised by the chondrocytes. These proteoglycans trap water with the result that the water content of cartilage can be as high as 80%. It is important to realise that cartilage is avascular and that its nutrition comes from the synovial fluid; this helps explain its inability to have a normal inflammatory response and its slow healing ability. In addition, a lack of innervation means that articular damage is not directly related to pain.

Joint inflammation (arthritis) can arise from injury to any of the structures of the joint and can be divided into two categories depending on the location of the injury that initiates the signs of pain (Pool *et al* 1980a).
1 *Intra-articular joint disease.* In this category are included primary osteoarthritis (osteoarthris) in which there is no known predisposing cause and in which a number of joints are possibly involved, and secondary osteoarthritis that arises as a result of damage to the structure and function of the joint, e.g. trauma, intra-articular fractures, and infection. From studies in man (Mankin 1974, McKenzie *et al* 1976), and in the horse (Auer *et al* 1980, Pool

et al 1980a), the sequence of events occurring within articular cartilage have been elucidated. In the early stages, the superficial layer of the articular cartilage has multifocal areas of chondrocyte degeneration and de-aggregation and loss of the proteoglycans and collagen brought about by the release of enzymes from the chondrocytes (Dingle 1978). According to Pool *et al* (1980a), these early changes are a very common finding in joints of thoroughbreds examined at necropsy. These degenerative changes can take place without clinical signs because of the absence of pain receptors in the cartilage. Continued trauma can lead to further progressive and more pronounced damage to the articular cartilage, subchondral bone sclerosis, remodelling of articular margins, synovial abnormalities, and periarticular osteophyte production (Pool *et al* 1980a). The early and late changes within cartilage can result in the release of substances, including proteoglycans, into the synovial fluid and it is believed that these are irritant to the synovial membranes and initiate the inflammatory response. One of the resultant changes in the synovial fluid is its decreased viscosity, and this will lead to an increase in friction between cartilage surfaces and to possible further mechanical injury to the cartilage.

2 *Periarticular joint disease.* In these conditions, pain and lameness can result from injury to supportive soft tissues around joints including tendons, ligaments and synovium without articular cartilage damage. These may or may not lead to the development of a synovitis.

Therefore, depending on the aetiology of the damage, intra-articular therapy may have varying effectiveness. To ascertain whether the pain and lameness is due primarily to a synovitis, the response to an intra-cellular injection of a local anaesthetic is ascertained. Radiographic examination should also be used to determine if the inflammation is due to chip fractures or osetoarthritis. However both conditions may be difficult to detect.

Corticosteroids

These agents, which are relatively inexpensive, have been used in the treatment of equine arthritis since the mid 1950s (Wheat 1955). Today numerous preparations are available which vary in potency and duration of action within the joint. The major advantage of the newer, more potent agents is that smaller volumes can be injected. As the short-acting steroids, e.g. hydrocortisone acetate, are rapidly cleared from the joint cavity within a few hours, being taken up by the synovial cells and by the capillaries into the systemic circulations, long-acting preparations which remain in the synovium for several days are now generally used. Combinations of compounds are also available to give both prompt activity and prolonged effect. A combination of betamethasone phosphate–betamethasone diproprionate has been reported to give quicker and more prolonged action than the commonly used methyl prednisolone acetate (Vernimb *et al* 1977). With the former preparation, the blood eosinophil count (an index of the presence of systemic corticosteroids) was depressed for between 14 and 21 days, whilst for methyl prednisolone acetate this occurred only for about four days. The favourable use of a number of other corticosteroid preparations has also been described (Van Pelt *et al* 1970, 1971). The procedure involved in the intra-articular injection of corticosteroids and other drugs, and the necessary precautions, are described by Adams (1974).

Although corticosteroids are undoubtedly very effective in alleviating stiffness and pain by reducing the inflammatory response thus enabling the joint to be used more freely, their use for this purpose is controversial both in human and equine sports medicine. The main reason for this is that they are often used to return the athlete or horse to competition before the lesion has resolved and healing has occurred, thus risking further and possibly more serious injury. It has been argued that, although such treatment is not curative when chronic lesions are present, the horse's useful working life is prolonged (McKay & Milne 1976). Depending on the cause of synovitis, intra-articular corticosteroids can lead indirectly or directly to deleterious effects.

Indirectly. The injection of a corticosteroid without an appropriate period of rest can lead to exacerbation of the condition and eventual complete breakdown. Pool *et al* (1980a) suggested that carpal injections — by encouraging increased use of the joint — can precipitate a pathological chip fracture.

Directly. In addition to their anti-inflammatory activity these compounds lead to a number of other reactions.

1 *Post-injection flare,* which refers to an inflammatory response in the joint several hours after injection. This is only of a very low incidence and generally persists for a few hours to several days, although Pool *et al* (1980a) describe a case which continued for 13 days following methyl prednisolone acetate injection.

2 Inadvertent injection of long-acting preparations into the periarticular tissue may result in *metaplastic bone formation* — or soft tissue calcification.

3 *Septic arthritis,* can develop if proper aseptic techniques are not used at the time of injection or organisms are already present within the joint. Schurman *et al* (1975) have shown that the number of organisms needed to cause a joint infection is decreased following either intra-articular or systemic corticosteroid therapy.

4 *'Steroid arthropathy'.* It has been claimed by many investigators that

repeated administration of corticosteroids leads to degenerative changes within the joint (Meagher 1970, Gabel 1977), although McKay & Milne (1976) and Marcoux (1977) concluded that repeated intra-articular injections of corticosteroids can be carried out with relative impunity. Pool *et al* (1980a) reported that both in-vitro and in-vivo studies of cartilage exposed to corticosteroids indicated that degenerative changes occurred, with loss of proteoglycans; the lesions being most severe where stresses were greatest in weight bearing and joint extension. They also concluded that the lesions seen following multiple corticosteroid injections were similar to those occurring in the later stages of degenerative joint disease, with no lesion being pathognomic for corticosteroid arthropathy.

These pathological findings have been supported by a number of laboratory investigations. Even a single injection of a corticosteroid leads to depression of chondrocyte metabolism (Mankin & Conger 1966). Repeated injections were found to cause a progressive degeneration of articular cartilage in rabbits (Behrens *et al* 1975). Initially a rapid and profound depression of synthesis of collagen and proteoglycan occurs followed by a linear drop in proteoglycans concentration of the matrix. In non-weight-bearing joint regions this change in stiffness of the cartilage has little effect, but in the weight-bearing areas the cyclic compression causes fissure formation at the surface and cystic degeneration in the middle zone. As Pool *et al* (1980a) point out, these lesions may be more severe in rabbits than other species as the proteoglycans have a considerably shorter half-life in rabbits than in man; half-life data are presently unavailable in the horse. In another study, the recovery after repeated corticosteroid injections was investigated (Behrens *et al* 1976): although there was a marked increase in synthesis of collagen and protoglycans, proteoglycans concentration took up to six months to return to normal. In-vitro studies have also demonstrated that hyaluronic acid synthesis by fibroblasts is inhibited by low concentrations of corticosteroids (Saarni & Hopsu-Havu 1978).

Indications and contraindications for local therapy with corticosteroids

From the evidence now available, indications and contraindications for use of these compounds within joints can now be suggested. Corticosteroids should only be used in decreasing the pain and swelling resulting from injury to either the periarticular soft tissues or synovial membrane where articular cartilage has not been damaged. This can be assessed by synovial fluid particle analysis (Nizolek & White 1981). If used for this purpose, an adequate period of rest is essential (Van Pelt *et al* 1970, Owen 1980, Nizolek & White 1981) which will be considerably longer if the arthritis results from ligament damage rather than direct trauma to the synovial membrane. The contraindications for corticosteroid injections are summarised by Nizolek & White (1981) as being 1 sepsis existing within or around a joint; 2 presence of intra-articular fracture; 3 damage to articular cartilage; 4 extensive degenerative bony lesions; 5 previous injections being ineffective; and 6 the possibility of overexercise of the joint.

Local injections of corticosteroids have also been employed in the treatment of tendinosynovitis and bursitis. Recent work by Pool *et al* (1980b) in examining tendon changes after corticosteroid (methyl prednisolone) injection into normal tendons and the examination of bowed tendons after corticosteroid therapy, has indicated that, as well as causing calcification, focal areas of necrotising inflammation result. These workers concluded that local injection exacerbates the condition as well as retarding the fibrous connective tissue component of the repair process.

In contrast to the damage that can be caused using intra-articular or tendon injections of corticosteroids, it appears that their local application into bursae can be very effective without any risks of side-effects.

Hyaluronic acid

As already described, this substance is found within the synovial fluid and in the cartilage matrix in combination with proteoglycans. Since, in arthritis, there is often a decrease in viscosity of the synovial fluid which can lead to further cartilage damage, the use of hyaluronic acid as a therapeutic agent has been investigated. Preparations extracted from rooster combs are now commercially available and, although an expensive means of treatment, a number of favourable results have been reported in the horse. Exactly how exogenous hyaluronic acid exerts its effect when injected intra-articularly is presently unknown. The limited data available from studies in a number of species are reviewed by Nizolek & White (1981). As a glycoprotein and not hyaluronic acid is considered to be the main cartilage lubricant, a favourable protective action by this means is unlikely. Auer *et al* (1980) have suggested that the injected hyaluronic acid is partially incorporated into the cartilage and binds proteoglycans. This might serve to improve the quality of the joint surface and prevent its further destruction, thereby interrupting the chain of events leading to synovitis and pain. In addition hyaluronic acid may cause aggregation of proteoglycans released by damage into the synovial fluid and this would prevent their irritant activity. An advantage of hyaluronic acid over corticosteroids is that it augments natural healing tendencies rather than inhibiting them.

The general consensus from both experimental and clinical investigations on the use of hyaluronic acid is that it has a beneficial effect greater than would be expected following conventional treatment. Since the initial report by Rydell *et al* 1970) that a greater response was seen when hyaluronic acid was injected in combination with a corticosteroid than a corticosteroid alone, studies by Asheim & Lindblad (1976), Rose (1979), Gingerich *et al* (1979), Irwin 1980, Phillips (1980) and Auer *et al* (1980) have all found that an excellent response was obtained in the majority of animals, with a rapid return to normal movement. In an experimentally-induced arthritis, Gingerich *et al* (1979) found a marked improvement within 3–7 days. Phillips (1980) reported that, following treatment, mean time to a return to racing or training was 9.5 days (range 1–60 days). In treatment generally, only a single intra-articular injection (20–40 mg) is required (Gingerich *et al* 1981).

Synovial fluid transfusion

With respect to therapy of arthritis, a preliminary report (Rulcker & Lindholm 1981) has indicated that synovial fluid transfer (4–10 ml) from a sound joint to an arthritic joint resulted in a very favourable response. In horses examined 4 and 60 days following treatment complete recovery was recorded in 81% and 71% of cases respectively. The reason for the effectiveness of this form of treatment is not known but Rulcker & Lindholm (1981) suggested that it might be due to the hyaluronic acid transferred. For best results these workers also suggested a convalescent period of 10–14 days. If further trials substantiate these favourable effects, a relatively cheap but effective method of treatment will be available.

Orgotein

This compound which has been introduced recently for commercial use is a water-soluble metalloprotein extracted from bovine liver (Huber *et al* 1968). It has a molecular weight of about 30 000 and contains copper and zinc ions which are considered important for its activity. It can be used both systemically and locally, the latter being the more common.

Although Faull *et al* (1976) suggest that its anti-inflammatory activity is due to a number of actions, there is little evidence to substantiate this as published data on this compound are sparse. However, one action that may contribute to its beneficial effect is that this group of compounds acts enzymically as superoxide dismutases, and therefore are able to destroy the superoxide radicals released during injury (McCord 1974). Superoxide radicals have been shown to cause the depolymerisation of hyaluronic acid with a resulting decreased viscosity and ability to form a 'mucin clot' of synovial fluid. Such superoxide radicals are produced by phagocytising polymorphonuclear cells when they emigrate to an injured area and are released into the surrounding tissue. McCord (1974) has demonstrated a strong correlation between decreased viscosity of the synovial fluid and the number of polymorphonuclear cells present. Therefore its beneficial action when injected into joints may be by preventing depolymerisation of hyaluronic acid, and therefore enhancing the maintenance of normal hyaluronic acid within the synovial fluid, and also possibly within articular cartilage.

It has also been shown that orgotein exerts an anti-inflammatory effect on soft tissue injuries following intramuscular injection of small amounts (5–10 mg). In these instances no explanation for their mechanism of action is available. Smith & Ford-Hutchinson (1979) have suggested that, because of the small quantities injected, orgotein may be acting as a homeopathic remedy.

In the clinical trials that have been conducted with orgotein for joint, tendon, and soft tissue injuries (Cushing *et al* 1973, Faull *et al* 1976, Linton 1976, Ahlengard *et al* 1978, Coffman *et al* 1979), beneficial results have usually been found. However, unfortunately, the clinical assessment and follow-up studies in evaluating the response to orgotein have not been generally as rigorous as in the studies of hyaluronic acid. The most extensive study with orgotein is that carried out in Sweden by Ahlengard *et al* (1978) in the treatment of clinical cases of aseptic arthritis in one or more joints of 134 horses. In these cases, 5 mg orgotein was injected into the affected joint(s) on 1–4 occasions (mean 2.5) at weekly intervals. On the basis of follow-up information, these workers reported a 94% recovery where lameness had been present for less than two months prior to treatment and 49% recovery in those lame for longer than two months. Treatment of soft tissue injuries with orgotein involves a series of deep intramuscular injections, and in some cases local injection at a dosage of 5–15 mg.

No adverse side-effects have been reported following intramuscular injection of orgotein (Carson *et al* 1973). However Ahlengard *et al* (1978) reported a 5% incidence of transient side-effects following intra-articular injection, including increased lameness, overproduction of synovial fluid, and swollen joint capsules.

Glycosaminoglycan polysulphate (Arteparon)

This compound is used in Europe for the treatment of degenerative joint disease and is being presently tested in the USA (Nizolek & White 1981). It is a compound of approximately 10 000 molecular weight, and is classified as an 'oversulphated heparinoid', with a similarity to chondroitin sulphate.

Information on the use and possible mode of action of this compound is reviewed by Nizolek & White (1981). It appears that this compound is deposited within cartilage and preferentially in diseased cartilage, probably due to its similarity to natural proteoglycans. It also exerts an effect on synoviocytes leading to increased production of hyaluronic acid, and an increase in viscosity of synovial fluid. Other possible actions are described by Nizolek & White (1981).

The drug can be administered either intra muscularly or intra-articularly with equal effectiveness. A dose of 125–250 mg is used and this is repeated at weekly intervals for up to 10–15 weeks. No side-effects from its use have been reported. In a study in the horse, Kubitza (1966) reported a 67% success rate in the treatment of articular disease.

References

Adams O. R. (1974) *Lameness in Horses,* 3rd ed. Lea & Febiger, Philadelphia.

Ahlengard S., Tufvenson G., Petterson H. *et al* (1978) Treatment of traumatic arthritis in the horse with intra-muscular orgotein (palosein). *Eq. Vet. J.* **10,** 122.

Asheim A. & Lindblad G. (1976) Intra-articular treatment of arthritis in racehorses with sodium hyaluronate. *Acta Vet. Scand.* **17,** 379.

Auer J. A., Fackelman G. E., Gingerich D. A. *et al* (1980) The effect of hyaluronic acid in naturally occurring and experimentally-induced osteoarthritis. *Am. J. Vet. Res.* **41,** 568.

Bachmann K. A. & Burkman A. M. (1975) Phenylbutazone–warfarin interactions in the dog. *J. Pharm. Pharmacol.* **27,** 832.

Behrens F., Shepard N. & Mitchell N. (1975) Alteration of rabbit and articular cartilage by intra-articular injections of glucocorticoids. *J. Bone Joint Surg.* **57**-A, 70.

Behrens F., Sheperd N. & Mitchell N. (1976) Metabolic recovery of articular cartilage after intra-articular injections of glucocorticoid. *J. Bone Joint Surg.* **58**-A, 1157.

Blackwell G. J., Carnuccio R., Di Rossa M. *et al* (1980) Macrocortin: a polypeptide causing the anti-phospholipase effect of glucocorticoids. *Nature* **287,** 147.

Busse W. N. (1979) Histamine: mediator and modulator in inflammation. In *Chemical Messengers of the Inflammatory Process,* ed. Houck J. C. p. 1. Elsevier/North Holland, Amsterdam.

Carson S., Vogin E. E., Huber W. *et al* (1973) Safety tests on Orgotein, an anti-inflammatory protein. *Toxicol. Appl. Pharmacol.* **26,** 184.

Chapman D. I., Moss M. S. & Whiteside J. (1977) The urinary excretion of synthetic corticosteroids by the horse. *Vet. Rec.* **100,** 447.

Coffman J. R., Johnson J. H., Tritschler L. G. *et al* (1979) Orgotein in equine navicular disease: A double-blind study. *J. Am. Vet. Med. Assoc.* **174,** 261.

Conner G. H., Riley W. F., Beck C. C. *et al* (1973) Arquel (Cl-1583) A new non-steroidal anti-inflammatory drug for horses. *Proc. Am. Assoc. Eq. Pract.* **19,** 81.

Cushing L. S., Decker W. E., Santos F. K. *et al* (1973) Orgotein therapy for inflammation in horses. *Mod. Vet. Pract.* **54,** 17.

Davis L. E. & Westfall B. A. (1972) Species differences in biotransformation and excretion of salicylate. *Am. J. Vet. Res.* **33,** 1253.

Decker W. E., Edmondson A. H., Hill H. E. *et al* (1974). *Mod. Vet. Pract.* **55**, 773.

Dingle J. T. (1978) Articular damage and its control. *Ann. Intern. Med.* **88**, 821.

Dunn S. P. (1972) A clinician's view on the use and misuse of phenylbutazone. *Eq. Vet. J.* **4**, 63–5.

Eberhardson B., Olsson G., Appelgren L-E *et al* (1979) Pharmacokinetic studies of phenylbutazone in cattle. *J. Vet. Pharmacol. Therap.* **2**, 31.

Eyre P. (1972) Release of 5-Hydroxytryptamine release from calf-lung *in vitro* by specific antigen and by compound 48/80. *Arch. Int. Pharmacodyn. Ther.* **192**, 347.

Eyre P. (1980) Pharmacological aspects of hypersensitivity in domestic animals: A review. *Vet. Res. Comm.* **4**, 83.

Eyre P., Elmes P. J. & Strickland S. (1979) Corticosteroid-potentiated vascular responses of the equine digit. A possible pharmacologic basis for laminitis. *Am. J. Vet. Res.* **40**, 135.

Faull G. L., Baker De B., Walt H. S. *et al* (1976) Clinical trials with orgotein (palosein) *J. S. Afr. Vet. Assoc.* **47**, 39.

Ferriera S. H. & Vane J. R. (1979) Mode of action of anti-inflammatory agents which are prostaglandin synthetase inhibitors. In *Anti-inflammatory Drugs,* eds. Vane J. R. & Ferreira S. H., p. 348. Springer-Verlag, Berlin.

Flower R. J. & Blackwell G. J. (1979) Anti-inflammatory steroids induce biosynthesis of a phospholipase A₂ inhibitor which prevents prostaglandin generation. *Nature* **278**, 456.

Flower R. J. (1981) Glucocorticoids, phospholipase A₂ and inflammation. *Trends Pharmacol. Sci.* **2**, 186.

Gabel A. A. (1977) Corticosteroids — side effects and toxicity. *Proc. Am. Assoc. Eq. Pract.* **23**, 393.

Gabel A. A., Tobin T., Ray R. S. *et al* (1977) Phenylbutazone in horses: A review. *J. Eq. Med. Surg.* **1**, 221.

Gabriel K. L. & Martin J. E. (1962) Phenylbutazone short-term versus long-term administration to Thoroughbred and Standardbred horses. *J. Am. Vet. Med. Assoc.* **140**, 377.

Gandal C. P., Dayton P. G., Werner M. *et al* (1969) Studies with phenylbutazone, oxyphenbutazone and para-para-dichlorophenylbutazone in horses. *Cornell Vet.* **59**, 577.

Gerring E. L., Lees P. & Taylor J. G. (1981) Pharmacokinetics of phenylbutazone and its metabolites in the horse. *Eq. Vet. J.* **13**, 152.

Ghadially F. N. (1978) Fine structure of joints. In *The Joints and Synovial Fluid,* vol. 1, ed. Sokoloff L. Academic Press, New York.

Gingerich D. A., Auer J. A., & Fackelman G. E. (1979) Force plate studies on the effect of exogenous hyaluronic acid on joint function in equine arthritis. *J. Vet. Pharmacol. Therap.* **2**, 291.

Gingerich D. A., Auer J. A. & Fackelman G. E. (1981) Effect of exogenous hyaluronic acid on joint function in experimentally-induced equine osteoarthritis: dosage titration studies. *Res. Vet. Sci.* **30**, 192.

Hanna C. J., Eyre P., Wells P. W. *et al* (1982) Equine immunology 2: Immunopharmacology-biochemical basis of hypersensitivity. *Eq. Vet. J.* **14**, 16.

Houck J. C. (1979) *Chemical Messengers of the Inflammatory Process.* Elsevier/North Holland, Amsterdam.

Houdeshell J. W. & Hennessey P. W. (1977) A new non-steroidal, anti-inflammatory analgesic for horses. *J. Eq. Med. Surg.* **1**, 57.

Houghton E., Dumasia M. C. & Wellby J. K. (1981) The use of combined high performance liquid chromatography negative ion chemical ionization mass spectrometry to confirm the administration of synthetic corticosteroids to horses. *Biomedical Mass Spectrometry* **8**, 558.

Huber W., Schulte T. L., Carson S. *et al* (1968) Some chemical and pharmacological properties of a novel anti-inflammatory protein. *Toxicol. Appl. Pharmacol.* **12**, 308.

Irwin D. H. G. (1980) Sodium hyaluronate in equine traumatic arthritis. *J. S. Afr. Vet. Assoc.* **50**, 231.

Jenny E., Steinijans V. W. & Seifert P. (1979) Pharmacokinetic interaction of isopropylamino-phenazone and phenylbutazone in the horse. *J. Vet. Pharmacol. Therap.* **2**, 101.

Jones E. W. & Hamm D. (1978) Comparative efficacy of phenylbutazone and naproxen in induced equine myositis. *J. Eq. Med. Surg.* **2**, 341.

Jouany J. M., Boudene C., Belegaud J. *et al* (1979) Oral administration of aspirin to horses. In *Third International Symposium on Equine Medication Control,* eds. Tobin T., Blake J. E. & Woods W. E., p. 31. International Equine Medication Control Group, Lexington.

Kampmann E. & Frey H. (1966) Serum concentration of phenylbutazone in tests for anti-phlogistic activity and under clinical treatment. *Nature* **209**, 579.

Kilian J. G., Jones E. W., Hamm D. *et al* (1974) The efficacy of equiproxen (naproxen) in a unique equine myositis model. *Proc. Am. Assoc. Eq. Pract.* **20**, 201.

Kubitza G. (1966) The treatment of degenerative articular disease in horses and dogs. *Tierartzl. Umsch.* **8**, 420.

Kurz H. & Friemal G. (1967) Artspezifische unterocheide der Bindung an Plasmaproteine. *Arch. Exp. Path. Pharmakol.* **257**, 35.

Lambert M. B., Evans J. A. & Miller J. (1979) The pharmacokinetics of ibuprofen in the horse and greyhound. In *Third International Symposium on Equine Medication Control,* eds. Tobin T. Blake J. W. & Woods W. E., p. 381. International Equine Medication Control Group, Lexington.

Lehmann W., Wintzer H-J. & Frey H. H. (1981) Kinetik einiger analgetisch-antiinflammatorischer arzneimittel in serum und synovia beim pferd. *Dtsch. Tierarztl. Wschr.* **88**, 218.

Linton J. A. M. (1976) The use of orgotein in the treatment of soft tissue injuries of the horse. *Irish Vet. J.* **30**, 53.

Mankin H. G. & Conger K. A. (1966) The effect of cortisol on articular cartilage of rabbits. 1. Effect of a single dose of cortisol on glycine-C^{14} incorporation. *Lab. Invest.* **15**, 794.

Mankin H. J. (1974) The reaction of articular cartilage to injury and osteoarthritis. *New Engl. J. Med.* **291**, 1285–92.

Marcoux M. (1977) The effects of methylprednisolone and blood on equine articular structures. *Proc. Am. Assoc. Eq. Pract.* **23**, 333.

McCord J. M. (1974) Free radicals and inflammation: Protection of synovial fluid by super-oxide dismutase. *Science* **185**, 529.

McKay A. G. & Milne F. J. (1976) Observations on the intra-articular use of corticosteroids in the racing Thoroughbred. *J. Am. Vet. Med. Assoc.* **168**, 1039.

McKenzie L. S., Horsburgh B. A., Ghosh P. *et al* (1976) Effect of anti-inflammatory drugs on sulphated glycosaminoglycan synthesis in aged human articular cartilage. *Ann. Rheum. Dis.* **35**, 487.

Meagher D. M. (1970) The effects of intra-articular corticosteroids and continued training on carpal chip fractures of horses. *Proc. Am. Assoc. Equine Pract.* **16**, 405.

Moffat A. C. (1978) In *Drug Metabolism in Man,* eds. Garrod J. W. & Beckett A. H., p. 1. Taylor and Francis, London.

Moore P. K. & Hoult J. R. S. (1980) Anti-inflammatory steroids reduce tissue PG synthetase activity and enhance PG breakdown. *Nature* **288**, 269.

Moss M. S. (1976) The metabolism and urinary and salivary excretion of drugs in the horse and their relevance to detection of dope. In *Drug Metabolism from Microbe to Man.* Taylor and Francis, London.

Moss M. S. & Haywood P. E. (1973) Persistence of phenylbutazone in horses producing acid urines. *Vet. Rec.* **93**, 124.

Muylle & Oyaert (1973) Lung function tests in obstructive pulmonary disease in horse. *Eq. Vet. J.* **5**, 37.

Nizolek D. J. & White K. K. (1981) Corticosteroid and hyaluronic acid treatment in equine degenerative joint disease. A Review. *Cornell Vet.* **71**, 355.

Owen R. (1980) Intra-articular corticosteroid therapy in the horse. *J. Am. Vet. Med. Assoc.* **177**, 710.

Palmoski M. & Brandt K. (1976) Hyaluronate-binding by proteoglycans. Comparison of mildly and severely oesteoarthritic regions of human femoral cartilage. *Clin. Chem. Acta* **70**, 87.

Phillips M. W. (1980) Intra-articular sodium hyaluronate in the horse: A clinical trial. *Proc. Am. Assoc. Eq. Pract.* **26**, 389.

Phillips M. W., Salyer G. & Ray R. S. (1980) Equine metabolism and pharmacokinetics of indomethacin. *Equine Pract.* **2**, 45.

Piferno E., Ellis D. J., Getty S. M. *et al* (1968) Plasma and urine levels of phenylbutazone in the horse. *J. Am. Vet. Med. Assoc.* **153**, 195.

Pool R. R., Wheat J. D. & Ferraro G. L. (1980a) Corticosteroid therapy in common joint and tendon injuries of the horse. Part I, Effects on joints. *Proc. Am. Assoc. Eq. Pract.* **26**, 397.

Pool R. R., Wheat J. D. & Ferraro G. L. (1980b) Corticosteroid therapy in common joint and tendon injuries of the horse. Part II. Effects on tendons. *Proc. Am. Assoc. Eq. Pract.* **26**, 407.

Pratt G. W. & O'Connor J. T. Jr. (1976) Force plate studies. *Am. J. Vet. Res.* **37**, 1251.

Purohit R. C. & McCoy M. D. (1980) Thermography in the diagnosis of inflammatory processes in the horse. *Am. J. Vet. Res.* **41**, 1167.

Riley W. F., Romane W. M., Ellis D. J. *et al* (1971) Preliminary report on a new non-steroidal anti-inflammatory agent in the horse. *Proc. Am. Assoc. Eq. Pract.* **17**, 293.

Riley W. G., Conner G. H. & Beck C. C. (1975) Arquel as a treatment for equine laminitis. *Proc. Am. Assoc. Eq. Pract.* **21**, 115.

Rose R. J. (1979) The intra-articular use of Na hyaluronate for treatment of osteo-arthritis in the horse. *N.Z. Vet. J.* **27**, 5.

Robert A. (1974) Effects of prostaglandins on the stomach and the intestine. *Prostaglandins* **6**, 523–532.

Rocha e Silva M. (1978) A brief history of inflammation. In *Inflammation,* eds. Vane J. R. & Ferriera S. H., p. 6. Springer-Verlag, Berlin.

Rulcker C. & Lindholm A. (1981) Preliminary trials of synovial fluid transfer for treating joint lameness in Standardbreds. *Eq. Vet. J.* **13**, 264–65.

Ryan G. B. & Majno G. (1977) Acute inflammation. *Am. J. Path.* **86**, 185.

Rydell N. W., Butter J. & Balazs E. A. (1970) Hyaluronic acid in synovial fluid. IV. Effect of intra-articular injection of hyaluronic acid on the clinical symptoms of arthritis in track horses. *Acta. Vet. Scand.* **11**, 139.

Saarni J. & Hopsu-Havu V. K. (1978) Decrease of hyaluronate synthesis by anti-inflammatory steroids *in vitro. Br. J. Dermat.* **98**, 445.

Samuelsson B. (1980) The leukotrienes: A new group of biologically active compounds including SRS-A. *Trends Pharmacol. Sci.* **1**, 227.

Schror K., Sauerland S., Kuhn A. *et al* (1980) Different sensitivities of prostaglandins–cyclo-oxygenases in blood platelets and coronary arteries against non-steroidal anti-inflammatory drugs. *Arch. Pharmacol.* **313**, 69.

Schurman D. J., Johnson B. L. & Amstutz H. C. (1975) Knee joint infections with *Staphylococcus aureus* and Micrococcus species. *J. Bone Joint Surg.* **57-A**, 40.

Shen T. Y. (1979) Prostaglandin synthetase inhibitors. In *Anti-inflammatory Drugs,* ed. Vane J. R. & Ferriera S. H., p. 305. Springer-Verlag, Berlin.

Smith M. J. H. & Ford-Hutchinson A. W. (1979) Anti-inflammatory agents of animal origin. In *Anti-Inflammatory Drugs,* ed. Vane J. R. & Ferriera S. H., P. 673, Springer-Verlag, Berlin.

Snow D. H. (1981) Non-steroidal anti-inflammatory agents in the horse. *In Practice* **3**,(5), 24.

Snow D. H., Baxter P. & Whiting B. (1981a) The pharmacokinetics of meclofenamic acid in the horse. *J. Vet. Pharmacol. Therap.* **4**, 147–156.

Snow D. H., Bogan J. A., Douglas J. A. *et al* (1979) Phenylbutazone toxicity in ponies. *Vet. Rec.* **105**, 26.

Snow D. H., Douglas T. A., Thompson H. *et al* (1981b) Phenylbutazone toxicosis in equidae: A biochemical and pathophysiologic study. *Am. J. Vet. Res.* **42**, 1754.

Snow D. H., Douglas T. A., Thompson H. *et al* (1982) Effect of non-steroidal anti-inflammatory agents on plasma protein concentration of ponies. *Vet. Res. Comm. In press.*

Sullivan M. & Snow D. H. (1981) Factors affecting absorption of non-steroidal anti-inflammatory agents in the horse. *Vet. Rec.* **110**, 554.

Swann D. A. (1978) Macromolecules of synovial fluid. In *The Joints and Synovial Fluid,* vol. 1, ed. Sokoloff L. Academic Press, New York.

Tobin T. (1981) *Drugs and the Performance Horse.* Charles C. Thomas, Springfield, Illinois.

Tobin T., Blake J. W. & Valentine R. (1977) Drug interactions in the horse: Effects of chloramphenicol, quinidine and oxyphenbutazone on phenylbutazone metabolism. *Am. J. Vet. Res.* **38**, 123.

Toothaker R. D. & Welling P. G. (1980) The effect of food on drug bioavailability. *Ann. Rev. Pharmacol. Toxicol.* **20**, 173.

Turk J. L. & Willoughby D. A. (1978) Immunological and paraimmunological aspects of inflammation. In *Inflammation,* eds. Vane J. R. & Ferriera S. H., p. 231. Springer-Verlag, Berlin.

Van Pelt R. W., Tillotson P. J. & Gertsen K. E. (1970) Intra-articular injection of betamethasone in arthritis in horses. *J. Am. Vet. Med. Assoc.* **156**, 1589.

Van Pelt R. W., Tillotson P. J., Gertsen K. E. *et al* (1971) Effects of intra-articular injection of flumethazone suspension in joint diseases in horses. *J. Am. Vet. Med. Assoc.* **159**, 739.

Vane J. R. & Ferriera S. H. (1978) *Inflammation.* Springer-Verlag, Berlin.

Vernimb G. D. & Hennessey P. W. (1977) Clinical studies on flunixin meglumine in the treatment of equine colic. *J. Eq. Med. Surg.* **1**, 111–16.

Vernimb G. D., Van Hoose L. M. & Hennessey P. W. (1977) Equine arthropathies. *Vet. Med/Small Anim. Clin.* **72**, 241.

Weaver A. D. (1981) *Lameness in Cattle,* 2nd ed. John Wright–Scientechnia, Bristol.

Wheat J. D. (1955) The use of hydrocortisone in the treatment of joint and tendon disorders in large animals. *J. Am. Vet. Med. Assoc.* **127**, 64.

Willis A. L. (1969) Release of histamine, kinin and prostaglandin during carrageenin-induced inflammation in the rat. In *Prostaglandins, Peptides and Amines,* eds. Montegazza P. & Horton E. W., p. 31. Academic Press, New York.

Wilhelmi G. (1974) Species differences in susceptibility to the gastroulcerogenic action of anti-inflammatory agents. *Pharmacology* **11**, 220.

<h1 style="text-align:center">20</h1>

<h1 style="text-align:center">Corticosteroids</h1>

A. J. TEALE

The corticosteroids, both in the natural form but more especially in the form of synthetic analogues, comprise an important part of the clinician's armamentarium. Their therapeutic potential, diversity of action, potency, and scope for misuse are great. There is no doubt that they are widely misused and that this stems from a lack of understanding of the basic physiological and pharmacological properties of this most interesting and, when used rationally, most valuable group of compounds.

In an effort to aid the clinician in deciding which compound or preparation to use, when to use it, and to what extent, this chapter reviews those properties of the corticosteroids that are relevant in reaching such decisions. Such a review must on occasion be relatively superficial but the reader will be directed to sources of information offering more depth should he feel any particular aspect of this vast subject is worthy of further investigation.

Origin and definition

Along with weak androgens, the corticosteroids are synthesised in the adrenal cortex from cholesterol. They differ from the androgens in that they are based on a 21-carbon molecular structure while the androgens possess a 19-carbon structure. Cholesterol, which can be regarded as the basic unit on which the adrenal cortex elaborates to produce the corticosteroids, can itself be synthesised from acetate in the cortex, but it is mostly derived from exogenous sources. Work on the human subject suggests that the corticosteroids are not stored to any great extent in the cortex and tend to be produced and secreted at short notice, to demand (Borkowski *et al* 1967).

Natural corticosteroids in a normal animal are involved in the regulation of fluid and electrolyte balance on the one hand, and carbohydrate metabolism on the other. Most corticosteroids are able to influence both systems to a greater or lesser extent and, on the basis of which they affect most, they are arbitrarily categorised as mineralocorticoids and glucocorticoids. The actions of the mineralocorticoids are extremely complex, but for practical

428

purposes they can be considered as being responsible for the regulation of body sodium levels. Compounds in this group include 11-desoxy-corticosterone and aldosterone. Hydrocortisone is the principal natural glucocorticoid. Corticosterone, however, is intermediate between these two groups and has significant mineralocorticoid and glucocorticoid activities. As far as the natural compounds are concerned therefore, aldosterone and hydrocortisone can be considered as being at opposite ends of a spectrum of physiological function. The synthetic corticosteroids have markedly extended the spectrum at the glucocorticoid end and hydrocortisone, as a result, could now be considered as intermediate in function.

Regulation of secretion

Glucocorticoids

These are produced by the adrenal cortex in response to stimulation by adrenocorticotrophic hormone (ACTH), which is itself secreted by the anterior pituitary in response to corticotrophin releasing factor (CRF) which has its origin in the hypothalamus. This system forms the hypothalamo–pituitary–adrenal axis (HPA). The system is to some extent self-regulating; raised circulating levels of glucocorticoids exerting a negative-feedback effect at hypothalamic level. This self-regulating mechanism can be over-ridden however in two ways. First, in most mammals, the basal ACTH release pattern follows a circadian cycle. In diurnal species, there is peak release during the first quarter of the day, and in nocturnal species this occurs during the third quarter of the day. Secondly, there is an HPA stress response which can occur at any time in a healthy subject in response to a variety of stimuli, which results in an increase in ACTH release. Stimuli capable of initiating this response include pain, fever, metabolic disturbances, fear, adverse environmental conditions and surgical interference. This override of the basic regulatory system, under some circumstances, is life-supporting.

Release of ACTH is in 'bursts' and it seems that an overall increase in secretion is achieved by lessening the interval between such bursts (Myles and Daly 1974). An important point as far as therapy with corticosteroids is concerned is that the peak ACTH productive phase within the circadian pattern is very sensitive to suppression by exogenous corticosteroids and, consequently, when a steroid is administered in the late evening or early morning it will have a profound suppressive effect in diurnal species. On the other hand, providing the action of the steroid is of short duration (see below), it will have a minimal suppressive effect when administered to a diurnal animal in the second quarter of the day. This phenomenon can be put to good use in prolonged treatment regimens, when short-acting preparations can be given in the morning only, or in some cases on alternate mornings (so-called alternate-day therapy), when the desired therapeutic effect may be quite sufficient whilst at the same time HPA suppression is minimal.

Mineralocorticoids

Increased mineralocorticoid production in the adrenal cortex is in response to increased activity of the kidney renin/angiotensin system. ACTH does have a stimulating effect on mineralocorticoid production, but by comparison it is a minor one.

Structure and structure/function relationships

The basic structure of the corticosteroids is the 21-carbon pregnane nucleus. By convention the carbon atoms are numbered and the four rings they form are lettered A–D as in Fig. 20.1.

The stereochemical arrangement is of prime importance to biological activity. The four rings form a virtually flat molecule with the side chains projecting above and below the plane in which they lie. Groups projecting above the plane are designated β and those below are designated α, the upper surface being that from which project the methyl groups at positions 10 and 13. If hydrocortisone is used as an example, it can be defined as 11β, 17α, 21-trihydroxy Δ^4 pregnene-3, 20-dione, where the 11 hydroxyl group projects above the plane of the rings and the 17 group, below. The Δ^4 refers to the double bond between carbon atoms 4 and 5 in the A ring.

Corticosterone differs from hydrocortisone in that it does not possess a

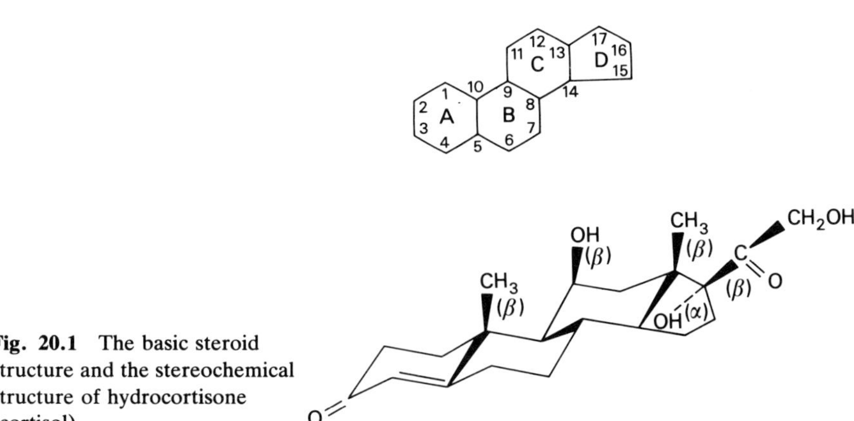

Fig. 20.1   The basic steroid structure and the stereochemical structure of hydrocortisone (cortisol).

17α hydroxyl group. 11-desoxycorticosterone lacks both the 17α and 11β hydroxyl groups. These reductions at the 11 and 17 positions produce compounds with an increased mineralocorticoid effect in comparison with hydrocortisone. Thus 11-desoxycorticosterone is a more potent mineralocorticoid than corticosterone which in its turn has more mineralocorticoid effect than hydrocortisone. Aldosterone, the most potent mineralocortocoid of all, however, does not appear at first sight to follow the general trend away from the hydrocortisone structure in that it possesses an 11β-hydroxyl group. This apparent anomaly is explained by the formation of the hemi-acetal form in the body, which possesses the mineralocorticoid activity.

As far as the glucocorticoids are concerned, certain basic features of the molecule are required for effect. These are:

A double bond between carbons 4 and 5 (Δ^4).

An 11-hydroxyl group. It is of interest to note that cortisone shows an apparent discrepancy in this regard, and indeed it is inactive *per se*. Activity is dependent on conversion to hydrocortisone in the body, mainly by liver enzymes.

A ketone group at the 3 position.

A 20 keto group.

A 21 methoxy group (CH_2OH) or derivative.

There are a few exceptions to this rule in that some progesterone-like compounds (with a 21 methyl group) have some glucocorticoid effect, especially if they also possess 9 or 12 fluoro groups. Clobetasol, which has a chloro group at the 4 position, is extremely active by topical application.

By making alterations to this basic glucocorticoid structure, function or more especially differential potency can be altered. In 1954 it was discovered that the introduction of halogen atoms into the molecule could greatly enhance biological activity. The fundamental discovery that 9-fluorocortisol had a greatly enhanced anti-inflammatory effect compared to cortisone and an even more markedly enhanced mineralocorticoid effect, opened the way to the production of a vast range of synthetic analogues. This is because it was realised that, by substitution and addition to the basic structure, function could not only be altered quantitatively but qualitatively also, i.e. the two basic properties of the corticosteroids could largely be separated. Thus:

1 The introduction of a double bond at C1–2 (Δ^1) results in increased gluconeogenic potency and prednisolone, which differs from hydrocortisone only in this respect, has four times the potency of hydrocortisone.

2 Substitution at the 6 and 9 positions in the B ring generally produces an increased gluconeogenic effect and decreased mineralocorticoid effect. Substitutions at 6 can be methyl, fluoro or chloro, and at 9, fluoro or chloro. The substitution at the 9 position must be α.

3 Certain C16 substitutions in the D ring increase gluconeogenic activity. Examples in common use in veterinary medicine are dexamethasone and betamethasone. Both have a methyl grouping at this position, but this is α in the case of dexamethasone and β in betamethasone. In comparison with hydrocortisone they have a markedly increased gluconeogenic potency and reduced mineralocorticoid activity. An α-hydroxyl group at the C16 position also markedly reduces sodium-retaining effect, e.g. triamcinolone. A point of particular relevance to large animal practitioners is that the ability to induce parturition with corticosteroids is very much associated with the methyl substitution at this position.

4 The introduction of a 17 hydroxy or substituted hydroxy group confers increased gluconeogenic effect.

These structural modifications probably produce alterations in biological activity in at least two ways: firstly by decreasing the rate of enzymic breakdown. Thus Δ^1 protects the 3 keto group and the Δ^4 double bond, 9α fluoro substitution protects the 11β hydroxyl group, and 16α substitutions protect the C_{20} position. Secondly by reducing plasma-protein binding. Generally, α substitutions have this effect so that more of the administered steroid is free to exert a pharmacological effect. (Some synthetic corticosteroids also show increased tissue binding.)

Although enormous efforts have been made and vast sums of money spent on finding, testing, developing and marketing the wide range of synthetic analogues now available, it is most important that those who administer corticosteroids should appreciate two fundamental points. Firstly, although it has proved possible to separate the gluconeogenic and mineralocorticoid effects, it has not been possible to dissociate anti-inflammatory potency from catabolic effects; secondly, increased potency results in increased suppression of the HPA axis. In veterinary medicine, the very potent analogues tend to be widely used, and this is probably justifiable when long term therapy is not involved. However, these compounds, although they may not circulate in the blood for very long periods, are capable of exerting intense effects, and effects which are prolonged even after a single administration. This residual effect is a feature of corticosteroid action in general and is not dependent on their continued presence. Furthermore, it tends to increase with increased gluconeogenic potency. Very importantly it reduces the HPA axis-sparing effect of 'alternate day therapy' even when these highly active analogues are used in their short-acting forms. For this type of regimen, therefore, hydrocortisone (especially in human medicine) and prednisolone and its derivatives are preferred to dexamethasone, betamethasone and flumethasone. The latter compounds have a valid place in veterinary medicine but there is as yet no 'corticosteroid for all seasons', and the choice of a particular steroid should be based on consideration of the desired effect, over what period this is required, and whether HPA axis suppression is likely or acceptable.

Apart from the very specific modifications to the basic structure which have already been outlined, other changes can be made to achieve certain desired results in the final product for specific uses. Thus, increased aqueous solubility can be achieved by the production of the sodium phosphate and succinate esters which are particularly suitable for intravenous administration. Generally these must be converted back to the parent molecule within the body before they can exert their effect. For those compounds not administered intravenously, the rate of release from the injection site can be considerably reduced by increasing the size of the substituent group at the C17 or 21 positions, e.g. adamantoate, phenylpropionate, acetate, trimethylacetate, etc., which makes them particularly suitable where a prolonged effect is required. The butyrates and valerates lend themselves to topical application.

Transport, metabolism and excretion

Of the naturally-circulating corticosteroids, by far the largest proportion is reversibly protein-bound in plasma. Two proteins are involved: corticosteroid-binding globulin which has a high affinity but a low capacity for steroids, and albumin which has a low affinity but high capacity. Under normal circumstances, most is bound to globulin so that when a corticosteroid is administered there is an increase in the non-bound fraction and in the albumin bound fraction (Seal & Doe 1956).

The breakdown of corticosteroids is complex but basically it involves reduction to hydroxyl of the 4 and 3 ketone entities and also reduction of the 20 ketone group. This occurs for the most part in the liver but to some extent in kidney also. The 3 hydroxyl group is then conjugated, e.g. sulphated prior to excretion in the urine (Siegel 1965). The biliary system is also a significant excretion route for endogenous steroids in some animals. The synthetic steroids undergo much less metabolism than their endogenous counterparts (as might be expected from their molecular structures) and appear in greater proportions unchanged in the urine.

Cellular effects of corticosteroids

It is not known with absolute certainty how the corticosteroids exert their effects at a cellular level, but several mechanisms have been proposed, some or all of which may indeed operate. One such proposal based on good evidence is that corticosteroids are able to de-repress transcription of DNA to mRNA in the target cell nucleus. This is based on the theory that all body cells are multipotential and have the genetic capability of producing every protein in the organism as a whole. Cell specialisation is made possible by use only of limited parts of this genetic information, and hence only some of the complete range of proteins are produced in a given type of cell. These proteins could be enzymes and therefore potent expressors of the genetic information used. It is thought that the parts of the information which are not being used at any one time are 'locked-up' by repressor proteins attaching to specific parts of the DNA chains. After combination initially with a cytoplasmic receptor and then with a nuclear receptor, the steroids are able to disrupt the binding of such repressor proteins to DNA and so release genetic information. This allows transcription of the DNA to mRNA which is then translated in the process of protein synthesis (Tomkins & Martin 1970, Tomkins & Gelehrter 1972).

Action at this fundamental level would indeed explain how the same hormone can have such wide-ranging, and often apparently opposite, effects in different tissues of the same animal. It may even be that some of the proteins, the synthesis of which is made possible by steroids, are themselves either positive or negative in function, i.e., initiate or inhibit subcellular processes depending on the particular protein or cell involved (Makman *et al* 1971). The growth-suppressing effect of corticosteroids could also be explained by the binding of steroid-receptor complexes to chromatin.

Other mechanisms proposed for steroid action include a boosting of cellular levels of cyclic AMP, this being made possible by steroid inhibition of phosphodiesterases which would otherwise metabolise this very active compound (Myles & Daly 1974), and membrane-stabilising effects including those of lysosomes (Weissman 1969). Nijkamp *et al* (1976) amongst others, suggest that at least some of the anti-inflammatory activity of corticosteroids could be due to inhibition of prostaglandin synthesis by suppression of the release of arachidonate, the precursor, from cell membranes (*see also* p. 414).

Physiology and pharmacology

It must be emphasised in any discussion of the action of corticosteroids that much of what is known is based firstly on observations of disease states such as Cushing's syndrome and Addison's disease in animals, and especially in man, and secondly on the effects of exogenous hormones administered to animals, isolated tissues and organs, cell cultures and cell components. Extrapolation from one system to another should be done with caution. To illustrate this point, a great deal has been learned of the effects of the corticosteroids in the laboratory rat. However, the steroids given have on occasion been administered in high doses, and it is now known that the rat is not typical in certain of its responses to exogenous steroid administration. Much of what follows in this section is therefore of a general nature and should be viewed as background information. There is a very large amount of published material on this aspect of the corticosteroids and readers are referred to the further reading section at the end of this chapter.

Effects on electrolyte and water balance

Potencies of the various steroids, as judged by their ability to maintain life in adrenalectomised animals, closely parallel their sodium-retaining activity. Thus an adrenalectomised dog requires approximately $10\mu g$/day aldosterone or 5000 μg hydrocortisone. As well as the retention of sodium, associated particularly with mineralocorticoids but also to some extent with glucocorticoids, these compounds cause an increase in potassium excretion. Further, mineralocorticoids play a very important role in the distribution of electrolytes between the various body compartments. As far as glucocorticoids are concerned the enhanced potassium excretion is a more consistent effect than sodium retention and prolonged administration of high doses can result in hypokalaemia. A frequent clinical observation is the diuresis which occurs on occasion in association with glucocorticoid therapy. This is probably due to an increase in glomerular filtration rate and possibly also in part to a direct effect on the renal tubule. This is consistent with the fact that in hypoadrenocorticism there is an inability to excrete a free water load but this is responsive to substitution therapy with glucocorticoids.

In addition to causing sodium retention and potassium excretion, corticosteroids also promote hydrogen ion and calcium excretion. The latter effect, combined with an antagonistic effect on intestinal absorption of calcium, is consistent with the osteoporosis which is seen at least in human cases of Cushing's syndrome and during long term steroid therapy. In this case, however, other mechanisms may also be operating such as a general catabolic effect on bone metabolism producing an interference with the connective tissue matrix of bone.

Effects on carbohydrate, protein and lipid metabolism

The overall effects of the glucocorticosteroids are to increase gluconeogenesis in the liver, to increase glycogen storage, and to promote lipolysis and protein mobilisation. All these effects are connected and some may be mediated indirectly. For instance, it is possible that the glycogen synthesis that occurs in response to glucocorticoid administration is an insulin effect, insulin secretion having been enhanced in response to the raised blood glucose levels caused by the steroid. Except in this regard however, the glucocorticoids may be considered as anti-insulin in their effect on carbohydrate metabolism.

It is true that body fats in some tissues, expecially in some species, increase in response to glucocorticoid administration over prolonged periods. This again may be an insulin rebound effect. The result is therefore an apparent redistribution of body fat in many cases, with the direct steroid effect dominant in certain areas of the body and the secondary insulin effect holding sway in others.

The effect of corticosteroids on protein metabolism, like that on fat metabolism, is catabolic. There is decreased incorporation of amino acids into protein and increased protein breakdown. The amino acids produced with the glycerol from fat metabolism are used as fuel for the gluconeogenic activity of the liver.

Effects on the cardiovascular system

Corticosteroids have a profound effect on blood volume through their effects on body water and electrolyte levels. They also have three other very important actions with regard to blood volume which, as will be seen in a later section, assume great significance in the 'shocked' animal. The first is a protective effect on capillary integrity, the second is that they tend to inhibit the vasomotor response peripherally to vasoconstrictor substances, and the last that there is a positive inotropic effect on cardiac function in shocked animals. As far as therapy is concerned, when these properties are to be utilised, dosage rate is of paramount importance and will be dealt with in more detail in the relevant section on therapeutics.

Effect on skeletal muscle

There is a tendency to decrease muscular power in both hyper- and hypo-adrenocortical state. In the former case this can largely be accounted for by muscle wasting, and in the latter by a decreased efficiency of the circulatory system (Gilman *et al* 1980).

Effects on CNS

Direct effects of steroids on the CNS are well known and indeed some steroids are in common use as general anaesthetics in both the human and veterinary fields. The sedative effects of progesterone-like compounds are well recognised particularly in feline medicine. It would therefore not be surprising if the corticosteroids also had some direct effect on CNS function. Hydrocortisone does seem to help maintain a sense of well being in human hypoadrenocortical patients. Desoxycorticosterone acetate (which has been used with hydrocortisone in such cases as the mineralocorticoid) does not have this effect. There is also some evidence that glucocorticoids in high doses lower the threshold to convulsive seizures in man.

Haematological effects

Administration of glucocorticoids results in increased numbers of circulating polymorphonuclear leucocytes and a decrease in the numbers of other circulating leucocytes. The lymphocytopenia may be due to redistribution rather than destruction. As a general rule, the glucocorticoids tend to cause an increase in haemoglobin levels and an increase in numbers of circulating erythrocytes.

Effects on the immune system and inflammation

Lymphoid tissue varies between species in its sensitivity to corticosteroids. Generally, corticosteroid effects on lymphoid tissue are catabolic. Rats and mice show the most dramatic responses, and in these species administration of corticosteroids is followed quite rapidly by actual destruction of lymphocytes and a marked effect on thymic tissue. Conversely, man, monkey, ferret and guinea pig are relatively resistant to these effects of the corticosteroids and to some extent the small rodents (in which much of the work on the effects of the corticosteroids has been carried out) are exceptional.

In the same way that there appears to be little effect in many species on the numbers of cells involved in the immune response, there also seems to be little effect on the levels of circulating immunoglobulins. However, there is no doubt that exogenous corticosteroids are capable of suppressing the immune response in disease and in the normal animal. Indeed, this is a valuable effect in the treatment of many disease conditions, but on occasions it is a disastrous side-effect. Their level of activity seems to be on the development of effects of immune system activation. As an example, they have been shown to suppress the effect of lymphokines (produced by lymphocytes in response to antigen stimulation) on macrophages.

With regard to the anti-inflammatory properties of the glucocorticoids, they are able to suppress both the cardinal signs of acute inflammation regardless of cause and the long term effects of inflammation, such as fibrin deposition and scar tissue formation. The non-selectivity of these steroids in this respect is both useful and potentially misleading. It is useful in any situation where inflammation or the effects of the immune response are life threatening. The clinician need not concern himself initially with the cause when he administers a suitable steroid in high doses, whether the case is acute inhalation pneumonia or acute respiratory distress syndrome of the anaphylactic type. In some circumstances, however, inhibition of an inflammatory response may be counter-productive in that it may be necessary for recovery or it may be necessary to alert the clinician to an underlying disease process.

The mechanism by which the glucocorticoids exert an anti-inflammatory effect is complex and certainly cannot be totally explained by stabilisation of lysosomal membranes. Though this protection against the various mediators of the inflammatory response which are formed under the influence of lysosomal enzymes does play a part, there is increasing evidence for a direct suppressive effect on prostaglandin synthesis, possibly by a block on the release of arachidonate, which is the prostaglandin precursor, from cell membranes (Nijkamp *et al* 1976). Suppression of prostaglandin synthesis is a property shared with other anti-inflammatory agents such as salicylates, indomethacin and mepacrine. It is of interest to note that the relative potencies of the various glucocorticosteroids in this system closely parallel their anti-inflammatory potencies.

Effects on growth and cell division

There is evidence for a suppressive effect of the corticosteroids on growth and cell division. In practice, this is probably of little importance in the veterinary field. The mechanism of this effect is poorly understood although it is thought that there is a direct action on DNA metabolism. Certainly, the effect on growth is not universal and bone marrow and gut cell turnover seem to be spared, which is not the case with classical antimitotic agents. Also it appears that the presence of corticosteroids is necessary for the synthesis of such things as surfactant in foetal lung, myelin and some proteins (Myles & Daly 1974).

Therapeutic uses

Therapy with corticosteroids can be either specific or non-specific. Specific therapy is substitution therapy in cases of adrenocortical insufficiency and as such has little application at the present time in veterinary medicine. However, cases have been described in various species including the horse (Kirk 1974) and the dog (Feldman *et al* 1977). All other types of therapy with corticosteroids are of a non-specific nature which highlights a very important and fundamental fact about corticosteroid administration: that other lines of treatment should be considered and possibly effected simultaneously. The use of a corticosteroid as the sole means of therapy is rarely justified.

As will be appreciated from a knowledge of the pharmacology of the corticosteroids, they have very many therapeutic uses. For this reason subsequent sections will merely illustrate the basic points of therapy with a number of examples.

The use of corticosteroids as anti-inflammatory agents

This is the area in which the corticosteroids are most used in veterinary medicine. The indications for use are many and varied, possibly because the corticosteroids are capable of suppressing the inflammatory response in several ways and irrespective of cause.

Musculoskeletal disorders

Such disorders are very often responsive to corticosteroids administered orally, parenterally or locally. Consideration of their widespread and sometimes profound effects when they are administered orally or parenterally suggests that local therapy be undertaken whenever possible. This principle is generally sound, but great care is required in administration by injection into lesions or localised affected areas such as joints, tendon sheaths, etc. Technique should be aseptic as far as possible and, when injecting into well defined spaces such as joints, care should be taken to remove an equivalent amount of fluid beforehand (Gallagher 1977). Care should also be exercised in the selection of the steroid preparation given locally, for not all preparations may be suitable. Such information is readily available from manufacturers.

A great deal of attention has been focussed on the horse in this context, since the indications for corticosteroid treatment of musculoskeletal disorders are more numerous in this species than in farm animals. Flumethasone in particular has been studied in detail for the effects on healthy joints following intra-articular injection (Van Pelt 1973a). A mild synovitis occurs seven days after injection which Van Pelt considers is caused by the microcrystalline nature of the flumethasone suspension used. He also found a decreased synovial effusion and increased relative viscosity of joint fluid in comparison with control joints. There were additionally mild degenerative changes in the synovial membranes but there was no inflammatory reaction. It must be emphasised that all these changes were subclinical. There is some evidence of decreased hyaluronidase activity in joints injected repeatedly and this is especially associated with the use of hydrocortisone preparations.

McKay & Milne (1976) made a valuable contribution to the discussions surrounding the injection of anti-inflammatory agents into equine joints and, although they reported a single case of a severe joint lesion of a productive/destructive nature which was considered to be corticosteroid-induced, most of their patients appeared to benefit from therapy.

Two conditions which merit special attention in this section are laminitis and navicular disease. Colles & Jeffcott (1977) have suggested that, if treatment of laminitis is to be undertaken with corticosteroids, it should be restricted to the first 24 hours of the syndrome because of a possible interference with the healing processes after that time. For navicular disease, Colles (1979) suggests that local therapy with corticosteroids may be more damaging than beneficial.

Some attention has also been given to the treatment of degenerative joint diseases of cattle with corticosteroids (Van Pelt 1973b, 1975). The general principles of therapy are the same as those relating to the horse.

Hypersensitivity

All types of hypersensitivity reaction can be suppressed by the proper use of corticosteroids. A very important group of conditions which fall into this category are some entities of the so-called bovine 'acute respiratory distress syndrome' (ARDS). This includes Fog Fever which, in this context, can be defined as acute respiratory distress of adult cattle at pasture in the late summer and autumn. Another example is milk allergy which occurs most often in heifers of dairy breeds which suffer acute respiratory distress very often when they are actually being walked in for milking.

These two conditions particularly demand very prompt attention if there is to be even a chance of a successful outcome. There is no doubt that properly considered steroid therapy can be life-saving in these cases. However, for rapid availability of the drug at target sites in the respiratory system, one needs very high doses of water-soluble preparations, administered intravenously. It is difficult to overdose these conditions and quantities of suitable preparations should be measured in bottles per animal and not in millilitres. Even the mildest case justifies a minimum dose of 100 mg dexamethasone sodium phosphate or equivalent. It is possible that the corticosteroids are particularly efficacious in these cases because of their ability to suppress prostaglandin synthesis and it may be that other inhibitors would also be effective in treatment.

Bovine farmer's lung and certain types of urticaria and sweet itch in horses can also be considered for corticosteroid therapy. However, all three conditions illustrate the non-specific nature of therapy, because in each case other approaches could obviate the need for corticosteroids.

Photosensitisation

It is likely that corticosteroids in high doses will give a certain measure of protection against the development of severe lesions, but probably in most cases of photosensitisation administration is too late because they are not presented until the skin changes are well advanced. However, provided the basic principles of corticosteroid therapy are observed, administration of a single high dose is justified on the grounds that little harm is likely to result and, if nothing else, the systemic effects could well be beneficial to an animal suffering pain and possible secondary circulatory problems and ion imbalances (especially hyperkalaemia).

Infections

Glucocorticoids are commonly used as an adjunct to antibiotic therapy in a number of conditions involving infection. As a general rule it is probably wise to avoid the use of steroids except in those instances where a secondary inflammatory response of life-threatening proportions is present or a systemic toxic effect is produced. Infections of the lower respiratory tract where cellular proliferation and effusions occur are frequently treated with steroids. However, Christie *et al* (1977) reported a survey of infectious respiratory disease cases in feedlot cattle where treatment was either with oxytetracycline and an antihistamine, or with oxytetracycline, antihistamine and 20 mg dexamethasone. They found that the recovery rate was better in those animals not given the steroid and also that the relapse rate was higher in those that were.

Mastitis in various species is another condition frequently treated with corticosteroids. The reasons for this are four-fold. First, corticosteroids are sometimes present in proprietary intramammary preparations in conjunction with an antibiotic in order to protect the udder tissue from the irritant action of some of the constituents of the preparation itself. It can be argued that such usage is fully justified. Secondly, they are used in an effort to reduce the long term effects of inflammation such as fibrosis; in this case they may be administered both locally and parenterally. It is unclear whether results justify the administration of corticosteroids for this purpose. Thirdly, they are given to reduce acute inflammatory changes, which are obviously distressing for the animal. In this context caution is needed, for, although the short term result may be apparently beneficial, it must be borne in mind that the inflammatory process is in many ways protective and an integral part of the animal's defence system. If antibiotics were wholly efficient in the treatment of mastitis, there would be no need for caution, but this is certainly not the case. Moreover, many of the antibiotics used in mastitis therapy are bacteriostatic and an efficient immune system is a prerequisite for their use. The ability of glucocorticoids to inhibit macrophage aggregation and activity is worthy of some consideration when they are given in cases of acute mastitis. Fourthly, they are used to reduce the impact of toxins (produced in the udder by micro-organisms). In this circumstance the glucocorticoids may well have a valuable role to play in mastitis therapy, particularly in those cases where *E. coli* is thought to be involved and systemic effects are marked. Indeed it can be argued that, in these circumstances, corticosteroid therapy is more helpful than antibiotic therapy since maintenance of circulatory function is of prime importance and the anabolic effects of the glucocorticoids on liver function probably play a part in their overall therapeutic effect.

Another syndrome involving *E. coli* endotoxin is that produced by the proliferation of certain serotypes of *E. coli* in the calf. Again the pathogenesis seems to involve the systemic effects of toxin.

The use of corticosteroids in the treatment of metabolic disorders
(see also Chapter 16)

Since Hatziolos & Shaw (1950) demonstrated the efficacy of glucocorticoids in the treatment of bovine ketosis, these compounds have found wide acceptance as therapeutic agents for this syndrome. This is certainly justifiable and a good cure rate can be achieved by a single administration of one of the very potent fluorinated analogues such as betamethasone or dexamethasone which are particularly active promoters of gluconeogenesis. Flumethasone and fluoroprednisolone are also commonly used for the treatment of acetonaemia.

The mechanism of action of the glucocorticoids in this condition is far from clear and it certainly cannot be dismissed as a simple gluconeogenic effect, for a number of reasons. Firstly, many cows with ketosis have blood glucose levels within the normal range, although after glucocorticoid administration there is an hyperglycaemic response. Secondly, the glucocorticoids increase lipolysis and protein catabolism and this will tend to exacerbate ketosis/acidosis. Thirdly, increased gluconeogenesis in itself could only be beneficial if the glucose produced was then available for energy production and a marked effect of the glucocorticoids is the stimulation of glycogenesis from glucose in the liver, at least in monogastric animals.

Baird and Heitzman (1971) have shed some light on the mechanism of action of corticosteroids in bovine ketosis by studying the levels of citric acid cycle intermediates and relevant liver enzymes both in normal and ketotic animals and in response to glucocorticoid administration. Their work suggests that there is an increased influx of citric acid cycle substrates and raised levels of cycle intermediates without a corresponding increase in gluconeogenesis, resulting in a net increase in energy production and reduced ketogenesis. They also suggest that this effect may be peculiar to ruminants.

The administration of corticosteroids to lactating cows tends to reduce milk production, and the easing of the energy requirement of the animal in this way may also be contributory to the therapeutic effect in these cases. Bovine ketosis is a good example of a condition responsive to corticosteroid therapy which may be treated by one, or a combination, of several alternatives. There is little doubt that exercise, the provision of grazing, the administration of high energy feeds, etc. all help in the management of these cases and may obviate the need for corticosteroids.

Pregnancy toxaemia (twin lamb disease) of sheep is a related condition which is also treated with glucocorticoids. The situation in this case is not so satisfactory however, and adequate responses to treatment are not so frequent or marked. Nevertheless, it is fair to say that no other class of therapeutic agent currently available offers a better alternative in the treatment of a well established pregnancy toxaemia, although some recent developments with anabolic steroids may prove fruitful. There seem to be no contraindications to the use of glucocorticoids in this condition (providing adequate antibiotic cover is maintained, particularly where dead lambs might be involved). If the glucocorticoid used is able to induce parturition, this could well be decisive in bringing about a recovery and possibly this should be the aim of glucocorticoid therapy in these cases.

From what is known of the effects of the glucocorticoids on intermediate metabolism of ruminants, it really is not surprising that they are not very effective in the treatment of pregnancy toxaemia of sheep. What is more surprising is their particularly good record in the treatment of bovine ketosis.

Two equine conditions which can be considered in this section are azoturia and neonatal maladjustment syndrome (NMS). Both involve degrees of acidosis which may well respond to glucocorticoid therapy. In the case of azoturia there is also breakdown of muscle tissue with release of myoglobin into the general circulation and, theoretically at least, the steroids may moderate this process by virtue of their membrane stabilising effect. In cases of NMS, as well as acidosis, there is a degree of cerebral oedema in many affected foals. An important use of glucocorticoids in both human and veterinary fields is in the treatment of cerebral oedema secondary to physical trauma and cardiac arrest, so it is not surprising that they do find a use in the treatment of this condition.

The use of corticosteroids to induce parturition

The induction of parturition was originally considered an undesirable side-effect of corticosteroid therapy. It has subsequently been put to good use. The effect is particularly associated with the C16-substituted corticosteroids such as betamethasone, dexamethasone and flumethasone, but for the purpose of avoiding unwanted induction it should be assumed that all the corticosteroids have this potential. Different species react differently to corticosteroid usage in this regard. Ruminants tend to be very susceptible to parturition induction with the steroids, whereas horses are more refractory. They will therefore be considered separately.

Cattle (*see also* Chapter 13)

It is worthwhile considering firstly the indications for parturition induction in cattle, because the indication can have some bearing on the choice of steroid preparation used. The indications include:
1   Illness or injury of the dam.
2   Hydropic conceptus.
3   The avoidance of absolute or relative foetal oversize.
4   Maintenance of seasonal calving patterns.
5   Udder oedema.
6   Convenience, i.e. avoidance of calvings at holiday times, weekends, etc.
   The avoidance of oversize problems by the induction of parturition before too great a disparity in foetal and birth canal dimensions develops has become increasingly important in the UK in recent years with the more frequent use of large, continental-breed bulls for crossing with dairy cows of indigenous type. In these cases induction can often be delayed until the last few days of a normal gestation period because daily foetal weight gains gradually increase as the final trimester advances. Such daily gains can be of the order of several kilograms in the last few days of pregnancy. Therefore, if pregnancy is shortened by just one week, much can be gained in terms of reduced foetal size at parturition.
   There are two approaches to induction with corticosteroids: induction after day 260 of pregnancy and induction prior to day 260. The avoidance of oversize therefore falls into the first category. The alleviation of problems associated with excessive periparturient oedema of the udder (which is particularly common in primiparous cattle) likewise calls for interference in the terminal stages of pregnancy.
   Induction after day 260 is usually effected easily with a single administration of a C16-substituted corticosteroid in a short-acting formulation, such as the free alcohol or soluble ester (e.g. betamethasone and dexamethasone sodium phosphate, respectively). The period from injection to parturition is

dependent on the individual animal, the preparation used, and the dose; however, the use of the short-acting steroids at this stage of gestation usually results in parturition within a few days. Generally, as drug administration approaches full term, the latent period becomes shorter. In the purebred Charolais for instance, an intramuscular injection of 30 mg dexamethasone sodium phosphate after day 280 usually results in parturition in 28–40 hours. There is a possibility of a breed resistance to induction with betamethasone in the case of the Maine-Anjou. Plenderleith (1974) reported this when 20 mg of the steroid were given; however, there was no apparent resistance at higher dose levels.

The major problem associated with parturition induction in this manner is retention of the afterbirth (Grunert *et al* 1975, Tervit 1976), although Plenderleith (1974) did not encounter this difficulty in his series of inductions with betamethasone in beef heifers in-calf to continental breed bulls. Several workers have attempted to alleviate this problem by administering oestrogens and calcium solutions either together or separately, at the time of steroid administration. In a very few cases there were apparent successes (Grunert *et al* 1975), when very large doses of stilboestrol were given in combination with calcium borogluconate. However, direct comparisons of different series of inductions should be made with caution because it does seem that, the closer to term the induction is performed, the less likely it is that afterbirth retention will be a problem with the short-acting steroids.

It is worth noting that, despite the potential afterbirth problem in this category of inductions, there is general agreement that subsequent fertility is not affected. Furthermore, induction after day 260 is not associated with decreased immunoglobulin content of colostrum (Beardsley *et al* 1976, Hoerlein & Jones 1977), and absorption of immunoglobulins by the calf is not apparently reduced (Hoerlein & Jones 1977, Langley & O'Farrel 1976). It is perhaps not surprising therefore that the calf survival rate after induction in this manner is not significantly different from that of full-term controls. Beardsley *et al* (1976) found that, after induction with betamethasone in combination with an oestrogen given on day 273 of gestation, milk yield was reduced in the first nine weeks of the subsequent lactation and body weight loss was reduced over the same period in comparison with controls.

Induction in the period prior to day 260 of gestation calls for a different approach. The main indication is the maintenance of seasonal calving patterns and, although this is not common practice in most UK systems of management, it is a widely adopted procedure in some other countries, notably New Zealand. As a general rule, induction becomes progressively more difficult to achieve the earlier in the last trimester it is attempted; for this reason, a single injection of a short-acting steroid is rarely successful prior to day 260, although there are wide variations between individuals and there are exceptions to this rule. For this reason, the longer-acting formulations such as dexamethasone trimethyl acetate are usually used alone or in combination with other steroids for these earlier inductions. There is a significant delay (sometimes of weeks) between administration and induction with these compounds and the end result is by no means as certain as with induction after day 260 with the short-acting steroids.

Calf mortality, as might be expected, can be a significant problem. Attempts have been made to reduce this by the administration of a second steroid, usually of the short-acting type, 6–12 days after the depot injection (Welch *et al* 1977). Nevertheless, although these regimens do seem to meet with some success, mortality rates have still been higher than in calves allowed to go to full term. Dexamethasone trimethyl acetate has been used in combination with progesterone (O'Farrel & Crowley 1974), but calf mortality rates were still high and a high incidence of vulval and mammary swelling was reported. By comparison with early induction with the long-acting preparations, induction after day 260 with the short-acting preparations is more predictable and is associated with lower calf mortality and a higher incidence of afterbirth retention (Grunert *et al* 1975).

With the increased usage of the prostaglandins in veterinary medicine it is perhaps worth comparing their performance as inducers of parturition with that of the corticosteroids in cattle. The available evidence suggests that they offer no real advantages over the steroids, and in some respects they do not perform so well. Kordts & Jochle (1975) compared flumethasone with prostaglandin F2α (PGF$_2\alpha$), given between days 267 and 270 of gestation. Induction was more rapid after the corticosteroid and, at the dose rate used (20 mg PGF$_2\alpha$), there were no induction failures with the steroid whereas the prostaglandin was not invariably successful in inducing parturition. The subsequent interval from calving to conception was marginally shorter in those cows given prostaglandin. There is some evidence that the incidence of dystocia in Charolais and Normand cattle is higher in association with the use of cloprostenol by comparison with dexamethasone (Bosc *et al* 1975). Bosc *et al* suggested that the degree of pelvic ligament relaxation was less in those cases induced with the prostaglandin. Beal *et al* (1976) found that PGF$_2\alpha$ appeared to hasten the onset of labour in those cows which were still uncalved 40 hours after the administration of 20 mg dexamethasone sodium phosphate. In those cows receiving the prostaglandin at this stage, the average induction time after the initial steroid injection was 44 hours, compared to 52.6 hours in those late-responding animals which received steroid alone.

Sheep

Corticosteroids have been proven useful in the tightening of lambing patterns (Lucas & Notman 1974, Penning & Gibb 1977). The short-acting preparations are normally used and, when administered in the final week or so of gestation, they give induction periods of $1\frac{1}{2}$–2 days (Harrison 1982). After day 138 of gestation there appears to be no evidence of poor lamb viability, poor lactation, or retained afterbirths (Emady *et al* 1974).

Horses

Horses are considerably more resistant than ruminants to parturition induction with the corticosteroids, and require doses of the order of 100 mg dexamethasone daily for 3–4 days. Jeffcott & Rossdale (1977) compared a corticosteroid with oxytocin and fluprostenol for parturition induction performance and concluded that, after the use of the corticosteroid, first stage labour was unduly short — causing a non-acceptable incidence of foetal malposture and neonatal deaths when compared with the other agents.

Because of this relative resistance of the horse to the induction of parturition with corticosteroids, there would appear to be less cause for concern when steroids are administered during pregnancy, providing daily dose rates are not very high and dosing is not prolonged. Burns (1973) stated that normal therapeutic doses will not produce parturition in the horse when given either intravenously or intramuscularly. (It is, however, difficult to define a 'normal therapeutic dose'.) He pointed out that the equine oestrogens, equilin and equilinin, are unusual in that they have an unsaturated B ring, and that levels of these particular oestrogens increase during the second half of pregnancy. Furthermore, their production seems to be independent to a large extent of that of the classic oestrogens and so may be unaffected by corticosteroid administration.

The use of the corticosteroids in the treatment of shock

For the purpose of this discussion, shock may be defined as acute, progressive, circulatory collapse, irrespective of the initial triggering factor (Fig. 20.2). Benefit may be derived from corticosteroid therapy irrespective of cause.

To focus attention on the types of conditions for which corticosteroids may be of some value as part of a shock therapy regimen, it is perhaps worthwhile reviewing some potential causes of the shock syndrome. These include haemorrhage (surgical and non-surgical), cardiac failure, infection, toxaemia, anaphylaxis, and adrenal failure.

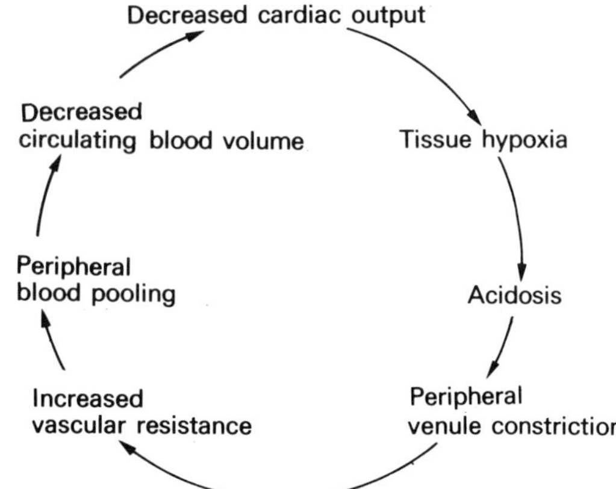

Fig. 20.2 The shock circle.

Exactly how the corticosteroids benefit a shocked patient is not known although many possible actions have been suggested. Some of the more obvious of these include: stabilisation of lysosomal membranes, maintenance of endothelial integrity. suppression of anaphylotoxin production which results from antigen/antibody/complement interaction, prevention of platelet aggregation, inhibition of vasoconstrictor substances, and a vasodilator effect on arterioles and venules. Other mechanisms have been proposed and some or all of these may well be important.

As far as the use of corticosteroids in the management of a shock case is concerned, the type of preparation used is important. The beneficial effects are attributable to glucocorticoid rather than mineralocorticoid activity. Furthermore, shock is a life-threatening emergency and, as such, speed of onset of action is of the essence in therapy. Therefore, a glucocorticoid should be chosen which will become readily and rapidly available in target tissues and sites. For these purposes the water-soluble esters or free alcohols are required, e.g. betamethasone, dexamethasone, sodium phosphate and methyl prednisolone sodium succinate — all of which may be given intravenously.

A second factor of major significance is the dose rate. In the treatment of shock, very large doses indeed should be given if possible. In man, methylprednisolone sodium succinate has been recommended at a dose rate of 30 mg/kg given intravenously over a period of ten minutes (Hankes 1976). In dogs, dose rates of 4–11 mg/kg dexamethasone sodium phosphate have achieved good results. In these terms, quantities required for the treatment of large farm animals become prohibitively large, but in very valuable young stock such therapy may be felt to be justified.

A final point to bear in mind in the treatment of shock, as in other situations when corticosteroid therapy is instituted, is that there are often other measures which should be taken. The maintenance of circulating blood volume with intravenous infusions of blood or plasma expanders, and measures to correct acidosis such as the infusion of lactated Ringer's solution and/or sodium bicarbonate can mean the difference between success and failure.

General points in corticosteroid therapy

1 The correct dose for each patient for many conditions is found only by trial and error and should be periodically re-evaluated in prolonged therapy.
2 A single dose, even a very large one, is virtually without harmful effect. This justifies the use of the corticosteroids in any major crisis.
3 The incidence of harmful side-effects increases with prolongation of therapy above substitution level.
4 Except in the treatment of adrenal insufficiency, therapy is only palliative.
5 Abrupt cessation of therapy after prolonged use at high dose rates can be life-threatening because of adrenal insufficiency.
6 Glucocorticoids should not be used in ruminants in the last third of pregnancy unless termination of pregnancy is desired or acceptable.
7 Specific therapy, when indicated, should not be overlooked.

References

Baird G. D. & Heitzman R. J. (1971) Anti-ketogenic action of glucocorticosteroids in the cow. In *The Application of Corticosteroids in Veterinary Medicine*. Glaxo Laboratories.

Beal W. E., Graves N. W., Dunn T. G. *et al* (1976) Induction of parturition with $PGF_{2\alpha}$ following dexamethasone. *J. Anim. Sci.* **42**, 1564.

Beardsley G. L., Muller L.D., Garverick H. A. *et al* (1976) Initiation of parturition in dairy cows with Dexamethasone. II Response to dexamethasone in combination with Estradiol benzoate. *J. Dairy Sci.* **59**, 241.

Becker M. J., Helland D. & Becker D. N. (1976) Serum cortisol (hydrocortisone), values in normal dogs as determined by radioimmunoassay. *Am. J. Vet. Res.* **37**, 1101.

Borkowski A. J., Levin S., Delcroix C. *et al* (1967) Blood cholesterol and hydrocortisone production in man: quantitative aspects of the utilisation of circulating cholesterol by the adrenals at rest and under adrenocorticotrophin stimulation. *J. Clin. Invest.* **46**, 797.

Bosc M. J., Feure J. & Fontaubert Y. U. de. (1975) A comparison of induction of parturition with dexamethasone or with an analog of prostaglandin $F_{2\alpha}$ (A–PGF) in cattle. *Theriogenology* **3**, 187.

Burns S. J. (1973) Clinical safety of dexamethasone in mares during pregnancy. *Equine Vet. J.* **5**, 91.

Christie B. M., Pierson R. E., Braddy P. M. *et al* (1977) Efficacy of corticosteroids as supportive therapy for bronchial pneumonia in yearling feedlot cattle. *Bovine Practit.* **12**, 115.

Colles C. M. (1979) Ischaemic necrosis of the navicular bone and the treatment. *Vet. Rec.* **104,** 133.

Colles C. M. & Jeffcott L. B. (1977) Laminitis in the horse. *Vet. Rec.* **100,** 262.

Emady M., Noakes D. E., Hadley J. C. *et al* (1974) Corticosteroid-induced lambing in the ewe. *Vet. Rec.* **95,** 281.

Feldman E. C., Ettinger S. J. E. & Peters G. (1977) Hypoadrenocorticism in a dog. *Mod. Vet. Prac.* **58,** 433.

Gallagher K. (1977) Use of corticosteroids in the equine. *Am. Assoc. Equine Practit.* Newsletter No 2.

Grunert E., Ahlers D. & Jochle W. (1975) Effects of a high dose of diethylstilboestrol on the delivery of the placenta after corticoid-induced parturition in cattle. *Theriogenology* **3,** 249.

Hankes G. M. (1976) Therapy of Shock: The corticosteroid question. *Vet. Clin. N. Am.* **6,** 277.

Harrison F. A. (1982) Dexamethasone-induced parturition in sheep. *Br. Vet. J.* **138,** 402.

Hatziolos B. C. & Shaw J. C. (1950) An approach to the problem of the aetiology of ketosis in dairy cows. *J. Dairy Sci.* **33,** 387.

Hoerlein A. B. & Jones D. L. (1977) Bovine immunoglubulins following induced parturition. *J. Am. Vet. Med. Assoc.* **170,** 325.

Jeffcott L. B. & Rossdale P. D. (1977) A critical review of current methods for induction of parturition in the mare. *Equine Vet. J.* **9,** 208.

Kirk M. D. (1974) Field diagnosis and treatment of secondary adrenocortical insufficiency in the horse. *Vet. Med.* **69,** 1383.

Kordts E. & Jöchle W. (1975) Induced parturition in dairy cattle: a comparison of a corticoid (flumethasone) and a prostaglandin ($PGF_{2\alpha}$) in different age groups. *Theriogenology* **3,** 171.

Langley O. H. & O'Farrel K. J. (1976) Immune status of dairy calves following induced parturition. *Vet. Rec.* **99,** 187.

Lucas J. M. S. & Notman A. (1974) The use of corticosteroids to synchronise parturition in sheep. *Br. Vet. J.* **130,** 1.

Makman M. H., Dvorkin B. & White A. (1971) Evidence for induction by cortisol in utero of a protein inhibitor of transport and phosphorylation in rat thymocytes. *Proc. Nat. Acad. Sci.* (USA) **68,** 1269.

McKay A. G. & Milne F. J. (1976) Observations on the intra-articular use of corticosteroids in the racing thoroughbred. *J. Am. Vet. Med. Assoc.* **168,** 1039.

Myles A. B. & Daly J. R. (1974) *Corticosteroid and ACTH treatment.* Edward Arnold, London.

Nijkamp F. P., Flower R. J., Moncada S. *et al* (1976) Partial purification of rabbit aorta contracting substance releasing factor and inhibition of its activity by anti-inflammatory steroids. *Nature* **263,** 479.

O'Farrel K. J. & Crowley J. P. (1974) Some observations on the use of two corticosteroid preparations for the induction of premature calving. *Vet. Rec.* **94,** 364.

Penning P. D. & Gibb M. J. (1977) The use of corticosteroid to synchronise parturition in sheep. *Vet. Rec.* **100,** 49.

Plenderleith R. W. J. (1974) Induction of parturition in heifers using betamethasone. *Vet. Rec.* **95,** 160.

Seal U. S. & Doe R. P. (1956) Vertebrate distribution of corticosteroid binding globulin and some endocrine effects on concentration. *Steroids* **5: 6,** 827.

Siegel E. T. (1965) Determination of 17-hydroxycorticosteroids in canine urine. *Am. J. Vet. Res.* **26,** 1152.

Tervit M. R. (1976) Techniques and hazards of embryo manipulation and induction of parturition. *N.Z. Vet. J.* **24,** 74.

Tomkins G. M. & Martin D. W. (1970) Hormones and gene expression. *Ann. Rev. Genet.* **4,** 911.

Tomkins G. M. & Gelehrter T. D. (1972) The present status of genetic regulation by hormones. In *Biochemical Actions of Hormones,* ed. G. Litwack, vol. 2. Academic Press, New York.

Van Pelt R. W. (1973a). Intra-articular injection of flumethasone suspension in normal joints in horses. *Equine Vet. J.* **5,** 162.

Van Pelt R. W. (1973b) Idiopathic tarsitis in post-parturient dairy cows: Clinico-pathological findings and treatment, *J. Am. Vet. Med. Assoc.* **162,** 284.

Van Pelt R. W. (1975) Intra-articular treatment of tarsal degenerative joint disease in cattle. *J. Am. Vet. Med. Assoc.* **166,** 239.

Weissman G. (1969) The effects of steroids and drugs on lysosymes. In *Lysosymes in Biology and Pathology,* eds J. T. Dingle and H. B. Fell, vol. 1. North Holland, Amsterdam.

Welch R. A. S., Crawford J. E. & Duganzich D. M. (1977) Induced parturition with corticosteroids: a comparison of four treatments. *N.Z. Vet. J.* **25,** 111.

Zolovich A., Upson D. W. & Eleftheriou B. E. (1966) Diurnal variation in plasma glucocorticosteroid levels in the horse. *J. Endocrin.* **35,** 249.

Further Reading

Gilman A. G., Goodman L. S. & Gilman A. (1980) *Goodman and Gilman's The Pharmacological Basis of Therapeutics,* 6th edn. Macmillan, New York.

Hankes G. M. (1976) Therapy of shock: The corticosteroid question. *Vet. Clinics N. Amer.* **6,** 277.

Myles A. B. & Daly J. R. (1974) *Corticosteroid and ACTH treatment.* Edward Arnold, London.

21

Chemical restraint of large animals

P. LEES & M.J. MEREDITH

Terminology and nomenclature

In this chapter the term 'chemical restraint' is used to refer to drugs, other than volatile or gaseous general anaesthetics, which have been used to restrain animals by their effect on the peripheral or central nervous systems. Eight classes of drug will be considered (Table 21.1). It will be seen that only one group, the peripherally-acting muscle relaxants, acts on the peripheral nervous system; all others act to depress (or sometimes to stimulate) some part of the CNS.

The first three groups of drugs are all classified as sedatives, two of these also are hypnotics. Some explanation is clearly called for. First, it should be noted that the classification is based on the *type* of action produced rather than the *mode* or *site* of action on the nervous system. Thus, agents in group 1 are the well known phenothiazine and butyrophenone ataractics. In human medicine, their principal use is as antipsychotic agents and the presence of a sedative action constitutes an undesirable side-effect. For veterinary use on the other hand, sedation is the action required to produce a calm, tractable animal and drugs are therefore selected which possess significant sedative properties. Compounds in group 2 are also sedatives but they differ in several ways from those in group 1. At high dose rates the sedative-anaesthetics produce loss of consciousness, relaxation of voluntary muscle, and (at the very least) a light plane of general anaesthesia. In contrast, the tranquilliser-sedatives do not produce general anaesthesia even at very high dose rates. Rather, in laboratory animals, high doses produce catalepsy— the state of waxy rigidity in which consciousness is retained while muscle tone is increased so that limbs will remain in unusual postures when so placed (the 'plastic limb' syndrome). In general, sedative-anaesthetic agents will blunt the arousal response to sensory stimulation. This will normally be sluggish and delayed in character, the patient quickly lapsing back into a sedated state. With tranquilliser-sedative drugs, however, animals may respond normally to sensory stimulation and a violent, exaggerated reaction involving increased excitability can even occur.

452

Table 21.1 Classification of agents used in chemical restraint.

Group	Examples	Features
1 Tranquilliser-sedative (ataractic)		Calming, quietening action
a. phenothiazines	acepromazine	
b. butyrophenones	azaperone	
2 Sedative-anaesthetic (classical sedative)	chloral hydrate xylazine diazepam	Calming, quietening action
3 Sedative-anaesthetic (injectable general anaesthetic)	thiopentone pentobarbitone metomidate saffan	General (non-selective) CNS depressants usually producing sedation and ataxia at low dose rates but almost invariably used at higher doses to give a light plane of general anaesthesia
4 Dissociative anaesthetic	ketamine tiletamine phencyclidine	Loss of consciousness, analgesia, commonly maintain or increase voluntary muscle tone, retention of many reflexes
5 Peripheral, non-competitive muscle relaxant (depolarising neuromuscular blocker)	suxamethonium	Voluntary muscle paralysis caused by maintained depolarisation of motor end plate receptors on skeletal muscle
6 Central muscle relaxant	glyceryl guaicolate	Voluntary muscle paralysis caused by blockade of spinal interneurones
7 Narcotic-analgesic (sedative-analgesic)	morphine fentanyl etorphine	Analgesia (elevation of pain threshold) mediated by action on central opiate receptors; sedation in some species
8 Neuroleptanalgesic	etorphine + acepromazine	State of altered CNS activity in which animal is immobilised by actions of a narcotic-analgesic and tranquilliser-sedative; major species' differences in actions

There are two further distinctions that can be made between sedative compounds in groups 1 and 2. First, the consistency with which a satisfactory sedative response is obtained is generally high with the latter group, whereas compounds in group 1 may produce a response ranging from no observable effect to deep sedation: they are thus less predictable in their actions. Secondly, the lack of significant respiratory depressant actions of phenothiazine and butyrophenone tranquillisers probably explains why they possess a higher therapeutic index than most sedative-anaesthetics in laboratory animal tests. Their sparing effect on respiration probably accounts also for the wide safety margin that is generally ascribed in clinical use to phenothiazines and butyrophenones.

The reason for subdividing sedative-anaesthetic agents into two groups is more straightforward: group 2 compounds are usually used at subhypnotic dose rates (i.e. as sedatives), while those in group 3 are normally given in sufficient amounts to produce light surgical anaesthesia, both as single and repeat doses for induction and maintenance, respectively. A further group of injectable anaesthetics, the dissociative agents (group 4), are administered in amounts sufficient to permit minor surgical operations to be performed. To the clinician, a separate grouping for these drugs might therefore seem unnecessary, but to the pharmacologist the differences between agents in groups 3 and 4 are considerable, involving both central and peripheral effects (*see* p. 472).

When the degree of restraint required by the clinician involves complete immobilisation of an animal, this can be achieved either by anaesthetic doses of agents in groups 2–4 or, more selectively, by compounds which act peripherally (group 5) or centrally (group 6) to produce paralysis of skeletal muscle.

Drugs in group 7, the narcotic-analgesics, are being used increasingly for the chemical restraint of farm animals. However, there are species variations in response to these drugs. The overall effect is sedative in some animals (man, monkey, dog, rabbit, rat and bird), while in others (horse, cow, pig and sheep) it is less predictable and may involve a weak sedative effect or even an excitatory reaction.

Finally, the last 15 years has seen the introduction of drug combinations comprising a narcotic-analgesic together with a tranquilliser-sedative (neuroleptic) agent from group 1. This explains the cumbersome term, neuroleptanalgesia, which is used to describe the effects of these drug mixtures. Neuroleptanalgesia is sometimes referred to as a form of anaesthesia which, in our opinion, it is not. It may be more appropriate to regard it as a state equivalent (but not equal) to a light plane of anaesthesia, although even this definition is a gross oversimplification. Because of the species differences in the actions of analgesic drugs, the state of neuroleptanalgesia in the horse, for example, is very different from neuroleptanalgesia in the dog.

1   Tranquilliser-sedatives

Phenothiazines

General pharmacology

The general pharmacology of phenothiazines has been adequately described in standard texts. For present purposes it is sufficient to note that phenothiazines exert many side-effects, the intensity of which varies from compound to compound. Actions of phenothiazines include antihistamine, anti-5HT, ganglion blocking, α-adrenoceptor blocking, atropine-like, quinidine-like and spasmolytic effects. In addition, they produce hypothermia by their central and peripheral effects and they possess anti-pruritic, anti-inflammatory and local anaesthetic properties.

All phenothiazines are hypotensive (an action which is probably caused principally by their α-adrenoceptor blocking property) and all are therefore potentially toxic in hypovolaemic animals. They are also all subject (in all species) to considerable variation in sedative effect. This disadvantage cannot be entirely overcome by increasing the dose rate, because the sedative action is not closely related to the dose administered. However, side-effects are appreciably more pronounced with increasing dosage. In addition, high dose rates can further increase the long duration of action, while very high dose rates can induce either profound depression or excitement.

Acepromazine is one of the most potent phenothiazines and can therefore conveniently be given in small volumes to large animals. It appears to be associated with fewer problems in clinical use than other phenothiazines and has been accepted as the phenothiazine of choice for large animal species.

Applied pharmacology

Horse. For chlorpromazine, dose rates of up to 2.5 mg/kg have been recommended, but it is probably advisable to restrict dosage to 0.4 mg/kg. Larger doses may induce a panic-like reaction (Owen & Neal 1957) which is not due to the drug's hypotensive action (Hall 1960) but may be related to muscle weakness or to some unknown central action. It has been suggested that absorption of intramuscular injections of chlorpromazine may be irregular (Hall 1971), which is an additional reason why chlorpromazine is now used infrequently in horses. Other phenothiazines also tend to be unpredictable in their sedative actions and are capable of causing panic in a minority of horses.

At recommended dose rates the onset of action of most phenothiazines is slow (30–60 minutes after intramuscular injection). However, acepromazine is exceptional in that absorption is more rapid and onset of sedation is quicker (15–30 minutes). For all these drugs, the duration of action is in the region of 4–6 hours, although slight residual effects can last for 24 hours. Characteristic features of phenothiazine-induced sedation in the horse are the adoption of a quiet, standing posture, with head drooping, partial ptosis and disinterest in the surroundings.

A common side-effect of phenothiazines in the horse is a partial or complete prolapse of the penis, commencing at the onset of sedation. Retraction of the penis into the prepuce often commences during the later stages of sedation and is usually complete by the time that sedation is no longer apparent. Occasionally, however, prolapse of the penis persists, leading to permanent paralysis (Wheat 1966, Bolz 1970). The cause of this reaction is not known.

A related, but possibly distinct, phenomenon has been reported by Pearson & Weaver (1978). Two horses premedicated with acepromazine prior to induction of anaesthesia with thiopentone, and five horses given a neuroleptanalgesia combination (etorphine with acepromazine) developed priapism (persistent penile engorgement and turgidity simulating an erection) and were unable to withdraw the penis into the prepuce (paraphimosis). In most cases, amputation of the organ became necessary because of soiling and trauma to the integument. Lucke & Sansom (1979) recommended that drug-induced priapism is treated by anaesthetising the horse and applying manual compression from the glans to force blood out of the penis until it can be reduced back into the prepuce.

Several groups of investigators have described the cardiovascular effects of phenothiazine tranquillisers in the horse. Kerr *et al* (1972b) reported a mild tachycardia and a moderate hypotension in response to a dose rate of 0.066 mg/kg of acepromazine intravenously. Experiments in our laboratory have confirmed and extended these findings (Hillidge & Lees, unpublished data). We have demonstrated that the hypotension produced by doses of 0.1 mg/kg acepromazine, administered intravenously, was initially due entirely to a decrease in total peripheral resistance. However, by 15 minutes, cardiac output was also reduced and subsequently made an increasing contribution to the hypotension, while the effect of decreased peripheral resistance declined.

Occasionally there is collapse, followed by rapid recovery, when phenothiazines are given by rapid intravenous injection. This may be due to the suppression of myocardial conductivity caused by exposure of the heart to a high drug concentration. The effects of the negative dromotropic action of phenothiazines can be avoided if the injection is administered slowly over at least 30 seconds.

Phenothiazines reduce packed cell volume and haemoglobin concentration (Martin & Beck 1956, de Moor & van den Hende 1968). These effects are probably caused by increased splenic storage of erythrocytes. Muir & Hamlin (1975) have studied the respiratory effects of acepromazine (0.065 mg/kg intravenously) and found that the principal change was a decrease in respiratory rate; however, this was compensated for by an increase in tidal volume, so that minute volume was little changed. Using a somewhat higher dose rate of acepromazine (0.1 mg/kg intravenously), we have recorded slight respiratory depression (Hillidge & Lees, unpublished data), as indicated by decreased arterial oxygen tension.

Pig. Recommended intramuscular dose rates usually provide sufficient sedation to allow intravenous injection of an anaesthetic some 30–60 minutes later, but, as Vaughan (1961) points out, sedation is always inadequate in a proportion of subjects. Phenothiazines give a more consistent effect when administered intravenously, but the injection should be made slowly to minimise the risk of cardiac arrhythmias. With chlorpromazine, very dilute solutions should be used to avoid the risk of thrombosis (Hall 1971).

We have investigated the clinical pharmacology of acepromazine in six Göttingen miniature pigs and one Large White pig (Lees & Meredith, unpublished data). A dose rate of 0.1 mg/kg intramuscularly gave good sedation, reduced rectal temperature by 1°C, increased heart rate by up to 50 beats/minute (for no more than 30 minutes), and reduced mean arterial pressure by as much as 40 mmHg. The hypotension was more persistent than the tachycardia. Packed cell volume was not significantly affected and respiratory function was also unchanged.

Cattle. Phenothiazines can provide a limited but useful degree of restraint when, for example, operations are to be performed under local anaesthesia. On the other hand, they are not recommended for premedication because they are unnecessary (recovery excitement from anaesthesia is unusual) and infact undesirable (their action in prolonging anaesthesia increases the risk of anaesthetic complications). Moreover, Jones (1972) has suggested that phenothiazines may increase the incidence of regurgitation of rumen contents. Maximum sedation is achieved after 30–60 minutes and is maintained for 4–6 hours, with slight residual actions persisting for up to 24 hours.

According to Jones (1972), the administration of phenothiazines to cattle by the intravenous route is contraindicated, because a number of deaths have occurred. This author also comments on the variable nature of the response when phenothiazines are administered intravenously to cattle.

Azaperone

General pharmacology

Azaperone is the only tranquilliser-sedative of the butyrophenone group which has been used extensively in large animals. Laboratory animal studies indicate that azaperone possesses a pronounced sedative action and a wide safety margin with relatively few side-effects. The cardiovascular effects of the drug seem to derive principally from its α-adrenoceptor blocking action, which has been demonstrated both *in vivo* and *in vitro* (Hapke & Prigge 1972).

In large animals azaperone is used to produce tranquillisation or, at higher dose rates, sedation and it can also be used in conjunction with the hypnotic, metomidate, to produce general anaesthesia.

Applied pharmacology

Pig. After intramuscular administration, the first signs of sedation are observed at 3–10 minutes. Peak effects occur after approximately 15 minutes in young pigs, and after 30 minutes in adults. The duration of action increases with dose and ranges from 1 to 6 hours (Marsboom & Symoens 1968). At low dose rates (0.4–1.0 mg/kg) there is a tranquillising or slight sedative effect: the pig is somewhat indifferent to its environment, but can be driven without difficulty. With doses of 2 mg/kg or more, the pig is deeply sedated and adopts a position of sternal recumbency for approximately two hours. Doses of 8 mg/kg produce immobilisation in lateral recumbency, but recovery is prolonged.

Sensory stimulation should be avoided while azaperone is taking effect. Even in the absence of overt stimulation, some individuals pass through a restless phase at 5–10 minutes after intramuscular administration but, if pigs are disturbed at this time, there may be loss of sedative effect and/or a period of violent excitable behaviour.

The effects of azaperone on the cardiovascular and respiratory systems have been studied by Clarke (1969). Blood pressure was reduced to between 70 and 84% of control values. Clarke also observed a heavy breathing pattern in sedated pigs and the impression that respiration was stimulated was confirmed by decreases in arterial carbon dioxide tensions. The cause of respiratory stimulation has not been determined but it may be related to the hypotensive action of the drug, since carotid and aortic chemoreceptors are known to increase their firing rates when arterial pressure falls.

Recently attention has been drawn to the possibility of injury to the penis when azaperone is used on young entire male pigs (Darnley 1980). A proportion of such pigs developed protrusion of the penis and in some cases this led to traumatic injury. To avoid the risk of penile injury, it is now recommended that entire male pigs should not be given doses in excess of 1 mg/kg.

Horse. Roztočil *et al* (1971b) obtained a reliable sedative effect in horses from 1 mg/kg azaperone administered intramuscularly. Serrano & Lees (1976) also achieved an excellent and consistent sedative action with intramuscular doses of 0.8 mg/kg. The level of sedation was greater than that achieved with acepromazine (0.1 mg/kg intramuscularly) but the onset of action was quicker and the duration of action was shorter (approximately four hours for azaperone). Arterial oxygen and carbon dioxide tensions were unchanged but heart rate was increased slightly for up to 60 minutes and a moderate degree of hypotension occurred for at least four hours (Lees & Serrano 1976). Other side-effects include sweating, muscle weakness and tremor, prolapse of the penis, and a small decrease in body temperature — but these were believed to be relatively unimportant. However, in view of the deep sedation induced by azaperone, caution is required when using it as a premedicant. It is necessary to reduce the induction doses of agents such as thiopentone and methohexitone, otherwise prolonged apnoea may result (Hillidge *et al* 1977).

MacKenzie & Snow (1977) also evaluated azaperone (0.7 mg/kg) in the horse and concluded that, at the dose rates used, it was more effective than acepromazine (0.5 mg/kg) and xylazine (2.0 mg/kg) in minimising responses to mildly stressful procedures. Unfortunately, the intravenous use of azaperone is contraindicated in the horse since several groups of investigators have described excitatory and ataxic reactions.

2/3   Sedative-anaesthetics

Chloral hydrate

General pharmacology

At low dose rates chloral hydrate produces sedation, at moderate dose rates it produces basal narcosis, and at high dose rates it produces general anaesthesia. As one would expect from a drug which has been in use for such a long period, it has a wide safety margin in animals when used under clinical conditions. This probably does not reflect a low toxicity of chloral hydrate *per se,* but is more likely attributable to the technique of administration.

Although it is readily soluble in water it has a low potency and solutions are irritant. Hence, a large volume of dilute solution has to be given and administration will inevitably be slow. If the intravenous infusion is stopped when sufficient drug has been given to induce recumbency, then overdosing is easily avoided. The advantages of chloral hydrate as a sedative or general anaesthetic are said to include consistency of response, absence of excitement during induction or recovery in most animals, and absence of post-anaesthetic malaise (Hall 1971).

In spite of its safety in clinical use in large animals, chloral hydrate has been largely superseded by other sedatives, basal narcotics or anaesthetic agents. The large volumes of solution that have to be handled are very inconvenient, the solution must be prepared freshly before use, and the slow induction of anaesthesia can lead to practical difficulties. A further disadvantage of chloral hydrate lies in the nature of the recovery phase: when anaesthetic doses have been given this may be relatively prolonged ($1\frac{1}{2}$–2 hours) and may be accompanied by involuntary excitement, especially in the horse. Finally, chloral hydrate resembles the barbiturates in lacking significant analgesic activity at subanaesthetic dose rates.

Chloral hydrate is an example of a pro-drug, i.e. it is converted in the body to another compound (in this case trichloroethanol) which accounts for most of the pharmacological activity.

$$CCl_3CH(OH)_2 \rightarrow CCl_3.\ CH_2OH \rightarrow CCl_3.\ CH_2OH\text{–glucuronide}$$

Chloral hydrate,   trichloroethanol,   urochloralic acid

Trichloroethanol is conjugated by liver microsomal enzymes with glucuronic acid. The glucuronide (also known as urochloralic acid) is polar and hence readily excreted in the urine. Some is also excreted in bile.

Applied pharmacology

Horse. Hall (1971) considers that chloral hydrate is still the best basal narcotic for the horse. The intravenous doses recommended for producing medium and deep narcosis are 80–100, and 100–120 mg/kg, respectively. Narcosis of medium depth implies a very heavy degree of sedation since horses normally become recumbent with a dose of 80–100 mg/kg. The anaesthetic dose is 130–140 mg/kg. When medium depth narcosis has been induced, recovery to the standing position takes 30–45 minutes, while, with deep narcosis, it is usually 60 minutes or so before the animal stands. Recovery may take two hours when anaesthetic doses have been given.

Gabel *et al* (1964) have studied the cardiovascular effects on horses of an intravenous sedative dose (37 mg/kg) of chloral hydrate. At this dose rate (which is less than half the amount recommended by Hall for medium narcosis) blood pressure and cardiac output were not significantly altered while heart rate was increased by 5–15 beats per minute.

Cattle. Chloral hydrate may be administered orally or intravenously, but it has now been superseded to a large extent by xylazine.

Pigs. Dose rates for administration by intravenous or intraperitoneal injection or by stomach tube have been described by Hall (1971).

Xylazine

General pharmacology

The sedative-anaesthetic agent xylazine has been used in veterinary medicine for more than ten years. It is an organic base, of simple structure, which is administered as an aqueous solution of the hydrochloride salt.

Xylazine is used extensively in cattle and is now generally regarded as the sedative of choice for this species. It is also used in goats and sheep and to some extent in horses. The dose rate for horses is between 10 and 20 times higher than that for cattle, so that it is a relatively expensive agent for the horse. In the pig, for some reason dose rates 20–40 times greater than those for cattle produce virtually no effect (Sagner *et al* 1969) so xylazine is not used in this species.

General advantages of xylazine include the possibility of either intramuscular or intravenous administration, and the small volume of solution required for ruminants. According to most authors there is no marked irritation when the intramuscular route is used and, in contrast to phenothiazine tranquillisers, xylazine does not seem to cause any manifestation of excitability either during onset of action or recovery. The type of sedation induced by xylazine has been said to resemble that produced by chloral hydrate rather than that of the phenothiazines. In addition to its sedative action, a number of reports ascribe analgesic and muscle relaxant properties to xylazine (Hoffman 1974, Sagner *et al* 1968, 1969). However, some authors deny that significant analgesia is attained at the usual dose rates (Bollwahn *et al* 1970, Clarke & Hall 1969).

Xylazine does not possess any major side-effects, although animals may be very sensitive to noise during recovery, some sweating may occur and a number of cardiovascular effects have been reported. Xylazine is contra-indicated in the last month of pregnancy (except at the time of parturition) because it stimulates uterine contractions and this may lead to premature delivery, at least in cattle.

Applied pharmacology

Cattle. An early report on xylazine in cattle recommended the use of 0.05–0.20 mg/kg by intravenous or intramuscular injection (Clarke & Hall 1969). These dose rates produced effects ranging from sedation, through 'chloral hydrate-type' narcosis, to complete anaesthesia. However, other workers claim that true anaesthesia is never achieved, even with high dose rates (Sagner *et al* 1969). In the study of Clarke & Hall (1969) analgesia was present only in the most deeply sedated animals, so that supplementation with a general or local anaesthetic was required for surgery. Initial effects of xylazine are usually apparent within five minutes of intramuscular administration and the maximum response occurs after approximately 15 minutes. When doses of 0.20 mg/kg or greater are used, a residual drowsiness may persist for several hours.

Side-effects of xylazine in cattle are relatively few. Mitchell (1972) has noted that loss of rumen tone commonly leads to tympany. Such distension can occur in both standing and sternally recumbent animals and is prevented by passing a needle through the abdominal wall into the rumen. Hall (1971) advises keeping a close watch on cattle recovering from the effects of xylazine, since animals which have stood and seem to be fully conscious can relapse to a posture of lateral recumbency and become tympanitic. He recommends disturbing the animal so that eructation occurs.

Low doses of xylazine do not markedly depress respiration, but accidental overdosage may cause respiratory failure. The cardiovascular effects of xylazine (0.35 mg/kg) in cattle were said to include a temporary decrease of 15–20% in mean arterial pressure and either a slight reduction or no change in heart rate (Sagner *et al* 1969). On the other hand, using doses of 0.05–0.1 mg/kg, Fess (1970) noted decreases in heart rate of 30–40%.

As noted above, one complication is an increased tendency for premature births to occur when xylazine is given after the 270th day of gestation. This was noted in six of 14 animals and all calves survived (Ahlers *et al* 1969). Xylazine has an ecbolic action throughout pregnancy but it does not produce complications in the first eight months, although it can make diagnosis of early gestation more difficult.

Sheep and goat. Green (1979) and Straub (1971) recommend xylazine as the sedative of choice for sheep. A dose rate of 1 mg/kg intramuscularly produces deep sedation within 10–15 minutes, which is maintained for a further 30 minutes. It has also been used intravenously by Green (1979) at a lower dose rate (0.05 mg/kg) in combination with the dissociative agent, ketamine. The same author encountered marked cardiac arrhythmias when doses of 0.05 mg/kg xylazine were given intramuscularly to goats, and recommended that this dose rate should never be exceeded in this species.

Horse. Xylazine doses of 0.5–1.1 mg/kg intravenously or 1–2 mg/kg intramuscularly are commonly recommended for the horse, although Clarke & Hall (1969) recommended 2–3 mg/kg intramuscularly. Some care may be required when the drug is given intravenously, since Clarke & Hall (1969) produced collapse and death in a 54 kg pony which received 150 mg xylazine (i.e. approximately three times the recommended maximum dose). The manufacturers now recommend that a maximum of 1 mg/kg should be given intravenously over a period of 1–2 minutes.

Xylazine has a rapid onset of action: 1–3 minutes after intravenous and approximately 5 minutes after intramuscular injection. Maximum effects are obtained at 15–20 minutes after administration and sedation persists up to 30–60 minutes after intravenous, or up to 120 minutes after intramuscular injection. The general characteristics of xylazine sedation in the horse include apparent indifference to the surroundings, lowering of the head, drooping of the lower lip and eyelids, and slight prolapse of the penis. In contrast to phenothiazine tranquillisers, however, xylazine does not seem to produce paraphimosis or priapism (McCashin & Gabel 1971). In most horses xylazine produces sweating around the ears and poll region. Other reported side-effects of xylazine have mainly concerned cardiovascular function. Arterial blood pressure rises immediately, but transiently, following intravenous injection, while heart rate decreases and, in some animals, sinoatrial block or second degree atrioventricular block occurs (Clarke & Hall 1969, Garner *et al* 1971, Kerr *et al* 1972a). These effects on the heart are probably attributable to a reflex increase in vagal tone, because they usually occur only whilst arterial pressure is raised and can be prevented by premedication with atropine (Kerr *et al* 1972a, 1972b).

In the study of Clarke & Hall (1969), intramuscular injections of 3 mg/kg xylazine increased blood pressure in one horse and reduced it in two others, while heart rate remained within normal limits. Kerr *et al* (1972b) also recorded a moderate degree of hypotension and a slight degree of bradycardia in response to 2.2 mg/kg. In contrast, McCashin & Gabel (1975) failed to detect any change in blood pressure but they did record cardiac arrhythmias (second degree AV block or SA block) in 5 of 12 horses within 1–3 minutes of administering 2 mg/kg xylazine intramuscularly.

Barbiturates

General pharmacology

The barbiturate anaesthetics have been available for more than 40 years and several (thiopentone, thiamylal, thialbarbitone, pentobarbitone and methohexitone) are still used extensively for inducing light-to-medium planes of surgical anaesthesia in large animals.

In standard pharmacological texts, barbiturates are classified, according to duration of action, as long-acting (phenobarbitone), intermediate-acting (pentobarbitone) and short- or ultra-short-acting (thiopentone, thiamylal, thialbarbitone, methohexitone). This classification is valid for man and for most small animals but, in many farm animal species, pentobarbitone has only a short duration of action due to its more rapid metabolism by the mixed function oxidase enzyme system of farm animals.

As the salts of weak acids (pKa = approx. 7.5), the sodium salts are alkaline in solution (pH 9–11) and, to varying degrees, irritant to tissues when injected perivascularly. This is particularly true of thiobarbiturates when used in the high concentrations generally recommended to minimise the administration volume for large animals. Tissue necrosis usually follows perivascular injection of thiobarbiturates, although the severity of the reaction can be minimised by infiltration of the area with normal saline, 1% lignocaine hydrochloride and/or hyaluronidase.

Aqueous solutions of the sodium salts of barbiturates are physically incompatible with acidic solutions: the barbiturate will be precipitated. Solutions should not, therefore, be mixed in the syringe with atropine, D-tubocurarine, suxamethonium, phenothiazine, tranquillisers, analgesics or adrenaline.

The pharmacological effects of barbiturates have been documented extensively, so only the essential details will be summarised here. As anaesthetics, all barbiturates are said to be poor analgesics and weak muscle relaxants. Good analgesia and relaxation therefore require the production of dangerously deep levels of anaesthesia with severe respiratory depression and some cardiovascular depression. However, barbiturates are still used extensively alone at lower dose rates for minor surgery and, in combination with other agents, for major surgery. Anaesthetic doses of barbiturates generally depress the rate and depth of breathing in direct proportion to the depth of anaesthesia. With overdosage, the usual cause of death is a failure of central respiratory control mechanisms.

Barbiturates also exert a number of depressant effects on the cardiovascular system although, in cases of acute overdosage, the heart usually continues to beat for up to 5 minutes after the onset of apnoea. This provides a reasonable period in which to commence resuscitation. Respiratory depression is therefore more significant than cardiovascular depression.

The safety margin of barbiturates, as indicated by measurements of therapeutic index in rats and mice, is in the region of 4–8, which is low in comparison with some of the newer injectable anaesthetics such as saffan, metomidate and ketamine. The clinical significance of a low therapeutic index may be slight in healthy, normovolaemic animals. However, in poor-risk patients, hypovolaemic animals and those with cardiovascular disease, barbiturates must be used with great care. This applies also to animals in states of existing or incipient shock where the administered dose and the rate of injection must be reduced.

Although all barbiturates exert similar actions on the body, there are major differences in their distribution, metabolism, and duration of effect. These differences are, in part, attributable to differences in their lipid solubility. Thiopentone and methohexitone cross the blood–brain barrier quickly and attain effective concentrations in the time taken for one 'vein to brain' circulation; with pentobarbitone, peak levels in the CNS are achieved more slowly, while for barbitone and phenobarbitone, they are attained so very slowly that these drugs have no clinical value as anaesthetic agents. Thiopentone and methohexitone can be used in the 'bolus injection' technique to produce a period of anaesthesia which is rapid in onset and of short duration. The success of this technique depends not only on high lipid solubility of the drugs but also on the physiological fact that distribution of blood from the left ventricle is disproportionately high to several organs, including the brain. As the circulating concentration decreases, these drugs are able to leave the CNS with the same ease that they entered, so the anaesthesia only lasts for a few minutes. Re-distribution away from the brain is therefore the major factor which terminates anaesthesia with short-acting barbiturates.

The factors determining the next phase of the recovery period differ for oxybarbiturates and thiobarbiturates (compounds containing a sulphur atom). The latter drugs are metabolised slowly by the liver (approx. 15% of the administered dose per hour, for thiopentone) but the fall in plasma level is also due to uptake, initially by muscle and later by adipose tissue. However, for oxybarbiturates, biotransformation is much more significant.

Barbiturates are readily absorbed from the gastrointestinal tract and from the peritoneal cavity. However, administration by these routes does not give a predictable anaesthetic effect. The route of choice for achieving rapid effect, quick recovery and predictable level of anaesthesia is the intravenous one. In large animals, barbiturates which cross the blood–brain barrier rapidly (thiobarbiturates and methohexitone) are usually given by the bolus injection technique to achieve a rapid, smooth induction. Induction is usually followed by a period of apnoea of up to 90 seconds, after which normal respiration is resumed as the CNS concentration falls. With these drugs, large animals can be cast efficiently and humanely and minor surgery can be undertaken or anaesthesia can be maintained by another (usually volatile) agent. Pentobarbitone, because of its slower penetration of the blood–brain barrier, is not used in this way in horses and adult cattle, but it is still administered frequently to other farm animals by slow intravenous injection, either 'to effect' or as a calculated dose.

Applied pharmacology

Horse. With thiobarbiturates the induction of anaesthesia is usually smooth and the horse falls within 40 seconds. Occasionally, induction excitement may occur in which the horse rears and falls awkwardly to lie in lateral recumbency making violent paddling movements. To prevent this reaction a small dose of suxamethonium (0.15 mg/kg) may be given intravenously immediately after the barbiturate. During recovery from barbiturate anaesthesia, excitement is common and sometimes extreme (Grono 1966, Ford 1951). However, this can be largely controlled by premedicating with a sedative drug (such as acepromazine or xylazine) and by minimising sensory stimulation.

The period of induction apnoea with thiopentone averaged 39 seconds in one study (Tavernor & Lees 1970) and rarely exceeds 90 seconds. It is usually preceded by one or two deep breaths and clinical problems from respiratory embarrassment are uncommon. With thiopentone the period of surgical anaesthesia is brief (3–5 minutes) and the horses are generally well coordinated after one hour, although slight residual depression can persist for up to 24 hours. Tyagi *et al* (1964) have studied the clinical pharmacology of dose rates of 9–17 mg/kg thiopentone in horses. They detected hyperglycaemia, leucopenia, decreased cardiac output and tachycardia, but there was little change in arterial pressure. Tavernor & Lees (1970), using 10 mg/kg, also reported moderate, transient tachycardia and absence of electrocardiographic changes (except for transient reversal of the T wave).

Pig. For pigs it is usually recommended that barbiturates should be given intravenously 'to effect', e.g. half of the calculated dose of thiopentone should be injected rapidly to induce a light plane of anaesthesia, and the remainder administered slowly to effect (Booth 1977).

Pentobarbitone is believed to provide safe and effective anaesthesia for pigs weighing less than 50 kg but, in larger animals, it has a poor reputation for safety and should be administered slowly. Recommended doses are 24 mg/kg for pigs up to 100 kg, and up to 20 mg/kg for larger pigs (Booth 1977). Hall (1971) proposed a higher dose rate of 30 mg/kg for pigs weighing up to 50 kg and warned that lower dose rates would be required for larger pigs and greater variations in susceptibility would be encountered.

The cardiovascular and respiratory effects of pentobarbitone (20 mg/kg intravenously) on miniature pigs premedicated with azaperone (2 mg/kg intramuscularly) have been investigated in our laboratory (Lees & Meredith, unpublished data). Packed cell volume was decreased and an initial mild tachycardia was followed by a slight decrease in heart rate. Respiratory depression and hypotension occurred and in some animals these effects were profound.

Cattle. Thiopentone (10 mg/kg in a 10% solution by rapid intravenous injection) gives rapid and satisfactory anaesthesia of 3–4 minutes' duration. The hazards of tympany, regurgitation and inhalation of rumen contents which can occur are common to most injectable anaesthetics. The problems of perivascular and intracarotid injection are similar to those arising with thiopentone in the horse. In contrast to the horse, however, emergence excitement is not a problem, so premedication with a phenothiazine sedative is not necessary and is in fact contraindicated because it prolongs anaesthesia and increases the risk of tympany.

Calves less than two weeks' old should not be anaesthetised with thiopentone because the period of anaesthesia is likely to be prolonged. High dose rates of thiopentone (15–22 mg/kg) have been recommended (by dosing 'to effect' over five minutes) for calves over this age (Booth 1977). Light surgical anaesthesia is said to last for 10–12 minutes with full recovery within two hours.

Methohexitone has been found to be a satisfactory anaesthetic for adult cattle when up to 2.5 g was given slowly 'to effect', however the effect of rapid injections was unpredictable (Hall 1971). The dose rate of methohexitone for young calves is 1 mg/kg (Tavernor, Pers. Commun.).

Though rarely used as a general anaesthetic for adult cattle, small doses of pentobarbitone (2–6 mg/kg intravenously) may be used to produce sedation or to prolong chloral hydrate basal narcosis. In calves, the dose range producing surgical anaesthesia is 20–29 mg/kg but the drug is contraindicated in animals less than one month of age, because narcosis can persist for more than two days (Hall 1971).

Sheep. Both thiopentone and thialbarbitone provide a rapid, smooth induction and an excitement-free recovery. The recovery is more rapid after thialbarbitone. Methohexitone also produces anaesthesia of short duration in sheep. Pentobarbitone has a short duration of action as well and Harrison (1964) has recommended an average dose rate of 24 mg/kg (range 11–54 mg/kg) administered slowly 'to effect'. The short half-life of pentobarbitone in sheep (67 minutes) has been attributed to rapid metabolism of polar metabolites, such as hydroxypentobarbitone, which are mainly excreted in the urine (Dos Santos & Bogan 1974).

Experimental investigations by Waterman & Livingston (1978a, 1978b) demonstrated that, in sheep, 20 mg/kg of pentobarbitone reduced arterial oxygen tension to less than 60 mmHg for approximately 8 minutes. Even at a dose level of 10 mg/kg there was a marked, though transient, fall in arterial blood pressure and a prolonged decrease in cerebral blood flow.

Metomidate

General pharmacology

Metomidate (formerly known as metoxymol) is a weak organic base of simple structure based on imidazole. It is used as the hydrochloride salt, which dissolves readily in water. An outstanding property of metomidate, which distinguishes it from almost all other induction agents, is its relative freedom from depressant effects on respiration and cardiovascular function. Clinical dose rates of metomidate produce little or no change in blood pressure, cardiac output or arterial tensions of oxygen and carbon dioxide. This probably explains the high therapeutic index of the drug in laboratory animals and its wide safety margin in clinical use. Metomidate does, however, possess a number of potential disadvantages. First, a muscle tremor or spasm and involuntary limb movements are relatively common during recovery from anaesthesia, even when animals have been premedicated with tranquilliser-sedatives such as azaperone. Secondly, aqueous solutions of metomidate hydrochloride are highly acidic and very irritant. If injected perivascularly, tissue necrosis may occur (Meredith & Lees 1979). Thirdly, a slight degree of intravascular haemolysis occurs when metomidate is administered intravenously (Allsup *et al* 1973).

Applied pharmacology

Pig. When metomidate is used alone, analgesia is poor and there can be problems from spontaneous movements during anaesthesia or excitement during recovery. However, premedication with azaperone results in a state of anaesthesia of approximately 30 minutes duration, which is characterised by excellent analgesia and muscle relaxation.

The manufacturers' recommended dose rate and route of administration vary with the size of the animal and the reason for anaesthesia. They recommend that pigs weighing less than 50 kg are premedicated with azaperone intramuscularly (2 mg/kg) then given metomidate intra-peritoneally (9 mg/kg) either immediately after the azaperone or 10–15 minutes later. For pigs heavier than 50 kg, the recommendation is intra-muscular premedication with azaperone (2 mg/kg) followed by intravenous administration of metomidate (4 mg/kg), 15–20 minutes later.

After intravenous administration of metomidate, induction is very rapid (less than 30 seconds), while intraperitoneal injections produce loss of consciousness within 3–4 minutes. Recovery is slower with the intraperitoneal route, although in both cases pigs normally regain consciousness after 60 minutes and are capable of standing within 2–3 hours.

There are some doubts about the efficacy of metomidate when it is administered intraperitoneally. For example, anaesthesia was said to be poor in all animals receiving 10 mg/kg metomidate and in 10% of pigs receiving 15 mg/kg or more (Dimigen & Reetz 1970). Failure to induce anaesthesia occurred in 9% of cases according to Callear & van Gestel (1973), while Cox (1973) reported a somewhat higher failure rate and noted that analgesia was inadequate for all but minor surgical interferences. Studies in our laboratory (Meredith & Lees 1979) have drawn attention to the difficulty of ensuring that supposedly intraperitoneal injections do in fact enter the peritoneal cavity. When metomidate solution was inadvertently administered retroperitoneally, or into the intestinal lumen, there was no anaesthetic effect.

In contrast to these difficulties, there are several clinical reports which indicate that intravenous metomidate gives a smooth induction and it is probably the agent of choice for intravenous anaesthesia of pigs (Dimigen 1972, Callear & van Gestel 1973, Roztočil *et al* 1971a). The principal side-effects with the intravenous route seem to be: peripheral vasoconstriction, slight haemolysis, and tissue necrosis if the drug is injected perivascularly. Rapid intravenous injection of metomidate can produce transient apnoea but respiratory function is subsequently well maintained. Respiratory rate is usually decreased but the depth may be increased and consequently there is little change in arterial blood tensions of oxygen and carbon dioxide (Orr *et al* 1976). Orr *et al* have also reported moderate decreases in heart rate, arterial blood pressure and cardiac output. Experience in our laboratory confirms these findings, although we have noted a small degree of respiratory depression in the first few minutes after induction: the mean decrease in arterial oxygen tension was 17 mmHg.

Horse. Rapid and smooth induction of anaesthesia is obtained when metomidate is administered intravenously (3.0–3.5 mg/kg) to horses which have been premedicated with azaperone (Hillidge & Lees 1971a, Roztočil *et al* 1972a). The premedication dose used by these authors was 0.2 mg/kg intravenously, and there was some muscle tremor, spasm and movement. However, these effects were greatly reduced when the dose was 0.5 mg/kg intravenously or 0.8 mg/kg intramuscularly, although recovery was more protracted (Hillidge *et al* 1973). Varying degrees of excitement occurred during the recovery period and it was concluded that the use of metomidate

should preferably be restricted to induction of anaesthesia prior to maintenance with halothane. Metomidate is probably unsuitable for use in
thoroughbreds and other large breeds because of the high incidence of
excitatory phenomena (Marsboom, Pers. Commun.). Azaperone/metomi-
date anaesthesia has been reported to produce only slight effects on cardiovascular function and respiration (Hillidge *et al* 1975).

Saffan (formerly CT1341)

General pharmacology

The history of steroid anaesthesia began with the report of Hans Selye in
1941 that certain steroid hormones, when administered intraperitoneally at
dose rates in excess of physiological levels, produced deep and reversible
anaesthesia in rats. These findings were not put to practical use until 1955
when the pregnanedione derivative, hydroxydione sodium, was introduced
as an injectable anaesthetic agent. Hydroxydione had the merits of a wide
safety margin, minimum depression of cardiovascular function and respiration, little excitement during induction or recovery, and absence of hormonal activity. Unfortunately, these properties were offset by several
disadvantages which were solved by the introduction of a new steroid
anaesthetic in 1971. This was known commercially as Saffan (the veterinary
product) or Althesin (the identical human product), and contained a mixture of two pregnanedione-derived steroids — alphaxalone and alphadolone
acetate.

The final solution is slightly viscous and froths if shaken because of the
presence of the non-ionic surfactant, Cremophor EL (polyoxyethylated
castor oil). The latter is used as a solubilising agent for the main active
constituent, alphaxalone, which is very insoluble in water. The second
steroid, alphadolone acetate, is approximately half as potent as alphaxalone
and, being present in a lesser amount, it accounts for only one-eighth of the
anaesthetic activity of the product. In fact, alphadolone is included not for its
anaesthetic activity but because it improves the solubility of alphaxalone
more than threefold. The final solution is of approximately neutral pH and,
since it seems to be non-irritant to tissues, it does not cause thromboph-
lebitis.

Saffan is generally held to possess a wide safety margin in clinical use and
this is probably attributable to less depression of respiration compared with
most other injectable anaesthetics. A notable side-effect in some species is
histamine release from mast cells and a resulting vasodepression. The
release of histamine was originally ascribed to the action of the surfactant
component Cremophor EL and, although the latter is undoubtedly impli-

cated, several recent studies have shown that there are other interacting factors.

In contrast to thiobarbiturates such as thiopentone, Saffan is not dependent on uptake by adipose tissue for termination of its activity. It is metabolised in the liver and the highly polar metabolites are then secreted in the bile. This explains the lack of cumulation with Saffan and is clinically relevant, since it allows anaesthesia to be maintained for prolonged periods by the administration of incremental doses (or by intravenous infusion) without unduly prolonging the recovery period (Child *et al* 1972).

The active constituents of Saffan cross the blood–brain barrier rapidly so there is minimal delay between administration and loss of consciousness. This occurs in little more than one vein-to-brain circulation time. Both induction and recovery are normally smooth and excitement-free and muscular relaxation is fair to good, so that the quality of anaesthesia is generally satisfactory. However, these findings do not apply in the horse (see p. 472).

Profound hypotension has occurred when Saffan has been injected intravenously after barbiturates (Clarke & Hall 1975) or chloralose. It is probably unwise, therefore, to use Saffan in combination with other injectable anaesthetics.

Applied pharmacology

Pig. Clarke & Hall (1975) produced anaesthesia of 10–15 minutes' duration with doses of 3–6 mg/kg Saffan intravenously and Cox *et al* (1975) used azaperone or atropine to premedicate pigs before inducing anaesthesia with 2.0–3.0 mg/kg Saffan intravenously. They reported an excellent induction effect with only slight respiratory depression, good muscle relaxation, and an absence of marked excitement during recovery. These authors also achieved a satisfactory sedative effect when doses of 6.0 and 8.0 mg/kg Saffan were injected intramuscularly. It is likely that Saffan could be very valuable for chemical restraint in small pigs (Green 1979) but the large volumes of solution required both for sedation and anaesthesia will render its use impractical and expensive in large pigs.

Glen *et al* (1978) have studied the effects of repeated doses of Saffan in miniature pigs. After a second dose of the drug they observed skin flushing, cyanosis, raised plasma histamine concentration and a marked fall in polymorph count. This 'hypersensitivity' reaction occurred when the interval between first and second dose was 1–2 weeks but not when the interval was only four days.

Horse. Preliminary studies (Hall 1972) indicated that doses of 1.20–1.34

mg/kg Saffan intravenously produced a satisfactory anaesthetic induction but there were violent paddling and galloping movements during the recovery phase. These excitatory effects were abolished by premedication with xylazine. In a more detailed study, Eales (1976) selected 1.9 mg/kg Saffan as the optimum dose, but induction was associated with excitement, muscle relaxation was poor, and there was marked hyperaesthesia to tactile and audible stimuli during recovery. The excitement in recovery could not be prevented by acepromazine or xylazine premedication but it was almost completely prevented by blindfolding and plugging the external ear canals.

Sheep, goat, cow. Hall (1972) reported the use by Stowe of single doses of 2.2 mg/kg Saffan as an induction agent in sheep. There was a decrease in heart rate, cardiac output and arterial blood pressure and a rise in left ventricular end-diastolic pressure. Waterman & Livingston (1978a, 1978b) have also studied the cardiovascular effects of Saffan in sheep. A dose of 2.2 mg/kg intravenously produced an immediate fall in blood pressure to 50% of the control level, followed by a return to normal within 10 minutes.

Clarke & Hall (1975) have produced satisfactory surgical anaesthesia in sheep and goats with doses of Saffan from 1.2 to 2.4 mg/kg, and in calves up to one year of age with 2.4 mg/kg. Anaesthesia lasted for 5–20 minutes and recovery was uneventful. Saffan, therefore, appears to be a useful intravenous anaesthetic in all farm animal species, although the high cost and large volumes required preclude its extensive use.

4   Dissociative anaesthetics

General pharmacology

General properties. Dissociative anaesthesia may be defined as a state of altered CNS activity, involving both stimulant and depressant components. Thus, in summarising the effects of dissociative agents in animals, Chen (1973) indicated that with increasing doses the progressive central effects were excitation, ataxia, catalepsy, general anaesthesia and convulsions. Dissociative anaesthesia is produced by a group of synthetic organic bases derived from phenylcyclohexylamine which includes phencyclidine, tiletamine and ketamine. Phencyclidine is the most potent and possesses the longest duration of action, while ketamine is the least potent and acts for the shortest period. Ketamine is the most commonly used dissociative agent both in animals and man.

Although there are some similarities between the states of dissociative and general anaesthesia, there are also many differences. For example, muscle tone may be maintained or even increased by dissociative anaesthetics, to give a state of cataleptoid immobility. Also several reflexes which are abolished by injectable general anaesthetics are retained. These include pharyngeal and laryngeal reflexes (though these may be abolished with high doses) and palpebral and corneal reflexes which are present and vigorous throughout anaesthesia. Dissociative agents may also produce other characteristic ocular effects: the eyelids remain open, the pupil is dilated and nystagmus is commonly present. Hypnotic doses of general anaesthetics (e.g. barbiturates) usually give little analgesia, subhypnotic doses give none. In contrast, dissociative agents provide good somatic analgesia, which makes them particularly suitable for superficial surgical procedures. However, visceral analgesia is poor.

Respiration is said by most workers to be well maintained during dissociative anaesthesia and this presumably explains the high therapeutic indices of dissociative agents in laboratory animal studies and the wide safety margins in clinical use. In addition, dissociative anaesthetics alter the character of respiration in a distinctive way: it becomes apneustic (i.e. breath-holding on inspiration) and jerky (the expiratory phase taking the form of a series of short and irregular components). In man, a number of psychic effects during the recovery phase have been reported and these may be accompanied by severe motor activity. It is uncertain whether or not psychic effects occur in animals, but in the absence of firm evidence to the contrary it would seem wise to assume that they may. Certainly, catatonia and bizarre behaviour patterns have been observed in animals. From the clinical viewpoint it is important to note that recovery excitement may be minimised by avoiding unnecessary sensory stimulation (noise, touch, light, etc.) and by premedication with a sedative.

Many investigators have described the use of supplementary agents for minimising the hypertonus, tremor, clonic activity and psychic effects which can occur with dissociative anaesthetics. Thus, Green (1979) has established dose rates of diazepam and xylazine for use with ketamine in many animal species. A combination product (CI/744) containing a 1:1 ratio by weight of the benzodiazepine, zolazepam, with tiletamine, has been described for use in dogs, cats, zoo animals and sheep (Conner *et al* 1974, Ward *et al* 1974).

The central effects of dissociative agents include a stimulant action on centres controlling outflow in efferent sympathetic nerves. This explains several peripheral effects such as mydriasis, bronchodilation, hyperglycaemia and a number of cardiovascular responses. Increased sympathetic tone tends to increase heart rate and constrict blood vessels. Increased peripheral resistance and cardiac output both contribute to the rise in arterial blood pressure and, since cerebral vessels do not participate in the general constrictor reaction, cerebral blood flow is increased.

Sympathoadrenal activation is not the only way in which dissociative anaesthetics affect cardiovascular function. Their direct action on the heart is the usual dose-related negative inotropic action which all anaesthetics possess. At high dose rates this direct myocardial depression may override the sympathetic effects to give a reduction in arterial blood pressure. Such an effect is likely to occur shortly after ketamine has been administered by rapid intravenous injection.

In contrast to their effects on the sympathetic nervous system, dissociative anaesthetics do not induce a comparable general increase in parasympathetic nervous activity. However, they do increase salivation in most species and this can be controlled by premedication with atropine.

Ketamine possesses anticonvulsant properties, although some types of seizure (e.g. those induced by strychnine) are not suppressed. This action, like the antiarrhythmic effect of ketamine on the heart, may be explained by a general stabilising effect on membranes since dissociative agents are known to possess local anaesthetic properties. A stabilising action on membranes would account for the bradycardia and arrhythmias that have been reported after intravenous administration of phencyclidine (Green 1979).

Dissociative agents are recommended for administration by intravenous and intramuscular routes. When the latter is used, anaesthesia is achieved 3–6 minutes after the injection. Intravenous administration gives a more rapid induction, although this is definitely a little slower than the induction time with thiobarbiturates.

Studies of the metabolism of ketamine in several species have shown that at least four metabolites (a demethylated product, a cyclohexene derivative and two hydroxylated compounds) may be formed. Relatively little unchanged ketamine is excreted in the urine. Biotransformation in the liver probably constitutes the principal means of terminating the activity of ketamine, although uptake by adipose tissue may also be involved. In view of the importance of biotransformation in terminating the action of ketamine, it is not surprising that clinical evidence of tolerance has been reported following repeated use in monkeys (Bree *et al* 1967). That this is probably caused by induction of liver enzymes is indicated by the findings of Livingston & Waterman (1978) in rats. These authors found that the tolerance induced by daily administrations of ketamine was accompanied by lower blood and brain levels of ketamine and higher levels of the oxidation metabolite.

Applied pharmacology

Pig. The first dissociative agent to be used in veterinary medicine was phencyclidine. It was introduced by Tavernor (1963, 1964a) for chemical restraint of the pig. The optimum intramuscular dose rate was 2 mg/kg in adults and 4–6 mg/kg in young pigs (Perry 1964). The principal advantages were the ease of administration (small volumes intramuscularly), the rapid onset of action and the uneventful recovery. Side-effects included paddling movements, hyperthermia, tremor and excessive salivation.

Unfortunately, phencyclidine has been withdrawn from use in the UK, but its successor, ketamine, has been evaluated in pigs. Roberts (1971), Thurman *et al* (1972) and Denny & Lucke (1977) have used ketamine intramuscularly at a dose level of 20 mg/kg. We have administered the drug both intravenously and intramuscularly, with and without azaperone pre-medication, in more than 100 pigs of various breeds (Lees & Meredith 1978). Doses of 5–15 mg/kg intravenously or 15–25 mg/kg intramuscularly produced a light plane of anaesthesia, which was suitable for minor surgery or as premedication for halothane anaesthesia. There was a useful degree of chemical restraint but the weak analgesic action and poor muscle relaxation preclude its use as a sole anaesthetic agent for major surgery. Respiration was sometimes depressed (increased carbon dioxide tension and decreased oxygen tension in arterial blood) but this response varied widely from animal to animal. Tactile stimuli during induction or recovery sometimes provoked clonic convulsions.

Horse. Of the available dissociative agents, only ketamine has been fully evaluated in the horse. A light plane of anaesthesia with excellent analgesia has been achieved with a combination of ketamine (2.2 mg/kg) and xylazine (1.1 mg/kg) administered intravenously. The xylazine was administered either simultaneously with or prior to the ketamine (Muir *et al* 1977). In this study cardiovascular parameters remained within normal limits but there was a mild depression of respiration. Induction and recovery were generally smooth and free of excitement. Several anaesthetists regard xylazine–ketamine anaesthesia as a major advance.

Sheep. Satisfactory use of ketamine in sheep has been reported by Taylor *et al* (1972) and Britton *et al* (1974) using an intramuscular dose rate of 20 mg/kg. However, according to Green (1979) satisfactory use of ketamine intravenously requires premedication with xylazine or diazepam. Moreover, the latter author used a much lower dose of ketamine — an initial injection of 4 mg/kg followed by infusion of ketamine to effect or by maintenance with nitrous oxide. Thurman *et al* (1973) used doses of 22–44 mg/kg intra-venously or intramuscularly to provide short-lived periods of anaesthesia. Premedication with atropine to control salivation and with acepromazine to provide greater muscle relaxation and a longer duration of analgesia were recommended by these authors.

Waterman & Livingston (1978a, 1978b) studied the physiological effects of ketamine in sheep. Dose levels of 2–11.6 mg/kg intravenously produced initial dose-dependent falls in arterial pressure and cerebral flow and this was sometimes followed by a mild pressor phase and an increase in cerebral blood flow. Similarly, respiration was first depressed and then stimulated as indicated by blood gas measurements.

Cattle. Fuentes & Tellez (1974, 1976) administered ketamine intravenously (2 mg/kg) to produce a depth of anaesthesia which permitted laparotomy. Anaesthesia was maintained by infusion of ketamine at a rate of 20 mg/minute. Rapid recovery followed termination of the infusion.

Goat. Green (1979) has recommended a dose rate in goats of 4 mg/kg intravenously 15 minutes after premedication with diazepam (2 mg/kg intravenously). As in sheep, further ketamine is then infused intravenously to effect or the animals are anaesthetised with nitrous oxide:oxygen (1:1). Advantages of ketamine anaesthesia are rapid recovery and absence of respiratory depression, although ketamine alone provides insufficient muscle relaxation for surgery.

5 Peripheral muscle relaxants

Suxamethonium

General pharmacology

The only peripheral muscle relaxant of importance as a chemical restraining agent in veterinary medicine is suxamethonium (succinyldicholine). It is the ester formed by linking two choline molecules with one molecule of succinic acid. The neuromuscular blocking action of suxamethonium is short lived in comparison with that of most other skeletal muscle relaxants. Its action is terminated by the enzyme, pseudocholinesterase, which is present in plasma and in the liver. The plasma levels of pseudocholinesterase and the dose rates of suxamethonium vary considerably between the species. For example, the horse, pig and cat require relatively large doses of suxamethonium, while dogs, sheep and cattle are sensitive to small doses; the dose rates used by Hansson (1957) to cast horses and cattle were 0.17 and 0.02 mg/kg, respectively.

The following sequence of muscular paralysis is produced by agents acting at the neuromuscular junction, although exceptions may occur in individual animals (Hall 1971): **1** Within 30–60 seconds of intravenous injection, the muscles of the face, jaw and tail are paralysed. **2**   The distal limb and neck muscles are next affected, followed by the proximal limb muscles. **3**   The swallowing and phonatory muscles are paralysed. **4**   Finally, paralysis of the muscles of the abdominal wall, the intercostal muscles and the diaphragm occurs (in that order). The muscles usually regain function in the reverse order during recovery.

Applied pharmacology

In the period from 1954 to 1970 suxamethonium was used extensively in certain countries as an 'immobilising agent' in many species of game and also in large domesticated species, including horses, cattle and pigs. Some early reports referred to either intramuscular or intravenous administration, but the former was generally unsatisfactory because of excitement and ataxia which frequently preceded immobilisation. Use in domestic species other than the horse was also short lived. In cattle, for example, the margin of safety was found to be narrow and the risk of aspiration of rumenal contents presented a further hazard (Hansson 1957). Hence, the principal use of the drug became that of an intravenous casting agent in the horse.

Horse. Commencing from the early years of the last decade intravenous usage in the horse has also declined. There have been three principal reasons for this: **1** Several reports of the profound effects of suxamethonium on cardiovascular and respiratory function have demonstrated that there are strong reasons for discontinuing its use as a casting agent. **2** Veterinary anaesthetists have been most concerned that loss of the ability to stand, transient apnoea with larger doses, and fasciculations which are probably very painful, may combine to cause considerable distress in an animal that is not unconscious nor even sedated. Furthermore, the possibility that surgery might be performed on a conscious but immobilised animal has given cause for additional concern (Tavernor 1964b, Hall 1971). **3** The advent of other intravenous agents such as the thiobarbiturates and glyceryl guaicolate, which have fewer side-effects and which can be used to cast animals more humanely.

The main way in which suxamethonium is now used in chemical restraint is to inject a barbiturate and suxamethonium in rapid succession into the jugular vein. This technique ensures the horse sinks quietly to the ground, and thus overcomes the problems of induction excitement which occur with barbiturates in a small number of cases (Hall 1971).

6 Central muscle relaxants

Glyceryl guaicolate

General pharmacology

From what has been said concerning the effects of peripherally acting muscle relaxants when administered to conscious animals, it might be supposed that there would be no place in veterinary medicine for any drug which paralyses skeletal muscle in an animal which is not fully anaesthetised. This is not so. One such drug, glyceryl guaicolate (guaicol glycerol ether), is used extensively in the USA and in Europe both in the horse and to a lesser degree in cattle, sheep, pigs and dogs. Although there are some side-effects and disadvantages associated with the use of this agent, they are totally different from the toxic actions of suxamethonium, and the type of paralysis produced by the two agents is quite distinct. This account of the properties of glyceryl guaicolate should be read in conjunction with Table 21.2, which compares its actions with those of suxamethonium.

Glyceryl guaicolate is related to mephenesin both structurally and in its actions. Pharmacologically, both of these centrally acting muscle relaxants are more precisely described as interneuronal blocking agents: their principal action being blockade of impulse conduction across internuncial neurones in the spinal cord. These interneurones are concerned with the coordination of opposing muscle groups. Thus, when extensor muscle neurones are stimulated, their collateral nerves stimulate interneurones which release the inhibitory transmitter glycine. This hyperpolarises the postsynaptic membranes of flexor motor neurones and hence suppresses flexor muscle movement. Glyceryl guaicolate is believed to mimic the action of glycine. The paralysis produced by the glycerol ethers is 'curare-like' in nature. Thus, the loss of skeletal muscle tone causes flaccid paralysis and, in contrast to suxamethonium, initial muscle contraction and fasciculation are absent.

Applied pharmacology

Horse. Glyceryl guaicolate is used in two main ways: **1**   by intravenous infusion to produce casting prior to induction of anaesthesia with another agent or prior to surgery under local anaesthesia: **2**   admixed with a thiobarbiturate, the mixture being given by intravenous infusion to produce a light plane of surgical anaesthesia with muscle relaxation. In both instances it has been usual to premedicate the animal with a phenothiazine tranquilliser.

Table 21.2 Comparative pharmacology of suxamethonium and glyceryl guaicolate.

Property	Suxamethonium	Glyceryl guaicolate
Type of muscular paralysis	Depolarising block producing initial muscle contraction (fasciculation)	Flaccid paralysis, no initial stimulation or fasciculations
Muscles affected at clinical dose rates	All (possibly including diaphragm)	Limb muscles (respiratory muscles unaffected)
Onset of action	Rapid (25–40 sec)	Slow (1–4 minutes); peak response even slower
Duration of action	3–6 minutes, not entirely dose related	10–30 minutes depending on dose
Administration and usage	Rapid i.v. *injection* over 2–5 seconds (alone or immediately *following* a thiobarbiturate)	i.v. *infusion* over 1–4 minutes (alone or *with* a thiobarbiturate)
Respiratory effects	Apnoea for up to 2 min; marked decrease in P_{aO_2}, increase in P_{aCO_2}	Little or no effect with clinical doses; small decrease in P_{aO_2} but P_{aCO_2} unchanged
Cardiovascular effects	Profound tachycardia, various arrhythmias, including ventricular extrasystoles and possibly ventricular fibrillation; marked increase in arterial pressure	Negligible or slight tachycardia; mild hypotension
Haematological effects	Probably haemoconcentration resulting from expulsion of erythrocytes from spleen	No acute effects but leucocytosis noted at 24 hours; intravascular haemolysis with concentrations exceeding 10%
Central effects	None, animal fully conscious; molecule completely ionised therefore does not penetrate blood–brain barrier	Muscular relaxation, sedation or hypnosis, mild analgesia

When used alone, the usual procedure is to prepare a fresh 5% or 10% solution in warmed sterile water or dextrose solution. This is administered by infusion into a jugular vein at a dose rate of up to 160 mg/kg over 1–3 minutes. The animal usually becomes recumbent within 2–4 minutes. For a 500 kg horse, 1.6 litres of solution are required. This large volume, and the time required for its administration, constitute obvious practical disadvantages. Difficulties in administration will clearly be greatest in fractious animals and under field conditions. For use in combination with short-acting barbiturates, several dose rates have been recommended. Although most authors have preferred to use barbiturate–glyceryl guaicolate combinations when endotracheal intubation has to be carried out, it is possible to intubate under the influence of glyceryl guaicolate alone (Heath & Gabel 1970, Roberts 1968, Schatzman 1974). The duration of action of glyceryl guaicolate is dose dependent: the first recovery movements are usually seen after 10–30 minutes, although the time to standing can exceed 60 minutes with high dose rates.

The side-effects seem to be relatively few. Cardiovascular changes were reported by Tavernor (1970), Heath & Gabel (1970) and Jackson & Lundvall (1972). The first of these authors reported a small decrease in arterial pressure and slight increase in heart rate. Clinical dose rates of glyceryl guaicolate given alone seem to exert almost no effect on respiration. The small decrease in arterial oxygen tension noted by Tavernor (1970) was probably attributable to the physical effect of the change in posture from the standing position to lateral recumbency. On the other hand, two out of three studies (Tavernor 1970, Schatzman 1974) indicate that a distinct degree of respiratory depression occurs when glyceryl guaicolate is combined with barbiturates. In the third study (Jackson & Lundvall 1972) there were no changes in respiratory rate, arterial pH or carbon dioxide tension, and only a very small decrease in arterial oxygen tension.

In spite of many favourable reports on the clinical use of glyceryl guaicolate, the suspicion remains that use of this drug alone to cast horses may be inhumane because they are not anaesthetised. Thus, Schatzman (1974) observed that animals which were intubated after receiving a dose of 80–100 mg/kg '. . . appeared still to be conscious when connected to the anaesthetic apparatus'. Against this, it must be said that all authors consider the drug to be safe and satisfactory in clinical use. Moreover, the pronounced sedative effect and slight analgesic action ensure that the animal is at least not in a normal state of consciousness.

7 Narcotic-analgesics

General pharmacology

These drugs are *not* in fact widely used *alone* for chemical restraint, since they produce a combination of central stimulant and depressant actions. The predominance of stimulation or depression depends on several factors, including the particular drug used, the dose and route of administration, the species of animal and its pathophysiological status. For example, animals in pain are more likely to be sedated by morphine-like drugs than those which are not.

A brief account of the pharmacology of narcotic-analgesics and, in particular a consideration of species' differences in their actions, is required since one agent, etorphine, has been available for use as a combination product (with acepromazine) for use in large animals since 1969. The actions of morphine and related drugs were well described by Dun in 1895.

'In veterinary patients the prominent phenomena are agitation, unrest inco-ordinate, generally manege, movements, diminished sensibility to pain, indisposition for voluntary movement, and in toxic doses convulsions, coma, and death by respiratory arrest. Moderate doses diiate the blood-vessels and quicken heart action, and this is more notable in horses than in man . . . Horses, with less development of these higher brain centres, have relatively more development of the locomotor centres and of the reflex centres of the spinal cord, and upon these lower centres opiates in equine subjects exert their primary stimulant effects. Instead of sleep there are produced restless, involuntary movements of the head and limbs, pawing with one foot sometimes for half an hour, or walking continuously round the box; while large doses cause tetanic convulsions . . . Mr. A. E. Macgillivray, Banff, who has used morphine hydrochlorate hypodermically for years, states that in susceptible horses he has repeatedly found grs. iv. or grs. v. induce staring eyes, restlessness, prancing round the box, increased rapidity and threadiness of the pulse — symptoms which sometimes continue three to five hours (*Veterinarian, March 1881*) . . . Dogs exhibit effects intermediate between those observed in man and in horses. Relatively to their body-weight, they take eight or ten times the dose prescribed for man. They show more preliminary excitement than man, but less involuntary muscular movement than the horse, but during drowsiness and sleep muscular twitchings occur. Sleep, however, is never very profound; the dogs are easily awakened; they dream, and have hallucinations, and after full doses remain stupid for a day . . . Ruminants, like horses, are usually excited and restless. Cattle bellow, digestion is deranged, and tympanitis frequently supervenes. Sleep is not quickly or readily induced, excepting by full and repeated doses... Cats are as much excited as horses or cattle, more so than dogs, and hypnosis is produced with difficulty ... Swine receiving one or two drachms of opium become first lively and then dull and sleepy, their bowels constipated, and their skins hot.'

The spectrum of activity of drugs acting on opiate receptors ranges from drugs with 'pure' agonist activity through partial agonists (compounds with mixed agonist–antagonist properties) to 'pure' antagonists (Table 21.3). This progression is very relevant to chemical restraint because those drugs with purely or predominantly antagonist actions can compete with agonist drugs for both central and peripheral opiate receptors to terminate their pharmacological actions. Hence they may be used as 'reversing agents' for morphine-like drugs, either in cases of overdosage or simply to terminate the action of normal doses. Clinically, this has obvious attractions but there are drawbacks to the use of these drugs. The abrupt and complete transition from a state of deep narcosis to one of normal consciousness has been associated, in man, with undesirable behavioural symptoms (uneasiness, anxiety) and effects attributed to hyperactivity of the autonomic nervous system (tachycardia, hypertension, mydriasis, vomiting) (Tremblay *et al* 1976).

The only narcotic-analgesic which has been used extensively to restrain large animals is etorphine. Etorphine is a synthetic organic base, derived from thebaine. It is used as the water-soluble hydrochloride salt. The potency of etorphine (administered subcutaneously to laboratory animals) has been shown to be 150–80 000 times greater than that of morphine, depending on the test situation (Blane *et al* 1967). This is only partially explained by its twenty-fold greater affinity for opiate receptors. The fact that etorphine is 300 times more lipid soluble accounts for much of its high potency (because of efficient penetration of the blood–brain barrier), and also accounts for the rapid onset of action following administration to animals or after accidental self-administration in man.

Table 21.3 Classification of drugs acting on opiate receptors.

Property	Drugs
Strong agonist	Phenazocine
Agonist	Morphine, etorphine
Weaker agonist	Methadone
Mixed agonist–antagonist	Pentazocine, buprenorphine
Antagonist with weak agonist activity	Nalorphine, diprenorphine
Antagonist with no agonist activity	Naloxone

For large animal chemical restraint, narcotic-analgesics are usually used in combination with sedative drugs. These combinations take two forms. In the first a low dose of narcotic-analgesic is used to provide analgesia to supplement the mild physical restraint of the sedative. In the second type of combination (known as neuroleptanalgesia), the narcotic analgesic is given at a very high dose rate to provide both analgesia and a greater degree of restraint (immobilisation). With this combination, the main role of the sedative is to suppress undesirable side-effects of the analgesic and to provide persistent sedation after reversal of the immobilising action of the analgesic by a competitive antagonist.

Applied pharmacology

Horse. Recent studies (Muir *et al* 1978, Combie *et al* 1979) of the clinical pharmacology of narcotic-analgesics in domestic breeds of horse have confirmed and extended the early description of Dun (1895). Using analgesic dose rates of several analgesics (including morphine, methadone and pethidine) Muir *et al* (1978) subjectively assessed that an initial dysphoria (subjects ill at ease) was followed by euphoria (feeling of well being), the dysphoria being particularly notable with morphine. In addition, all three drugs increased heart rate by 15–30 beats/minute and mean arterial pressure by some 30 mmHg, possibly by stimulating central sympathetic centres. Another action of low doses of morphine and related drugs in the horse is the induction of ingestive behaviour (Combie *et al* 1979), but no sedative action is apparent. Intermediate doses (for morphine = 6–24 times the analgesic dose) of narcotic-analgesics produce dose-related increases in locomotor activity, which is only well coordinated at the lower doses within this intermediate range (Tobin 1978, Combie *et al* 1979). These findings suggest that sedation cannot be obtained with either small or intermediate doses of narcotic-analgesics and their value in the chemical restraint of large *pain-free* animals is therefore questionable. As indicated earlier, low dose rates of analgesics can be administered, together with sedatives, to provide chemical restraint for animals in pain, or to facilitate minor surgical procedures. For example, Král *et al* (1970) used intravenous xylazine (0.8 mg/kg) and methadone (0.15 mg/kg) with atropine (0.05 mg/kg subcutaneously) to provide sedation, analgesia and relaxation. However, this combination was ineffective in particularly fractious horses and increasing the dose levels also failed to provide adequate analgesia and sedation. Analgesic dose rates for other narcotic-analgesics in the horse are: morphine 0.12 mg/kg, pethidine 1.10 mg/kg, oxymorphone 0.03 mg/kg, and pentazocine 0.90 mg/kg (Muir *et al* 1978).

8 Neuroleptanalgesics

Etorphine with acepromazine

General pharmacology

Neuroleptanalgesia is a state of altered CNS activity involving both stimulant and depressant components (in differing degrees according to drugs, dosage, and species) which is produced by the combined administration of a narcotic-analgesic of the morphine type and sedative-tranquilliser (neuroleptic) from the phenothiazine or butyrophenone groupings. Three neuroleptanalgesic combinations (etorphine + methotrimeprazine, fentanyl + droperidol, fentanyl + fluanisone) have been available for more than ten years for use in the dog and some laboratory animal species, such as the rabbit and guinea pig, but only one mixture — *Large Animal Immobilon* (etorphine + acepromazine) — has been used extensively for the restraint of large, domesticated animals. It is administered intravenously or intramuscularly and the action of the analgesic component can be terminated by an intravenous or intramuscular injection of diprenorphine (*Large Animal Revivon*). This leaves the animal in a sedated state due to the continuing action of the acepromazine.

There are undoubtedly real differences between species in the actions of analgesics and these are reflected in the resultant states of neuroleptanalgesia. In the dog, for example, neuroleptanalgesia is characterised by deep sedation, muscle relaxation and parasympethetic predominance (hypotension, bradycardia, miosis). In contrast, in the horse there is increased muscle tone and fasciculation, tachycardia, hyperglycaemia, sweating, an initial rise in blood pressure, and other symptoms typical of generalised activation of the sympathetic nervous system.

Applied pharmacology

Horse. The early studies of Harthoorn (1965), Harthoorn & Bligh (1965) and King & Klingel (1965) established the effectiveness of etorphine for the chemical restraint of domestic ponies, donkeys and wild ungulates. Using dose rates of 2–20 μg/kg intravenously (in combination with hyoscine), Harthoorn (1965) produced a rapid collapse in donkeys accompanied by rigidity of the neck and limb muscles, increase in heart rate and decrease in respiratory rate. Respiration was stertorous in character and this was probably caused by prolonged exhalation through a partially closed glottis. King & Klingel (1965) administered etorphine (5.7 μg/kg intramuscularly) to Welsh Mountain ponies and recorded ataxia, salivation, lacrimation, tremors of head and forelimbs and resentment of handling. However, when the ponies received 49 µg/kg acepromazine in addition, they lay quietly in recumbency.

In 1969, Immobilon, a neuroleptanalgesic mixture of etorphine hydrochloride (22.5 µg/kg of the base) and acepromazine maleate (100 µg/kg of the base), was introduced for use in domestic breeds of horse by either intravenous or intramuscular route of administration. The dose rate of etorphine which is now recommended is higher than the dosages employed by early workers, although half the new dose rate is considered to be satisfactory for donkeys and sheep. The product is supplied together with an aqueous solution of the etorphine antagonist, diprenorphine (Revivon), which is to be administered intravenously in a volume equal to the volume of Immobilon originally given, the normal dose rate being 30 µg/kg. In a preliminary report, Hillidge & Lees (1971b) described their findings following the intravenous injection of Immobilon in ponies. A smooth fall to the ground after approximately 30 seconds was followed by a period of immobilisation in lateral recumbency with muscle tremor over the whole body and with the front legs held in rigid extension and the hind legs in spastic flexion. In some ponies the increased muscle tone subsided after 5–10 minutes. From the consistent and marked increase in heart rate (and in some animals cardiac arrhythmias), mydriasis, sweating and rises in haematocrit and blood glucose concentration, it was concluded that the drug combination caused activation of the sympathetic nervous system.

Jenkins *et al* (1972), reporting their clinical experiences with Immobilon, noted muscle tremor in 80% of cases, which made minor surgical interferences difficult, although they always were able to castrate animals. These authors used the intramuscular route and observed varying degrees of excitement in the period (3–6 minutes) before the horses became recumbent. It can be very difficult to control large horses in this period. In fact, the degree of excitement led these authors to increase the dose from 15 µg/kg etorphine to 22.5 µg/kg. Excitement was said to be minimal at the higher dose rate. Jenkins *et al* (1972) considered that the principal advantages of Immobilon were a consistently reliable effect, a reduction of the difficulties and dangers of handling horses when little or no skilled assistance was available, and a rapid reversibility of the action of etorphine. Other advantages are the opportunity for either intravenous or intramuscular administration, and the very small volume to be injected.

Early reports of the clinical pharmacology of Immobilon were made by Daniel & Ling (1972) and Schlarmann *et al* (1973). Both groups recorded marked tachycardia and hypertension. Tachycardia was greater following intramuscular injection than after intravenous administration, and the rise in blood pressure was only marked for the 20-minute period following administration.

More detailed cardiovascular and respiratory studies have been undertaken in our laboratory. The marked decrease in respiratory rate produced by Immobilon was accompanied by a moderate decrease in pH of arterial blood and an increase in carbon dioxide tension (Hillidge & Lees 1975a). Arterial oxygen tension was reduced from an average of 92 mmHg to less than 50 mmHg throughout the 30 minutes for which Immobilon was allowed to act. Despite the profound reduction in arterial oxygen tension, it was not clear whether or not Immobilon caused widespread tissue hypoxia, because the fall in oxygen tension was offset by two other factors. Firstly, haemoglobin concentration was increased, so arterial oxygen content was only slightly reduced. Secondly, cardiac output was increased, so oxygen flux (the product of arterial oxygen content and left ventricular output: a measure of the total quantity of oxygen supplied to organs by the left ventricle) was actually increased (Hillidge & Lees 1975b). We have reached the tentative conclusion that severe tissue hypoxia does not occur in Immobilon-treated ponies.

Some of the cardiovascular effects of Immobilon have been well defined. A marked tachycardia (heart rate sometimes increasing to about 200 beats/minutes) has been reported with both intravenous and intramuscular routes of administration by Hillidge & Lees (1971b), Daniel & Ling (1972) and Schlarmann *et al* (1973). The rapid, forceful heart beat can sometimes be heard from a distance of several feet. All three groups have also reported increases in arterial blood pressure, but usually these were not well maintained. In more detailed investigations, Lees & Hillidge (1975) and Hillidge & Lees (1976) reported a marked increase in heart rate and a significant reduction in stroke volume. However, the former response predominated sufficiently to cause a moderate rise in cardiac output. Total peripheral resistance was initially unchanged but, by 15 minutes after injecting Immobilon, it was reduced and this response persisted after reversing the state of neuroleptanalgesia with diprenorphine. Mean arterial pressure (the product of cardiac output and total peripheral resistance) reflected these changes. Thus, it was increased by an average of approximately 40 mmHg at 5 minutes, but had returned to the control level by 15 minutes.

To explain these cardiovascular changes, Lees & Hillidge (1975) have suggested that etorphine activates the sympathetic nervous system and that those sympathetic responses (e.g. vasoconstriction) which are mediated by α-receptors are at least partially antagonised by the α-receptor blocking action of acepromazine. Reduced vasomotor tone, resulting from α-receptor blockade, could also explain the hypotension and fall in total peripheral resistance which occurs after reversing the actions of etorphine by diprenorphine. These proposals have been substantiated by control experiments, in which etorphine and acepromazine have been administered separately to ponies (Bogan *et al* 1978, Hillidge & Lees, unpublished data).

Etorphine, administered alone, produced greater and more sustained rises in arterial blood pressure and haematocrit than did Immobilon.

A further side-effect of unknown, but probably low, incidence is the condition of priapism with possible consequences of penile injury, paraphimosis, and paralysis. Priapism has been reported by Pearson & Weaver (1978) in five horses which had received Immobilon, also in one horse given acepromazine and thiopentone, and in one which had received acepromazine, thiopentone and chloroform. Amputation of the penis had to be undertaken in five of these seven horses. Acepromazine alone can produce this reaction, but it is not clear whether or not other drugs, such as thiopentone and etorphine, can interact with acepromazine to increase the incidence of priapism.

There appear to be some breed and species differences in the response of equidae to Immobilon. Wild species of equidae seem to be less prone to manifest excitatory effects than do the domestic breeds. Dobbs & Ling (1972) have reported some distinct differences between horses and donkeys in the effects of Immobilon at the normal dose rate (1.0 ml/100 kg body weight). These differences (Table 21.4) were attributed to subtle variations in activity at the receptor level within the CNS. Great care is required when using etorphine and diprenorphine in donkeys, because of the greater intensity, higher incidence, and shorter latency of the post-diprenorphine excitement reaction. No more than half the normal dose of Immobilon for horses should be administered, and reversal is achieved with an equal volume of diprenorphine solution.

Excitement has been reported at various times in relation to the administration of Immobilon and Revivon to the horse and has taken several forms. The cardiovascular, sympathetic and skeletal muscle effects which occur both before and during recumbency have already been described.

Table 21.4 Effects of Immobilon in the horse and donkey (Dobbs & Ling 1972).

Effect	Horse	Donkey
Induction excitement after intramuscular injection	Possible	Usually absent
Interval from administration to recumbency	0.5–2 min (i.v.), 4–6 min (i.m.)	May be considerably longer
Skeletal muscle tone and activity	Increased tone, tremor	Excellent relaxation, tremor seldom observed
Heart rate	Marked increase	Within normal limits
Excitement following diprenorphine administration	Restlessness and excitement occur infrequently 6–8 hours later	Frequently, 1.5–2 hours later, there is incoordination, aimless wandering, sweating, tachycardia and sometimes immobilisation

Delayed excitement sometimes occurs 6–8 hours after administering Immobilon followed by Revivon. It can be reversed by further administration of diprenorphine and is probably due to enterohepatic recycling of etorphine (this is known to occur in laboratory animals) at a time when the initial dose of diprenorphine has ceased to act. Marked hyperexcitability (sweating, hyperaesthesia and purposeless movement) has also been reported within two minutes of administering diprenorphine. We have observed violent reactions in two ponies when given diprenorphine after an azaperone–etorphine combination (Hillidge & Lees, unpublished data). Excitement at this time may be an individual idiosyncrasy. In certain ponies we have recorded consistent increases in heart rate and in haemoglobin concentration within five minutes of administering diprenorphine (Hillidge & Lees 1978). A possible cause of this early excitement is the precipitation of an 'acute abstinence syndrome' by abrupt reversal of the actions of a large dose of etorphine. A sensible precaution when reversing the actions of etorphine would be to provide a quiet, dimly lit environment.

Pig. The recommended dose rate of Immobilon for the pig is identical to that for horses: 22.5 μg/kg of etorphine and 100 μg/kg of acepromazine. However, in pigs it is recommended that only the intramuscular route is used. At this dose rate, the drug combination was employed by Fraser (1971) to produce a state of 'deep somnolence', which permitted semen collection by electro-ejaculation.

There have been a number of reports of death following the administration of Immobilon to pigs. In one series, 6 of 36 pedigree Hampshires succumbed (Gardner 1971). No deaths occurred in 28 pigs receiving Immobilon in the report of Poyser (1971). Cox & Meese (1973) administered Immobilon on a total of 188 occasions to 116 young and 10 adult pigs, and recorded 3 deaths. They concluded that Immobilon was a useful agent for producing, under field conditions, rapid, effective and safe immobilisation with rapid recovery, especially for pigs between weaning and porker weight. They did not observe any evidence of recycling of etorphine. The restraint was classified as inadequate in 8% of the pigs and untoward sequelae occurred in 8 of the 188 administrations. These sequelae included apnoea, cardiac arrest (possibly caused by an air embolism when injecting diprenorphine), and three deaths. The authors acknowledge that factors other than drug administration may have been implicated in two of the fatalities. Cox & Meese (1973) concluded that Immobilon was safe in clinical use provided that cases of respiratory embarrasment were promptly recognised and treated.

Studies of the clinical pharmacology of Immobilon in Göttingen miniature pigs (Lees & Meredith 1978) have revealed that cardiovascular changes are intermediate between the depressant effects of neuroleptanalgesic drugs in dogs and the sympathetically mediated stimulant effects reported in the horse. In contrast to the marked reduction of respiratory rate in horses, the rate was increased in the pig. The decrease in arterial oxygen tension was also smaller and less persistent in the pig compared with the horse, however, in individual pigs respiratory depression was sometimes pronounced. This finding suggests that the deaths reported by earlier workers may have been due to hypoxia possibly exacerbated by hypotension.

Cattle. Dobbs & Ling (1973) administered Immobilon intramuscularly at the equine dose rate (22.5 μg/kg of etorphine and 100 μg/kg of acepromazine) to five Friesian bullocks aged 8–12 months. This produced recumbency in approximately six minutes which was preceded by a period of controllable excitement. Administration of Immobilon by the intravenous route reduced the time from administration to recumbency to less than one minute and abolished the excitement phase. All animals were insensitive to audible, visual and nociceptive stimuli, but muscle relaxation varied considerably. Maximum relaxation was usually achieved after 10–15 minutes. Bloat sometimes developed in laterally recumbent animals. Respiratory and heart rates were increased by Immobilon, as in the pig; however, detailed cardiovascular studies in cattle have not been reported.

Some bulls have died following single, recommended doses of Immobilon (Rafferty 1976, Scorer 1977). In these two case reports a common factor, and the probable cause of death, was respiratory embarrassment. An additional occasional complication of neuroleptanalgesia in cattle is the reapparance of excitement (trotting and bellowing) some eight hours after the initial administration of Immobilon and Revivon (Dobbs & Ling 1973). This was attributed to enterohepatic recycling of etorphine. These authors also stated that the minimum time which should elapse between an immobilisation/remobilisation cycle and a second dose of Immobilon is six hours.

Sheep, goat. The manufacturer's recommended dose rate for Immobilon in sheep is half that proposed for other large domesticated animals (11.3 μg/kg of etorphine and 50 μg/kg of acepromazine). As in cattle, positioning of sheep in sternal recumbency, with the head down, is advisable to facilitate drainage from the mouth. Pretreatment with atropine (4–8 mg subcutaneously per animal) is advisable, to reduce salivation.

Mitchell (1978) described the effects of Immobilon in sheep in the following terms: within 1–2 minutes of intramuscular administration the sheep become stiff and arch their backs; within 2–3 minutes they lie on their sides; marked analgesia develops but muscle tone is often increased; the limbs and thorax are very rigid and mechanical ventilation is poor; respiratory acidosis and marked bradycardia occur. Ducker & Boyd (1972) reported excitement, shallow breathing and tachycardia during the onset of action of Immobilon. They also referred to a critical period, just after immobilisation, when it was essential to ensure that breathing was regular. Mitchell (1978) considered that Immobilon has a place in the restraint of sheep, particularly in view of the ready reversibility achieved with Revivon.

Immobilon does not seem to have been used extensively in goats. The original report of Harthoorn (1965) established the effectiveness of doses of 0.05–5.0 mg etorphine per animal (by either intravenous or intramuscular injection) as an immobilising agent for this species. The goats were premedicated with either hyoscine or with acepromazine. The degrees of immobilisation and analgesia were sufficient to permit surgical insertion of rumen cannulae.

References

Ahlers D., Frerking H. & Treu H. (1969) Trial with the new anaesthetic Rompun in gynaecology and surgery of the udder in cattle. *Vet. Med. Rev.* No. **2**, 142.

Allsup F. C., Hillidge C. J., Lees P. *et al* (1973) Azaperone/metomidate anaesthesia in the horse. *Vet. Rec.* **93**, 498.

Blane G. F., Boura L. A., Fitzgerald A. E. *et al* (1967) Actions of etorphine hydrochloride (M99): a potent morphine-like agent. *Br. J. Pharm. Chemother.* **30**, 11.

Bogan J. A., MacKenzie G. & Snow D. H. (1978) An evaluation of tranquillisers for use with etorphine as neuroleptanalgesic agents in the horse. *Vet. Rec.* **103**, 471.

Bollwahn W., Vaske T. & Rojas M. R. (1970) Experiments and experiences with Bay Va 1470 (Rompun) in cattle of Rio Grande do Sul, Brazil. *Vet. Med. Rev.* No. **2**, 131.

Bolz W. (1970) The prophylaxis and therapy of prolapse and paralysis of the penis occurring in the horse after the administration of neuroleptics. *Vet. Med. Rev.* (Leverkusen) **4**, 255.

Booth N. H. (1977) Intravenous and other parenteral agents. In *Veterinary Pharmacology and Therapeutics* 4th ed.; eds. L. Meyer Jones, N. H. Booth and L. E. McDonald. The Iowa State University Press, Ames.

Bree M. M., Feller I. & Corssen G. (1967) Safety and tolerance of repeated anaesthesia with CI-581 (Ketamine) in monkeys. *Anesth. Analg. Curr. Res.* **46**, 596.

Britton B. J., Wood W. G. & Irving M. N. (1974) Sedation of sheep and patas monkeys with ketamine. *Lab. Anim.* **8**, 41.

Callear J. F. F. & Van Gestel J. F. C. (1973) An analysis of the results of field experiments in pigs in the UK and Eire with the combination anaesthetic azaperone and metomidate. *Vet. Rec.* **92**, 284–7.

Chen G. (1973) Sympathomimetic anaesthetics. *Canad. Anaesth. Soc. J.* **20**, 180.

Child K. J., Davis B., Dodds M. G. *et al* (1972) Anaesthetic, cardiovascular and respiratory effects of the new steroidal agent CT 1341: a comparison with other intravenous anaesthetic drugs in the unrestrained cat. *Br. J. Pharmacol.* **46**, 189.

Clarke K. W. (1969) Effect of azaperone on the blood pressure and pulmonary ventilation in pigs. *Vet. Rec.* **85**, 649.

Clarke K. W. & Hall L. W. (1969) 'Xylazine' — a new sedative for horses and cattle. *Vet. Rec.* **85**, 512.

Clarke K. W. & Hall L. W. (1975) New steroids in veterinary anaesthesia. *World Vet. Cong. Proc.* **2**, 1679.

Combie J., Dougherty J., Nugent E. *et al* (1979) The pharmacology of narcotic analgesics in the horse. IV. Dose and time response relationships for behavioural responses to morphine, meperidine, pentazocine, anileridine, methadone and hydromorphone. *J. Eq. Med. Surg.* **3**, 77.

Conner G. H., Coppock R. W. & Beck C. C. (1974) Laboratory use of CI-744, a cataleptoid anaesthetic, in sheep. *Vet. Med. S.A.C.* **69**, 479.

Cox J. E. (1973) Immobilisation and anaesthesia of the Pig. *Vet. Rec.* **92**, 143.

Cox J. E., Done S. H., Lees P. *et al* (1975) Preliminary studies of the actions of alphaxalone and alphadolone in the pig. *Vet. Rec.* **97**, 497.

Cox J. E. & Meese G. B. (1973) The use of Large Animal Immobilon in pigs. *Vet. Rec.* **93**, 354–8.

Daniel M. & Ling C. M. (1972) The effect of an etorphine–acepromazine mixture on the heart rate and blood pressure of the horse. *Vet. Rec.* **90**, 336.

Darneley A. H. (1980) Side effect of azaperone injection in young boars. *Pig. Vet. Soc. Proc.* **6**, 75.

Denny H. R. & Lucke J. N. (1977) Anaesthetic and surgical technique for bilateral adrenalectomy in stress sensitive pigs. *Res. Vet. Sci.* **23**, 372.

Dimigen J. & Reetz I. (1970) Versuche zur Schmerzausschaltung beim Schwein mit dem neuroleptikum azaperon und dem hypnotikum metomidat. 1. *Mitteilung, Dtsch. Tierärztl. Wschr.* **77**, 470.

Dimigen V. J. (1972) Die anaesthesie mit der Kombination Metomidat/Azaperon andaßlich der eberkastration. *Dtsch. Tierärztl. Wschr.* **79**, 102.

Dobbs H. E. & Ling C. M. (1972) The use of etorphine/acepromazine in the horse and donkey. *Vet. Rec.* **91**, 40.

Dobbs H. E. & Ling C. M. (1973) Reversible immobilisation and analgesia in the bullock. *Vet. Rec.* **93**, 11.

Dos Santos M. & Bogan J. A. (1974) The metabolism of pentobarbitone in sheep. *Res. Vet. Sci.* **17**, 226.

Ducker M. J. & Boyd J. S. (1972) The successful use of etorphine hydrochloride/diprenorphine hydrochloride in sheep. *Vet. Rec.* **91**, 458.

Dun F. (1895) *Veterinary medicines their action and uses,* 9th edn., p. 545–52. David Douglas, Edinburgh.

Eales F. A. (1976) Effects of Saffan administered intravenously in the horse. *Vet. Rec.* **99**, 270.

Fessl L. (1970) Clinical experiences with Bay Va 1470 (Rompun). *Vet. Med. Rev. No.* **3**, 199.

Ford E. J. H. (1951) Some observations on the use of thiopentone in large animals. *Vet. Rec.* **63**, 636.

Fraser A. F. (1971) Boar semen sampling by electro-ejaculation. *Vet. Rec.* **88**, 208.

Fuentes V. O. & Tellez E. (1974) Ketamine dissociative analgesia in the cow. *Vet. Rec.* **94**, 482.

Fuentes V. O. & Tellez E. (1976) Mid-line Caesarian section in a cow using ketamine anaesthesia. *Vet. Rec.* **99**, 338.

Gabel A. A., Hamlin R. & Smith E. (1964) Effects of promazine and chloral hydrate on the cardiovascular system of the horse. *Am. J. Vet. Res.* **25**, 1151.

Gardner P. L. (1971) The use of Immobilon in pigs. *Vet. Rec.* **89**, 148.

Garner H. E., Amend J. F. & Rosborough J. P. (1971) Effects of BAY VA 1470 on cardiovascular parameters in ponies. *Vet. Med. Small. Anim. Clin.* **71**, 1016.

Glen J. B., Davies G. E., Thomson D. S. *et al* (1978) Adverse reactions to intravenous anaesthetics in animals. In *Adverse Response to Intravenous Drugs,* J. Watkins and A. Milford Ward (eds.) Academic Press. New York.

Green C. J. (1979) *Animal Anaesthesia. Laboratory Animal Handbooks 8.* Laboratory Animals Ltd., London.

Grono L. R. (1966) Methohexital sodium anaesthesia in the horse. *Aust. Vet. J.* **42**, 398.

Hall L. W. (1960) The effect of chlorpromazine on the cardiovascular system of the conscious horse. *Vet. Rec.* **72**, 85.

Hall L. W. (1971) *Wright's Veterinary Anaesthesia and Analgesia,* 7th edn., Baillière Tindall, London.
Hall L. W. (1972) Althesin in the larger animal. *Postgrad. Med. J.* (Suppl. 2) **48,** 55.
Hansson C. H. (1957) Clinical observations on casting horses and cows with succinylcholine. *Nord. Vet. Med.* **9,** 753.
Hapke V. H. J. & Prigge E. (1972) Herz-und kreislaufwirkungen von azaperon (stresnil). *Dtsch. Tierärztl. Wschr.* **79,** 500.
Harrison F. A. (1964) The anaesthesia of sheep using pentobarbitone sodium and cyclopropane. In *Small Animal Anaesthesia,* p. 149, ed. O. Graham-Jones. Pergamon Press, Oxford.
Harthoorn A. M. (1965) The use of a new oripavine derivative for restraint of domestic hoofed animals. *J. S.Af. Vet. Med. Assoc.* **36,** 45.
Harthoorn A. M. & Bligh J. (1965) The use of a new oripavine derivative with potent morphine-like activity for the restraint of hoofed wild animals. *Res. Vet. Sci.* **6,** 290.
Heath R. B. & Gabel A. A. (1970) Evaluation of thiamylal sodium, succinylcholine, and glyceryl guaicolate prior to inhalation anaesthesia in horses. *J. Am. Vet. Med. Assoc.* **157,** 1486.
Hillidge C. J. & Lees P. (1971a) Metomidate azaperone anaesthesia in the horse: a clinical and pharmacological study. *Proc. Assoc. Vet. An. G.Br. and Ir.* **3,** 84.
Hillidge C. J. & Lees P. (1971b) Preliminary investigations of the actions of Immobilon in the horse. *Vet. Rec.* **89,** 280.
Hillidge C. J. & Lees P. (1975a) Influence of the neuroleptanalgesic combination of etorphine and acepromazine on the horse: blood gases and acid-base balance, *Eq. Vet. J.* **7,** 148.
Hillidge C. J. & Lees P. (1975b) Influence of neuroleptanalgesia on cardiovascular, respiratory and metabolic functions in the horse. *Proc. 20th World Vet. Cong.* p. 734.
Hillidge C. J. & Lees P. (1976) Influence of etorphine, acepromazine and diprenorphine on cardiovascular function in ponies. *Br. J. Pharmacol.* **56,** 375P.
Hillidge C. J. & Lees P. (1978) Actions of diprenorphine in ponies. *Proc. Assoc. Vet. Clin. Pharmacol. Therap.* **3,** 53.
Hillidge C. J., Lees P. & Serrano L. (1973) Investigations of azaperone/metomidate anaesthesia in the horse. *Vet. Rec.* **93,** 307.
Hillidge C. J., Lees P. & Serrano L. (1975) Influence of azaperone and metomidate on cardiovascular and respiratory functions in the pony. *Br. Vet. J.* **131,** 50.
Hillidge C. J., Lees P. & Serrano L. (1977) Chemical restraining agents in the horse. *Vet. Rec.* **101,** 174.
Hoffman P. E. (1974) Clinical evaluation of xylazine as a chemical restraining agent sedative and analgesic in horses. *J. Am. Vet. Med. Assoc.* **164,** 42.
Jackson L. L. & Lundvall R. L. (1972) Effect of glyceryl guaicolate–thiamylal sodium solution on respiratory function and various hematologic factors of the horse. *J. Am. Vet. Med. Assoc.* **161,** 164.
Jenkins J. T., Crooks J. L., Charlesworth C. *et al* (1972) The use of etorphine-acepromazine (analgesic tranquilliser) mixtures in horses. *Vet. Rec.* **90,** 207.
Jones R. S. (1972) A review of tranquillisation and sedation in large animals. *Vet. Rec.* **90,** 613.
Kerr D. D., Jones E. W., Huggins K. *et al* (1972a) Sedative and other effects of xylazine given intravenously in horses. *Am. J. Vet. Res.* **33,** 525.
Kerr D. D., Jones E. W., Holbert D. *et al* (1972b) Comparison of the effects of xylazine and acetylpromazine maleate in the horse. *Am. J. Vet. Res.* **33,** 777.
King J. M. & Klingel H. (1965) The use of the oripavine derivative M.99 for the restraint of equine animals and its antagonism with related compound M.285. *Res. Vet. Sci.* **6,** 447.
Král E. Nêmeĉek L. & Pavlica J. (1970) Rompun with Methadon in horse surgery. *Vet. Med. (Praha)* **15,** 401.
Lees P. & Hillidge C. J. (1975) Neuroleptanalgesia and cardiovascular function in the horse. *Eq. Vet. J.* **7,** 1.

Lees P. & Serrano L. (1976) Effects of azaperone on cardiovascular and respiratory functions in the horse. *Br. J. Pharmac.* **56,** 263.

Lees P. & Meredith M. J. (1978) Clinical pharmacology of azaperone/ketamine combinations in the pig. *AVCPT Proceedings* **3,** 62.

Livingston A. & Waterman A. E. (1978) The development of tolerance to ketamine in rats and the significance of hepatic metabolism. *Br. J. Pharmacol.* **64,** 63.

Lucke J. N. & Sansom J. (1979) Penile erection in the horse after acepromazine. *Vet. Rec.* **105,** 21.

Mackenzie G. & Snow D. M. (1977) An evaluation of chemical restraining agents in the horse. *Vet. Rec.* **101,** 30.

Marsboom R. & Symoens J. (1968) Azaperone (R 1929) as a sedative for pigs. *Neth. J. Vet. Sci.* **1,** 125.

Martin J. E. & Beck J. D. (1956) Some effects of chlorpromazine hydrochloride in horses. *Am. J. Vet. Res.* **17,** 678.

McCashin F. B. & Gabel A. A. (1971) Rompun — a new sedative with analgesic properties. *Proc. Am. Assoc. Equine Pract.* 111.

McCashin F. B. & Gabel A. A. (1975) Evaluation of xylazine as a sedative and preanaesthetic in horses. *Am. J. Vet. Res.* **36,** 1421.

Meredith M. J. & Lees P. (1979) Problems associated with the intraperitoneal administration of metomidate in the pig. *Pig. Vet. Soc. Proc.* **4,** 61.

Mitchell B. (1972) Personal communication to R. J. Bywater. Central nervous system depressants recently introduced for veterinary use. In *Vet. Annual* Grunsell C.S.G. and Hill F. W. G. eds. John Wright, Bristol.

Mitchell B. (1978) Chemical restraint in ruminants. *Proc. AVCPT* **3,** 55.

de Moor A. & van den Hende C. (1968) Effect of propionylpromazine, promethazine and atropine on packed cell volume and circulating red cell mass in horses and cattle. *Zbl. Vet. Med. A.* **15,** 544.

Muir W. W. & Hamlin R. L. (1975) Effects of acetylpromazine on ventilating variables in the horse. *Am. J. Vet. Res.* **36,** 1439.

Muir W. W., Skarda R. T. & Milne D. W. (1977) Evaluation of xylazine and ketamine hydrochloride for anaesthesia in horses. *Am. J. Vet. Res.* **38,** 195.

Muir W. W., Skarda R. T. & Sheenan W. C. (1978) Cardiopulmonary effects of narcotic agonists and a partial agonist in the horse. *Am. J. Vet. Res.* **39,** 1632.

Orr J. A., Manohar M. & Will J. A. (1976) Cardiopulmonary effects of the combination of neuroleptic azaperone and hypnotic metomidate in swine. *Am. J. Vet. Res.* **37,** 1305.

Owen L. N. & Neal P. A. (1957) Sedation with chlorpromazine in the horse. *Vet. Rec.* **69,** 413.

Pearson H. & Weaver B.M.Q. (1978) Priapism after sedation, neuroleptanalgesia and anaesthesia in the horse. *Eq. Vet. J.* **10,** 85.

Perry J. S. (1964) Anaesthesia of the adult sow. In *Small Animal Anaesthesia,* O. Graham-Jones (ed.), p. 155 Pergamon, Oxford.

Poyser M. R. (1971) Prevention of excitement in pigs. *Vet. Rec.* **89,** 676.

Rafferty G. C. (1976) Immobilon/Revivon in the bull. *Vet. Rec.* **98,** 18.

Roberts D. (1968) The role of glyceryl guaicolate in a balanced equine anaesthetic. *Vet. Med. Small Anim. Clin.* **63,** 157.

Roberts F. W. (1971) Anaesthesia in pigs: intramuscular ketamine as an induction agent. *Anaesthesia* **26,** 445.

Roztočil V., Němeĉek L. & Pavlica J. (1971a) The use of the sedative stresnil and the hypnotic hypnodil for operations in pigs. *Vet. Med. (Praha)* **16,** 591.

Roztočil V., Němeĉek L. & Pavlica J. (1971b) Stresnil as a sedative in horses. *Vet. Med. (Praha)* **16,** 613.

Roztočil V., Němeĉek L., Pavlica J. *et al* (1972) Effects of the combination of stresnil and hypnodil in the horse. *Acta Vet. Brno.* **41.** 271.

Sagner G., Hoffmeister S. & Kronenberg G. (1968) Pharmakoligische Grundlagen eines neuartigen Präparates fur die Analgesie, Sedation and Relaxation in der Veterinarmedizin (Bay Va 1470). *Dtsch. Tierärztl. Wschr.* **75**, 565.

Sagner G., Hoffmeister F. & Kronenberg G. (1969) Pharmacological principles of a new preparation for analgesia, sedation and relaxation in veterinary medicine (Bay Va 1470). *Vet. Med. Rev.* No. **3**, 226.

Schatzman U. (1974) The induction of general anaesthesia in the horse with glyceryl guaicolate. Comparison when used alone and with sodium thiamylal (Suritol). *Eq. Vet. J.* **6**, 164.

Schlarmann B., Görlitz B. P., Wintzer M. J. *et al* (1973) Clinical pharmacology of an etorphine-acepromazine preparation: experiments in dogs and horses. *Am. J. Vet. Res.* **34**, 411.

Scorer J. W. (1977) Death of a bull under Immobilon. *Vet. Rec.* **100**, 326.

Serrano L. & Lees P. (1976) The applied pharmacology of azaperone in ponies. *Res. Vet. Sci.* **20**, 316.

Straub O. C. (1971) Anaesthesie beim schaf durch Rompun. *Dtsche. Tierärztl. Wschr.* **78**, 537.

Tavernor W. D. (1963) A study of the effect of phencyclidine in the pig. *Vet. Rec.* **75**, 1377.

Tavernor W. D. (1964a) The use of phenylcyclohexylpiperidine hydrochloride in the pig. In *Small Animal Anaesthesia*. Pergamon, Oxford.

Tavernor W. D. (1964b) Muscle relaxants in veterinary practice. *Vet. Rec.* **76**, 718.

Tavernor W. D. & Lees P. (1970) The influence of thiopentone and suxamethonium on cardiovascular and respiratory function in the horse. *Res. Vet. Sci.* **11**, 45.

Tavernor W. D. (1970) The influence of guaicol glycerol ether on cardiovascular and respiratory function in the horse. *Res. Vet. Sci.* **11**, 91.

Taylor P., Hopkins L., Young M. *et al* (1972) Ketamine anaesthesia in the pregnant sheep. *Vet. Rec.* **90**, 35.

Thurman J. C., Nelson D. R. & Christie C. J. (1972) Ketamine anaesthesia in swine. *J. Am. Vet. Med. Assoc.* **160**, 1325.

Thurman J. C., Kumar A. & Ling R. P. (1973) Evaluation of ketamine hydrochloride as an anaesthetic in sheep. *J. Am. Vet. Med. Assoc.* **162**, 293.

Tobin T. (1978) Pharmacology review: narcotic analgesics and the opiate receptors in the horse. *J. Eq. Med. Surg.* **1**, 397.

Tremblay E., Colombel M. C. & Jacob L. (1976) Precipitation et prévention de l'abstinence chez le Rat la Souris en etat de dépendence aiguë. Comparison de la naloxone, de la naltrexone et de la diprenorphine. *Psychopharmacol.* **49**, 41.

Tyagi R. P. S., Arnold T. P., Usenik E. A. *et al* (1964) Effects of thiopental sodium (Pentothal sodium) anesthesia on the horse. *Cornell Vet.* **54**, 584.

Vaughan L. C. (1961) Anaesthesia in the pig. *Br. Vet. J.* **117**, 383.

Ward G. S., Johnsen D. O. & Roberts C. R. (1974) The use of CI-744 as an anaesthetic for laboratory animals. *Lab. Anim. Sci.* **24**, 737.

Waterman A. & Livingston A. (1978a) Some physiological effects of ketamine in sheep. *Res. Vet. Sci.* **25**, 225.

Waterman A. & Livingston A. (1978b) The influence of ketamine and other intravenous anaesthetic agents on cerebral blood flow in sheep. *J. Vet. Pharmacol. Ther.* **1**, 205.

Wheat J. D. (1966) Penile paralysis in stallions given propiopromazine. *J. Am. Vet. Med. Assoc.* **148**, 405.

22

Effects of drugs on performance of the horse

J. SANFORD

Discussion of the effect of drugs on performance often involves two assumptions: firstly that the performance is competitive and secondly that drugs are administered with intent. These assumptions are too narrow to cover the current situation, where drugs may be given inadvertently and where performance may be materially altered other than at a race or competitive event — at the time of sale for instance.

It is also necessary to differentiate between substances which can be expected to modify performance in a pharmacological or clinical sense and substances which racing authorities, such as the Jockey Club, consider to be able to affect performance. The basis of the Jockey Club concept will be considered later, but in essence their list includes all substances which could, when given in appropriate amount, affect performance, irrespective of the quantity actually detected. Virtually all substances foreign to the body, some endogenous hormones used therapeutically and some constituents of feedstuffs are included in the list.

Possible means of improving performance by drugs

Improvement in competitive performance may be either an improvement in speed, an improvement in agility and co-ordination, or a combination of the two. Improved speed may involve also a lessening in fatigue or a more speedy recovery between events, while improvement in agility and co-ordination could confer a variety of practical advantages: easier starting from stalls, better jumping, better control at dressage, less disturbance during travelling and so on.

If, as is so often the case, a horse develops some minor disability, better performance may consist essentially of overcoming this defect. This is particularly the case for the musculoskeletal system and the extensive use of phenylbutazone in show jumpers underlines the importance of this corrective therapy. It has been argued that administration of drugs for this purpose should be ethically acceptable and, in the USA, some state racing

495

boards have permitted medication in specified horses, which are then tested to show the presence rather than the absence of drugs.

Improving performance by the use of drugs may involve actions both on the central nervous, the cardiovascular or the respiratory system and to improve metabolism, particularly in the skeletal muscles and liver. These effects will now be discussed in detail.

Central nervous system

Stimulants

The use of stimulants of the CNS is traditionally associated with doping to improve performance and experimental work has been carried out with amphetamine and similar compounds. Running speed in various tests has been increased by amphetamine and methylamphetamine (Stewart 1972b, Aitken *et al* 1973, Sanford 1974), methylphenidate (Sanford 1974), pemoline (Sanford 1974), and caffeine (Fujii *et al* 1972, Sanford 1974).

Other CNS stimulants which have been shown to have cardiovascular stimulant effects but no clear associated increase in running speed include ephedrine, etamiphylline and nitroglycerin. The latter has been examined as it formed one of the ingredients of a traditional doping mixture which also included strychnine.

Procaine has been shown to have stimulant effects when infused intravenously (Tobin *et al* 1977a) but is is doubtful whether this compound would have much practical use as a doping agent. Theobromine, which has given rise to several Stewards' enquiries in recent years, may be suspected of stimulant properties but, in the author's hands, it failed to produce any significant effect in oral doses up to 8 mg/kg.

Depressants

A wide variety of CNS depressants may be used effectively to depress performance. The phenothiazine tranquillisers (Carey & Sanford 1966, Stewart 1972b, Fujii *et al* 1975) have been studied extensively and have been shown to reduce running speed and co-ordination if given in sufficient doses. The butyrophenone tranquillisers, such as azaperone, have similar effects. Barbiturates, as would be expected, reduce speed although Fujii *et al* (1975) found that phenobarbitone had no demonstrable effect in their tests in subcutaneous doses up to 3 g (approximately 6 mg/kg).

Morphine and etorphine show evidence of increasing speed in low doses but they impair speed and co-ordination as the dose is increased. The author has found that prednisolone has a variable effect on speed and co-ordination and was able to find no evidence for a so-called euphoric effect of this corticosteroid.

The locomotor activity of horses dosed with narcotic analgesics has been studied by Tobin and his colleagues (Combie *et al* 1981). Locomotion was assessed by counting steps over a two minute period with the subject contained in a 16 m² box stall. Using this technique it was found that morphine (2.4 mg/kg i.,v.) and fentanyl (0.02 mg/kg i.v.) both gave an increase in activity which was antagonised by naloxone. Although these tests give useful information on the effects of various classes of compound on spontaneous activity in a confined space, they can in no way be regarded as indicative of changes in racing performance.

Cardiovascular system

Many drugs may affect heart rate and blood pressure but these actions do not in themselves imply an improvement in cardiovascular function during exercise. The rate of deceleration of heart and respiratory rates after strenuous exercise has been used as a measure of the state of fitness of the horse and of the effects of drugs during exercise (Bannister & Purvis 1968, Mackay Smith 1968, Stewart 1972a, Aitken *et al* 1973). Reports on the effects of drugs on physiological changes during exercise have been reviewed by Sanford & Aitken (1975). It was concluded that, in general, effective stimulants cause increases in heart and respiratory rates proportional to their effects on running speed. Only caffeine showed evidence of increased speed without a prolongation of recovery time, although Fujii *et al* (1972) noted some retardation of post–exercise deceleration with this compound. Many compounds including amphetamine, methylphenidate, etorphine and acepromazine affect heart rate before and during exercise, but the significance of such changes in terms of differences in performance is not known.

Musculoskeletal system

Drugs affecting this system include corticosteroids and the non-steroidal anti-inflammatory agents. These compounds are used to restore normal performance in horses debilitated by some injury to joints, tendons, or muscles and their effect is achieved by an anti-inflammatory action and, to some extent in the case of many of the non-steroidal agents, by the relief of pain. The short-term efficacy of such treatment is not in any doubt, although the long-term merits are more questionable. The cynical comment that corticosteroids allow the patient to walk to the post-mortem room is an overstatement, but it is always pertinent to ask whether the affected joint or muscle would not benefit more from the rest it would be given if treatment were not applied.

Non-steroidal anti-inflammatory agents, particularly phenylbutazone, are in wide use in show jumpers and there are many people who believe that such use is justified. In racing, on the other hand, no exemption is made in the rules for this group of drugs, although phenylbutazone is permitted by some state racing boards in the USA.

It is not profitable to consider here the ethics of this situation, involving, as it does, a critical examination of the whole edifice of competitive sport where what is or is not permissible is largely a matter of opinion. There are few, however, who would not condemn the use of anti-inflammatory agents to mask unsoundness in a horse offered for sale.

Corticosteroids

Corticosteroids are usually given either by intramuscular injection to exert a systemic effect, or by direct intra-articular injection to obtain a local effect within an inflamed joint. A wide variety of compounds and formulations may be used, giving effects which may last from a few hours to several weeks.

Water-soluble salts, such as prednisolone sodium phosphate, are short-acting and undergo rapid metabolism and excretion. Esters such as acetates and propionates have a much more persistent action due largely to retention at the site of injection. The plasma half-life of free corticosteroids is not more than a few hours and persistence of effect, with continued presence in urine, is due to retention both at sites of injection and at sites of action. Extensive protein binding also contributes to corticosteroid persistence in the body.

Houdeshell (1969) examined the effects of a mixed preparation given by intra-articular injection to 181 horses. The preparation contained a rapidly-acting soluble salt, betamethasone sodium phosphate (3 mg/ml), and a long-acting soluble ester, betamethasone acetate (12 mg/ml). Relief of pain was apparent within 12 hours and the effects lasted for three weeks or more. The same mixture was used by Van Pelt *et al* (1970) in eight horses. These authors stressed that the action was essentially palliative and that therapy should include rest with the avoidance of any further trauma. With proper use, beneficial effects might persist for several months before a further injection was needed. The persistence in urine of various corticosteroid metabolites has recently been reviewed by Chapman *et al* (1977).

Non-steroidal anti-inflammatory agents

These compounds produce similar beneficial effects to those of the corticosteroids. Since they are well absorbed from the gut they are usually given orally as a powder in the feed. There is no pharmacological advantage in administration by injection and binding to muscle protein at the site of injection will lead to more prolonged but less predictable effects. Elimination will also be prolonged (Moss 1972).

Although phenylbutazone is the drug most commonly used in horses, several other compounds of this class produce similar effects. These include sodium meclofenamate, naproxen, and flunixin (recently introduced in the UK for equine use) and indomethacin. There is no good evidence to suggest that phenylbutazone and related drugs can improve performance in a sound horse, their action depending entirely on their anti-inflammatory and pain-relieving properties. The action of phenylbutazone persists for as long as the compound is present at the site of inflammation at an effective concentration. This may be longer and more consistent than plasma levels would suggest (Duggan *et al* 1972).

Some years ago the practical possibility of using an anti-inflammatory agent to mask unsoundness in a horse at the time of sale led to demands for a blood test for phenylbutazone and to offers to perform such a test. It was pointed out at the time that blood was less suitable than urine for the detection of this compound and also that a test which only detected phenylbutazone would hardly be adequate to cover the large number of compounds available to a potential 'doper'. Discussions led to the conclusion that the effects of medication were likely to wear off within a few days of sale, and that samples could be discarded if no unsoundness had developed after ten days of normal work (*see* correspondence in *Vet. Rec.*, Jan–Feb 1972).

Local anaesthetics

Local anaesthetic agents may also be used to improve performance by the relief of musculoskeletal pain. In the horse, procaine or lignocaine may be used to produce nerve blocks or injected directly into inflamed joints (Tobin *et al* 1977b). Tobin *et al* (1977a) have shown that, whether administered as a local anaesthetic or as procaine penicillin, the subsequent fate of procaine in the body is similar and it is therefore impossible to distinguish between these two uses on the basis of a single blood or urine sample. The persistence of procaine penicillin suspension at the site of injection makes it likely that procaine in this form will be present in the body for longer than when it is administered as the hydrochloride —the usual salt used in local anaesthetic preparations.

Muscles and metabolism

It seems possible that increased performance could be obtained by improving muscular function during exercise. This might be achieved either by promoting greater activity or by increasing efficiency and so delaying the onset of fatigue. It may also be possible to increase muscle mass by the use of anabolic agents in addition to the normal training programme.

Muscle metabolism

Anderson (1975a) has examined muscle metabolites produced in the horse during exercise. These are influenced by diet, both carbohydrates and free fatty acids acting as fuel for exercising muscle. Provision of additional energy-giving substrates might be expected to aid performance, but to be effective these must be given shortly before racing. Infusions of red blood cells to increase the oxygen-carrying capacity of the blood during severe exercise may also be given, although the value of this practice is doubtful.

Strenuous exercise, particularly if prolonged, results in the release into the bloodstream of muscle enzymes, including creatine phosphokinase, lactic dehydrogenase, and aldolase (Anderson 1975b). It has been shown (Wagner & Critz 1968) that prednisolone reduces the loss of cellular enzymes during exercise in dogs. Anderson demonstrated a similar effect of prednisolone in the horse following intramuscular injection (0.3 mg/kg) two hours before running. It is not known whether such treatment would aid performance, but it might benefit a debilitated or poorly trained horse.

An increase in energy-producing substances in the blood follows the injection of catecholamines (Anderson & Aitken 1977). Isoprenaline produced large increases in lactate and free fatty acids, but no change in blood glucose; adrenaline increased all three substrates. These effects are accompanied by tachycardia and profuse sweating and it should not be concluded that injections of catecholamines would necessarily aid performance.

Further studies of the metabolic actions of adrenoceptor agonists and antagonists have been carried out more recently by Snow (1979a). This author examined the effects of various antagonists in modifying the actions of infused adrenaline. He concluded that lipolysis and hyperglycaemia were mediated through β-adrenoceptors; this finding was in contrast to that of Anderson & Aitken (1977) who obtained no hyperglycaemic response to the injection of the β agonist isoprenaline. In an investigation of the effects of the β-adrenoceptor blocking drugs, propranolol and metoprolol in exercised horses, Snow *et al* (1979) found that both compounds reduced exercise-induced tachycardia and also reduced gallop speeds. Exercise-induced rises in plasma glucose, glycerol and lactate were also reduced by these compounds. Snow (1979b) also noted that horses appeared more lethargic under the influence of these β-antagonists, which he attributed to a central effect.

Apart from the value of this work in furthering our understanding of the role of adrenoceptor mechanisms during exercise, some agents having effects on these systems are now being used in horses. These compounds, terbutaline and clenbuterol, are classed as β_2 agonists and may be employed to increase bronchodilatation and to reduce exercise-related bronchospasm. Snow (1979b) concluded that such compounds were unlikely to be of value in normal subjects.

There is experimental evidence that xanthines, particularly theophylline and caffeine, diminish muscle fatigue and this may contribute to an improvement in performance (Huidobro 1945).

Anabolic agents

These agents have been widely used to enhance performance although the mode of action and effectiveness of this therapy are still not clear. Primarily the anabolic action should result in an increase in skeletal muscle mass, but the extent of this effect is likely to be small in healthy mature horses. It has also been suggested that there may be a secondary central stimulant effect related to the androgenic nature of these compounds. Effects appear to be greatest in growing animals. Evidence suggests that much of the increase in muscle size is due to increased water content, rather than to an actual increase in muscle protein. Reports by Stihl (1968) and Dietz *et al* (1974) suggest that performance of treated horses is increased. Stihl also noted increases in body weight and raised RBC count and haemoglobin. Dietz *et al* (1974) recorded changes in muscle mass but not in blood cells.

Although central stimulant effects of anabolic androgens have been suggested, limited studies carried out at Glasgow (Aitken 1974, unpublished data) with testosterone in geldings showed no change in performance or behaviour. Single doses of 50–100 mg/kg gave peak plasma levels greater than those considered normal in stallions in 0.5–2 hours; testing was carried out one hour after intramuscular injection. There was no consistent effect on speed and no behavioural changes were noted. These limited experiments are obviously inconclusive and it is possible that repeated doses over a period of several days or weeks may be needed to produce an effect.

From the evidence available at the time Snow *et al* (1977) concluded that anabolic agents have no appreciable effect in improving performance. Their use may, however, have a general beneficial effect in helping a horse to withstand the stresses of a racing season and may promote more rapid recovery from minor injuries. Recently these workers have studied the effects of eleven, once weekly, injections of nandrolone phenylpropionate on mature thoroughbred geldings in training (Snow *et al* 1982). No improvement in performance was obtained but virilising effects were noted, persisting for up to six weeks after the final injection. Detailed examination of skeletal muscle obtained by biopsy showed a lack of any marked effect of the anabolic steroid. These authors concluded that the beneficial effects which have been claimed for anabolic steroids in horses are probably not due to a myotrophic effect.

Miscellaneous agents

Prevention of epistaxis

Preparations which will effectively prevent the development of epistaxis during racing can be used to improve the performance of horses suffering from this condition. A variety of agents have been tried for this purpose but recently some success appears to have followed the prophylactic use of frusemide (furosemide), a sulphonamide-derivative diuretic. Although its mode of action in preventing epistaxis is not fully understood, it is said to reduce oedema in the lungs and airways (Veterinary-Chemist Advisory Committee 1977). Some racing authorities in the USA permit the use of frusemide shortly before a race, but it has been found (Roberts *et al* 1976) that the diuretic effect of this drug will greatly reduce the urinary concentration of phenylbutazone. If given more than four hours before racing, however, it does not appear to affect the ability to detect other drugs, including phenylbutazone.

Some years ago the author was asked to examine a styptic mixture preparation which was recommended for the prevention of epistaxis. It was not possible to comment on its efficacy for this purpose but no evidence could be found that the active ingredients, which included the alkaloids hydrastine and berberine, had any effect on the performance of healthy horses.

Vitamins and tonics

There is no good evidence that vitamins alone have any beneficial effect on performance except in states of deficiency. Possible effects on running speed following the administration of thiamine (5 mg/kg i.v.) were examined by Stewart (1972b). No consistent effect was observed on speed or on heart and respiratory rates, confirming earlier observations by Irvine & Prentice (1962).

Possible effects of mixed vitamin and tonic preparations may be due less to their vitamin content than to the other agents which they contain. One well known preparation, much used in stables, contains more than 1% caffeine as well as a small quantity of nux vomica. It is hardly surprising that such a mixture sometimes causes problems for trainers.

Tests for the examination of effects on performance

Most tests have concentrated on the measurement of speed, either by timing over a measured distance (Stewart 1972a, Fujii *et al* 1972) or by measuring speed over a set time (Aitken *et al* 1973). In most tests, horses were ridden, but in some experiments to assess changes in heart rate they were lunged in a circle. After much trial and error a series of tests were evolved which, it was believed, would give a sensitive indication of the effects of drugs on performance (Carey & Sanford 1966, Aitken *et al* 1973, Sanford 1973, 1974). A test scheme for the evaluation of the effects of centrally-acting drugs on behaviour was also devised (Aitken & Sanford 1972) but was never fully evaluated.

Tests

Racecourse test

This was run on a racecourse over a distance of 800 or 1000 metres. Horses were run singly or up to four together in a simulated race. Although this test was affected by several variables, including the weather, it proved practicable for comparative tests over short periods (4–8 days). Speed was timed over the whole length and separately over the last 200 metres.

Short gallop test

Horses were run singly over 200 or 400 metres from a flying start. The gallop was repeated after an interval of about five minutes during which the horse returned to the start at a trot or slow canter. Pulse and respiratory rates were measured before and after each run.

Indoor performance test

This was carried out in a covered riding school providing an oval circuit of approximately 100 metres circumference. Each horse ran two circuits on each rein at collected and extended trots and at a canter. Horses were run singly, circuits were timed and pulse and respiratory rates measured before and after the test. Running tests were followed by a co-ordination test which involved traversing a line of six cavalletti at walk and trot, and trotting along a lane formed by a double line of cones. After passage in each direction the cones were moved closer together to make the lane narrower. Faults were scored by counting the number of times obstacles were hit, point scores being greater when they were further apart.

Lunge test

Each horse cantered on a lunge rein in a circle approximately 17 metres diameter in the riding school. Cantering continued for 20 minutes, 10 minutes on each rein, to give a total distance of 5–5.5 km according to speed. Time per circle was recorded and the handler attempted to maintain a minimum speed for each horse without preventing it from running faster of its own accord. Respiratory rates were recorded before and for up to 50 minutes after exercise. ECGs were recorded by radiotelemetry over the same period and, in some cases, also during the period of exercise (Aitken *et al* 1973).

Methods

Each horse served as its own control and adequate training periods were allowed before the start of an experiment. Tests were carried out blind, neither riders nor observers knowing on which days drugs were given. Doses were selected which produced no obvious changes in behaviour or function since such changes would inevitably lead to withdrawal of a horse from a race. Administration before tests was aimed at obtaining peak effect at the time of the test.

Results

Racecourse tests

Methylamphetamine, 0.2 mg/kg i.m., increased speed over 800 metres in two of three horses tested. Methylphenidate, 0.5 mg/kg subcutaneously, also increased speed in two of three horses over 800 metres but only one horse maintained this improvement over the full kilometre. The third horse given methylphenidate was slower over the whole distance. Caffeine given orally at 4.0 mg/kg had no effect. It is unwise to draw firm conclusions from these tests since they were few in number and subject to wide variations in weather conditions, but the results do suggest that improvements in perfor-

Table 22.1　Gallop test 2 × 200 metres. Compounds increasing speed significantly ($p<0.05$).

Compound	Dose (mg/kg)	Route	No. tested
Methylamphetamine	0.1	i.m.	3
	0.2	i.m.	1
Methylphenidate	0.25	s.c.	4
	0.5	s.c.	4
Pemoline	4.0	Oral	4
	8.0	Oral	4
Caffeine	2.0	Oral	3
	4.0	Oral	3
	8.0	Oral	1
Phenylbutazone	6.6	i.m.*	4

*Injection made 23 hours before test.

mance may be very variable. Dosed horses were more excitable and tended to be more difficult to control at the start. Such changes in behaviour might not be apparent to those not familiar with the horse's normal temperament.

Gallop tests

Methylamphetamine, methylphenidate, pemoline and caffeine all increased speed in this test (Table 22.1). Rather surprisingly phenylbutazone also increased speed when given i.m. on the day preceding the test, although variable results were obtained when the injection was made nearer to testing. It is possible that this result indicated a degree of latent unsoundness in the test subjects.

Performance tests

Results obtained for various drugs in performance tests are shown in Table 22.2. Methylamphetamine, methylphenidate and pemoline all gave increases in speed at one or more paces but caffeine had no clear effect, although horses dosed with this substance appeared more excitable. Promazine (0.2–0.8 mg/kg i.m.) and acepromazine (0.02–0.08 mg/kg i.m.), as expected, both reduced speed in these tests. Extensive tests were not carried out with other depressants of the central nervous system as interest was primarily in compounds which might improve performance. Morphine (0.8 mg/kg s.c.) and etorphine with acepromazine (0.8 μg/kg etorphine and 3.3 μg/kg acepromazine i.m.) all increased speed in these tests.

Co-ordination was not significantly affected by stimulants but was impaired by tranquillisers and other depressants. Unexpectedly, two or

Table 22.2 Performance test. Effect of CNS stimulants on speed at trot and canter.

Compound	Dose (mg/kg)	Route	No. tested	Effect on speed at trot and canter
Methylamphetamine	0.05	i.m.	4	+ in 2/4 at extended trot
	0.1	i.m.	4	+ in 2/4 at collected trot
				+ in 4/4 at extended trot
				+ in 2/4 at canter
Methylphenidate	0.25	s.c.	4	+ in 4/4 at all paces
	0.5	s.c.	4	+ in 4/4 at all paces
Pemoline	4.0	Oral	3	+ in 3/3 at all paces
	8.0	Oral	3	+ in 3/3 at all paces
Caffeine	2.0	Oral	3	No consistent effect
	4.0	Oral	3	No consistent effect

+ = increased speed

three horses dosed with prednisolone intramuscularly showed significant improvement in co-ordination tests although this steroid had no clear effect on running speed.

Lunge tests

In these tests methylphenidate and pemoline both increased cantering speed, but cardiac deceleration time was also increased. Tests on other compounds have been reported previously (Aitken *et al* 1973). They showed that methylamphetamine had a similar action. Only caffeine increased speed without prolonging cardiac deceleration. Results are summarised in Table 22.3.

In general these tests confirm the impression that the degree of tachycardia during and after exercise is dependent on the speed of running (Sanford & Aitken 1975). It does not appear to be directly influenced by drugs in the doses used in these tests. Measurement of heart rate after

Table 22.3 Lunge test. Effects of drugs on speed and cardiac deceleration.

Compound	Dose (mg/kg)	Route	Effect on speed	Effect on cardiac deceleration time
Methylphenidate	0.5	s.c.	+	+
Pemoline	4.0–8.0	Oral	+	+
Methylamphetamine	0.4	i.m.	+	+
Caffeine	8.0	Oral	+	0
Ephedrine	4.0	Oral	$\bar{0}$	0

+ = increase, 0 = no effect, − = decrease

exercise is often confused by the development of cardiac arrhythmias when stimulant drugs have been given. Such changes have been noted for caffeine (Fujii *et al* 1972), amphetamine (Stewart 1972b), and methylphenidate.

Problems arising from drug therapy

In spite of a general awareness of Jockey Club Rules, problems still arise from unexpected positive urine samples in horses which have been treated prior to racing. With the wide range of preparations available and the increasing sensitivity of methods of detection it is difficult to suggest a clearance period which may be generally applied with confidence. Many factors affect the rate of elimination of a drug from the body so that, even when a clearance period is specified for a particular product, considerable latitude must be allowed. These factors have been reviewed with details of clearance times for a number of compounds by Moss & Clarke (1977). However cautious and qualified a general statement may be, it leads to a false sense of security which may prove unjustified.

With existing rules relating to the administration of a substance which could affect performance, it is not necessary to demonstrate (or even to believe) that the concentration of the offending substance present in the horse was high enough to exert a pharmacological effect. It is only necessary clearly to identify the presence of the substance and/or its metabolites in a sample of urine. Although the Jockey Club has been consistent in this approach for many years, the situation is still misunderstood by some trainers and their veterinary surgeons. To avoid unnecessary problems attention should be paid to the following:

1   The persistence of a drug and/or its metabolites in the urine and *not* its duration of action determines whether or not the rules have been infringed.

2   When a drug undergoes a complex pattern of metabolism, when enteric recirculation occurs, or when there is extensive binding to body tissues, individual variations in clearance times may be greater than anticipated.

3   Suspensions or oily solutions given by injection may persist for long periods at the site of injection with consequent slow elimination from the body.

4   Clearance times depend on the form, formulation, and method of administration of a preparation as well as on the active principle which it contains.

5   Local application, such as topically or intra-articularly, can give rise to detectable concentrations in urine which may then persist for longer than when the same compound is given systemically.

6   Clearance times may be altered by changes in food and water intake which may affect absorption, hepatic metabolism and renal elimination.

7 Co-administration of two or more drugs may lead to interactions delaying the clearance of any or all of them.

8 Tonics and foodstuffs may contain pharmacologically active ingredients. Caffeine and theobromine have proved particularly troublesome in this respect.

In the author's experience problems with some of the following agents recur regularly. This suggests that the possibility of their occurrence is not fully appreciated.

Procaine

The presence of procaine may result from injections of procaine penicillin used to treat infections. Tobin *et al* (1977b) have shown that procaine from this source is cleared from the body in exactly the same way as procaine hydrochloride which might be administered as a stimulant or as a local anaesthetic. Thus the use of procaine penicillin in horses in training should obviously be avoided wherever possible.

Caffeine and theobromine

Caffeine is present in a number of beverages and in a widely used equine tonic. Theobromine is present in cocoa bean meal which may be used as a constituent of concentrate feeds. Since caffeine is metabolised partially to theobromine, the authorities are often reluctant to accept the presence of the latter alkaloid at its face value, but may regard it as a possible indication that caffeine was given some days previously. Caffeine-containing tonics should not be given to horses in training.

Phenylbutazone

Traces of this compound or its metabolites can often be detected in the urine for some time after its beneficial action may be considered to have ended. This is particularly the case when phenylbutazone is given by intramuscular injection.

Conclusions

Stimulants of the central nervous system can improve performance but, apart from caffeine, they are unlikely to be given inadvertently. Anabolic steroids, corticosteroids and non-steroidal anti-inflammatory agents are likely to cause the greatest ethical problems for veterinary surgeons and the extent to which it is justifiable to use these agents in horses engaged in competitive events will continue to be a matter of opinion. Veterinary surgeons whose clients may face an official enquiry should try to obtain clear factual evidence of the following:

1 How large a dose of drug was given.

2 How many doses were given.

3 When the last dose was actually given (this may be different from when it was supposed to be given).

Finally, in estimating safe clearance periods it is sensible to adopt an empirical rule of allowing *twice* the stated clearance time for the product in question.

References

Aitken M. M. & Sanford J. (1972) Comparative assessment of tranquillisers in the horse. *Proc. Assoc. Vet. Anaes.* no. 3, 20–8.

Aitken M. M., Sanford J. & McKenzie G. (1973) Factors influencing deceleration of heart and respiratory rates after exercise in the horse. *Equine Vet. J.* **5**, 8–14.

Anderson M. G. (1975a) The effect of exercise on blood metabolite levels in the horse. *Equine Vet. J.* **7**, 27–33.

Anderson M. G. (1975b) The influence of exercise on serum enzyme levels in the horse. *Equine Vet. J.* **7**, 160–5.

Anderson M. G. & Aitken M. M. (1977) Biochemical and physiological effects of catecholamine administration in the horse. *Res. Vet. Sci.* **22**, 357–60.

Banister E. W. & Purvis A. D. (1968) Exercise electrocardiography in the horse by radiotelemetry. *J. Am. Vet. Med. Assoc.* **152**, 1004–8.

Carey F. M. & Sanford J. (1966) The effect of tranquillisers on performance in the horse. *J. Physiol.* **187**, 21P.

Chapman D. I., Moss M. S. & Whiteside J. (1977) The urinary excretion of synthetic corticosteroids by the horse. *Vet. Rec.* **100**, 447–50.

Combie J., Shults T., Nugent E. C. *et al* (1981) Pharmacology of narcotic analgesics in the horse: selective blockade of narcotic-induced locomotor activity. *Am. J. Vet. Res.* **42**, 716–21.

Dietz O., Mill J. & Teuscher R. (1974) Experimentelle untersuchungen zur anwendung anaboler Steroide bei Sportpfeerden. *Monatsschr. Veterinamed* **29**, 938–40.

Duggan D. E., Hogans A. F., Kwan K. C. *et al* (1972) The metabolism of indomethacin in man. *J. Pharmacol. Exp. Therap.* **181**, 563–70.

Fujii S., Inada S., Yoshida S. *et al* (1972) Pharmacological studies on doping drugs for race horses II. Caffeine. *Jap. J. Vet. Sci.* **34**, 135–41.

Fujii S., Inada S., Yoshida S. *et al* (1975) Pharmacological studies on doping drugs for race horses: IV chlorpromazine and phenobarbital. *Jap. J. Vet. Sci.* **37**, 133–9.

Houdeshell J. W. (1969) Field trials of a new long-acting corticosteroid in the treatment of equine arthropathies. *Vet. Med.* **64**, 782–4.

Huidobro F. (1945) A comparative study of the effectiveness of 1,3,7, trimethylxanthine and certain dimethylxanthines against fatigue. *J. Pharmacol. Exp. Ther.* **84**, 380–6.

Irvine C. H. G. & Prentice N. G. (1962) The effect of large doses of thiamine on the horse. *N.Z. Vet. J.* **10**, 86–8.

Mackay-Smith M. P. (1968) TPR evaluation. *Light horse* **17**, 484.

Moss M. S. (1972) Uses and misuses of anti-inflammatory drugs in racehorses II. *Equine Vet. J.* **4**, 69–73.

Moss M. S. & Clarke E. G. C. (1977) A review of drug 'clearance times' in racehorses. *Equine Vet. J.* **9**, 53–6.

Roberts B. L., Blake J. W. & Tobin T. (1976) Effects of furosemide on plasma and urinary levels of pheylbutazone. *Res. Comm. Chem. Pharmacol.* **15**, 257–66.

Sanford J. (1973) Drugs and performance in the horse. *Proc. HBLB Conf. Res. Workers* 40–1.

Sanford J. (1974) Doping of racehorses. *Br. J. Sports Med.* **8**, 176–80.

Sanford J. & Aitken M. M. (1975) Effects of some drugs on the physiological changes during exercise in the horse. *Equine Vet. J.* **7**, 198–202.

Snow D. H. (1979a) Chemistry, metabolism and action of adrenergic agonists and antagonists in the horse. *IIIrd Int. Symp. on Equine Medication Control* (Lexington), eds. Tobin T., Blake J. W. & Woods W. F. 351–66.

Snow D. H. (1979b) Metabolic and physiological effects of adrenoceptor agonists and antagonists in the horse. *Res. Vet. Sci.* **27**, 372–78.

Snow D. H., Munro C. D. & Nimmo M. (1977) Anabolic steriods in equine practice. *Proc. 23rd Conf. Am. Assoc. Equine Practit. Ann.* 411–18.

Snow D. H., Munro C. D. & Nimmo M. (1982) The effect of nandrolone phenylproprionate in the horse. *Equine Vet. J.* (in press).

Snow D. H., Summers R. J. & Guy P. S. (1979) The actions of the β-adrenoceptor blocking agents propranolol and metoprolol in the maximally exercised horse. *Res. Vet. Sci.* **27**, 22–9.

Stewart G. A. (1972a) Drugs, performance and responses to exercise in the racehorse. 1. Physiological observations on the cardiac and respiratory responses. *Aust. Vet. J.* **48**, 537–43.

Stewart G. A. (1979b) Drugs, performance and responses to exercise in the racehorse. 2. Observations on amphetamine, promazine and thiamine. *Aust. Vet. J.* **48**, 544–47.

Stihl Von H. G. (1968) Uber die Anwendung eines anabolen Steroides in der Pferdepraxis. *Berl. Munch. Tieraztl. Wschr.* **81**, 378–82.

Tobin T., Blake J.W., Sturma L. *et al* (1977a) Pharmacology of procaine in the horse; pharmacokinetics and behavioural effects. *Am. J. Vet. Res.* **38**, 637–47.

Tobin T. Tai C. Y., O'Leary J. *et al* (1977b) Pharmacology of procaine in the horse; evidence against the existence of a 'procaine-penicillin' complex. *Am. J. Vet. Res.* **38**, 437–42.

Van Pelt R. W., Tillotson P. J. & Gertsen K. E. (1970) Intra-articular injection of betamethasone in arthritis in horses. *J. Am. Vet. Med. Ass.* **156**, 1589–99.

Veterinary Chemist Advisory Committee NASRC (1977) Report. In *J. Am. Vet. Med. Assoc.* **170**, 1399.

Wagner J. A. & Critz J. B. (1968) The effect of prednisolone on the serum creatine phosphokinase response to exercise. *Proc. Soc. Exp. Biol. Med.* **128**, 716–20.

23

Equine colic: causes, diagnosis and treatment

E. L. GERRING

Colic is acute abdominal pain whose characteristic is to wax and wane in concert with smooth muscle contractile activity. This broad definition of colic is narrowed in this context to pain emanating from the gastrointestinal tract. The clinical features of alimentary pain in the horse show a wide diversity of type and this reflects the underlying pathogenesis. Colic may be broadly classified into five types: *spasmodic* in which there is an increase in bowel motor activity; *impactive* in which motility is reduced and the lumen becomes obstructed with dry fibrous contents; *obstructive* in which the passage of ingesta is prevented by major injury to the bowel often resulting from strangulation of the vascular supply from a variety of causes; *flatulent* in which the accumulation of gas in the bowel also gives rise to pain; and finally *idiopathic* in which there are no obvious lesions, even at laparotomy, to account for the pain experienced by the horse.

This unusual predeliction of the alimentary tract to conditions giving rise to serious illness is unique to the equine species. Most horses will recover from an episode of colic with medical treatment, but this condition is still the largest single cause of death in horses (Baker & Ellis 1981, Tennant *et al* 1972). The role of infection with the red worm *Strongylus vulgaris* in the pathogenesis of colic is difficult to evaluate. While almost all horses carry a strongyle burden, the incidence of emboli in resected operative specimens is low (Pearson *et al* 1971). It may be that the lesions are present in the terminal vascular tree within the gut wall rather than more obviously in the larger vessels supplying the bowel. However, Kester (1975) believes that thrombo-embolic lesions arising directly from strongyle damage to vessel walls, notably the cranial mesenteric artery, are the root cause of most colic episodes.

The life cycle of *S. vulgaris* is complex (Ogbourne & Duncan 1977). Eggs hatch on pasture to produce first stage larvae, which then moult to produce second stage larvae and the process is repeated to produce the infective third stage larvae. The infective larva loses its sheath in the small intestine and migrates to the cranial mesenteric artery as the fourth stage. From this site they return to the caecum, where they moult to fifth stage larvae in the wall and then enter the lumen of the large bowel to become adults. Effective control of this parasite with drugs will therefore require that the anthelmintic has larvicidal properties in addition to activity against the adult worms.

Diagnosis of colic

History. The history can often be helpful — recent uncontrolled access to grain or fermented food suggesting gastric impaction. A history of vague discomfort and bouts of moderate pain over several days may indicate large intestinal impaction, whereas sudden onset of severe pain with sweating and a continually rising pulse rate often signify a small intestinal obstruction.

Age. Retained meconium affects foals in the first 2–3 days of life. Young animals from a few months to 2–3 years may be affected by massive strongyle larvae migrations damaging the gut wall, while arterial lesions are often implicated in older animals. Old horses with dental problems leading to ineffective mastication often present with large bowel impactions.

Clinical examination. All cases of colic are in pain. This may range from vague unease, lifting the hind feet alternately and looking at the flanks, to violent kicking and rolling on the floor. The degree of pain will also be reflected in the pulse rate. An increasing rate with time usually signifies a major condition requiring surgery. Surgery should certainly be undertaken if a pulse rate of 80 beats per minute is reached and maintained. Other useful indicators of the state of the circulation are the appearance of mucous membranes, especially the mouth, and the capillary refill time. Mucous membranes progress from pink through brick red to cyanotic purple. Capillary refill greater than three seconds suggests gross circulatory disturbance. Auscultation of the abdomen low on each flank will allow examination of the large colon. Caecal sounds are heard in the right sublumbar fossa; frequently the high pitched 'tinkling' of a fluid–gas interface can be detected. While greatly increased intestinal sounds are heard in spasmodic colic, there are few sounds in large bowel impaction and a silent abdomen accompanies major obstruction.

Rectal examination. Rectal examination can yield much valuable information to the experienced clinician but to less skilled veterinarians there are often only three likely conclusions. Firm impaction of the pelvic flexure of the large colon is readily identified and may be continued along the large bowel. Gas-filled coils of small intestine in the right sublumbar fossa can usually be detected in cases of obstruction proximal to the ileo-caecal valve.

Occasionally it is possible to palpate an intussusception or a tense band of mesentry associated with strangulation. In many cases, however, no firm conclusions can be drawn to aid diagnosis.

Gastric intubation. Passage of a nasogastric tube gives positive evidence either of gastric flatus or of fluid accumulation. A flow of gas from the tube confirms flatulent colic and the gastric decompression gives immediate relief of pain. When fluid flows back up the tube, it is very likely that an obstruction is present proximal to the caecum. The nasogastric tube also permits the administration of medicaments.

Packed cell volume (PCV). Probably the only simple and rapid haematological test likely to be available in field conditions is a PCV estimation. Normal values seldom exceed 45%. Increases in this parameter in cases of colic indicate dehydration. Values above 50% urgently require fluid therapy, while animals with a PCV exceeding 70% seldom survive. Serial estimations of PCV are a useful guide to the efficacy of fluid therapy.

Abdominal paracentesis. A technique for the collection of peritoneal fluid was described by Bach & Ricketts (1974). The normal pale yellow appearance of the fluid may change to amber or pink in cases of infarction, but colour changes tend to lag behind clinical features. The colour changes reflect an increasing number of polymorphonuclear cells and then haemolysis of extravasated blood. Blood and gut contents will be present where bowel rupture has occurred.

An accurate diagnosis early in the course of the disease is likely in only a small proportion of cases. Spasmodic colic, large bowel impactions, and over-eating of grain are usually readily diagnosed, but in other cases the response to initial medical treatment is a valuable aid to refining diagnosis. Those cases which do not show an improvement with medical treatment over the succeeding 3–5 hours should be referred for surgery.

Medical treatment of colic

The major factor in the management of colic is the control of pain. In addition to humanitarian needs, the horse suffering colicky pain may sustain considerable injury as a result of its violent activity. In some cases, analgesics may be required before a clinical examination can be carried out.

With the exception of spasmodic colic, when spasmolytic drugs are indicated, the further medication is less certain and depends upon the stage to which the condition has progressed. A practical system of management is

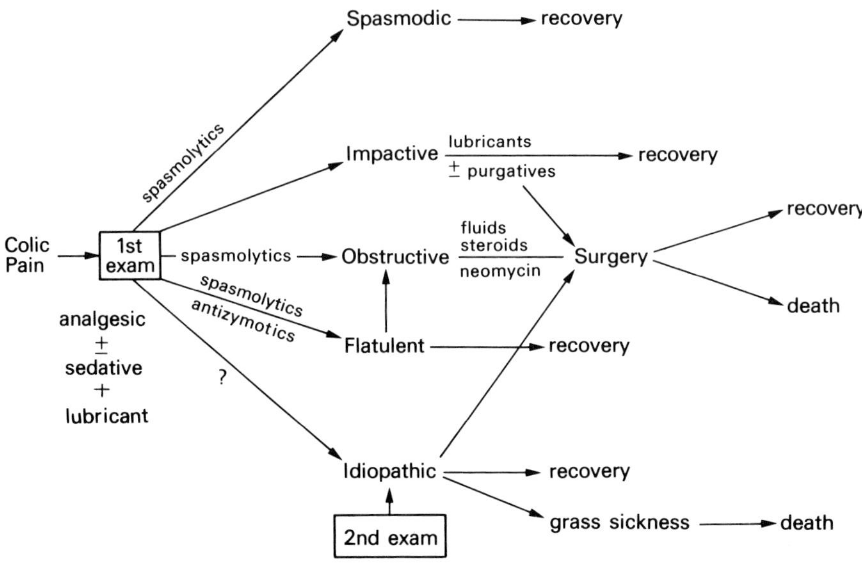

Fig. 23.1 A practical system for managing a colic case.

suggested in Fig. 23.1. At the first examination, analgesics are given with or without the addition of a sedative and a lubricant in cases where a definitive diagnosis has not been possible. At a second examination 2–4 hours later, additional information deriving from the initial treatment will often allow the case to be assigned to one of the five categories of colic and subsequent action thereby determined. Analgesic or lubricant therapy may be repeated or referral for surgery may be decided.

Good nursing is important in all colic cases. The animal should be kept warm with rugs and stable bandages, additional heat being supplied from infra red lamps if necessary. A warm bran mash should be offered and gentle walking exercise given for 5–10 minutes in every hour. The horse should not be discouraged from lying down in a deep straw bed, but should be prevented from rolling over (Seckington 1972).

Among traditional medicaments which have stood the test of time, magnesium sulphate (250 g) in 3–4 l of water, and turpentine (60 ml) with spirit of nitrous ether (30 ml) in 450 ml of linseed oil given at the first examination via the nasogastric tube are still widely used (Seckington 1972).

<h2 style="text-align:center">Drug treatment of colic (Table 23.1)</h2>

Analgesics and sedatives

Both centrally and locally-acting analgesics are used. The synthetic

Table 23.1 Drugs used in treatment of colic.

Drug classification	Agent used	Dose and route of administration	Comments
Narcotic–analgesics	Pethidine	2 mg/kg i.v. or i.m.	Short duration
	Methadone	0.1 mg/kg i.v. or i.m.	3–6 hours analgesia
	Pentazocine	1–2 mg/kg i.v. or i.m.	1–2 hour analgesia
Sedatives	Acepromazine	0.05–0.1 mg/kg i.v. or i.m.	Hypotension with higher doses
	Xylazine	1 mg/kg i.v.	Good analgesia
	Chloral hydrate	30 g in water orally	Several hours effect
Non-steroidal anti-inflammatories (NSAIDs)	Phenylbutazone	2–4 g orally or i.v.	Injectable formulation available
	Meclofenamic acid	2.2 mg/kg orally	
	Flunixin	1.1 mg/kg orally or i.v.	
Spasmolytics	Atropine	10–40 mg i.v. or i.m.	Often combined with an NSAID
	Methindizate	25–50 mg i.v. or i.m.	
	Chloradyne	6–8 ml orally	An analgesic to relax pylorus
	Lignocaine 2%	15–45 ml orally	
Lubricants	Liquid paraffin	4–8 litres orally	Via nasogastric tube
	D.O.S.S.	7–30 g orally	
Antizymotics	Chloral hydrate	10–30 g orally	May be given in water or
	Turpentine oil	30–60 ml orally	in 450 ml of raw linseed oil
	Spirit of nitrous ether	30 ml orally	
	Formalin	30 ml orally	
	Neomycin	4–8 g orally	
Purgatives	Magnesium sulphate	250 g in water orally	Only used after lubricants
	Dihydroxyanthroquinone	10–20 g	have been given
Anthelmintics	Ivermectin	200 μg/kg i.m.	Every 6–8 weeks
Crystalloid fluids	Hartmann's solution	50% of calculated deficit i.v.	Warm to body temperature before use
	0.15% NaCl + 4.5% dextrose	Subsequent maintenance i.v.	
	4.2% Sodium bicarbonate	2 m mol/kg i.v. (i.e. 2 ml/kg)	
Plasma volume expanders	Low molecular weight dextran (Rheomacrodex)	Up to 20% of blood volume i.v. but 2–3 litres often sufficient	Give some crystalloid fluid before volume expanders
	Gelatin polymer (Haemaccel)		Blood volume is approximately 8% of body weight
Corticosteroids	Betamethasone	250 mg i.v.	One large single dose not harmful,
	Dexamethasone	250 mg i.v.	can be lifesaving

morphine-like drugs, pethidine, methadone and pentazocine, act by raising the central pain threshold. Pethidine is approximately one-tenth as potent as morphine and is rapidly excreted by the kidney. Its duration of action in the horse is short; in an experimental colic model in ponies the mean duration was only 21 minutes (Lowe 1969). The maximum recommended dose is 2 mg/kg, since higher doses may result in excitement. Methadone is more potent than morphine and less likely to cause excitement in the horse (Davis & Knight 1977). It is longer-acting than pethidine — 3–6 hours analgesia resulting from a dose of 0.1 mg/kg. Pentazocine has also been used at a dose rate of 0.5–2 mg/kg and its duration of effect appears to be intermediate between pethidine and methadone (Lowe 1969).

In a recent study the actions of pethidine, methadone, acepromazine and a proprietary mixture of metamizole and hyoscine (Buscopan) were com-

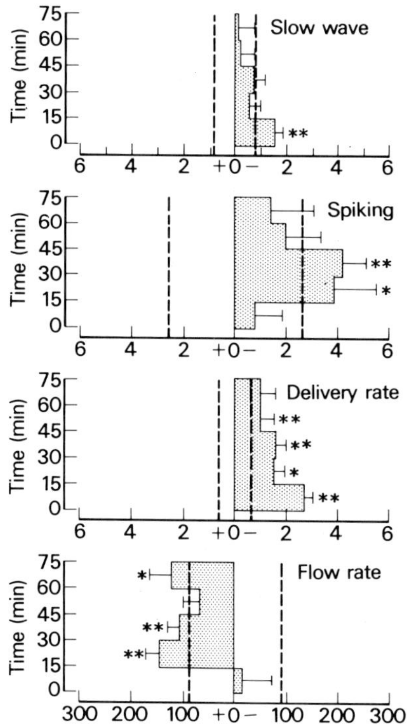

Fig. 23.2 The effect of pethidine on small intestinal motility in the horse. *Slow wave* — change in the elctrical slow wave frequency (cycles/5 min). *Spiking* — change in the incidence of spike action potentials superimposed on the slow wave. *Delivery rate* — change in the rate of delivery jets of a fluid test meal. *Flow rate* — change in the rate of transport of a test meal (ml). Each solid bar represents change per unit time from pre-injection control mean values. Vertical hatched line = s.e. of control mean. Bars = s.e.m. Injection given at time 0. *$p < 0.1$, ** $p < 0.05$. Mean results from three experiments in each of three ponies.

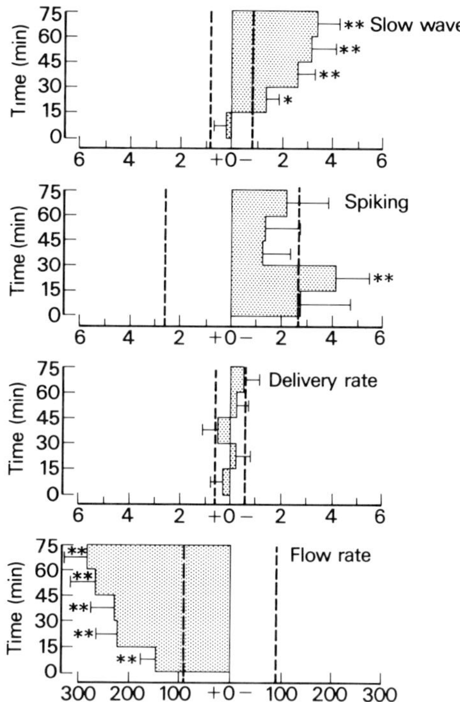

Fig. 23.3 The effect of acepromazine on small intestinal motility in the horse. Details as Fig. 23.2

pared in ponies fitted with a Thiry–Vella loop of terminal jejunum. Motor activity of the loop was recorded as spike potentials by means of paired electrodes sited close to strain gauge transducers at intervals along the loop. The T–V loop was fed from a constant head of fluid and the frequency of delivery jets and the volume of the fluid transported were recorded (Gerring & Davies 1982).

This study showed that pethidine significantly decreased motor activity but increased the transport of fluid in the loop (Fig. 23.2). A similar but more marked effect was obtained with methadone, suggesting that, in the small intestine, these drugs reduce spasm and increase transport along the gut. Buscopan had little effect upon the electrical activity of the gut and reduced both delivery jets and fluid transport.

Acepromazine had the most marked effect in this model (Fig. 23.3). Electrical slow wave activity was reduced and transport was markedly increased, suggesting an antispasmodic action. Although this experimental study was confined to the small intestine, it does suggest that acepromazine may be the drug of choice, particularly at the initial stage of treatment.

Considerable care is required in dosage, however, since acepromazine has potent α-adrenoceptor blocking actions and it may produce marked hypotension, particularly if shock subsequently supervenes. The recommended dose is 0.05 mg/kg intravenously. Significantly greater sedation is not achieved by increasing dosage but hypotension may become much more profound.

Chlorodyne, a tincture of chloroform and morphine, is used in doses of 15–45 ml in water and given orally to control pain and intestinal spasm.

Xylazine is included in this group since results in an experimental colic model, in which a balloon was inflated within the caecum of ponies via a caecostomy, suggest it to be an excellent analgesic (Lowe 1969). Doses of 2.2 mg/kg produced an hour of good analgesia. However, the drug is usually employed clinically at intravenous doses not exceeding 1.1 mg/kg. Even at these dose rates xylazine also has cardiovascular effects (Clarke & Hall 1969). Atrioventricular block and an initial hypertension are followed by hypotension, which may be due to catecholamine depletion from peripheral noradrenergic nerve endings.

Chloral hydrate produces central depression and analgesia. Given orally or intravenously in doses of 15–30 g it is metabolised to trichloroethyl alcohol and excreted by the kidney as the glucuronide conjugate, urochloralic acid. It is still a useful drug in the management of colic, its effect lasting several hours. Proquamezerine is a phenothiazine sedative which also possesses smooth muscle relaxant properties.

Non-steroidal anti-inflammatory drugs produce local analgesia by inhibiting the enzyme prostaglandin synthetase (cylco oxygenase) which is responsible for the local production of prostaglandins from arachidonic acid. Phenylbutazone, meclofenamic acid, flunixin and naproxen can be used. The former and flunixin have the advantage for colic therapy that an intravenous formulation is also available. A further member of the class, metamizole, is combined with spasmolytics in two commonly used proprietary preparations (Buscopan and Isaverin).

Spasmolytics

Drugs in this class are specific for the treatment of spasmodic colic, where pain is due to increased muscular activity and spasm of intestinal muscle. They are widely used to treat other forms of colic, but clear evidence for a beneficial action in such cases is lacking. Antispasmodics are often combined with an NSAID, two popular products containing metamizole.

Atropine (the racemic form of hyosycamine) 30–40 mg has been recommended (Seckington 1972) and hyosycamine may also be combined with metamizole (Buscopan). Methindizate is another spasmolytic used in combination with metamizole (Isaverin).

Lubricants

The most important aspect of the treatment of impactions is the use of lubricants. They are also commonly given for other types of colic in the early stages in the hope of hastening the passage of irritant material through the gut. Liquid paraffin (mineral oil) in doses of 3–8 l is given by nasogastric tube. In cases of meconium retention in new born foals, 200 ml is an appropriate dose. This is usually combined with an enema. In cases where there is no obstruction of the bowel lumen, liquid paraffin can usually be detected in rectal faeces 4–8 hours after administration. An anionic wetting agent, dioctyl sodium sulphosuccinate (DOSS), can also be used as a lubricant in doses of 7–30 g per horse. The upper limit of this dose range should not be exceeded, since toxic damage to the gut wall may occur with dehydration and death.

Antizymotics

A reduction in normal bowel motility, regardless of cause, will normally lead to accumulation of gas derived from bacterial action on the contained ingesta. For this reason suppression of the bacterial flora is particularly indicated in cases of flatulent colic. A variety of agents have been used: chloral hydrate (15–30 g), turpentine oil (15–30 ml), spirit of nitrous ether (15 ml), and formalin (15–30 ml) all have antizymotic action. They are often administered in 450 ml of raw linseed oil or liquid paraffin.

In conditions of altered metabolism within the bowel due to stasis, the growth of pathogenic toxin-producing bacteria may be favoured and this may lead to severe systemic toxaemia. Neomycin 4–8 g given orally has been shown to be effective in inhibiting bacterial multiplication and may be of value in cases of intestinal infarction prior to surgical treatment.

Purgatives

Purgatives have a very limited application in the medical management of colic and in cases of intestinal obstruction they are contraindicated since they may lead to rupture of the bowel. Impaction of the large colon and caecum can prove intractable to treatment and a mild purgative may be effective, but only after thorough lubrication and softening of the mass by liquid paraffin. Magnesium sulphate 200 g or dihydroxyanthroquinone 10–20 g are usually effective in 12–24 hours.

Parasympathomimetic drugs, such as carbachol and neostigmine, are best avoided since by their stimulant action these drugs exacerbate the pain of colic and the intensity of their action has been known to produce rupture of the bowel.

When the horse will eat, wheat bran soaked in boiling water with the addition of 30 g of sodium chloride and allowed to cool makes a safe and effective laxative.

Fluids and electrolytes

In cases of intestinal obstruction, particularly when it is proximal to the ileo-caecal valve, large amounts of fluid can be sequestered in the bowel and also be present in the peritoneal cavity. The effect is to produce dehydration and a serious reduction in circulating volume, with accompanying deficits of sodium, potassium, and bicarbonate ions. Effective fluid therapy requires the administration of very large volumes of fluid for the horse (a deficit of 50 l is common) and is an essential prerequisite of successful surgery. This subject is discussed further in Chapter 17 and has been reviewed by Rose (1981) but is briefly described here.

The total fluid deficit can be calculated from the PCV value, but rests upon several assumptions: firstly that the horse was not anaemic prior to the colic episode, secondly that red cell volume remains constant with increasing water loss, and thirdly that the blood volume is normally 88 ml/kg body weight. These factors inevitably introduce considerable errors. Red cell volume for instance does not remain constant; in water deficiency, the cells shrink and PCV therefore rises more slowly than predicted, while in a sodium deficit the reverse will occur. PCV can, however, be used as a useful guide to the volume required and serial estimations of this parameter can be used to assess the efficacy of treatment.

Reasonable approximation can be made by a formula, modified after Hall (1967) and based upon PCV as follows:

$$\text{total fluid deficit} = 10.5 \left(100 \cdot \frac{4500}{\text{PCV}}\right) \text{body weight (in kg)}$$

For example a PCV of 50% in a 450 kg horse indicates a 47 l deficit. The initial repair of the deficit is best made by intravenous infusion. A 14 gauge plastic catheter in one or both jugular veins will permit rapid infusion. The first 20% of the calculated deficit can be given as rapidly as the system allows, subsequent infusion rate should be adjusted to ensure that central venous pressure does not rise more than 5 cmH_2O above the pre-infusion value.

Clinical situations do not allow measurement of individual electrolyte concentrations. The most suitable fluid to use therefore is one in which the electrolyte components closely approximate to those in plasma. Polyionic solutions such as Hartmann's are the usual choice (Rose 1981). As a clinical guide, 50% of the deficit can be repaired with Hartmann's solution and the remainder with 0.15% sodium chloride made isotonic with 4.5% dextrose. Colic cases are frequently suffering from a metabolic acidosis. The infusion of 2 mmol of bicarbonate per kg body weight can be given on an empirical basis.

It is vitally important to restore the circulating plasma volume rapidly and plasma volume expanders will greatly assist by retaining the infusion fluid within the vascular space. Low-molecular-weight dextran 40 (Rheomacrodex) or a gelatin polymer colloidal solution (Haemaccel) can be valuable.

The efficacy of treatment can be assessed by serial measurements of PCV and fluid therapy must be continued until an oral intake adequate to maintain fluid balance is restored. A approximation of the daily fluid requirement for maintenance is 50 ml/kg body weight per 24 hours.

Fluid loss occurs mainly as a result of greatly increased capillary permeability. Very large doses of corticosteroids, up to 250 mg dexamethasone or betamethasone, can be very effective in reversing the increased permeability and may be life saving.

These recommendations are suggested purely as guidelines for emergency situations in clinical practice where time and facilities for sophisticated measurements are not available. They represent approximations and rely heavily on restoration of adequate renal perfusion to facilitate electrolyte regulation; however, they have a firm foundation in practice.

Other drugs

Where colic symptoms are associated with palpable aneurysmal lesions of the cranial mesenteric artery, Greatorex (1977) has shown beneficial results from repeated therapy over a period of weeks with low-molecular-weight dextran 70 solutions.

The close association of colic with strongyle infections suggests that an effective control programme associated with modern larvicidal anthelmintics such as Ivermectin (Slocombe & McCraw 1981) should be much more widely practised; however, Ivermectin is not yet marketed for use in the horse (see Chapter 12).

The management of colic cases presents a difficult clinical problem particularly since little is known of the aetiology of these conditions. Accurate diagnosis is seldom possible at an initial examination and the response to treatment forms an important part of the diagnostic process. For this reason a planned approach to each case (as in Fig. 23.1) is suggested. This will allow accumulated experience to be best used. The decision to refer the case to surgery should be taken in good time, and not 18–24 hours after the onset of the condition. Abdominal surgery in the horse is a routine procedure, but to have a reasonable chance of success it must be undertaken before irreversible shock has supervened.

The use of drugs in colic is largely empirical. Comparative trials of drugs are not feasible in clinical practice due to the poorly understood nature of colic and the variety of types presented. A better understanding of drug action may result from the careful use of colic models (Lowe 1969, Gerring & Davies 1982), but more research is required on the aetiology before major strides are likely in the management of this condition.

References

Bach L. G. & Ricketts S. W. (1974) Paracentesis as an aid to the diagnosis of abdominal disease in the horse. *Equine Vet. J.* **6**, 116.

Baker J. R. & Ellis C. E. (1981) A survey of post mortem findings in 480 horses 1958–80: (I) Causes of death. *Equine Vet. J.* **13**, 43.

Clarke K. W. & Hall L. W. (1969) Xylazine — a new sedative for horses and cattle. *Vet. Rec.* **85**, 512.

Davis L. E. & Knight A. P. (1977) Review of clinical pharmacology of the equine digestive system. *J. Equine Med. Surg.* **1**, 27.

Gerring E. L. & Davies J. V. (1982) Spasmolytic drugs and small intestinal function in the horse. In press.

Greatorex J. C. (1977) Diagnosis and treatment of verminous aneurysm formation in the horse. *Vet. Rec.* **101**, 184.

Hall L. W. (1967) In *Fluid Balance in Canine Surgery*, p 93. Ballière Tindall, London.

Kester J. (1975) Strongylus vulgaris — the horse killer. *Mod. Vet. Prac.* **56**, 569.

Lowe J. E. (1969) Pentazocine for the relief of abdominal pain in ponies — a comparative evaluation with description of a colic model for analgesia evaluation. *Proc. 15th Conv. AAEP*, 31.

Ogbourne C. P. & Duncan J. L. (1977) Strongylus vulgaris in the horse: its biology and veterinary importance. Commonwealth Agricultural Bureaux Miscellaneous Publication, no. 4.

Pearson H., Messervy A. & Pinsent P. J. M. (1971) Surgical treatment of abdominal disorders in the horse. *J. Am. Vet. Med. Assoc.* **159**, 1344.

Rose R. J. (1981) A physiological approach to fluid and electrolyte therapy in the horse. *Equine Vet. J.* **13**, 7.

Seckington I. M. (1972) Treatment of colic from a practitioner's point of view. *Equine Vet. J.* **4**, 188.

Slocombe J. O. D. & McCraw B. M. (1981) Controlled tests of Ivermectin against migrating strongylus vulgaris in ponies. *Am. J. Vet. Res.* **42**, 1050.

Tennant B., Wheat J. D. & Meaghen D. M. (1972) Observations on the cause of acute intestinal obstruction in the horse. *Proc. 18th Conv. AAEP*, p. 251.

24

Agents acting on the cardiovascular system of the horse

J.R. HOLMES

At the outset it is necessary to pose the question: what conditions are important in equine cardiology? They fall essentially into two main groups: arrhythmias and turbulent flow, and they may coexist.

Often in equine practice it is not a question of whether an abnormality might be treatable, but whether treatment is desirable. Horses are generally kept to work. Nowadays there is little haulage and farm work and the areas of work include the racecourse, hunting field, show jumping ring, three day event course and polo ground. Horses taking part in such activity must have an efficient circulatory system, for a rider is also often at risk. So important is this fact, that only in certain cases is treatment undertaken.

Common arrhythmias

First and second degree partial AV block (PAVB), Sinus node exit block (SA block, SAB)

The former condition is relatively common, the latter less so but not uncommon in many apparently normal horses with slow resting heart rates. The majority of cases probably represent the influence of vagal activity and are not clinically significant. The arrhythmia usually disappears when heart rate increases.

Both these arrhythmias may also occur immediately after the end of exercise when a rapid heart rate begins to fall. This post-exercise arrhythmia is transient and probably not significant; rhythm soon becomes regular as heart rate continues to fall. Again, it probably represents the effect of excessive vagal action as the vagus assumes its role in heart rate slowing.

These irregularities call for no treatment.

Sinus arrhythmia

Unlike the resting dog, in which sinus arrhythmia is commonly observed, the resting horse exhibits this arrhythmia relatively rarely. It sometimes occurs

523

transiently immediately after exercise and is probably not of any clinical significance. No treatment is necessary.

Ectopic beats

These may be of atrial or ventricular origin. Despite the fact that they are premature with a bizarre myocardial activation pathway, only when very frequent are they likely to be associated with any symptoms. Rarely, but occasionally, parasystole may occur but more often these premature beats occur unpredictably and with variable frequency even in the same animal. When they occur infrequently, no treatment is called for. When they occur frequently, the best treatment is probably a period of rest—this being one of the few conditions in equine cardiology in which rest is desirable as a form of treatment. Depending on the work load of the horse and the circumstances, this could vary from 3–6 months' complete rest.

Atrial fibrillation

The one arrhythmia which does call for treatment is atrial fibrillation. However, treatment of all cases of atrial fibrillation is not justified and the criteria of importance in deciding whether to advocate treatment are as follows:

1 The duration of the condition. There is accumulating evidence that the sooner the treatment is begun after the onset of arrhythmia, the better is the prognosis for successful restoration to sinus rhythm. In some cases it is possible to relate the onset to a particular event but in others there may be nothing in the history to explain its appearance.

2 The presence of any other cardiac abnormality, particularly murmurs or ectopic beats. In atrial fibrillation, the left AV valve is the one most often showing pathological change (Else & Holmes 1971) and murmurs may persist even if sinus rhythm is restored.

3 The work, age, and sex of the horse. In older horses and brood mares which may be used for breeding, treatment may not be warranted.

4 The value of the horse. Treatment is expensive; the drug generally used is quinidine sulphate and, in addition to its cost, it has to be administered by mouth (usually by stomach tube) which necessitates professional attention. The drug may not prove effective and, even if sinus rhythm is restored, relapse may occur. Glendinning (1965) reported a success rate of 60% in 12 horses.

Some horses with atrial fibrillation have severe atrial myocardial pathology (particularly left atrium) but others have no obvious gross or microscopic lesions (Else & Holmes 1971). There is no way of distinguishing the two on clinical examination. Thus, all cases of atrial fibrillation are potentially serious, although some work apparently normally with fibrillating atria. It would however, be unwise to advocate the continuing use of a known case of atrial fibrillation; owners who work these horses must do so at their own risk.

Quinidine therapy

Mode of action

The aim of treatment must be to restore sinus rhythm and the drug used in the horse is quinidine sulphate. Quinidine is the dextro isomer of quinine. This drug is relatively insoluble in water (1 in 90) and is bitter to the taste so it is usually given by stomach tube. After oral administration, absorption is almost complete, peak plasma levels being reached in 1–2 hours. Metabolism occurs in the liver and some 20–50% of the administered dose is excreted unchanged in the urine. The $t\frac{1}{2}$ for elimination of quinidine is 6–8 hours. Naylor (1975) listed its actions at the cellular level as follows:

1 It increases the electrical threshold of excitability. Quinidine does not affect the transmembrane resting potential nor the intracellular sodium and potassium concentrations. It probably acts by reducing the rate of entry of sodium ions into the cell during the rapid depolarisation phase (phase 0) thus restricting the sodium-dependent component of the inward current during the rapid depolarisation phase.

2 It slows the rate of rise of the cardiac action potential (phase 0), particularly at high rates of contraction. A minimum rate of depolarisation is necessary to propagate an action potential. Therefore fewer are transmitted, leading to a slowing of heart rate (Fig. 24.1).

3 It increases the duration of the refractory period, i.e. the time after a response before another potential can be propagated.

4 It slows the rate of propagation of a stimulus through the specialised conduction tissues (negative chromotropic action).

In addition to these direct effects on excitability, conductivity, and refractory period, quinidine possesses an atropine-like action. This may contribute to the effectiveness of the drug in cases of atrial fibrillation, since atropine and similar drugs also prolong the atrial refractory period.

Aetiology

There are a number of theories about the aetiology of atrial fibrillation and it is likely that any of them could explain such an arrhythmia (Holmes *et al*

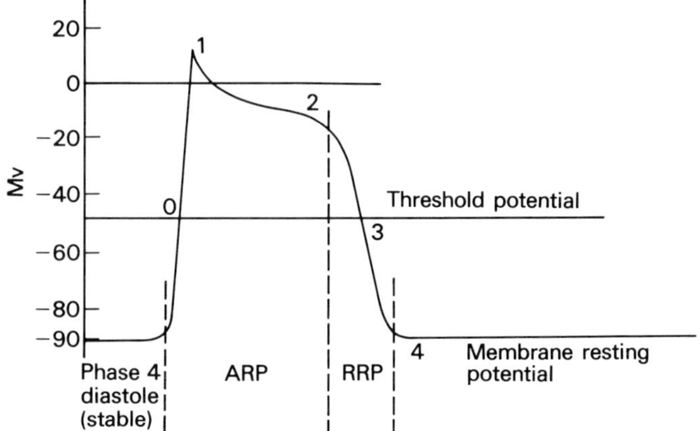

Fig. 24.1 Transmembrane action potentials of a non-pacemaking cell. Membrane resting potential during diastole is stable. Stimulation induces rapid depolarisation followed by repolarisation. (Compare with Fig. 24.3.) 0 = rapid, depolarisation, 1 = early, rapid repolarisation, 2 = slow repolarisation (plateau), 3 = terminal, rapid repolarisation. ARP = absolute refractory period, RRP = relative refractory period.

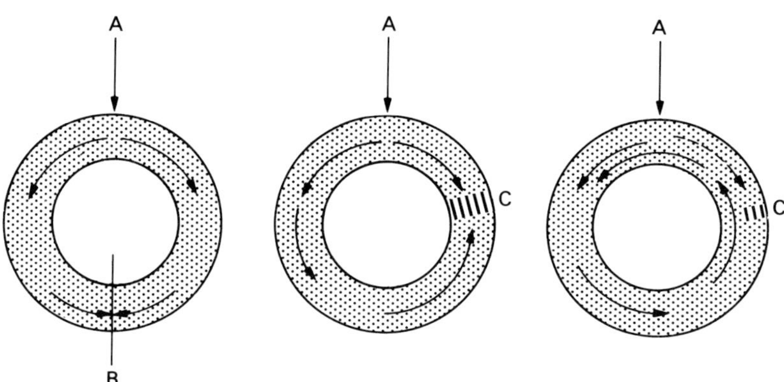

Fig. 24.2 The establishment of a 'circus movement' can be explained on the basis of a ring of muscle. If all the muscle is responsive, a stimulus applied at A will be transmitted in both directions and will be extinguished at B where refractory muscle will obstruct each wavefront (*left*). However, if at C there is initially an area of refractory muscle, then the clockwise wavefront will be extinguished. The anticlockwise stimulus will proceed around the ring (*middle*). If, by the time it arrives at C, this area is now responsive, it is possible to establish a continuous anticlockwise wave of activity which always finds responsive muscle ahead of it (*right*). In the atrium it is unlikely that the circus wavefront always follows the same path but it must always find some responsive tissue ahead of it to allow the activation to continue. To extinguish the circus movement it is necessary to increase the refractoriness of the muscle ahead of the wavefront.

1969). One attractive proposal is the concept of a circus movement first put forward by Lewis in 1920. This can be explained by a ring of muscle (Fig. 24.2) in which the sinus node is replaced by a mobile wavefront always able to find responsive muscle ahead of it. In a somewhat similar way, multiple atrial ectopic foci or an atrial parasystolic focus may induce perpetual atrial activation. Quinidine, by prolonging the refractory period, tends to suppress this type of activity. Of course there are risks in using quinidine sulphate: if atrial fibrillation is abolished, the sinus node or other potential pacemaking sites may be unable to sustain an adequate supraventricular rhythm. Experience in the horse indicates that either the animal responds and sinus rhythm is re-established (sometimes followed by relapse) or the fibrillation persists. It is usual not to exceed ten days of continuous treatment.

Treatment

Glendinning (1965) described the use of quinidine sulphate in the treatment of twelve horses with atrial fibrillation. The protocol involved initial use of digitalis then quinidine as follows:

Day　1　　　40 grains digitalis (Pulv. B. P.) b.i.d. on food
Day　2　　　30 grains digitalis (Pulv. B. P.) b.i.d. on food
Days 3 & 4　20 grains digitalis (Pulv. B. P.) b.i.d. on food
Day　5 up to 7–10 days after sinus rhythm was restored
15–20 grains daily
Day　5　　　Test dose 5 g quinidine sulphate
Day　6　　　10 g
Day　7　　　20 g
Day　8　　　30 g
Day　9　　　40 g　　In up to five doses at intervals during the day by
Day 10　　　50 g　　stomach tube (sometimes using an indwelling
Day 11　　　60 g　　stomach tube, which not all horses will tolerate).
Day 12　　　70 g
Day 13　　　80 g

As soon as sinus rhythm was established quinidine sulphate administration was stopped.

Side-effects

In man, quinidine may have untoward side-effects, including anaphylactic reactions, and it is usual to give a test dose before beginning a course of treatment. This procedure is also generally adopted in the horse, although there is no report of any such untoward reaction in this species. Increasing doses, both in man and animals, may produce marked symptoms of toxicity including depression, colic, anorexia, and incoordination; however, the drug is not cumulative and symptoms soon disappear when treatment is stopped. Other toxic effects, such as laminitis and oedema of the nasal mucosa have been reported elsewhere.

Administration

Quinidine sulphate is usually given by stomach tube and many horses (and it is usually large horses which develop fibrillation) begin to resent the frequent passage of a tube. To overcome this disadvantage and also to produce a more rapid response with less drug administered, Gerber *et al* (1971) reported the use of 10% dihydroquinidine glyconate intravenously. Six hours after an initial test dose of 3 g a horse was given 10 g diluted in 500 ml of saline intravenously over 15 minutes. Sinus rhythm was re-established and persisted. The intravenous form of quinidine is not presently available for use in the UK.

Monitoring and precautions

With both oral and intravenous therapy, careful monitoring of the heart is necessary during treatment; with the latter route this usually means continuous electrocardiography. Some have claimed that it is necessary to digitalise the heart prior to the introduction of quinidine therapy. Quinidine usually decreases the rate of impulse formation but, because of its vagolytic action, it may shorten AV nodal refractory period and increase the number of impulses which are conducted to the ventricles so that there is a risk of abnormally rapid ventricular contractions. This situation may arise because the reduction in atrial rate reduces any repetitive concealed conduction of atrial impulses in the AV node so that more of them succeed in activating the ventricles. One role of pretreatment digitalisation would be to increase the refractory period of the AV node and thus to protect the ventricles. However, it would appear that concealed conduction may not be important in every case. Certainly if treatment is to be attempted in cases showing a high average ventricular rate and/or the presence of a true jugular pulse and peripheral oedema, it would be rational first to use digitalis. However, where these features are not present it is questionable whether digitalis is necessary and results with quinidine alone would probably be just as good.

In man and the dog, the daily dose of quinidine is generally divided into four or more aliquots, the objective being to maintain a constant plasma quinidine level. In equine practice, this regimen poses difficulties and may not be really necessary since single large daily doses have proved quite effective in treating cases in the field, as the following case histories illustrate.

Eight-year-old hunter gelding

In the present owner's possession for two years. Heart found normal at time of purchase (December 1976). Bought for training for three day eventing; did some show jumping, one day events, and hunter trials in first season and was satisfactory.

January 1978: Brought in and started work. Began to show dyspnoea after jumping. Period of shivering and anorexia three weeks prior to examination at which atrial fibrillation was diagnosed on pulse palpation and auscultation and confirmed by electrocardiography. No murmurs were observed on auscultation and treatment with quinidine sulphate was advised.

12.4.1978: Bright. Alert. Eating well. Marked arrhythmia.

Treatment each day at 9.0 a.m. after cardiac auscultation.

13.4.1978: 10 g quinidine sulphate (test dose).

14/15.4.1978: 20 g quinidine sulphate.

16/17.4.1978: 30 g quinidine sulphate.

18.4.1978: 40 g quinidine sulphate.

Horse now depressed, complete anorexia, slight incoordination, heart still arrhythmic.

20.4.1978: 40 g quinidine sulphate. ⎫ Continued depression and
21/22.4.1978: 50 g quinidine sulphate. ⎭ anorexia.

23.4.1978: 60 g quinidine sulphate. Rhythm regular.

25.4.1978: 20 g quinidine sulphate.

Total dose: 370 g

4.5.1978: Rhythm regular. Horse in light work.

The practitioner noted that depression and anorexia were very marked in the early evening after the 9.0 a.m. doses but by the following morning these symptoms were much less marked. This observation corresponds with the absorption and physiological half-life of this drug.

Seven-year-old thoroughbred gelding

20 grains digitalis Pulv. daily for three days, then 20 grains digitalis Pulv. and 20 g quinidine sulphate daily for eight days. This was followed by 20 grains digitalis Pulv. and 50 g quinidine sulphate daily for four days. On 13th day rhythm returned to normal. 20 grains digitalis Pulv. and 40 g quinidine sulphate were continued for four days.

Dose to restore regular rhythm: 360 g quinidine sulphate.
Total dose: 520 g.

This horse returned to chasing, won two chases then fractured a shoulder and had to be destroyed.

Six-year-old thoroughbred gelding

30 grains digitalis Pulv. daily for three days, then 30 grains digitalis Pulv. and 30 g quinidine sulphate daily for ten days. This was followed by 20 grains digitalis Pulv. and 40 g quinidine sulphate daily for four days. Rhythm became regular. 20 grains digitalis Pulv. and 40 g quinidine sulphate daily were continued for three days.

Dose to restore regular rhythm: 460 g quinidine sulphate.
Total dose: 580 g.

This horse returned to racing and the heart rhythm was still regular years later.

In another example, after nine days treatment with 20 grains digitalis Pulv. per day and a total dose of 220 g of quinidine sulphate, rhythm became regular only to relapse 14 days later. Sinus rhythm again returned after two 30 g doses of quinidine sulphate plus digitalis. Relapse for the second time occurred 7 days later. Seven further days' treatment using a total of 270 g quinidine sulphate was again followed by relapse and the development of a systolic murmur.

Dosage

The results from single daily doses are as good as those where the dose is divided; and, in addition treatment is certainly much simpler. Recently Glazier (1981) has obtained good results using an initial dose of 15 g quinidine sulphate followed by 15 g of the drug every two hours until either sinus rhythm is restored or signs of toxicity occur. This method has the great advantage of speeding up treatment and allowing frequent monitoring. The ease of absorption and relatively short biological half-life of the drug make this method particularly attractive and could significantly reduce the cost of treatment by completing a course of therapy within one day. In the future the long-acting preparations of quinidine, such as quinidine polygalacturonate and quindine gluconate, which are reported to produce fewer gastrointestinal side-effects in man, might be worth trying in the horse.

Procainamide also possesses very similar anti-arrhythmic properties to quinidine. It also must be given by mouth. Intravenously it must be given by very slow infusion. It is not generally used in equine practice.

Bradycardia

Whilst at rest some horses may have very slow heart rates, marked bradycardia may occur at a rate of less than 25 beats/minute and this allows the appearance of several types of arrhythmia which are very commonly rate related. In the horse, bradycardia is often accompanied by a mixture of varying degrees of sinus node exit block, second degree partial AV block and, sometimes, atrial premature beats.

Automaticity of a pacemaker automatic fibre can be altered by: changing the slope of phase 4 depolarisation; altering the value of the threshold potential; or altering the value of the maximum diastolic potential. The effect of atropine at the cellular level is to increase the slope of the phase 4 depolarisation, causing enhancement of automaticity of the sinus pacemaker and thus increasing heart rate (Fig. 24.3).

The effect of atropine in a horse with bradycardia and arrhythmia is illustrated in the following example.

Ten-year-old thoroughbred × Dartmoor pony gelding

The pony was used for show jumping and eventing. There was bradycardia with the ventricular rate averaging 20–24/minute at rest. Marked arrhythmia was present with occasional periods of transient tachycardia. The irregular rhythm was associated with varying degrees of sinus node exit block and

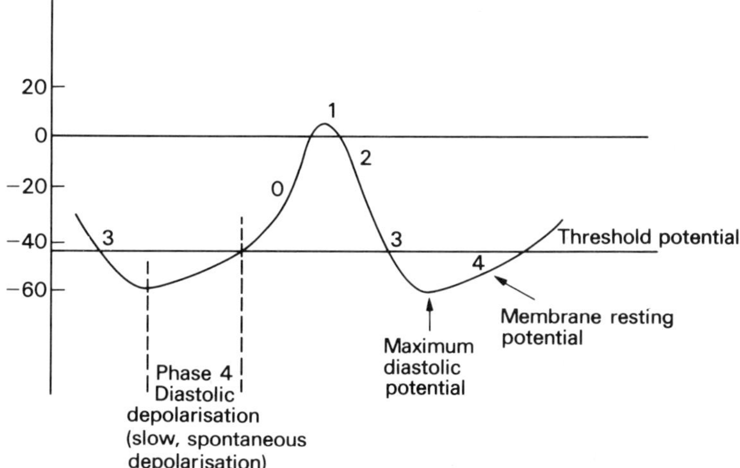

Fig. 24.3 Transmembrane action potentials of a pacemaking cell. During diastole membrane resting potential undergoes progressive slow, spontaneous depolarisation. Once threshold potential is reached there follows more rapid depolarisation. Rate of automaticity is influenced by the value of the maximum diastolic potential, the slope of diastolic depolarisation (phase 4) and the level of the threshold potential. (Compare with Fig. 24.1.)

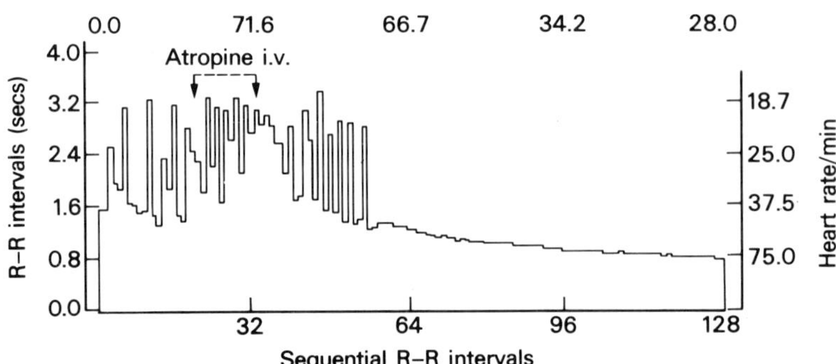

Fig. 24.4   Plot of 128 sequential heart beat intervals (ECG R–R intervals). There was initially marked arrhythmia with varying long and short R–R intervals with an average heart rate of 27 per minute. The long periods were due to varying degrees of sinus node exit block. The shorter intervals were caused by premature beats of atrial origin. 6 mg atropine sulphate was injected intravenously during the period of 34.5 seconds marked by the arrows. Following the injection, 52.28 seconds elapsed before tachycardia began to develop in association with a regular rhythm. Values at the top of the chart are times (seconds) for 32 beat intervals.

premature atrial systoles. After light exercise, premature beats of ventricular origin were also observed adding to the chaotic rhythm. After the administration of 6 mg atropine intravenously the ensuing tachycardia was associated with regular rhythm (Fig. 24.4).

In this case, therefore, the sinus node responded to atropine, providing evidence of its functional capacity and illustrating the potential use of atropine as a diagnostic agent.

Turbulence and murmurs

Flow in the arterial system is pulsatile but normally it approximates to laminar flow and is silent. When laminar or streamline flow is disrupted, turbulence develops, creating vibrations which are transmitted to the body surface and recognised as murmurs. These may arise from changes in blood velocity, the shape of the chambers, or blood viscosity. A fall in blood viscosity may be due to anaemia; this probably occurs most commonly in young animals with heavy parasite infestations. Murmurs from this cause will disappear when the anaemia is corrected following the use of appropriate parasiticides.

Typically, myocardial failure is characterised by an increase in heart rate, peripheral congestion (including jugular pulsation and/or pulmonary congestion), and peripheral oedema. Such manifestations are rare in horses even when loud murmurs are present on auscultation. This is probably because cardiac lesions are generally non-septic and develop slowly. Consequently the heart compensates, not only at rest but also, in many cases, at work. The ability of heart muscle to recover and to compensate following injury must always be remembered. For this reason discovery of a murmur does not necessarily indicate the need for any treatment; nor will it necessitate complete rest because this will discourage compensation. The objective here must be to facilitate compensation by keeping the horse at some work, the level of which relates to the fitness and work history of each individual. The possibility of failure to compensate always exists: even the physiological response to graded exercise characterised by left ventricular hypertrophy may, if it becomes marked, lead to a degree of myocardial ischaemia at exercise. Because failure to compensate, or the breakdown of the compensatory mechanism, may occur relatively rapidly, there are certain abnormalities in flow pattern which justify such a grave prognosis that the horse is unfit and/or unsafe to work. Horses are generally kept for work and, in these cases, treatment which might prolong life is of no importance. For this reason, in these animals diagnosis and especially prognosis are more important than therapy.

There are, however, occasions when horses with murmurs present signs of circulatory impairment on inspection. Atrial fibrillation is probably the commonest finding in these cases, the fibrillation being accompanied by valvular lesions. Such cases are rarely treated, because the underlying lesions remain, even if normal rhythm is restored.

Other drugs which are used in the treatment of cardiovascular disorders include xanthine derivatives and vitamin E, but the rationale for the use of these agents has not been clearly established.

References

Else R. W. & Holmes J. R. (1971) Pathological changes in atrial fibrillation in the horse. *Equine Vet. J.* **3**, 56–64.

Gerber H., Chuit P. & Schatzmann H. J. (1971) Treatment of atrial fibrillation in the horse with intravenous dihydroquinidine glyconate. *Equine Vet. J.* **3**, 110–13.

Glendinning S. A. (1965) The use of quinidine sulphate for the treatment of atrial fibrillation in twelve horses. *Vet. Rec.* **77**, 951–60.

Hoffman B. F., Rosen M. R. & Wit A. L. (1975) Electrophysiology and pharmacology of cardiac arrhythmias. VII Cardiac effects of quinidine and procaine amide. *Am. Heart J.* **89**, 804–8.

Holmes J. R., Darke P. G. G. & Else R. W. (1969) Atrial fibrillation in the horse. *Equine Vet. J.* **1**, 212–22.

Lewis T. (1920) Observations upon flutter and fibrillation. IV Impulse flutter; theory of circus movement. *Heart* **7**, 293.

Naylor W. G. (1975) The cellular basis for antiarrhythmic therapy. In *Cardiac Arrhythmias*, Krikler D. M. & Goodwin J. F. (eds.) W. B. Saunders, Philadelphia.

Therapy of diseases
of the equine respiratory system

P.M. DIXON, JILL R. THOMSON & D.H. SNOW

Diseases of the respiratory system are amongst the most common conditions seen in equine practice. In a British survey in 1962–63, 10.3% of horses attended by veterinarians suffered from respiratory disease (BEVA 1965). There are many causes of equine respiratory disease, some of which may occur in epizootic form (e.g. strangles or equine influenza) and others of which may occur sporadically (e.g. guttural pouch mycosis). Although a number of these diseases are life threatening (e.g. bacterial pneumonias), most equine respiratory diseases exert their ill effects by inhibiting respiratory function and so causing reduced exercise tolerance. In this chapter, these conditions and the recommended therapies will be discussed. Conditions which are primarily corrected by surgery are not included. The second part of the chapter is devoted to a discussion of the pharmacological actions of these therapeutic agents and to a consideration of the possible application of some of the newer agents.

Aids to the diagnosis of respiratory diseases

Besides a thorough clinical examination at rest and (if appropriate) after exercise, there are a number of other procedures which can assist in establishing an accurate diagnosis and so allow selection of the most appropriate therapy.

Haematology

A leucopenia and increased percentage of myeloid leucocytes often occurs in the early febrile stages of viral respiratory infections but can later revert to a leucocytosis if secondary bacterial infection occurs. Primary bacterial respiratory infections are normally accompanied by a leucocytosis and neutrophilia, although in longstanding pyaemic conditions (e.g. guttural pouch empyaema or sinusitis), the white cell picture will sometimes revert to normal limits.

Virus isolation

In viral respiratory infections, virus can often be isolated from nasopharyngeal swabs provided that samples are taken during the early febrile stages of the disease, are immediately placed in suitable virus transport medium, are kept cool, and are transported to a specialised equine virus isolation laboratory within 24 hours of collection. Where equine herpes virus 1 (EHV1) infection is suspected, a herparinised blood sample for virus isolation should also be taken at this stage.

Bacteriological examinations

Samples for bacteriological culture and for subsequent antibiotic sensitivity testing of isolates can be obtained from the nasopharynx by using a sheathed swab but tracheal sputum cultures have been shown to give a more representative picture of the bacterial status of the lower respiratory system (Hajer 1979). Tracheal samples can be obtained by transtracheal aspiration (Schatzmann *et al* 1972), although this frequently causes a transient pneumomediastinum (Farrow 1976); these samples are thus best obtained through the biopsy channel of a flexible endoscope.

The more commonly accepted bacterial pathogens of the adult equine respiratory tract include *Streptococcus zooepidemicus*, *Streptococcus equi*, *Actinobacillus equiluus*, *Corynebacterium equi*, and *Bordetella bronchiseptica* (Hajer 1979). However, the mere isolation of these bacteria (particularly *Strep. zooepidemicus*) is not necessarily significant. A transient bacteraemia may occur during the early stages of bacterial pneumonias even though, in some cases, the causal bacteria cannot be cultured from sputum at this stage. A blood culture can indicate the aetiological bacteria (Cumming & Semple 1980).

Endoscopy

The use of the flexible fibre-endoscope has greatly facilitated equine respiratory examinations, particularly that of the upper respiratory tract. Details of its use are given by Cook (1974a) and Lane (1981).

Radiology

Despite the increasing use of endoscopy to visualise many upper respiratory disorders, radiology is still an essential tool for a complete upper respiratory examination. It is particularly useful in the examination for the presence of alveolar infections in cases of maxillary sinusitis and for more complete assessment of ethmoid haematoma, maxillary cysts, upper respiratory tumours, and guttural pouch disorders.

Thoracic radiology is very useful in foals and, together with a barium swallow, can be used to assess diaphragmatic hernias in adults. Although the use of newer, higher powered radiographic equipment and 'fast films' allows standing lateral thoracic radiography in adult horses, the resulting superimposed lung fields are often difficult to interpret unless gross abnormalities, such as hydrothorax, are present.

Tracheal sputum cytology

Tracheal sputum cyctology can be useful in the differential diagnosis of pulmonary disease (Schatzmann *et al* 1972). In cases of lungworm infection with low patency, an occasional *Dictyocaulus arnfieldi* embryonated larva may be recovered from tracheal sputum, even though repeated faecal examinations are negative. In the absence of any larvae, large numbers of eosinophils in sputum can indicate non-patent lungworm infection (Mackay & Urquhart 1979). Surprisingly in chronic obstructive pulmonary disease (COPD), where respiratory hypersensitivity is known to occur, the predominant sputum cells are neutrophils.

Respiratory function tests

As patient cooperation is required for many respiratory function tests, only a restricted range can be used in veterinary medicine. We do not know enough about the aetiology and the physiological changes that occur with many types of chronic equine respiratory disease, and respiratory function tests cannot yet be used to physiologically classify and subsequently diagnose such disorders.

An exception to this is COPD where respiratory function tests have been widely used (Gillespie & Tyler 1969, Sasse 1971, McPherson 1978). McPherson *et al* have shown that, in this disease, maximum intrapleural pressure changes of 6 mmHg and greater occur along with arterial oxygen partial pressures of 82 mmHg or lower. These parameters can be used to differentiate COPD from other clinically similar forms of chronic pulmonary disease. These tests also have the advantage of allowing one to objectively assess the degree of disease and response to treatment. Arterial blood gases and pH measurements have also been used to assess neonatal pneumonias (Rose & Love 1979), neonatal maladjustment syndrome (Rossdale 1970), and idiopathic laryngeal hemiplegia.

Antigen intradermal and inhalation tests

Intradermal and inhalation tests with certain antigens (e.g. *Micropolyspora faeni*) can aid the diagnosis of early or asymptomatic cases of COPD which are not showing overt signs. Intradermal tests with these antigens may provide a guide to the aetiological antigen in any given case.

Animals with respiratory hypersensitivity to the selected antigens will develop or show an exacerbation of the disease 4–8 hours after inhalation challenge.

Serology

A retrospective diagnosis of viral respiratory infections can be established by serological testing of paired serum samples, the first sample taken in the early febrile stage of the disease and the second (convalescent sample) usually taken 2–3 weeks later. Serology can also be used to help identify the aetiological agents of COPD (Lawson *et al* 1979). Precipitins to *Aspergillus fumigatus* are often found in cases of guttural pouch mycosis.

Lymphocyte stimulation tests

As the immunological response to infection with some micro-organisms may be mainly by cell-mediated immunity (CMI) rather than by humoral factors, lymphocyte stimulation tests to assess CMI have been used, particularly in EHV1 infection (Pachiarz & Bryans 1978) and in *Corynebacterium equi* infection (Prescott *et al* 1980).

Faecal lungworm larvae

Unlike donkeys, most cases of lungworm infection in horses are non-patent. Faecal larvae examination therefore is usually unrewarding in horses.

Some equine respiratory diseases and their treatment

General considerations in the treatment of equine respiratory disease

The stresses of training, competition and transport can exacerbate many respiratory conditions and so complete rest is probably the most important treatment for the majority of equine respiratory conditions. For primary viral infection it is normally all that is required. It is also important to consider the environment. Whilst removal from contact with hay and straw is a specific therapy for equine COPD, as a general rule all horses with respiratory disease, and indeed all horses, should be kept in a well ventilated stable with adequate airspace. Cases of infectious diseases should be isolated as effectively as possible. One should avoid dusty environments and sudden exposure to cold in horses, especially thoroughbreds, which are unaccustomed to such temperature fluctuations.

Equine viral respiratory infections

Although these diseases are frequently referred to as upper respiratory infections because of the prominence of upper respiratory clinical signs, it must be recognised that (with the possible exception of picornavirus infections) most also involve the lower respiratory system. In general the clinical signs of all these viral respiratory infections are similar even though they are caused by a variety of agents. These signs include fever, anorexia, dullness, serous to mucopurulent nasal discharge, and submandibular lymphadenitis. As no specific treatments for viral diseases are yet widely available, the main treatment for these infections is complete rest. Stress can affect the severity, duration and even the outcome of these diseases. The use of anti-inflammatory drugs to mask the clinical signs of viral infections is contra-indicated. The use of corticosteroids in particular is contraindicated because they can suppress the onset of immunity and may even cause recrudesence of latent viral infections (Martens 1980). Antibiotics are not indicated for primary viral infection because suppression of the normal respiratory bacterial flora may even be harmful (Martens 1980).

Equine influenza

This is one of the most important equine respiratory diseases and is caused by influenza A/equi 1 or influenza A/equi 2 viruses. Epizootics of equine influenza often occur at about three-year intervals, particularly in concentrated horse populations (Powell *et al* 1978). The very rapid spread, the frequency of a dry cough at rest, and a high temperature are characteristic though not pathognomonic for this disease. Consequently, for a definitive diagnosis, virus isolation or serology is required.

Killed vaccines containing antigens of both A/equi 1 and A/equi 2 are widely used. Whilst the efficacy of vaccination has been well shown it is however short lived, particularly in the case of A/equi 2 (Burki 1978). Thus booster vaccinations should preferably be given for more complete protection at 3–4 monthly intervals, rather than annually as most manufacturers recommend.

Equine herpes virus 1 (EHV1) infection

EHV1 respiratory infection, or rhinopneumonitis, is also one of the commonest causes of equine respiratory disease, particularly where large groups of young horses come together. Certain strains of this virus can also cause abortion or, less commonly a paraplegic syndrome. With EHV1 respiratory disease, the clinical signs frequently include a submandibular lymphadenitis. Secondary bacterial infection occurs commonly after EHV1 respiratory infections; it causes a profuse purulent nasal discharge and prolongs the course of the disease (Bryans 1980).

A variety of vaccines, primarily for protection against EHV1 abortion, have been developed. An inactivated EHV1 vaccine of tissue culture origin (Pneumabort K, *Fort Dodge Laboratories Inc.*) is now licensed in many countries and offers some protection against respiratory infection. As immunity to respiratory infection in young animals is short lived (i.e. only 2–3 months' duration, even after virulent field EHV1 infection), the use of a killed vaccine cannot be expected to even offer this short degree of protection (Thomson *et al* 1978).

Equine picornavirus (rhinovirus) infections

At least four types of picornaviruses are associated with respiratory infections in horses. These infections are usually subclinical or mild but occasionally may cause severe pharyngitis with pyrexia (Holmes 1980).

Equine adenovirus infection

Infection with this virus is very common in horses. It is of low virulence and usually causes mild or subclinical disease. However, in immunodeficient animals, particularly arab foals with congenital combined immunodeficiency, this infection is normally fatal (McChesney & England 1978).

Other respiratory infections

In common with other species, in very many apparent outbreaks of equine infectious respiratory disease there is no laboratory confirmation of infection with known agents. It appears likely therefore that other, as yet unidentified agents including possibly Mycoplasma spp. (Poland & Lemcke 1978) may also be involved in such outbreaks.

Strangles

Strangles is an acute suppurative pharyngitis caused by *Streptococcus equi*.

In susceptible animals, epizootics may occur which can affect all in-contact horses. Clinically it is characterised by pyrexia, dullness, profuse bilateral purulent nasal discharge, often a temporary functional pharyngeal paralysis, and virtually always the pathognomonic discharging submandibular lymph nodes.

Even though *S. equi* is sensitive to penicillin, the role of antibiotic therapy in its treatment is debatable. Antibiotics if used, should only be given in the earliest states of the disease, but it is generally preferred to allow the horse to overcome the disease naturally using its own immune response. This is said to permit the development of a fuller immunity and is also alleged to reduce the incidence of secondary abscesses elsewhere in the body. Although *Strep. zooepidemicus* is ubiquitous in the equine upper respiratory system (Woolcock 1975), it may on occasions be associated with acute suppurative pharyngitis. A nasopharyngeal culture is required to positively differentiate this condition from a strangles. Treatment is with penicillin G.

Sinus empyaema

This empyaema is caused primarily by dental disease, most commonly apical periodontitis with abscess formation, infundibular necrosis, tooth fracture and periodontal disease of the posterior upper cheek teeth (Baker 1979). Because of its poor anatomical drainage, primary sinus empyaema may also occur after infectious upper respiratory disease. It also occurs secondary to sinus tumours, facial fractures, and maxillary cysts — particularly after surgical interference. Clinical signs include an intermittent foul smelling unilateral nasal discharge, heat, swelling and pain over the affected sinus and unilateral epiphora. Systemic illness is unusual. Radiography of the cheek teeth roots on the affected side should be performed and, with the animal under general anaesthesia, the last four cheek teeth should be carefully examined.

Treatment should be directed at the primary cause, e.g. teeth repulsion if tooth fracture or severe infundibular necrosis is present. With primary cases of empyaema where no underlying disease is observed and with most cases of periodontal abscess formation, the problem is basically one of poor anatomical drainage and so treatment involves correcting this by repeatedly irrigating the affected sinus through a small trephine hole. Large volumes of luke-warm water are usually all that is required for this infusion.

Where this treatment is ineffective due to inspissated pus, irrigation with hydrogen peroxide may, by its mechanical action, speed up resolution. The local use of proteolytic enzymes (e.g. streptokinase, 30 000 IU, or trypsin) which should be infused into the sinus daily for 3–4 days and allowed to remain there, is also useful if inspissated pus is present. In all cases of sinusitis, flushing should be continued until a few days after all purulent material disappears; in many cases this will take weeks. If alveolar abscess formation is present, a simultaneous course of penicillin G for 1–2 weeks may speed up resolution.

Guttural pouch empyaema

This is frequently associated with strangles, due to abscess formation and drainage of the retropharyngeal lymph nodes into the guttural pouches. As with sinus empyaema, guttural pouch empyaema is often primarily a problem caused by poor natural drainage. Clinical signs include copious intermittent unilateral or bilateral purulent nasal discharge, particularly when the head is lowered. In severe cases, swelling of the parotid region and dysphagia or even dyspneoa may occur.

Some cases of guttural pouch empyaema can be cured by feeding the horse at ground level. This simple feature will promote natural drainage. If this treatment is not effective the guttural pouch may be irrigated via its pharyngeal orifice using a Nielson catheter or by an indwelling Foley catheter. Dilute hydrogen peroxide or dilute iodine solutions can be used to irrigate the guttural pouch. Approximately 100–150 ml should be infused daily and the horse encouraged to lower its head for some minutes afterwards to promote drainage.

Refractory cases are often caused by inspissated pus or chondroid formation and require surgical drainage.

Guttural pouch mycosis

This condition is associated with the growth of *Aspergillus fumigatus* on the roof of the guttural pouch which causes damage to underlying structures including blood vessels and nerves. Clinical signs include massive, often fatal, epistaxis, pharyngeal and laryngeal paralysis, Horner's syndrome, parotid pain, abnormal head posture, facial paralysis (Cook 1968), and less commonly encephalitis, and infections of the middle and external ear and atlanto-occipital joint.

For many reasons the treatment of guttural pouch mycosis is unsatisfactory. Often irreversible nerve damage may already be present. Also, as the condition may not be a primary mycotic infection, even if effective antimycotic therapy were available, this might be insufficient. Because of the lack of effective, non-toxic, parenteral, antimycotic agents, therapy is usually local. As the lesion is dorsal in the guttural pouch, local irrigation will tend to pool ventrally and will not reach the lesion. Contact with the fungal plaque can be achieved by administering the drug by nebulisation, by powder insufflation, or by liquid irrigation with the horse in dorsal recumbency under general anaesthesia. The agents used include nystatin, natamycin, and dilute iodine solutions. Even if these agents are brought in contact with the fungal plaque it is unclear whether they will penetrate it sufficiently to achieve the therapeutic concentrations at the mucous membrane surface where the damage is occurring.

Parenteral therapy used for this disease includes 30 g sodium iodide i.v. at weekly intervals, 10 g potassium iodide orally per day, or thiabendazole at normal therapeutic doses daily for many weeks; however, the efficacy of these treatments has not been shown. Severe epistaxis is usually due to erosion of the internal carotid artery and, if this occurs, surgical ligation of the affected vessel is indicated (Owen & McKelvey 1979).

Follicular pharyngitis (Follicular pharyngeal hyperplasia, pharyngeal lymphoid hyperplasia)

This condition, characterised by the presence of nodules of lymphatic tissue on the dorsal and lateral aspects of the nasopharynx, has been increasingly recognised with the use of flexible endoscopes. In younger horses the condition is so common that it must be considered physiological. However, in some cases, because of the size, appearance, numbers, and widespread distribution of these follicles, it is called follicular pharyngitis and Raker & Boles (1978) suggest some guidelines for its classification.

Follicular pharyngitis is often found in racehorses which have reduced performance and increased and harsh respiratory noises during exercise. Often, closer examination will show the presence of lower respiratory disease, i.e. tracheal exudate and coughing. Therefore in some animals the follicular pharyngitis may be secondary to some other respiratory condition and this underlying disease should be diagnosed and treated. Treatment of cases with no evidence of other respiratory disease (i.e. 'primary' cases of follicular pharyngitis) is empirical and has included local and parenteral corticosteroids or antibiotic administration, local DMSO, and even reversion to the barbaric practices of counter irritation, by local thermocautery or abrading the pharynx with iodine solutions.

Pulmonary haemorrhage (exercise-induced pulmonary haemorrhage)

This condition usually occurs during strenuous exercise and is associated with loss of performance. The predominant clinical sign is a slight unilateral or bilateral epistaxis which occurs during or shortly after the exercise. In some cases blood is not detected at the external nares but endoscopy after exercise will demonstrate blood in the trachea. A large proportion of normal horses show some blood in the trachea after exercise. Pulmonary haemorrhage must be differentiated from epistaxis associated with guttural pouch mycosis, ethmoid haematoma, upper respiratory tumours, trauma, etc. (Cook 1974b) which do not necessarily occur with exercise. In the UK pulmonary haemorrhage affects mainly older horses and most show evidence of chronic pulmonary disease (Cook 1974b). The actual site and mechanism of pulmonary haemorrhage are unknown but it has been suggested that pulmonary hypertension associated with hypoxaemia might predispose to this haemorrhage. In this respect the diuretic furosemide has been widely used particularly in the USA (Hamlin 1975). Muir *et al* (1976) suggested that its limited haemodynamic side-effects, by decreasing blood pressures, could provide a mode of action in preventing pulmonary haemorrhage. However Dixon (1980) found that this drug did not decrease pulmonary hypertension significantly in horses with COPD. It has been conjectured by Robinson & Sorenson (1978) that, in chronic pulmonary disease, small airway obstruction combined with the anatomically poor collateral airways in horses could result in large regional pressure variations in the lung, which could cause capillary haemorrhage.

Because of the lack of knowledge about the cause of pulmonary haemorrhage, treatment is empirical. It seems logical that if evidence of pulmonary disease is present, it should be diagnosed and treated.

Pneumonia

As previously noted, the viruses of equine influenza and EHV1 can cause pneumonia, particularly in foals, as also does equine adenovirus in immuno-deficient foals. Secondary bacterial pneumonias can follow these viral infections.

Many primary bacterial pneumonias are associated with neonatal septicaemia and are caused by a wide range of bacteria. This condition is frequently associated with inadequate colostral immunoglobulin transfer. Signs include pyrexia, severe depression, markedly increased respiratory rate, adventitious lung sounds and purulent nasal discharge. Evidence of intercurrent illness (e.g. navel or joint infection) may also be present.

Pneumonia associated with foreign body inhalation is also found in foals. In older foals (2–6 months), a specific suppurative pneumonia with multiple large pulmonary abscess formation is caused by *Corynebacterium equi*. It is most commonly recorded in thoroughbred stud farms. Signs of respiratory involvement may not become obvious until the condition is well advanced and these signs include coughing, widespread loud and musical rales, and sometimes a purulent nasal discharge.

With the possible exception of foreign body pneumonia, other types of pneumonia are uncommon in adult horses. Occasionally horses that are stressed (e.g. by prolonged transportation) develop a severe pneumonia which may be accompanied by pleuritis.

For the treatment of pneumonia, broad spectrum antibiotics should be administered parenterally and this treatment should continue until several days after all signs disappear. Drugs used include combinations of penicillin and streptomycin, trimethoprim and sulphonamide, or ampicillin. Gay *et al* (1981) have used high doses of benzylpenicillin (1 mega unit/foal/every 8 hours) with some success. Intranasal oxygen has been advocated during the acute stages of neonatal pneumonias. Treatment for *C. equi* respiratory infections and foreign body pneumonias are usually unsuccessful as irreversible damage is usually present by the time the disease is diagnosed.

Chronic obstructive pulmonary disease (COPD)

COPD, also known as heaves, broken wind, or emphysema, is a respiratory hypersensitivity to moulds such as *Micropolyspora faeni* which occur in hay, straw, and stable dust. After exposure to these agents, susceptible horses develop a widespread exudative bronchiolitis along with airway spasm. Despite its previous nomenclature of 'pulmonary emphysema', anatomical emphysema is uncommon (Nicholls 1978). The clinical signs of this airway obstruction include poor work performance, increased respiratory effort (manifested as a double expiratory effort), and a chronic cough. Pulmonary function tests will show increased intrapleural pressures and lower arterial oxygen levels. The prognosis for COPD-affected horses is good as the condition is potentially reversible in most cases. Treatment involves maintaining the affected horses in an environment relatively free from dust and moulds and with adequate ventilation. Stables should be bedded with shredded paper, peat moss, or wood shavings, and horses fed a complete cubed diet. Alternatively, horses may be kept at grass.

Drug treatment may be indicated when horses are in severe respiratory distress. In such cases, bronchodilator drugs or corticosteroids provide temporary symptomatic improvement and their administration in conjunction with environmental control will speed the remission of clinical signs. If unavoidable exposure to antigens is anticipated (e.g. during transportation), prophylactic administration of sodium cromoglycate to asymptomatic animals is effective (Thomson & McPherson 1981).

Lungworm (Dictyocaulus arnfieldi)

Donkeys are thought to be the natural hosts of this parasite and horses usually become infected through grazing with infected donkeys (Round 1976). In horses, the infection is seldom patent but inhibited fifth stage larvae in the bronchi and bronchioles give rise to coughing, increased respiratory rate, and adventitious lung sounds. The disease is usually non-patent in horses and tracheal cytology or sometimes a therapeutic diagnosis may have to be resorted to. Mebendazole 15 mg/kg/day for five days is an effective treatment (Clayton & Trawford 1981) (*see also* Chapter 11).

Ascariasis

Parascaris equorum infection is common in foals and yearlings. The presence of respiratory symptoms corresponds to the period of larval migration from the lungs to the gastrointestinal tract via the trachea.

Prevention and treatment depend on a strict control programme to minimise the number of ascarid eggs in stables and fields. This consists of cleaning and disinfecting foaling boxes and allowing mares with foals to graze on the cleanest paddocks. It is recommended that all horses be treated with anthelmintics every 4–6 weeks, commencing from one month of age in foals in order to prevent further contamination of the environment. Benzimidazole drugs are effective and pharmacologically different anthelmintics should be employed periodically to prevent the development of helminth resistance (Clayton 1978) (*see also* Chapter 11).

Actions of therapeutic agents used in the treatment of respiratory disease

Antibiotics

Antibiotics are used extensively in the treatment of respiratory conditions in the horse. Mansmann (1975) has discussed the use of antimicrobial therapy for respiratory conditions, whilst Knight (1975) and Baggot (Chapter 3) have discussed antimicrobial therapy in horses in general. In the treatment of respiratory conditions, antibiotics may be administered parenterally or locally. As noted above many chronic upper respiratory infections, e.g. guttural pouch empyaema or sinusitis, will not respond to antibiotic therapy as these are essentially caused by poor anatomical drainage.

Where possible, antibiotic sensitivity tests should be performed to select the appropriate agent. In antibiotic therapy of the lower respiratory tract, the distribution of the drug into the tissues and bronchial secretions should be considered. If the location of the organism is inaccessible (e.g. within a *C*.

equi pulmonary abscess) to the antimicrobial agent, bacterial growth will continue. Antibiotics differ in their capacity to cross the broncho–alveolar barrier. In man, the excretion of ampicillin, cephalothin (a cephalosporin), and gentamicin in bronchial secretions were compared to concentrations found in plasma (Wong *et al* 1975). These workers found that the concentration of ampicillin in bronchial secretions was less than 10% of that in serum, while the relative figures for cephalothin and gentamicin were 25% and 40% respectively. The type of infection was not found to influence the drug secretion. Although ampicillin concentration was low, it was still effective against Gram-positive organisms but ineffective against Gram-negative respiratory pathogens. The broad spectrum penicillin, amoxycillin, has been found to attain greater concentrations than ampicillin in bronchial secretions (May & Ingold 1974). Recent studies in the horse have shown ampicillin levels in bronchial secretions to be about 15% of serum levels (Galbraith, Pers. Commun.).

The use of antibiotics in purulent conditions warrants special consideration. It is well established that the presence of pus can interfere with the action of certain antibiotics either by inactivating the compound or by preventing its access to the organisms. The administration of certain broad spectrum antibiotics to horses in a stressed condition should be viewed with caution. Several authors (Cook 1973, Baker & Leyland 1973) have reported dullness, diarrhoea, and death in horses after treatment with oxytetracycline. Owen (1975) postulated that colitis X may be part of the same syndrome.

For bacterial infections of the respiratory tract in adult horses, penicillin is generally considered to be the antibiotic of choice, because of predominance of *Steptococcus zooepidemicus* in such infections. The absorption rate and plasma levels of penicillin vary according to the form used. To ensure that suitable initial therapeutic levels are attained, the use of soluble sodium benzylpenicillin is best employed in conjunction with procaine penicillin which provides lower but more prolonged plasma levels (English 1965). A single intramuscular injection of benzathine or benethamine penicillin can provide detectable penicillin levels for up to five days; however, these levels are not bactericidal after 24 hours. Where a broad spectrum penicillin is required ampicillin or amoxycillin are the drugs of choice. These compounds have to be administered daily by either subcutaneous or intramuscular injection.

The use of sulphonamides in combination with trimethoprim is considered of value, particularly in conditions of the lower respiratory tract. These drugs have been found to reach high concentrations in the lungs, but whether they are excreted in high amounts in bronchial secretions does not appear to have been investigated. The expectorant properties of the sulphonamide compounds may also be beneficial.

Chloramphenicol is used in the treatment of lower respiratory infections, particularly foal pneumonia. A notable disadvantage is that chloramphenicol has an extremely short half-life in the horse and so it may be difficult to maintain adequate blood levels (Pilloud 1973). Ideally, horses should be treated every 4–6 hours to ensure therapeutic levels. A further consideration is the possible development of bacterial resistance to chloramphenicol through its widespread use. In this respect, the Swann Committee in 1969 recommended that chloramphenicol should be used only when no other effective antibiotic is available.

As previously noted, the use of antibiotics in viral respiratory infections would appear to be of little value in altering the course of the disease and as a routine measure should be avoided (Smith 1977).

Antifungal agents

The use of antimycotic agents in the treatment of respiratory conditions in horses has not been well documented and is mostly limited to the treatment of guttural pouch mycosis which has been previously discussed. Aspergillosis of the turbinates may occur secondarily to tumours and turbinate necrosis, the absence of which should be confirmed before any antimycotic therapy of lesions in this area is undertaken, especially in older horses.

Nystatin, amphotericin B, and natamycin are all products of Streptomyces spp. and have useful antifungal properties, but are not antibacterial. Nystatin and natamycin are not absorbed, are poorly soluble, and their use is restricted to topical application. Amphotericin B is used intravenously in human medicine. Diffusion of the drug is good and depletion of the plasma levels occurs slowly over a day after injection. It should, however, be used with great caution as it has toxic properties and may be hazardous to life. It is advisable to dilute the drug in an intravenous saline drip which is administered slowly while observing any ill effects.

Corticosteroids

Corticosteroids administered parenterally are used in the treatment of some respiratory conditions. These compounds, like antibiotics, are often abused. Their pharmacological actions and the general principles governing their use have been considered in Chapter 20. Corticosteroid therapy may be applied in cases of pneumonia and COPD.

In cases of acute pneumonia, corticosteroids are sometimes used in conjunction with antibiotics to relieve respiratory distress and to improve the general well being of the animal. They exert these effects by reducing the general inflammatory response and, thereby, the amount of pulmonary effusion.

Systemic corticosteroid administration leads to suppression of the immune system (Tarr & Olsen 1978) and it is important therefore to provide adequate antibiotic cover for the duration of corticosteroid therapy and for at least 3–4 days thereafter. The selected antibiotic should have bactericidal rather than bacteriostatic properties, thereby minimising the recurrence of infection after cessation of antibiotic therapy. In general the use of corticosteroids is contraindicated in all but very severe cases of respiratory infections.

Corticosteroids have been advocated by several authors for the treatment of COPD in the horse, particularly in acute cases where horses show clinical improvement after treatment (Cook & Rossdale 1963, Gerber 1973). Unless there is a concurrent change in environment, clinical improvement will persist only as long as therapeutic levels of corticosteroids are maintained (Gfeller *et al* 1975). The long term use of corticosteroids is associated with a number of potentially serious hazards which include suppression of the pituitary adrenal axis; it is, therefore, contraindicated (O'Connor 1968).

Expectorants

Expectorants are substances which increase the volume and reduce the viscosity of respiratory secretions, thereby assisting the removal of mucus from the respiratory tract. Expectorants may be classified into two categories.

1 *Local expectorants* which act directly on the respiratory mucosa and may be administered by inhalation (e.g. benzoin and eucalyptus oil). This may be done by means of a face mask. Oral expectorants may be incorporated in the feed and in cough mixtures.

2 *Reflex expectorants* which act by stimulating nerve endings in the pharyngeal, oesophageal, and gastric mucosae, leading to a reflex which stimulates respiratory mucosal cells. The irritative action of the reflex expectorants may sometimes cause vomition and they are not advisable for use in the horse.

Mucolytic agents

It is claimed that these compounds decrease the viscosity of pulmonary secretions and, therefore, aid in their removal. Bromhexine hydrochloride (Bisolvon) is a compound which is reported to be mucolytic (Bruce & Kumar 1968) and antitussive, to increase the titre of antibodies in the respiratory mucus, and to aid bronchodilation (Amin & Mehta 1959). It has been successfully used in the treatment of a variety of respiratory conditions in the horse, namely virus infection (Sorel 1968), acute and chronic bronchitis, chronic cough, and glanders (Pradier 1969, Wormstrand 1969, Pearce *et al* 1978).

Antiseptics

Antiseptics are capable of destroying pathogenic micro-organisms, although they do not necessarily eliminate bacterial spores. In the respiratory system they may be employed in the irrigation of cavities, e.g. paranasal sinuses. They are usually germicidal at concentrations which do not harm tissue but, by virtue of their cytotoxic activity, tissue damage will occur if high concentrations are employed.

The following antiseptics may be used for irrigation.

Oxidising agents

A solution of hydrogen peroxide produces oxygen when in contact with tissue containing the enzyme catalase. The rapid production of oxygen causes an effervescence which aids the mechanical removal of pus and cell debris; in addition it has some antimicrobial and deodorant action. These functions persist only as long as oxygen is being produced. Therefore hydrogen peroxide may be extremely useful where there is an accumulation of purulent material in cavities.

Iodine is an oxidising agent and is an antiseptic in dilute solution; however it may be irritant and tends to retard healing. A solution of iodine (Lugol's) may be used up to concentrations of 0.2%. The iodophors which comprise iodine solubilised by surface-active agents are less irritant and less toxic than aqueous iodine solutions and for general antiseptic purposes 1% dilutions are suggested.

Organic compounds

Chlorhexidine hydrochloride and dequilinum chloride are highly active against many Gram-positive and -negative organisms and the presence of pus and tissue fluids does not diminish the activity. Solutions of 1:1000 may be used for irrigation purposes and local irritation is uncommon.

Bronchodilators

Bronchodilator drugs have limited application in the treatment of equine respiratory disorders. They can be used to temporarily alleviate dyspnoea in severe COPD cases and can be used as an adjunct in the treatment of pulmonary disorders (e.g. pneumonia in which removal of bronchial exudates may be facilitated through bronchodilation). The following bronchodilator drugs may be used in veterinary practice.

Parasympatholytics

In the respiratory tract, parasympatholytic agents, (e.g. atropine) reduce the volume of secretions and relax the bronchial and bronchiolar smooth muscle. Many authors have noted a marked clinical improvement in COPD-affected horses as a result of atropine treatment (Alexander 1959, Cook & Rossdale 1963, Sasse & Hajer 1977), however, the attendant side-effects (notably tachycardia, increased viscosity of bronchial secretions, and reduced bowel motility) preclude its use for horses with COPD other than for either temporary relief of dyspnoea in a severely affected case or as a diagnostic aid in the field (Cook 1976).

Sympathomimetics

Sympathomimetic amines act on adrenergic receptors which may be divided into α and β receptors (Ahlquist 1948). β receptors can further be divided into β_1, or cardiac receptors, and β_2, or smooth muscle receptors (Lands *et al* 1967). Specific β_2 stimulants will, therefore, produce bronchodilation with considerably fewer side-effects than the less specific sympathomimetic amines.

Two such β_2 sympathomimetic agents, terbutaline (Bricanyl) and salbutamol (Ventolin) are currently regarded as the bronchodilators of choice for the treatment of bronchial asthma in man (Formgren 1977). The administration of terbutaline and another β_2 sympathomimetic agent, clenbuterol (Ventipulmin), to horses affected with COPD brings about a marked improvement in clinical condition lasting 4–8 hours (Fig. 25.1) (Sasse & Hajer 1977, Murphy *et al* 1980). At therapeutic doses, there are usually no side-effects. In addition, clenbuterol has expectorant properties and is reputed, therefore, to enhance mucociliary clearance in the airways.

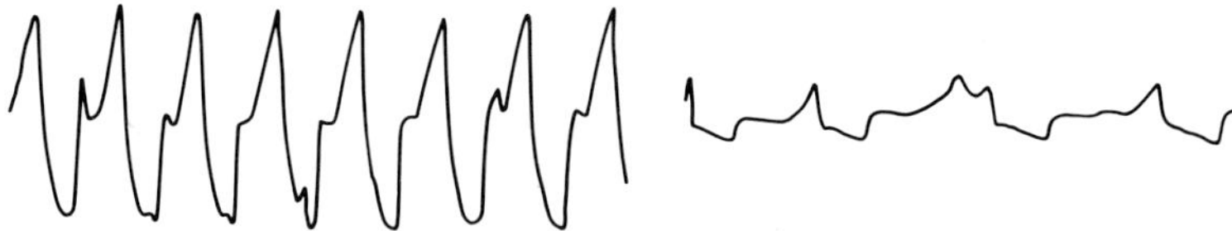

Fig. 25.1 Intrathoracic pressure measurements from a horse with chronic obstructive pulmonary disease before (*left*) and 20 minutes after (*right*) treatment with terbutaline.

Xanthine derivatives

Xanthine derivatives have a number of pharmacological actions, including central nervous system stimulation, myocardial stimulation, and bronchodilation. At the cellular level, the xanthine derivatives act as competitive inhibitors of cyclic nucleotide phosphodiesterase, an enzyme which catalyses the inactivation of cyclic 3′, 5′-AMP by conversion to 5′-AMP resulting in increased levels of cyclic AMP. Two of these compounds, aminophylline and etamiphylline, are thought to have more potent actions on the bronchioles, making them very effective bronchodilators (Pain 1973).

Sodium cromoglycate

This is a synthetic drug used in the prophylaxis and control of bronchial asthma in man and is administered by inhalation. It is not a bronchodilator and has no anti-inflammatory activity. The exact mode of action is not clear but it appears to act prophylactically, reducing the asthmatic response to allergen. Sodium cromoglycate is thought to act on the mast cells in the lung by maintaining membrane stability and inhibiting degranulation of sensitised mast cells which otherwise occurs after a challenge by antigen (Cox 1976) (Fig. 25.2). In controlled studies, this drug has been shown to be effective in preventing signs of COPD in affected horses when administered before antigen challenge (Murphy *et al* 1979).

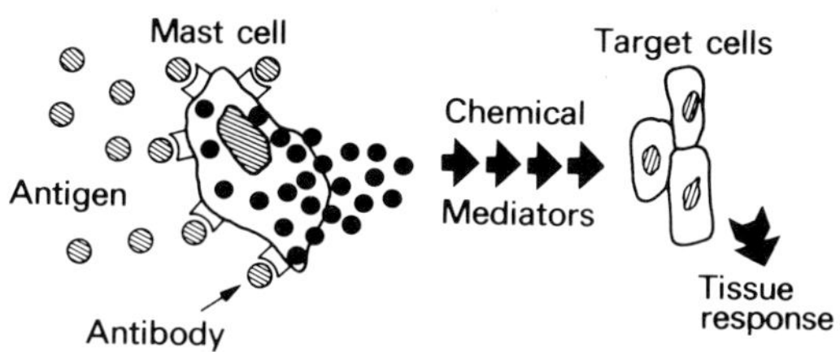

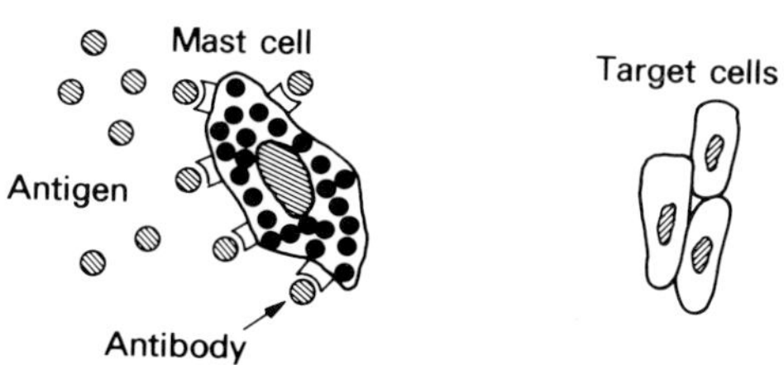

Fig. 25.2 Diagrammatic representation of the mode of action of sodium cromoglycate (SCG) in the lung. *Above* Antigen challenge without prior treatment with SCG — mast cell degranulates; *below* SCG given before antigen challenge — mast cell stabilised.

A linear response exists between the number of days treatment with this drug and the duration of remission of clinical signs of COPD, while horses are exposed to natural antigen challenge (dusty, mould-contaminated, straw bedding). A single daily dose (80 mg) on one day and on four successive days prevents clinical signs for a mean of 3 days and a mean of 24 days respectively (Thomson & McPherson 1981). Intermittent sodium cromoglycate treatment, e.g. two inhalations weekly, has been found to prevent the onset of clinical signs despite continuous exposure to natural antigen challenge (Thomson & McPherson, unpublished data) (Fig. 25.3).

Sodium cromoglycate is not effective in treating symptoms *following* exposure to antigen. Affected horses should initially be rendered asymptomatic through the use of a controlled environment and treated with sodium cromoglycate prior to any anticipated antigen exposure.

Non-steroidal anti-inflammatory agents

This group of drugs includes meclofenamic acid (Arquel) and acetylsalicylic

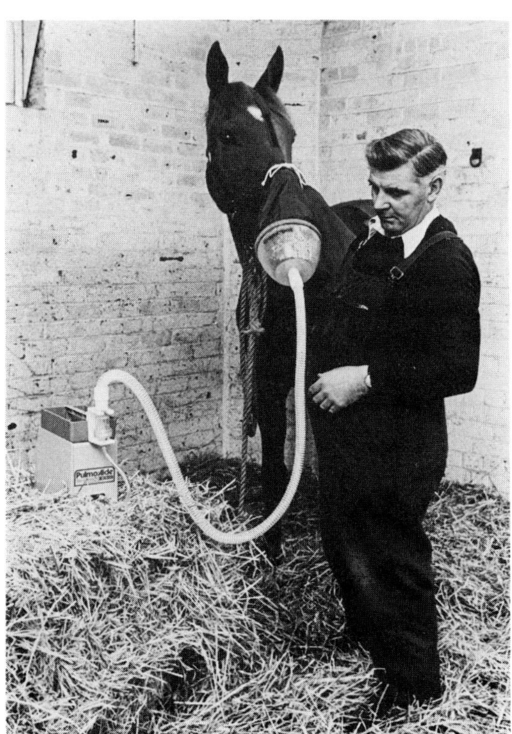

Fig. 25.3 A horse being inhaled with sodium cromoglycate using the Cromovet inhalation system.

acid and has been found to be effective in the treatment of experimentally induced anaphylaxis (Chand & Eyre 1977). These drugs inhibit the biosynthesis of kinins and prostaglandins and weakly block the biosynthesis of histamine and 5-hydroxytryptamine (serotonin). Furthermore, these agents pharmacologically antagonise kinins, prostaglandins and SRS-A and have been found to effectively control both respiratory and cardiovascular manifestations of hypersensitivity in horses. Although the role of the chemical mediators of anaphylaxis in the pathogenesis of COPD is unknown, the non-steroidal anti-inflammatory drugs may be found to be useful in the treatment of this condition (*see* Chapter 19).

Antihistamines

The antihistamines are not commonly used in the treatment of equine respiratory diseases. Although they were advocated for the treatment of COPD at one time, they have generally been found to be ineffective (Brion *et al* 1948, Sasse & Hajer 1977). In addition, antihistamines have a tendency to dry up bronchial secretions, making them more viscous and difficult to expel.

References

Ahlquist R. P. (1948) A study of the adrenotropic receptors. *Am. J. Physiol.* **153**, 586–600.

Alexander A. F. (1959) Chronic alveolar emphysema in the horse. *Am. Rev. Resp. Dis.* **80**, 141–6.

Amin A. H. & Mehta D. R. (1959) A bronchodilator alkaloid (vasicinone) from *Adhatoda vasica*. *Nature (Lond.)* **184**, 1317.

Baker G. J. (1979) Dental diseases in horses. *In Practice* **1**, 19–29.

Baker J. R. & Leyland A. (1973) Diarrhoea in the horse associated with stress and tetracycline therapy. *Vet. Rec.* **93**, 583–4.

B.E.V.A. Survey of Equine Diseases 1962/1963 (1965) *Vet. Rec.* **77**, 528–37.

Brion A., Pellerat J. & Castric M. (1948) L'histaminemie dans l'emphyseme pulmonaire du cheval. *C. R. Seanc. Soc. Biol.* **142**, 335–6.

Bruce R. A. & Kumar V. (1968) The effect of the derivative of vasicine on bronchial mucus. *Br. J. Clin. Pract.* **22**, 289–92.

Bryans J. T. (1980) Equine Herpesvirus 1. (Rhinopneumonitis). *Proceedings of the 1980 Invitational Workshop on Equine Viral Respiratory diseases and complications.* Columbus, Ohio.

Burki F. (1978) Serum antibody titres and nasal immunity following repeated parenteral influenza vaccinations in horses. *4th Int. Conf. Equine Infect. Dis.* 293–300.

Chand N. & Eyre P. (1977) Nonsteroidal anti-inflammatory drugs: a review. *Can. J. Comp. Med.* **41**, 233–40.

Clayton H. M. (1978) Ascariasis in foals. *Vet. Rec.* **102**, 553–6.

Clayton H. M. & Trawford A. F. (1981) Anthelmintic control of lungworms in donkeys. *Equine Vet. J.* **13**, 192–5.

Cook W. R. (1968) The clinical features of guttural pouch mycosis in the horse. *Vet. Rec.* **83**, 336–45.

Cook W. R. (1973) Diarrhoea in the horse associated with stress and tetracycline therapy. *Vet. Rec.* **93**, 15–17.

Cook W. R. (1974a) Some observations on diseases of the ear, nose and throat in the horse and endoscopy using a flexible fibroptic endoscope. *Vet. Rec.* **94**, 533–41.

Cook W. R. (1974b) Epistaxis in the racehorse. *Equine Vet. J.* **6**, 45–58.

Cook W. R. (1976) Chronic bronchitis and alveolar emphysema in the horse. *Vet. Rec.* **99** 448–51.

Cook W. R. & Rossdale P. D. (1963) The syndrome of broken wind in the horse. *Proc. R. Soc. Med.* **56**, 972–7.

Cox J. S. G. (1976) Disodium cromoglycate (cromolyn sodium) in bronchial asthma. In *Bronchial Asthma: Mechanism and Therapeutics,* pp. 805–836, E. B. Weiss & M. S. Segal (eds.). Little Brown, Boston.

Cumming G. & Semple S. J. (1980) *Disorders of the Respiratory System,* 2nd edn. Blackwell Scientific Publications, Oxford.

Dixon P. M. (1980) Effects of furosemide on pulmonary arterial pressures of normal horses and horses affected with chronic obstructuve pulmonary disease (COPD). *Equine Vet. J.* **12**, 28–9.

English P. B. (1965) The therapeutic use of penicillin: the relationship between dose rate and plasma concentration after parenteral administration of benzylpenicillin (penicillin G). *Vet. Rec.* **77**, 81–014.

Farrow C. S. (1976) Pneumediastinum in the horse: a complication of transtracheal aspiration. *J. Am. Vet. Radio. Soc.* **17** 192–5.

Formgren H. (1977) Broncho- and cardioselective B-receptor active drugs in the treatment of asthma patients. *Scand. J. Resp. Dis.* (Suppl.) **97.**

Gay C. C., Sloss V., Wrigley R. H. *et al* (1981) The treatment of pneumonia in foals caused by Rhodococcus (Corynebacterium) Equi. *Aust. Vet. J.* **57**, 150–1.

Gerber H. (1973) Chronic pulmonary disease in the horse. *Equine Vet. J.* **5**, 26–32.

Gfeller W., Spannring H. & Knusel F. (1975) Therapy of COPD in horses with opticortenol-S (Ciba-Geigy) *20th Wld. Vet. Congr.,* Summaries **2**, 955–6.

Gillespie J. R. & Tyler W. S. (1969) Chronic alveolar emphysema in the horse. *Adv. Vet. Sci.* **13**, 59–99.

Hajer R. (1979) Some aspects of the examination of sputum of horses with diseases of the respiratory tract. PhD thesis, Utrecht.

Hamlin R. L. (1975) Lasix and epistaxis in horses. *Proceedings of 21st Anim. Conv. Am. Ass. Equine Practit.* 277–80.

Holmes D. F. (1980) Equine Rhinoviruses I, II and III. *Proceedings of invitational workshop on Equine Viral Respiratory diseases and Complications.* Columbus, Ohio.

Knight H. D. (1975) Antimicrobial agents used in the horse. *Proc. 21st Ann. Conv. Am. Ass. Equine Practit.* 131–44.

Lands A. M., Arnold A., McAuliff J. P. *et al* (1967) Differentiation of receptor systems activated by sympathomimetic amines. *Nature* **214**, 597–8.

Lane G. (1981) Fibreoptic endoscopy. *In Practice* **3**, 24–30.

Lawson G. H. K., McPherson E. A., Murphy J. R. *et al* (1979) The presence of precipitating antibodies in the sera of horses with chronic obstructive pulmonary disease. *Equine Vet. J.* **11**, 172–6.

Mansmann R. A. (1975) Antimicrobial therapy in horses. *Vet. Clin. North Am.* **51**, 81–99.

Martens R. J. (1980) Management and treatment of acute viral respiratory infections. *Proceedings of the 1980 invitational workshop on equine viral respiratory diseases and complications.* Columbus, Ohio.

May J. R. & Ingold A. (1974) Amoxycillin in chronic respiratory infections. *Excerpta Med. I.C.S.* **236**, 130–4.

McChesney A. E. & England J. J. (1978) Equine adenoviral infection: pathogenesis of experimentally and naturally transmitted infection. *4th Int. Conf. Equine Infect. Dis.* 147–51.

MacKay R. J. & Urquhart K. A. (1979) An outbreak of eosinophilic bronchitis in horses possibly associated with *Dictyocaulus arnfieldi* infection. *Equine Vet. J.* **11**, 110–12.

McPherson E. A., Lawson G. H. K., Murphy J. R. *et al* (1978) Chronic obstructive pulmonary disease (COPD) in horses. Identification of affected horses. *Equine Vet. J.* **10**, 47–53.

Muir W. W., Milne D. W. & Skarda R. T. (1976) Acute haemodynamic effects of furosemide administered intravenously in the horse. *Am. J. Vet. Res.* **37**, 1177–80.

Murphy J. R., McPherson E. A. & Lawson G. H. K. (1979) The effects of sodium cromoglycate on antigen inhalation challenge in two horses affected with chronic obstructive pulmonary disease (COPD). *Vet. Immunol. & Immunopathol.* **1**, 89–95.

Murphy J. R., McPherson E. A. & Dixon P. M. (1980) Chronic obstructive pulmonary disease (COPD): Effects of bronchodilator drugs on normal and affected horses. *Equine Vet. J.* **12**, 10–14.

Nicholls J. M. (1978) A pathological study of chronic pulmonary disease in the horse. PhD thesis, University of Glasgow.

O'Connor J. T. (1968) Untoward effects of corticosteroids in equine practice. *J. Am. Vet. Med. Assoc.* **153**, 1614–17.

Owen R. (1975) Post stress diarrhoea in the horse. *Vet. Rec.* **96**, 267–70.

Owen R. R. & McKelvey W. A. C. (1979) Ligation of the internal carotid artery to prevent epistaxis due to guttural pouch mycosis. *Vet. Rec.* **104**, 100–7.

Pachiarz J. A. & Bryans J. T. (1978) Cellular immunity to equine rhinopneumonitis virus in pregnant mares. *4th Int. Conf. Equine Infect. Dis.* 115–27.

Pain M. C. F. (1973) The treatment of asthma. *Drugs* **6**, 118–26.

Pearce H. G., Wyburn R. S. & Goulden B. E. (1978) A clinical evaluation of Bisolvon for the treatment of some equine respiratory diseases. *N.Z. Vet. J.* **26**, 28–30.

Pilloud (1973) Pharmacokinetics, plasma protein binding and dosage of chloramphenicol in cattle and horses. *Res. Vet. Sci.* **15**, 231–8.

Poland J. & Lemcke R. (1978) Mycoplasmas of the respiratory tract of horses and their significance in upper respiratory tract disease. *4th Int. Conf. Equine Infect. Dis.* 437–46.

Powell D. G., Burrows R., Spooner P. R. *et al* (1978) A study of infectious respiratory diseases among horses in Great Britain 1971–76. *4th Int. Conf. Equine Infect. Dis.* 451–60.

Pradier P. (1969) Essais d'un broncho-secretolytique dans le traitement des affections respiratoires du cheval. *Bull. Mens. Soc. Vet. Prat. Fr.* **53**, 113–8.

Prescott J. F., Ogilvie T. H. & Markham R. J. F. (1980) Lymphocyte immunostimulation in the diagnosis of *Corynebacterium equi* pneumonia of foals. *Am. J. Vet. Res.* **41**, 2073–5.

Raker C. W. & Boles C. L. (1978) Pharyngeal lymphoid hyperplasia in the horse. *J. Equine Med. Surg.* **2**, 202–7.

Robinson N. E. & Sorenson P. R. (1978) Pathophysiology of airway obstruction in horses: A review. *J. Am. Vet. Med. Ass.* **172**, 299–303.

Rose R. J. & Love D. N. (1979) Intranasal oxygen in the treatment of staphylcoccal pneumonia in a foal. *Vet. Rec.* **104**, 437.

Rossdale P. D. (1970) Some parameters of respiratory function in normal and abnormal newborn foals with special reference to levels of PAO_2 during air and oxygen inhalation. *Res. Vet. Sci.* **11**, 270–76.

Round M. L. (1976) Lungworm infection (*Dictocaulus arnfieldi*) of horses and donkeys. *Vet. Rec.* **99**, 393–5.

Sasse H. H. L. (1971) Some pulmonary function tests in horses. PhD thesis, State University of Utrecht.

Sasse H. H. L. & Hajer R. (1977) Veterinary and clinical experience of the use of B_2-receptor stimulating sympatheticomimetic agent (NAB 365) in horses with respiratory diseases. *Tijdschr. Diergeneesk.* **102**, 1233–8.

Schatzmann U., Straub R. & Gerber H. (1972) Aspiration technique for bronchial secretion in the horse. *Sch. Arch. Tierheilk.* **114**, 395–403.

Smith H. (1977) *Antibiotics in Clinical Practice,* 3rd ed. Pitman Medical, Tunbridge Wells.

Sorel M. P. (1968) Experimentation d'un nouveau bronchosecretolytique chez le Pur-sang Anglais. *Bull. Zens. Soc. Vet. Prat. Fr.* **52**, 295–8.

Tarr M. J. & Olsen R. G. (1978) Suppression of the cell-mediated immune system of the horse by systemic corticosteroid administration. *J. Equine Med. Surg.* **2**, 129–34.

Thomson J. R. & McPherson E. A. (1981) Prophylactic effects of sodium cromoglycate on chronic obstructive pulmonary disease in the horse. *Equine Vet. J.* **13**, 243–6.

Thomson G. R., Mumford J. A. & Plowright W. (1978) Immunological responses of conventional and gnotobiotic foals to infectious and inactivated antigens of equine Herpes-Virus 1. *4th Int. Conf. Infect. Dis.*

Tobin T. (1978) Pharmacology review: chemotherapy in the horse — the penicillins. *J. Eq. Med. Surg.* **2**, 475–9.

Woolcock J. B. (1975) Epidemiology of equine streptococci. *Res. Vet. Sci.* **18**, 113–14.

Wong G. A., Pierce T. H., Goldstein K. S. *et al* (1975) Penetration of antimicrobial agents into bronchial secretions. *Am. J. Med.* **59**, 219.

Wormstrand A. (1969) Et nyttig middel mot hoste hos hast. *Medlemsbi. norske Veterinaerforen* **21**, 700–701.

Index

Page number prefixed by 't' indicates tabulated material

acepromazine t453, 455, 456, 485
  effects on performance of horse 497
  equine colic t515, 516–18
  Large Animal Immobilon 484, 485–90
  premedication of horse 466
  premedication of sheep 475
acetonaemia
  glucocorticoid therapy 442
  in cattle 326–30
acetylsalicylic acid 382, 402, 404, 552–3
active transport mechanisms 6–7
adjuvant *see* vaccine
albendazole
  fluke treatment 186
  for goats t189, 190
  for sheep t189, 190
  gastrointestinal nematode
     treatment 175, 180
  lungworm treatment 183
  solubility 7
aminophylline 551
amoxycillin 379, 546
amphetamine
  effects on performance of horse 496,
    497
  metabolism 25
  passive diffusion 9
amphotericin B 547
ampicillin
  dosage for horse 20
  equine endometritis 232
  equine respiratory disease 544, 546
  membrane penetration 48
  piglet diarrhoea 379
anabolic agents 501–2
  administration 334
  formulation 334, 336
  in cattle 338–41, 343–4
  in fish 342
  in pigs 341
  in poultry 342
  mode of action 347–9
  safety 342–7
  types t334, t335

anaesthesia 4
  barbiturate 34, 463–8
    methohexitone 464–7
    pentobarbitone 34, 453, 464–7
    thiamylal 464
    thiopentone 453, 468–7
  intravenous administration 13
  local 499
  metomidate 453, 468–70
  saffan 453, 470–2
anaphylaxis 152, 157
  from quinidine 527
  live vaccine induced 167
  slow reacting substance 398
Anoplocephala perfoliata 202
antagonism, drug 60
anthelmintics 174–98
  drug resistance 180–1, 205, 208
  prophylaxis 182–3, 195
  route of administration 181
  wide spectrum 174–9, 188
  see also cattle, sheep, goats, pigs
antibiotics
  appropriate use 138–9
  diarrhoea therapy 379–80
  horse 70–82, 231, 302
    gastrointestinal disease 76–7
    genitourinary disease 78–9
    limb infections 80–1
    racehorses 73
    respiratory disease 75, 545–7
    route 71
    side-effects 72
    skin disease 79–80
  see also feedingstuffs, mastitis, resistance
antibodies *see* immunoglobulins
antigen 145
  in vaccines 146
  resistance to infection 151–2
anti-inflammatory drugs
  cyclo-oxygenase inhibitors 402–13
  hyaluronic acid 420–1
  selection for local use 415–23
  synovial fluid transfusion 421